Date Due

RethinkHIV

Thirty years after the identification of the disease that became known as AIDS, humanitarian organizations warn that the fight against HIV/AIDS has slowed, amid a funding shortfall and donor fatigue. In this book, Bjørn Lomborg brings together research by world-class specialist authors, a foreword by UNAIDS founding director Peter Piot, and perspectives from Nobel Laureates and African civil society leaders to identify the most effective ways to tackle the pandemic across sub-Saharan Africa. There remains an alarming lack of high-quality data evaluating responses to HIV. We still know too little about what works, where, and how to replicate our successes. This book offers the first comprehensive attempt by teams of authors to analyze HIV/AIDS policy choices using cost-benefit analysis, across six major topics. This approach provides a provocative fresh look at the best ways to scale up the fight against this killer epidemic.

BJØRN LOMBORG is Adjunct Professor at Copenhagen Business School and Director of the Copenhagen Consensus Center. He is author of best-sellers *The Skeptical Environmentalist* (2001) and *Cool It* (2007), which challenged the effectiveness of standard responses to environmental challenges. He has been named one of the "top 100 global thinkers" by *Foreign Policy* in 2010 and 2011, one of the world's "100 most influential people" by *Time*, and one of the "50 people who could save the planet" by *The Guardian*. He is a sought-after speaker and opinion leader who frequently participates in debates on environmental and developmental policy choices.

RethinkHIV

Smarter Ways to Invest in Ending HIV in Sub-Saharan Africa

Edited by

BJØRN LOMBORG

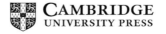

CAMBRIDGE UNIVERSITY PRESS
Cambridge, New York, Melbourne, Madrid, Cape Town,
Singapore, São Paulo, Delhi, Mexico City

Cambridge University Press
The Edinburgh Building, Cambridge CB2 8RU, UK

Published in the United States of America by Cambridge University Press, New York

www.cambridge.org
Information on this title: www.cambridge.org/9781107679320

First published 2012

Printed and Bound in Great Britain by the MPG Books Group

A cataloge record for this publication is available from the British Library

Library of Congress Cataloging in Publication data
RethinkHIV / [edited by] Bjørn Lomborg.
     p. ; cm.
Includes bibliographical references and index.
ISBN 978-1-107-02869-2 (hardback) – ISBN 978-1-107-67932-0 (pbk.)
I. Lomborg, Bjørn, 1965–
[DNLM: 1. RethinkHIV (Project)   2. Acquired Immunodeficiency Syndrome – prevention & control –
Africa South of the Sahara.   3. HIV Infections – prevention & control – Africa South of the Sahara.
4. Acquired Immunodeficiency Syndrome – economics – Africa South of the Sahara.   5. Cost-Benefit
Analysis – Africa South of the Sahara.   6. HIV Infections – economics – Africa South of the Sahara.
WC 503.6]
362.19697'9200967 – dc23   2012021834

ISBN 978-1-107-02869-2 Hardback
ISBN 978-1-107-67932-0 Paperback

Contents

List of figures   vii
List of tables   x
List of contributors   xiv
Acknowledgements   xvi
List of abbreviations and acronyms   xvii
Foreword   xix
Peter Piot

Introduction   1
Bjørn Lomborg

PART I   THE RESEARCH

1 Sexual transmission of HIV   11
   Jere R. Behrman and Hans-Peter Kohler
   ALTERNATIVE PERSPECTIVES
   1.1   *Damien de Walque*   49
   1.2   *Alan Whiteside*   61

2 Prevention of non-sexual transmission
   of HIV   74
   Lori A. Bollinger
   ALTERNATIVE PERSPECTIVES
   2.1   *Rob Baltussen and Jan Hontelez*   102
   2.2   *Mira Johri*   107

3 Treatment   125
   Mead Over and Geoffrey P. Garnett
   ALTERNATIVE PERSPECTIVES
   3.1   *Robert J. Brent*   151
   3.2   *John Stover*   178

4 Strengthening health systems   183
   *William P. McGreevey, with Carlos Avila
   and Mary Punchak*
   ALTERNATIVE PERSPECTIVES
   4.1   *Till Bärnighausen, David E. Bloom,
       and Salal Humair*   213
   4.2   *Nicoli Nattrass*   226

5   Social policy interventions to enhance the
     HIV/AIDS response in sub-Saharan
     Africa   238
     *Anna Vassall, Michelle Remme, and
     Charlotte Watts*
     ALTERNATIVE PERSPECTIVES
     5.1   *Tony Barnett*   281
     5.2   *Harounan Kazianga*   293

6   Vaccine research and development   299
     *Robert Hecht and Dean T. Jamison, with
     Jared Augenstein, Gabrielle Partridge,
     and Kira Thorien*
     ALTERNATIVE PERSPECTIVES
     6.1   *Steven S. Forsythe*   321
     6.2   *Joshua A. Salomon*   328

PART II   RANKING THE OPPORTUNITIES

7   Findings of the Nobel laureate economist
     expert panel   337
     *Ernest Aryeetey, Paul Collier, Edward C.
     Prescott, Thomas C. Schelling, and
     Vernon L. Smith*

7.1   Findings from African civil society   341
     *Bactrin Killingo, Nduku Kilonzo,
     Christiana Laniyan, Retta Menberu, and
     Ken Odumbe*

7.2   Conclusion   346
     Bjørn Lomborg

     Index   350

Figures

1.1 Subnational estimates of HIV prevalence among adults (age 15–59) in sub-Saharan Africa, 2001–2010. *page* 14

1.2 "Investment approach" to HIV prevention that combines community mobilization, synergies between program elements, and benefits of the extension of anti-retroviral therapy for prevention of HIV transmission. 16

1.3 Allocation of resources to HIV prevention in sub-Saharan Africa. 17

1.4 Male circumcision prevalence in sub-Saharan Africa, 2010. 24

1.5 Conceptual framework for the benefit-cost analyses of interventions to reduce the sexual transmission of HIV: Possible sequences for individual *i* starting at year *t*. 28

1.1.1 Percent condom use in a cohort of sex workers: Nairobi 1985–99. 51

1.2.1 Incidence by modes of HIV transmission (sexual). 67

2.1 HIV transmission by selected modes in five sub-Saharan African countries. 75

2.2 Schematic of the Goals model. 80

2.3 Percentage of men and women receiving a medical injection in the last year, by age group, various demographic and health surveys. 82

2.4 Percent of donated blood tested for HIV contamination in a quality-assured manner: countries with less than 100 percent coverage. 86

2.5 Number of blood units required per 1,000 population, data from countries attending 2010 UNAIDS-sponsored workshops. 87

2.2.1 Value for money of "component 3" pMTCT interventions in LMICs. 114

2.2.2 Impact of health system performance on childhood HIV infections. 117

2.2.3 Innovative "component 3" strategies to prevent mother-to-child transmission. 120

3.1 Schematic diagram of model for projecting the cost of anti-retroviral therapy, accounting for its prevention benefits. 129

3.2 Meta-analysis of studies of the cost per year of anti-retroviral therapy reveals heterogeneity within and between countries. 133

3.3 Average unit treatment budgets reported by PEPFAR for 2006–2008 show mild economies of scale. 134

3.4 Country-specific cost per person-year of treatment assumed in the projection model in 2012. 134

3.5   The five-year cost of various combinations of uptake rate and median CD4 at initiation.   136

3.6   Years gained by an individual patient from anti-retroviral therapy by CD4 at treatment initiation defined as the difference between life-expectancy at that CD4 count with and without treatment.   138

3.7   Zero uptake is a pessimistic counterfactual which avoids spending on AIDS treatment at the cost of millions of African lives.   139

3.8   Historical uptake expands treatment rolls and prolongs lives at the cost of an additional $15 billion per year by 2050, but total deaths rise almost as high as with zero uptake.   140

3.9   The high uptake scenario which costs $10 billion more than historical uptake greatly reduces unmet need and reduces the number of annual deaths in 2050 by about one million, but leads to an annual expenditure of almost $80 billion by the year 2050.   141

3.10 The universal access scenario increases the number on ART in early years and requires increasing investment by $30 billion over the next five years, but achieves a 25 percent reduction in people living with AIDS by the year 2050.   142

3.11 Cost per life-year saved at a range of discount rates.   143

3.12 Benefit to cost ratios for two $10 billion scenarios and one $30 billion scenario for two counterfactuals and two discount rates, assuming that a year of life is worth $5,000 and the prevention effect of ART is 70 percent.   143

3.13 Sensitivity of benefit to cost ratios to the prevention effect of ART, by counterfactual, discount rate, and scenario, assuming the value of a life-year is $5,000.   144

3.14 Benefit to cost ratios calculated identically to Figure 3.11, except that each year of life gained is valued at $1,000.   144

3.2.1 A model for tracking the effects of ART initiation at different CD4 counts.   180

4.1   NASA-identified total AIDS spending by type of expenditure, health systems strengthening, health sector, and non-health, nine low- and middle-income regions, 2006, percentage distribution.   187

4.2   Reaching the Abuja goal: by 2008, seven countries had, 38 had not.   204

4.1.1a Model that does not incorporate feedback due to reduced mortality because of ART.   219

4.1.1b Model that does incorporate feedback due to reduced mortality because of ART.   219

4.1.2 Human resources required to provide universal ART coverage for SSA, expressed as a function of population ART coverage.   220

4.2.1 Number of HIV-positive people in countries with 1 percent or more of the total sub-Saharan African HIV-positive population in 2009 (percent share indicated for the largest nine).   227

4.2.2 Responses to the Afrobarometer Survey (2005/6) to Question 66.   231

5.1   Hypothesized relationship between
        social factors being considered and
        HIV risk.   240

5.2   Steps in analysis.   249

6.1.1   Benefit to cost ratio based on
        variations in the unit cost of an
        AIDS vaccine.   322

6.1.2   Benefit to cost ratio based on
        variations in the effectiveness of an
        AIDS vaccine.   323

6.2.1   Components of costs and benefits
        for a new preventive HIV vaccine.   331

6.2.2   One-way sensitivity analyses
        on key assumptions and value
        choices.   331

6.2.3   Benefit to cost ratios for
        developing and delivering a
        preventive HIV vaccine under
        alternative assumptions about
        vaccination coverage.   333

Tables

1.1 HIV prevalence, HIV incidence, and number of persons living with HIV in sub-Saharan Africa, 2009. *page* 13

1.2 Cost per DALY and cost per infection averted for selected interventions in sub-Saharan Africa. 22

1.3 Benefits, costs, and benefit to cost ratios for three possible solutions to reduce sexual HIV/AIDS infections in SSA. 35

1.4 Costs per infection averted and costs per DALY for three possible solutions to reduce sexual HIV/AIDS infections in SAA. 38

1.5 Application to selected high- and medium-prevalence countries – Botswana and Mozambique. 40

2.1 Value of lifetime discounted ART and opportunistic infection treatment, $. 77

2.2 Value of life saved, by age, value of life year, and discount rate ($000). 78

2.3 Benefits associated with safe medical injections by discount rate, value of life year gained, and ART cost ($ million). 84

2.4 Benefit/cost ratios for safe medical injections by value of life year gained, discount rate, costs of ART, and unit cost of injection ($ million). 85

2.5 Benefits associated with safe blood transfusions by discount rate, value of life year gained, and ART cost ($ million). 88

2.6 Benefit to cost ratios of providing safe blood supply, by value of life year gained, discount rate, and cost of ART ($ million). 89

2.7 Benefits associated with pMTCT programs, by discount rate, value of life year gained, cost of ART, and different weights for life years gained ($ million). 91

2.8 Benefit to cost ratios of providing pMTCT programs, by discount rate, value of life year gained, cost of ART, and different life year weights ($ million). 92

2.9 Benefits associated with IDU interventions, by discount rate, value of life year gained, and cost of ART ($ million). 94

2.10 Sensitivity analysis of the benefits associated with IDU interventions, by discount rate, value of life year gained, cost of ART, and infections averted ($ million). 95

2.11 Benefit to cost ratios of providing IDU interventions, by discount rate, value of life year gained, and cost of ART ($ million). 95

2.12 Sensitivity analysis of the benefit to cost ratios of providing IDU interventions, by discount rate, value of life year gained, cost of

ART, and number of infections
averted ($ million).   96

2.13 Summary of benefits and costs
      associated with interventions to
      reduce non-sexual HIV
      transmission.   96

2.2.1 Comparison of recommended
      therapeutic options in women with
      CD4 >350 who do not require
      therapy for their own health.   112

2.2.2 Key indicators.   115

3.1   Cost per person-year in
      sub-Saharan Africa is modeled as
      varying by gross national income
      per capita, by drug regimen, and by
      scale of the national treatment
      effort.   135

3.2   Alternative scenarios for
      computing the benefit to cost ratio
      of additional AIDS treatment
      expenditure.   137

3.3   Parameters used in the AIDSCost
      projection program.   147

3.1.1 Benefits and costs for first-line
      treatment with 2012 costs and no
      externalities.   157

3.1.2 B/C ratios by CD4 count initiation
      and line of treatment with no
      externalities.   158

3.1.3 B/C ratios by CD4 count initiation
      and line of treatment with
      externalities.   160

3.1.4 Differences in life expectancy at
      birth without and with AIDS for
      selected sub-Saharan countries in
      2006.   162

3.1.5 B/C ratios for three prevention of
      MTCT programs.   163

3.1.6 Unmet need for family planning
      (FP) in the top 24 countries in SSA
      in 2009.   165

3.1.7 Benefits and costs when pregnant
      women are themselves treated
      and also prevent MTCT to
      four children.   167

3.1.8 B/C ratios for treating the pregnant
      mothers themselves with varying
      numbers of children.   168

3.2.1 Potential reductions in treatment
      cost per patient.   179

3.2.2 Years of survival on ART for a
      person starting treatment at age 35
      by CD4 count at initiation.   180

3.2.3 Discounted years of life gained,
      costs, and discounted cost per year
      of life gained by CD4 count at
      ART initiation.   181

4.1   Overview of solutions with
      potential impact on supply,
      demand, and price, and cost-benefit
      prospects.   186

4.2   Health spending ratios, major
      world regions, 2000, 2008.   187

4.3   Return on investment in the
      proposed UNAIDS framework.   188

4.4A Estimated benefits of saving lives,
      assuming adult DALYs valued at
      $1,000, and infant DALYs valued
      at $500, with discount rates of
      0, 3 percent, 5 percent, and
      10 percent, $000.   190

4.4B DALYs valued at $5,000 and infant
      DALYs valued at $2,500.   190

4.5   Disease statistics for HIV/AIDS
      infected population of South
      Africa, all sub-Saharan
      Africa.   200

4.6   Selected health benefits of health
      system strengthening.   202

4.7   Solutions with potential impact on
      supply, demand, b/c, cost per
      DALY, and cost per death averted.   206

4.8   Value of lives saved in infancy (where each year of an infant's life = 0.5 of an adult life-year), at age 22, and age 50, when value of current disability-adjusted life-year is $1,000 and $5,000, and discounted to present value at 3 percent, 5 percent, and 10 percent, $000.   207

4.9   Incremental B/C ratio ranging from 2 to 15, cost per DALY ranging from $320 to $444 for spending $2 billion to test, inform, and counsel all SSA adults on their HIV status, cutting expected new infections by 0.25 million annually to yield benefits of $6.25 billion (low) or $32 billion (high).   207

4.10   Benefits and costs to expand community health workers, $ billions, cost/DALY ($).   207

4.11   B/C ratio ranging from 4 to 25 for CRAG testing and treatment among 0.72 million in SSA, extending lives by 9 years at cost/DALY beyond age 22, B, C values in $ billions, C/DALY ($).   208

4.12   Incremental B/C ratios for spending an additional $29 billion on basic health system strengthening in 2015.   208

4.1.1   A framework for thinking about HSS interventions and the challenges they raise for cost-benefit analyses.   221

4.2.1   Development indicators for the nine countries highlighted in Figure 4.2.1.   227

4.2.2   Perceived most important problems facing governments (Afrobarometer 2005/6).   232

5.1   Sources of data used on current coverage of interventions: increasing alcohol taxes.   251

5.2   Sources of data used on current coverage of interventions: keeping girls in secondary school.   252

5.3   Sources of data used on current coverage of interventions: participatory gender and HIV training.   253

5.4   Sources of data used on current coverage of interventions: community mobilization.   253

5.5   Unit costs used in calculation of policy interventions: increasing alcohol taxes.   254

5.6   Unit costs used in calculation of policy interventions: keeping girls in secondary school.   255

5.7   Unit costs used in calculation of policy interventions: participatory gender and HIV training.   255

5.8   Unit costs used in calculation of policy interventions: community mobilization.   256

5.9   Key inputs used to estimate the impact of increases in taxation on HIV incidence.   257

5.10   Key inputs used to estimate the impact of adding HIV and gender training onto livelihood programs.   259

5.11   Key inputs used to estimate the impact of community mobilization.   259

5.12   DALY parameters.   260

5.13   Benefit to cost ratio of keeping girls in school, excluding HIV impact.   261

5.14   Parameters used in estimates of deadweight loss for alcohol tax.   262

5.15   Unit cost (mean/min/max), annual cost, and total cost (3%/5% discount rates) (2010 dollars).   264

5.16   Infections averted, DALYs averted, and cost savings (3%/5% discount rates) (2010 dollars).   264

5.17   Total cost, cost savings, DALYs
        averted incremental cost per DALY
        (2010 dollars).   264

5.18   Mean, minimum, and maximum
        incremental cost and cost per
        DALY per intervention (2010
        dollars).   266

5.19   Total cost, net health benefit, and
        benefit to cost ratio by intervention,
        using a 3% discount rate (2010
        dollars).   266

5.20   Total cost, net health benefit, and
        benefit to cost ratio by intervention,
        5% discount rate (2010 dollars).   266

5.21   List of countries where unrecorded
        consumption<50%, B/C ratio>1,
        and (HIV) CE threshold <3x
        GDP/cap.   267

5.22   Coverage by country (persons).   269

5.23   Infections averted and DALYs by
        country (3% discount rate).   271

5.24   Unit and total costs by country
        (2010 dollars).   272

5.25   Incremental cost per DALY by
        country (2010 dollars).   274

6.1   Annual investment in HIV vaccine
        R&D, 2000–2009.   303

6.2   Two scenarios for 2030 in
        sub-Saharan Africa (and globally) –
        numbers in millions.   305

6.3   Costs of AIDS vaccine program
        for sub-Saharan Africa
        ($ billions).   306

6.4   Benefits of averting 1,000
        infections: estimates by year and
        scenario (in $ millions).   308

6.5   Vaccine beneficiaries and
        infections averted (in a 25-year
        period after vaccine becomes
        available) in millions.   309

6.6   Total benefit of AIDS vaccine
        introduction in Africa
        ($ billion).   309

6.7   Benefit-cost ratios for AIDS
        vaccine development.   310

6.8   Hypothetical benefit-cost ratios
        from advancing time of vaccine
        availability.   311

6.9   Recent research advances.   313

6.10   Ongoing and completed Phase II
        and Phase III AIDS trials.   314

7.1   Expert economist panel outcome.   338

7.1.1   ICASA civil society outcome.   341

7.2.1   Global Fund-hosted event
        prioritization.   346

7.2.2   Addis Ababa youth forum
        prioritization.   347

7.2.3   Overview of prioritizations.   348

Contributors

Peter Piot Director and Professor of Global Health at the London School of Hygiene & Tropical Medicine.

Bjørn Lomborg Director of the Copenhagen Consensus Center and Adjunct Professor at Copenhagen Business School.

Jere R. Behrman W.R. Kenan, Jr. Professor of Economics and Director of Population Studies Center, University of Pennsylvania.

Hans-Peter Kohler Frederick J. Warren Professor of Demography, University of Pennsylvania.

Damien de Walque Senior Economist in the Development Research Group (Human Development and Public Services Team), World Bank.

Alan Whiteside Professor, Economic Research Unit; Director of Health Economics and HIV/AIDS Research Division, University of KwaZulu Natal in South Africa.

Lori A. Bollinger Vice President and Senior Economist, Futures Institute.

Rob Baltussen Health economics specialist and coordinator of NICHE – the Nijmegen International Center for Health Systems Research and Education, Radboud University Nijmegen Medical Center.

Jan Hontelez Assistant Professor, Erasmus University Rotterdam; Researcher at Nijmegen International Center for Health Systems Research and Education (NICHE), Radboud University Nijmegen Medical Center.

Mira Johri Associate Professor, International Health Unit (USI) and Department of Health Administration (DASUM), University of Montreal.

Mead Over Senior Fellow, Center for Global Development.

Geoffrey P. Garnett Professor of Microparasite Epidemiology, Imperial College London; Deputy Director Global Health – HIV, Bill and Melinda Gates Foundation.

Robert J. Brent Professor of Economics, Fordham University.

John Stover President, Futures Institute.

William P. McGreevey Associate Professor, Department of International Health, Georgetown University.

Carlos Avila Chief Strategy, UNAIDS, Geneva.

Mary Punchak Department of Biology, Georgetown University.

Till Bärnighausen Associate Professor of Global Health, Department of Global Health and Population, School of Public Health, Harvard University, and Senior Epidemiologist, Africa Centre for Health and Population Studies, University of KwaZulu-Natal.

David E. Bloom Clarence James Gamble Professor of Economics and Demography, Department of Global Health and Population, School of Public Health, Harvard University.

Salal Humair Research Scientist, Department of Global Health and Population, Harvard School of Public Health; Associate Professor, School of Science and Engineering, Lahore University of Management Sciences, Pakistan.

Nicoli Nattrass Professor, School of Economics, University of Cape Town.

Anna Vassall Lecturer, Economics of HIV, London School of Hygiene and Tropical Medicine.

Michelle Remme Research Fellow in Health Economics, London School of Hygiene and Tropical Medicine.

Charlotte Watts Professor, Social and Mathematical Epidemiology, London School of Hygiene and Tropical Medicine.

Tony Barnett Professor, London School of Economics.

Harounan Kazianga Assistant Professor, Spears School of Business, Oklahoma State University.

Robert Hecht Managing Director, Results for Development Institute.

Dean T. Jamison Professor, Global Health, University of Washington.

Jared Augenstein Yale School of Public Health.

Gabrielle Partridge Program Associate at the Results for Development Institute.

Kira Thorien Data Specialist, Results for Development Institute.

Steven S. Forsythe Senior Economist, Futures Institute.

Joshua A. Salomon Associate Professor of International Health, Harvard School of Public Health.

Ernest Aryeetey Vice Chancellor, University of Ghana.

Paul Collier Professor of Economics and Director of the Centre for the Study of African Economies, Oxford University.

Edward C. Prescott Nobel Laureate, W. P. Carey Professor of Economics, and the Director of the Center for the Advanced Study in Economic Efficiency at Arizona State University.

Thomas C. Schelling Nobel Laureate, Distinguished University Professor Emeritus at the University of Maryland.

Vernon L. Smith Nobel Laureate, Professor of Economics at Chapman University's Argyros School of Business and Economics and School of Law in Orange, California.

Bactrin Killingo Africa Program Manager of the HIV Collaborative Fund, a grants project of the International Treatment Preparedness Coalition (ITPC) and Tides Foundation.

Nduku Kilonzo Director of the Liverpool VCT, Care & Treatment.

Christiana Laniyan Managing Consultant at Strategic Development Initiatives (STRADIN) Consulting.

Retta Menberu Country Director, ActionAid, Ethiopia.

Ken Odumbe ActionAid International Regional HIV & AIDS coordinator for Africa.

David Young Project Manager and Head of Communications, RethinkHIV.

Kasper Thede Anderskov Project Manager and Economist, RethinkHIV.

Sibylle Aebi Communications Manager, RethinkHIV.

Sasha Beckmann Project Officer, RethinkHIV.

Sofie Findling Andersen Project Officer, RethinkHIV.

Acknowledgements

This book presents research from the *RethinkHIV* project, a collaboration between the Rush Foundation and the Copenhagen Consensus Center. This project was made possible to a large extent by funding and intellectual input from Kim Duncan and Marina Galanti of the Rush Foundation.

I am grateful for the commitment of staff members at the Copenhagen Consensus Center: Henrik Meyer, Ulrik Larsen, Sofie Findling Andersen, Sasha Beckmann, Sibylle Aebi, Sandra Andresen, and Zsuzsa Horvath. I would particularly like to thank the leaders of the project team for their exceptional dedication and enthusiasm: David Young and Kasper Thede Anderskov.

I would like to thank the Global Fund, the Gates Foundation, the Disease Control Priorities Network at the Department of Global Health at the University of Washington, the Ethiopian Government, the organizers of ICASA, Georgetown University, and Addis Ababa University for their collaboration. I thank Stef Bertozzi, King Holmes, Karl-Lorenz Dehne, Bernhard Schwartländer, David Wilson, Jeff Lazarus, and all of those who generously provided their time to reflect on the project and the application of its findings. The support and enthusiasm of Peter Piot has been of great assistance.

And, on behalf of the Rush Foundation and the Copenhagen Consensus Center, I would like to express my deep and sincere appreciation to each of the authors of the outstanding research in this volume, and to the remarkable members of the African Civil Society and Expert Economist panels.

Abbreviations and acronyms

ABCE	Goals and Allocation by Cost-Effectiveness model	FAO	Food and Agricultural Organization
ACT	artemisin combination therapy for malaria prevention and treatment	FP	family planning
		FSW	female sex worker
		GAVI	Global Alliance for Vaccines and Immunization
AGF	Abuja Goals Fund		
AMC	adult male circumcision	GF	The Global Fund to Fight AIDS, Tuberculosis and Malaria
AMI	acute myocardial infarction		
ANC	antenatal care		
ART	anti-retroviral therapy (three-drug combination therapy)	GHI	Global Health Initiative
		GNI	gross national income
		HC	human capital
ARV	any single or dual anti-retroviral drug regimen	HIA	HIV infection averted
		HICs	high-income countries
BCA	benefit-cost analysis	HIPC	Heavily Indebted Poor Countries Initiative of World Bank
BCC	behavioral change communication		
B/C ratio	benefit-cost ratio	HLT	High Level Taskforce on International Innovative Financing for Health Systems
CAR	Central African Republic		
CBA	cost-benefit analysis		
CCC	Copenhagen Consensus Center	HSS	health system strengthening = strengthening health systems
CCT	conditional cash transfer		
CEA	cost-effectiveness analysis	HSV-2	herpes
CHW	community health worker	HTC	HIV testing and counseling
CM	cryptococcal meningitis	IAC	International AIDS Congress
CMH	Commission on Macroeconomics and Health	IC	information campaigns
		ICD	infectious and communicable diseases
COD	cash on delivery		
CRAG	cryptococcal antigen	ICER	incremental cost-effectiveness ratio
DALY	disability-adjusted life year		
DCP2	Disease Control Priorities in Developing Countries, Second Edition	IDU	injecting drug user
		IHP+	International Health Partnership
DHS	Demographic and Health Surveys	IMAGE	Intervention with Microfinance for AIDS and Gender Equity
DMPPT	Decision Makers' Program Planning Tool	IOM	Institute of Medicine (USA)
		IPV	intimate partner violence
DOTS	directly-observed treatment, short course	IRR	internal rate of return; also, economic rate of return

LMICs	low- and middle-income countries	QALY	quality-adjusted life year
MBB	marginal budgeting for bottlenecks	RBF	results-based financing
		RCTs	randomized controlled trials
MC	male circumcision	R4D	Results for Development Institute
MD	medical doctor	SRH	sexual and reproductive health
MDG	Millennium Development Goal		
MDR-TB	multidrug resistant tuberculosis	SSA	sub-Saharan Africa
MMC	medical male circumcision	STI	sexually transmitted infection
MSF	Médecins Sans Frontières	TAC	Treatment Action Campaign
MSM	men who have sex with men	TB	tuberculosis
MTCT	mother-to-child transmission	TnT	treat and test
NASA	National AIDS Spending Assessment	UNAIDS	Joint United Nations Programme on HIV/AIDS
NCD	non-communicable diseases	UNGASS	United Nations General Assembly Special Session on HIV/AIDS (June 2001)
ODA	official development assistance		
OI	opportunistic infection		
OST	opioid substitution therapy	UNICEF	United Nations Children's Fund
PBI	performance-based incentives		
PDV	present discounted value	VCT	voluntary counseling and testing
PEPFAR	President's Emergency Program for AIDS Relief (USA)	VSL	value of a statistical life
		VSLY	value of statistical life year
pMTCT/PMTCT	prevention of maternal to child transmission	WHO	World Health Organization
		WTP	willingness to pay
POC	point-of-care	XDR-TB	extensively drug-resistant tuberculosis
PPP	purchasing power parity		
		YLL	years of life lost

Foreword

PETER PIOT

The emergence of the AIDS epidemic three decades ago represented an historic and unexpected development, upsetting the belief that the era of widespread infectious disease was coming to an end.

Since the beginning of the epidemic, almost 60 million people have been infected with HIV and 25 million people have died of HIV-related causes (UNAIDS and World Health Organization 2009). Yet, in that time an immense amount has been accomplished: scientific breakthroughs, unprecedented increases in global funding, and a new model for human rights and public health policy. Millions of lives have been saved.

At the end of 2010, five million people in sub-Saharan Africa had access to anti-retroviral treatment, whereas at the beginning of the millennium fewer than 100,000 had access (World Health Organization 2011).

The expansion of treatment has been one of several events that have recently changed the AIDS landscape. There have been positive research breakthroughs in demonstrating the effectiveness of male circumcision to prevent acquisition of HIV in men, and of treatment as prevention in serodiscordant couples. On the political side, the June 2011 United Nations Security Council Resolution on HIV/AIDS and General Assembly Political Declaration on HIV/AIDS reflect a promising level of renewed political engagement, as well as a changed strategy to focus on the populations that are at highest risk of HIV.

However, in an environment where aggregate funding is either declining or flat-lining, continuing with a "business-as-usual" approach will not work. The response to HIV needs to draw from lessons gained over the past thirty years, to identify greater efficiencies and establish a longer-term strategy.

We already know a considerable amount about the future of the epidemic. AIDS will remain an enormous global challenge. The disease will undoubtedly remain a major cause of death worldwide for years to come. In the worst affected countries in sub-Saharan Africa, AIDS will continue to undermine national economies, agricultural production, and community cohesion.

But there is much that remains uncertain – and dependent on decisions that we make in the next few years. The aids2031 Modeling Working Group showed (The aids2031 Consortium 2010) that tens of millions of lives can be saved over the next generation if efforts to tackle AIDS become smarter, more focused, more tailor-made, and more community-centered. However, if actions remain static or weaken, there will be millions of preventable new infections and deaths.

Although we talk about the so-called "global AIDS epidemic," in reality today there is a multitude of local epidemics that often differ markedly from one another among and within countries. While certain principles may apply universally in the fight against HIV – such as the importance of combating stigma, or of engaging affected communities – the variation teaches us that AIDS choices must address the unique settings of differing epidemics.

We must also learn to better reach the marginalized groups who experience the harshest effects of the HIV epidemic. Both globally and in sub-Saharan Africa, adult prevalence is considerably higher among people who inject drugs, men who have sex with men, and sex workers. Stigma, discrimination, and laws that criminalize these behaviors make it difficult for marginalized individuals in too many countries to seek health care, and to access preventative options.

Most importantly, we must acknowledge that AIDS is a generations-long challenge. Facing this reality requires us to adopt a longer-term, proactive mindset. Scaling up is vital, but it must be matched by an equal commitment to ensuring quality, efficiency, and sustainability.

This has profound implications for how we approach HIV. It would see us put more emphasis on investment in local capacity, identify greater synergies with other health and development needs, focus on locally adapted approaches rather than generic approaches, and introduce new prevention interventions in function of local needs.

Much of the knowledge that is needed to create radical reductions in the number of new HIV infections and AIDS deaths over the next generation is already available. The world possesses the research capacity to generate the new preventive and therapeutic tools that will be required.

However, AIDS research needs to evolve and develop. Whereas research for new interventions such as a vaccine microbicide or pre-exposure prophylaxis must continue, research in the real world into population level effectiveness must intensify, taking into account the effects of social marginalization, gender inequality, and management challenges of large-scale programs over a considerable period of time.

In translating new evidence, we should ask ourselves five questions to help to ensure that national strategies are based on more than received wisdom (Piot 2010):

- Does this work in the real world?
- Will people use it?
- What is the best way to deliver it?
- Can we afford it?
- Do the benefits warrant the costs?

RethinkHIV seeks to provide answers to each of those questions, and especially the last one. Prioritization based on establishing value for money is a different approach than the field of AIDS is accustomed to. The findings and implications from this first-ever, comprehensive effort to examine costs and benefits of the major HIV interventions across sub-Saharan Africa can be challenging and even confrontational. But the lessons from this field should be incorporated into our policy discussions and decisions, along with evidence from other scientific fields.

The *RethinkHIV* research captures human ingenuity and enterprise in the face of HIV, by outlining the considerable number of effective (and cost-effective) ways that have been found to respond to the epidemic. It is striking that the project asked researchers to focus on initiatives with benefit-to-cost ratios greater than one: In other words, each of the responses to the epidemic is, in itself, cost-effective. There are no silver bullets in the fight against HIV. But, as this research shows, there are many effective weapons in our arsenal.

It is also noteworthy that a number of the initiatives explored – such as financial incentives to keep girls in school, and efforts to reduce gender-based violence (Chapter 5) – have positive benefits that flow beyond HIV prevention. HIV does not exist within a vacuum, and responses that have broader impacts are commendable. Identifying areas of potential convergence between investment options will not only save costs, but may help to address other societal problems and strengthen health systems.

These chapters also underscore the considerable need for further intervention evaluation. It is vital that we generate more rigorous effectiveness studies, and engage in more research into structural interventions to reduce vulnerability to HIV.

However, the responsibility for building a sustainable long-term response to HIV does not just rest with the research community. Political courage and commitment need to increase.

As the aids2031 Consortium demonstrates, the magnitude and severity of the HIV pandemic can be reduced dramatically over the next generation if the global community brings the seriousness of purpose to this problem that it deserves. So far, some political leaders have outlined a bold vision. However, they have left an unfinished agenda.

True leadership is required to develop strong, evidence-based national responses. Among other actions, political leaders must prioritize rights-based approaches with respect to marginalized populations.

Globally, AIDS needs to remain high on the global political agenda, even among a proliferating array of challenges and issues – and against the backdrop of the economic crisis and AIDS "fatigue."

The response to AIDS needs to adapt to the changing environment. Funding demands will grow, but we can lower the long-term cost trajectory if wise policy choices are made today with attention paid to costs and benefits.

In highlighting effective responses, and shining a spotlight on prioritization and evidence-based decision-making, *RethinkHIV* adds to the body of information that can help to ensure smarter, sustainable decisions are made in the ongoing fight against HIV.

References

Piot, P. (2010). AIDS in Africa: Towards a new era. ICASA 2011 Keynote Speech. Addis Ababa: ICASA 2011.

The aids2031 Consortium. (2010). *AIDS: Taking a Long-Term View*. New Jersey: FT Press.

UNAIDS. (2010). *Global Report: UNAIDS Report on the Global AIDS Epidemic 2010*. Geneva: UNAIDS.

UNAIDS and World Health Organization. (2009). *Global Facts and Figures*. Geneva: UNAIDS.

World Health Organization. (2011). *Global HIV/AIDS Response: Epidemic Update and Health Sector Progress Towards Universal Access: Progress Report 2011*. Geneva: World Health Organization.

Introduction

BJØRN LOMBORG

There has been commendable progress in the fight against HIV/AIDS, but the time for a declaration of victory has not yet arrived. Humanity has struggled to eliminate diseases even when they are totally curable and preventable. AIDS – a disease which we do not yet know how to cure, and which we struggle to comprehensively prevent – has proven an immensely difficult adversary. It is still the biggest killer of women of reproductive age worldwide, and of men under the age of 40 in sub-Saharan Africa, where the pandemic is also responsible for 14 million orphans.

Sub-Saharan Africa continues to bear a disproportionate share of the HIV burden. With just 12 percent of the global population, the region accounted for a staggering 68 percent of all people living with HIV in mid-2010 (World Health Organization, UNAIDS, UNICEF 2011). While the number of new infections is decreasing, the 1.9 million people who became infected in 2010 represented 70 percent of all new cases globally (World Health Organization, UNAIDS, UNICEF 2011). For every person receiving anti-retroviral treatment, two others get infected, so HIV continues to exact an enormous socio-economic toll on a continent whose time is ripe for growth.

Today, the response to the epidemic is at a critical juncture. Following a decade of unprecedented increases in donor funding and a corresponding 17 percent decline worldwide in the number of new infections (UNAIDS and World Health Organization 2009), the fight against HIV is losing momentum.

An alarming 10 percent drop in funding was reported from 2009–10 (UNAIDS and Kaiser Family Foundation 2011). Meanwhile, US foreign aid outside the war zones of Iraq and Afghanistan has been cut by Congress (Cornwell 2011). There is a trend of reducing funding from European governments, owing both to financial crises and currency fluctuations (UNAIDS and Kaiser Family Foundation 2011). And in sub-Saharan Africa, few governments have made good their commitment a decade ago in the Abuja Declaration to increase health spending to 15 percent of GDP (World Health Organization 2011).

The considerable progress in recent years – including the 22-fold increase in the number of people receiving anti-retroviral drugs between 2001 and 2010 (UNAIDS 2011) – was due to scientific breakthroughs and to civil society's efforts to keep AIDS on the political agenda. But it is sobering to note that in sub-Saharan Africa and across all low- and middle-income countries globally, more than half of the people requiring treatment are not receiving anti-retroviral drugs. In western and central Africa, anti-retroviral therapy coverage is only 30 percent (World Health Organization, UNAIDS, UNICEF 2011).

Increasing treatment coverage is an imperative, not least because of its promise in preventing the spread of HIV. A breakthrough study in 2011 (Cohen *et al.* 2011) showed that when HIV-infected heterosexual individuals began taking anti-retroviral medicines while their immune systems were relatively healthy, they were 96 percent less likely to transmit the virus to uninfected heterosexual partners.

However, treatment remains expensive, and can be arduous for the individual. Stigma reduces the willingness of many to be tested in the first place. Such issues point to serious challenges to the sustainability of recent coverage increases. While we may hope for the situation to change, the truth is that right now we cannot simply treat our way out of the epidemic in Africa.

There remains an alarming lack of high-quality data evaluating responses to the HIV epidemic. As a result, we still know too little about what works, and how to replicate our successes elsewhere.

In a broad review of existing prevention interventions published in *Lancet* in 2011, Padian *et al.* noted that "until recently, HIV prevention lacked credibility with data from prevention trials showing little or no decrease in incident HIV. Furthermore, when successes were made public, explanations were often conflicting and lessons for application to other settings unclear" (Padian *et al.* 2011: 269).

We know that billions of dollars have been spent on abstinence campaigns without any reliable measure of the benefits they achieved. But this is not a unique problem. Even for mainstays of the response to HIV, like condom distribution and prevention information campaigns, there has been too little high-quality analysis of what benefits have been achieved at what cost.

As the aids2031 Consortium found in the book, *AIDS: Taking a Long-term View* (The aids2031 Consortium 2010: 64), "evidence on whether prevention programs are having any impact is typically lacking, and monitoring efforts generally focus more on counting the number of people who receive services than on measuring actual outcomes."

There are suggestions that this could be starting to improve. Padian *et al.* (2011: 269) argued that 2011 had marked "the end of this steady stream of disappointing results, and a concomitant change [that] is evident in public perception and the opinions of policy-makers."

Fiscal constraints today make it especially important for HIV prevention and treatment programs to be accountable. In making the case for funding to continue or increase, campaigners and donors need to be able to access and highlight clear evidence of the value that is delivered.

To add to the body of evidence is the overarching goal of this book. There is a strong moral case for providing better knowledge about the costs and benefits of competing ways to respond to HIV in the worst-affected region, sub-Saharan Africa.

The research project that led to *RethinkHIV* was proposed by the Rush Foundation in 2010 against the backdrop of the global financial crisis and amid growing fears about the sustainability of the fight against HIV in Africa.

The Rush Foundation is dedicated to providing effective funding for disruptive, innovative ideas in the fight against HIV in Africa. It complements its work on the ground by stimulating policy discussion and challenging thought leaders to work outside the existing frameworks of debate.[1]

The Rush Foundation approached the Copenhagen Consensus Center, which I am the director of, and proposed a major, year-long project utilizing teams of HIV specialist economists to create the first comprehensive cost-benefit analysis of HIV prevention and treatment interventions.

The Copenhagen Consensus Center is a think-tank based in Denmark that applies economic principles to analyze and prioritize opportunities to respond to global challenges. The Copenhagen Consensus Center's unique economic analysis framework has been used successfully to provide a comprehensive evaluation of the costs and benefits of climate change policy choices,[2] of Latin American development priorities,[3] and of ways to respond to ten global development problems.[4]

The Copenhagen Consensus Center's approach is founded on the belief that basic principles of economics can be used to improve the ability of any nation or organization to spend its money to achieve the most "good" possible.

Its past projects have been used by policy-makers and major philanthropic organizations, and have attracted attention from all around the world. The first-ever Copenhagen Consensus project in 2004 prompted the Danish government to increase HIV/AIDS spending to 500 million Danish kroner (Fogh Rasmussen 2008).

At the launch of the Copenhagen Consensus Center's flagship global development project in 2008,

---

[1] See: www.rushfoundation.org.

[2] The research is available in *Smart Solutions to Climate Change: Comparing Costs and Benefits* (Cambridge University Press, 2011).

[3] The research is available in *Latin American Development Priorities: Costs and Benefits* (Cambridge University Press, 2009).

[4] The research is available in *Global Crises, Global Solutions* (Cambridge University Press, 1st edn., 2005; 2nd edn., 2009).

Prime Minister Anders Fogh Rasmussen declared that, "because the results of Copenhagen Consensus are so concrete, and because they are based on solid knowledge, the results provide a valuable insight for politicians." In all, the Copenhagen Consensus Center has commissioned and published more than 100 research papers, which have been utilized by donors and international organizations.

This project set out to apply the Copenhagen Consensus methodology to responses to the challenges presented by HIV epidemics across sub-Saharan Africa, in a way that would provide academics, campaigners, politicians, and donors with fresh, robust analysis.

Part I of *RethinkHIV* presents the eighteen final research papers.

These chapters have been written by world-leading health economists, epidemiologists, and demographers examining responses to HIV/AIDS in sub-Saharan Africa under the following topics:

- prevention of sexual transmission
- prevention of non-sexual transmission
- treatment
- strengthening health systems
- social policy
- vaccine research and development efforts.

RethinkHIV marks the first time that cost-benefit analysis has been used systematically and comprehensively by teams of authors to analyze different possible responses to HIV/AIDS in Africa. The use of cost-benefit analysis allows us to establish – and compare – the overall benefits and costs to society of different responses to HIV.

As much as possible – and acknowledging the challenges posed by this being the first-ever effort – authors used the same set of broad assumptions and analytical tools to examine different interventions. This was designed to ensure the comparability of options. Also, authors were encouraged to identify and discuss potential synergies between different interventions, wherever possible.

Furthermore, authors identified where specific implementation issues exist for different interventions. Three research papers were commissioned for each topic in order to ensure a range of expert perspectives on what works, where, and why; and

to identify and highlight specific implementation issues.

Of course, this approach primarily leads to a broad-brush analysis. A natural next step is to focus more specifically on national and cultural-specific issues that modify the general findings of research papers.

The process of selecting the interventions for study involved a broad range of different inputs. First, input was gained from leaders in the fields of HIV medicine and economics on the project framework and on the options that should be examined. As many options as possible were added to a long list, and input was sought on how the overall subject should be divided into manageable topics.

The project's academic framework saw researchers asked to explore ways to allocate the same marginal amount of money, instead of reallocating the entire existing funding, which would be unrealistic and a less constructive input for donors and policy-makers.

To focus the researchers, they were asked to establish within one topic how an *additional* sum of $2 billion yearly could best be spent over the next five years. This hypothetical figure was selected after input from HIV experts and economists, because it is deemed enough to create meaningful effects, but is a limited and realistic sum, meaning that marginal analysis remains relevant.

Some readers may worry that evaluating ways to make spending smarter could be a proxy for an argument to reduce HIV funding. This could not be further from the truth. By making a compelling case for the effectiveness of one investment over another, we can make the argument for greater funding to go to the initiatives that need to be scaled-up and made sustainable.

At a time of funding constraints, this project's research could be a valuable source of intellectual material bolstering the case for increased funding.

Specialist HIV economist authors were approached for each topic and asked to use their expertise to identify quantifiable costs and benefits that would provide a meaningful input for policy-makers, even where data were scarce. In every case, it was left to the experts – the HIV authors – to draw the line as to how far the data could take us.

It is a striking feature of HIV intervention analysis that in some cases – even for mainstays of the HIV response – *RethinkHIV* authors concluded that there is simply too little reliable existing research to provide reliable numbers.

Therefore, one of the first-level, key conclusions that must be drawn from this pioneering project is the underscoring of a need for further analyses of intervention effectiveness, costs, and benefits, that are performed in specific settings and more broadly across regions.

This point is perhaps most obvious in the topic of prevention of sexual transmission (Chapter 1), where Jere Behrman and Hans-Peter Kohler highlight a startling absence of solid empirical evidence about the effectiveness, costs, and benefits of interventions and programs. They find sufficient data exists to compare just three approaches, pointing to a need for considerable empirical research into sexual prevention approaches.

Behrman and Kohler find strong empirical evidence of effectiveness from investment in male circumcision. While benefit-cost calculations are more speculative for HIV testing and counseling, they conclude that relatively comprehensive, repeated, home-based treatment and counseling is a realistic option in sub-Saharan Africa. And they point to studies showing that the efficacy of information campaigns can rise when more innovative program designs are used.

Two authors offer alternative perspectives on this topic. Damien de Walque (Alternative Perspective 1.1) supports Behrman and Kohler's selection of three interventions for analysis, and stresses the need for more and better impact evaluations of HIV/AIDS prevention interventions. De Walque argues that cost-effectiveness calculations should better integrate potential behavioral responses to prevention interventions, and discusses implications for cost-effectiveness of scaling-up interventions, especially male circumcision. He also reviews three additional solutions mentioned but not thoroughly analyzed in the previous chapter because they have been proposed and tested only recently and the evidence about their efficacy and effectiveness remains very limited: treatment as prevention, pre-exposure chemoprophylaxis for HIV prevention, and conditional cash transfers.

Alan Whiteside (Alternative Perspective 1.2) agrees that male circumcision is a good option, but notes that the analysis by Behrman and Kohler ignores the issue of men who have sex with men (MSM). No completed randomized controlled trial (RCT) has assessed whether circumcision could reduce transmission within this group.

Whiteside finds the cost-benefit evidence weakest for information campaigns, noting that there are numerous such programs but trying to evaluate them is extremely difficult and there are no RCTs or robust cost analyses. He proposes the novel idea of exploring the concept of a "sexual abstinence month" to reduce HIV incidence, a behavioral intervention where a population-wide "safe sex/no sex" effort for a set period of time could make a significant contribution to global prevention efforts. This is based on the idea that people have higher viral loads immediately after they are infected, and if they could avoid infecting others then the population viral load and infectivity would be reduced.

In Chapter 2, Lori Bollinger explores the topic of prevention of non-sexual transmission. She finds that there are cheap and effective ways to reduce or eliminate virtually every form of non-sexual transmission of HIV.

Bollinger finds that programs that prevent mother-to-child transmission are among the most cost-effective interventions available in the HIV/AIDS arsenal. But she finds that uptake of these programs is limited by low antenatal clinic attendance and hospital deliveries, and high levels of stigma associated with an HIV-positive diagnosis. She finds making blood transfusions safer the most attractive investment, with extremely high pay-offs for each dollar spent.

Bollinger also examines ways to make medical injections safer by ensuring an adequate supply of auto-disposable syringes, improving training for hospital staff, safe disposal of medical waste, and providing more information for the public. And she looks at ways to reduce risky injecting drug user behavior, but notes the difficulty of achieving a high level of coverage with programs targeting socially marginalized groups.

Baltussen and Hontelez (Alternative Perspective 2.1) draw attention to the issues associated with using a continent-wide analysis. While they are skeptical about the validity of some of Bollinger's estimates at an individual country-level, they agree that overall interventions to prevent non-sexual transmission are economically attractive, mainly due to their low cost and potential to prevent a large number of new infections.

Mira Johri (Alternative Perspective 2.2) focuses on mother-to-child transmission of HIV. She concludes that an analysis of a more comprehensive range of mother-to-child intervention options is required, including family planning, reproductive counseling, cotrimoxazole prophylaxis, early infant diagnosis, maternal ART for women requiring therapy for their own health, and other WHO Options (the guidelines of drug treatment provided by the World Health Organization) than "Option A," which Bollinger mainly looks at.

Johri examines four additional intervention strategies that she finds are likely to offer good value for money in some contexts and that have received less attention to date: interventions to improve health system performance, HIV screening in the labor ward, interventions to interrupt MTCT for HIV-positive women not delivering in a health facility, and the potential of an emerging "leapfrog" technology, multiplex point-of-care diagnostics.

In their examination of treatment (Chapter 3), Mead Over and Geoffrey Garnett find that an extra $10 billion over five years and proportionally sustained thereafter would have a dramatic impact on treatment coverage. They even look at the scale and resources needed to reach the Universal Coverage promised by world leaders.

Over and Garnett investigate a number of important trade-offs for discussion: should we invest in early or late treatment, first- or second-line drugs, cheaper or better quality drugs? Their findings suggest that the highest pay-offs can be obtained by treating people with the weakest immune system first with cheaper, first-line drugs.

Robert Brent (Alternative Perspective 3.1) sets forward an alternative analysis of costs and benefits of treatment scale-up, and suggests that Over and Garnett underestimated the benefits of treatment,

for example by not allowing for the fertility effects of treatment. Brent also points to doubts regarding Over and Garnett's assumption of falling average costs with treatment scale-up.

Brent explores the sensitivity of cost benefit ratios in the presence of a budget constraint. He recommends that the first $2 billion of the hypothetical additional funding of $10 billion should be devoted to the prevention of MTCT as this treatment intervention is likely to have the highest benefit to cost ratio of any treatment intervention.

In his analysis (Alternative Perspective 3.2), John Stover finds benefit to cost ratios to be higher than Over and Garnett. The difference is mainly due to different assumptions about the future costs of treatment per patient. Stover uses the assumptions of the Treatment 2.0 initiative (UNAIDS 2009) to project that improvements in drugs and service delivery will result in a 75 percent decrease in per patient costs. Stover also explores whether Over and Garnett's approach to simulating national epidemics is the best way to determine the impact of an additional $10 billion over five years.

William McGreevey *et al.* (Chapter 4) examine policy actions, interventions, and solutions that bridge the objective of strengthening health systems with that of continuing the fight against HIV/AIDS in sub-Saharan Africa.

McGreevey *et al.* evaluate four specific interventions, among them conditional cash transfers for HIV testing, and strengthening the community health worker base. They find that these interventions repay costs with substantial benefits in terms of better overall health indicators and reduction of HIV.

McGreevey *et al.* argue that HIV/AIDS spending already contributes to health system strengthening, but identifies two, key challenges. The first of these is that donors and African governments need to continue to raise their commitment to financing health care and strengthening the systems as a whole. The second is that greater efficiencies need to be developed, particularly in the effective extension of basic services to rural areas.

Among the options that McGreevey *et al.* explore in their chapter is the suggestion of using financial incentives to encourage sub-Saharan African governments to meet the target agreed in Abuja in 2001 to allocate 15 percent of their national budgets to the improvement of the health sector, with an adequate portion used for the fight against HIV/AIDS, tuberculosis (TB), and other related infectious diseases.

In an alternative take on this topic, Till Bärnighausen, David Bloom, and Salal Humair (Alternative Perspective 4.1) agree that the shift toward health system strengthening interventions has the potential to increase the effectiveness, efficiency, and sustainability of HIV programs. However, they question the static analyses utilized by McGreevey *et al.*, arguing that dynamic models incorporating unintended consequences and feedback are essential for a proper cost-benefit accounting of interventions.

Nicoli Nattrass (Alternative Perspective 4.2) raises two methodological concerns with the analysis by McGreevey *et al.*: their monetization of a human life year; and the way they extrapolate costs and benefits to the entire African continent without taking into account regional differences. Nattrass criticizes the way that incentives are designed by McGreevey *et al.*, arguing that this is based on conjecture, impossible to implement, and risks undermining other efforts to ensure people learn their HIV status.

Nattrass is also critical of McGreevey *et al.*'s proposal of an "Abuja Goals Fund." She argues that the *RethinkHIV* hypothetical budget would be best utilized if given to the international global infrastructure of the Global Fund to Fight AIDS, Tuberculosis and Malaria to carry on its current work, and specifically to help it build better health systems on the back of the AIDS response and to ensure that funding for patient advocate groups continues.

In their analysis of social policy levers (Chapter 5), Vassall, Remme, and Watts focus on interventions that seek to address key social drivers of HIV/AIDS vulnerability, and the social barriers to achieving a high coverage to proven HIV interventions. Economic and social factors continue to fuel HIV risk behaviors and undermine proven HIV interventions.

Vassall, Remme, and Watts propose using conditional cash transfers to keep girls in schooling longer as one response to the problem of transactional sex between young girls and older men, one of the main bridges of HIV infection from older sexually active men to uninfected, newly sexually active adolescent girls.

Widespread problematic alcohol use helps fuel engagement in risky sexual behaviors, and undermines core HIV prevention messaging. The authors cite research showing that pricing and tax policies can have a significant impact on problematic alcohol use.

They advocate "piggy-backing" training focusing on HIV and gender relationships onto livelihood interventions that have an income effect, in order to reduce gender inequalities and intimate partner violence which are both associated with an increased risk of HIV.

Finally, Vassall, Remme, and Watts look at programs to mobilize communities and reduce stigma which they argue is an important way to enable other core HIV prevention interventions.

Tony Barnett (Alternative Perspective 5.1) argues that the development of social policy interventions in response to the HIV/AIDS epidemic has been framed in the language of metaphors. He argues that three critical metaphors have been unexamined – the metaphor of "going upstream," the metaphor of a body undergoing treatment, and the idea of "drivers." These three metaphors have been important in framing the questions to be addressed by cost-benefit and cost-effectiveness analysis but their use obscures important problems which require working through before policy formulation. Barnett examines the flaws with using each metaphor and goes on to suggest a possible diagnostic tool which does away with the need for these metaphors: hope.

Harounan Kazianga (Alternative Perspective 5.2) offers insight into the potential challenges that policy-makers are likely to be confronted with when they wish to scale-up promising pilot studies in the field of social policy levers. Kazianga stresses the need for providing policy-makers with the tools and the information to move from promising pilot studies to full-scale projects. He also argues that cost-benefit calculations should better integrate changes in average costs that are likely to occur when going from a pilot study to full-scale project.

Finally, he proposes the tool of offering life insurance to adult individuals to stay HIV-free as a means for reducing risky sexual behavior and hence HIV transmission. Calibration exercises have suggested promising results, but randomized control trials would provide more credible evidence on the effectiveness of this policy.

In their examination of vaccine research and development (Chapter 6), Dean Jamison and Robert Hecht focus on vaccine research, but canvas the state of research into other options.

Based on interviews, they find a low probability of developing a drug to clear the body of HIV in the next twenty-five years. That said, they argue that research should continue. Other research efforts include those to create less expensive, more effective, and safer ARVs; better therapies for treating or preventing opportunistic infections; better diagnostics; and better barrier devices for transmission interruption. The interviews give good reason to believe that an effective vaccine will be possible within the next twenty years.

Jamison and Hecht find there to be a strong case, based on benefit-cost analysis, for increasing existing funding into vaccine research and development. Whether the vaccine is introduced in 2030 or in 2040, the investment appears to be compelling.

They explore the benefit associated with an increase of $100 million per year in research and development expenditure, spent outside existing institutional funding channels to increase the likelihood of an earlier discovery. This will likely shorten the time taken to achieve vaccine availability by half to one year, and would provide high potential benefits relative to costs.

Steven Forsythe (Alternative Perspective 6.1) notes that the decision to produce and manufacture an AIDS vaccine will not be made purely based on benefit to cost ratios, and there are many qualitative and non-economic issues which will need to be addressed by national and international policymakers.

Forsythe points out the tremendous uncertainty about the characteristics of an AIDS vaccine: economists don't know what an AIDS vaccine will cost, either for research and development or for manufacture; its effectiveness is unknown, along with its year of readiness; effects on disinhibition behaviors are not understood; the shape of the HIV epidemic in 2030 or 2040 is unclear.

He finds that there appears to be a strong case for developing an AIDS vaccine, but argues that it is important to recognize that resources are limited and therefore funds allocated to an AIDS vaccine will not be available for other interventions, such as the scale-up of male circumcision, an expanded distribution of condoms, or increased treatment.

Joshua Salomon (Alternative Perspective 6.2) notes that the analysis misses an exploration of the financial (as opposed to economic) implications of vaccination. A consideration only of the total cost misses the important lag between expenditures on vaccination and subsequent recovery of these costs through averted treatment, which means that even if a vaccine appears cost-saving based on the present value of expenditures in all years, that does not necessarily mean that it will be cost-saving in terms of the financial resources required in all specific budget periods. Rather, the largest component of the benefits provided is the social value of healthy life years gained and deaths averted.

Each of the eighteen research papers in Part I lays out a thoughtful evaluation of different ways to respond to HIV across Africa, with pioneering cost-benefit analysis for researchers, donors, and activists to grapple with.

Part II of this volume contains informed perspectives on the research. It is easy to say that we should do everything we can against the epidemic, all at once. That would be impossible even in the most optimistic funding scenario, let alone in a world of cutbacks. We lack the resources to scale up every intervention at once. It is much more difficult – but much more relevant – to ask: if we have limited resources, where should we first devote any additional funding?

That is the challenging question that the Rush Foundation and the Copenhagen Consensus Center posed to members of civil society, Nobel Laureate economists, senior representatives from HIV-focused international organizations, and other groups, in order to bridge the gap from this new research to debate and discussion that could inform policy decisions. Grappling with priorities forces us to consider more deeply the economic arguments put forward in each research paper.

Over the course of 2011, a panel of five expert economists, including three recipients of the Nobel Memorial Prize in Economic Sciences, read the *RethinkHIV* outlines and draft research papers, and conveyed feedback via the Copenhagen Consensus Center to authors. This group met at Georgetown University in September 2011 to interact with the researchers and to form their own prioritized list in answer to the question: where should additional funding be devoted first?

Their findings are presented here, along with the conclusions of a panel of African civil society members that gathered in Addis Ababa, Ethiopia, in December 2011. Members of the civil society panel attended the Georgetown University deliberations, and engaged with researchers there. In addition, the Copenhagen Consensus Center and the Rush Foundation conducted similar prioritizations with international institutional donors, students at Georgetown University, and students at the University of Addis Ababa School of Public Health. In the Conclusion, I will examine the similarities and differences between these groups' outcomes and other prioritization exercises completed for *RethinkHIV*, and explore potential next steps for this project.

I invite you to read the research and the viewpoints on priorities, and to form your own perspective on the best ways to continue to fight against this disease. This book clearly demonstrates that there are many investments that will do much more good than they cost. In a resource-constrained world, this is an important message. Moreover, it is my hope that this book will be used as powerful intellectual ammunition to make the case for ever-more effective action against HIV/AIDS in Africa.

References

Cohen, M. S. *et al.* (2011). Prevention of HIV-1 infection with early antiretroviral therapy. *New England Journal of Medicine*, 493–505.

Cornwell, S. (2011, December 19). *U.S. Foreign Aid Escapes Slashing Cuts in Fiscal 2012*. Retrieved January 10, 2012, from Reuters: www.reuters.com/article/2011/12/19/us-usa-aid-idUSTRE7BI1KO20111219.

Fogh Rasmussen, A. (2008, May 25). *Speech to Opening of Copenhagen Consensus Conference*. Retrieved January 12, 2011, from Website of the Prime Minister's Office: www.stm.dk/_p_11145.html.

Padian, N. S., McCoy, S., Karim, S., Hasen, N., Kim, J., Bartos, M., Katabira, E., Bertozzi, S. M., Schwartländer, B. and Cohen, M. S. (2011). HIV prevention transformed: the new prevention research agenda. *Lancet* **378**: 269–78.

The aids2031 Consortium. (2010). *AIDS: Taking a Long-Term View*. New Jersey: FT Press.

UNAIDS. (2009). *Treatment 2.0*. Geneva: UNAIDS and World Health Organization.

UNAIDS. (2011). *AIDS at 30: Nations at the Crossroads*. Geneva: UNAIDS.

UNAIDS and Kaiser Family Foundation. (2011). *Financing the Response to AIDS in Low- and Middle-Income Countries*. Geneva: UNAIDS and Kaiser Family Foundation.

UNAIDS and World Health Organization. (2009). *AIDS Epidemic Update*. Geneva: UNAIDS and World Health Organization.

World Health Organization. (2011, March 25). *The Abuja Declaration: Ten Years On*. Retrieved January 5, 2012, from www.who.int/healthsystems/publications/Abuja10.pdf.

World Health Organization, UNAIDS, UNICEF. (2011). *Global HIV/AIDS Response: Epidemic Update and Health Sector Progress Towards Universal Access: Progress Report 2011*. Geneva: World Health Organization.

PART I

The research

Sexual transmission of HIV

Assessment paper

JERE R. BEHRMAN AND HANS-PETER KOHLER

The purpose of *RethinkHIV* is to identify and highlight the most cost-effective responses to HIV/AIDS in sub-Saharan Africa (SSA) with economic analyses of the benefits and costs of specific interventions in six categories of responses to HIV/AIDS. This is the assessment paper on the first of the six topics: prevention of sexual transmission of HIV.

As is well-known, sexual infections are a major source of the spread of HIV/AIDS generally (UNAIDS 2010), and are thought to be by far the most important source of the spread of HIV/AIDS in SSA, though there also are other sources of spread of the disease, such as maternal-child infection and the use of contaminated blood or needles. Sexual interactions may directly result in the transmission of HIV, and they also may increase the vulnerability to the HIV virus through transmitting other sexually transmitted diseases. Interventions to reduce sexual infections broadly speaking can work through reducing the frequency of such interactions or through reducing the risks of sexual infection per sexual encounter. Selection of partners, including with respect to age and risk behavior of the partner, condom use or other risk reduction strategies with a specific partner, and biomedical interventions that affect HIV transmission can all affect HIV infection risks. Interventions have been proposed to work through both of these channels, though with greater emphasis probably on the latter.

In this assessment paper, we first discuss how we identified solutions through preventing sexual infections suggested by the literature. We then discuss benefit-cost analyses to help provide a framework for understanding what information is necessary for evaluating possible interventions. We then turn to assumptions for our estimated benefit to cost ratios for those solutions through preventing sexual infections suggested by the literature, and then present the estimated benefit to cost ratios and cost-effectiveness estimates for averting infections and per DALY.

The current debate about preventing HIV infections through sexual relations

Sexual transmission accounts for more than 80 percent of new HIV infections worldwide, with the rate in SSA being even higher. While paid sex is an important source of new HIV infections in SSA countries with relatively low prevalence, the vast majority of HIV infections in high prevalence countries is not related to paid sex. For example, while an estimated 32 percent of new HIV infections are attributed to paid sex in Ghana, where adult HIV prevalence is 1.8 percent, only about 10–14 percent of new infections are linked to sex work in Kenya and Uganda, where adult HIV prevalence is 6.3–6.5 percent. Urban data from Zambia suggests that 60 percent of people newly infected through heterosexual transmission acquired HIV within marriage or cohabitation, compared to 50–65 percent in Swaziland, 35–62 percent in Lesotho, and 44 percent in Kenya. Studies in eastern and southern Africa found that, among all couples tested who had at least one HIV-1 infected partner, the proportion of couples that were HIV-1-discordant varied by study sites from 36 to 85 percent, with an overall rate of 49 percent, indicating that discordant couples can succeed in effectively reducing HIV transmission to the uninfected spouses.

We gratefully acknowledge the many constructive comments that we have received from Damien de Walque, Alan Whiteside, Vernon Smith, Kasper Thede Anderskov and other members of the RethinkHIV Team, and Benjamin Armbuster and Stephane Helleringer.

The strategic goal of UNAIDS is to reduce sexual transmission by half, including among young people, by 2015 (UNAIDS 2010, 2011). While there is no doubt that the HIV/AIDS epidemic in SSA continues to be devastating, with about 1.8 million annual new infections in 2009, 20 million individuals living with HIV, constituting about two-thirds of the global total, rates of national adult prevalence ranging up to 25 percent in Swaziland, Botswana, and Lesotho (Table 1.1), and variance in regional prevalence being even higher (see Figure 1.1), there is also increasing evidence that the tide of the epidemic has shifted. UNAIDS (2010) for example points out that: (i) in SSA, the number of people newly infected with HIV fell from 2.2 million (1.9 million–2.4 million) people in 2001 to 1.8 million (1.6 million–2.0 million) in 2009; (ii) in twenty-two SSA countries, the HIV incidence rate declined by more than 25 percent between 2001 and 2009; (iii) among the five SSA countries with the largest HIV epidemics in terms of the numbers of infected individuals, four – Ethiopia, South Africa, Zambia, and Zimbabwe – reduced new HIV infections by more than 25 percent between 2001 and 2009, while Nigeria's HIV epidemic stabilized. HIV prevalence in Kenya fell from about 14 percent in the mid-1990s to 5 percent in 2006, and since 2001, HIV prevalence in Uganda has stabilized between 6.5 percent and 7 percent; and HIV prevalence in West and Central Africa remained relatively low in 2009, at or under 2 percent in twelve countries.

Based on these trends and recent progress in prevention strategies, the thirtieth anniversary of HIV coincides with a new optimism about the available mix of policies and interventions that aim at reducing HIV infections, and in particular, reducing the sexual transmission of HIV. *The Economist* recently heralded "The end of AIDS?", concluding that "Thirty years on, it looks as though the plague can now be beaten, if the world has the will to do so" (The Economist 2011). Padian *et al.* (2011) argue that "we have entered a new area in HIV prevention," where a rapidly changing landscape of HIV prevention suggests a new path of interventions that focus on efficient combination strategies to turn the tide in the HIV epidemic. Medical male circumcision (MC) has been shown in several randomized controlled trials in SSA to reduce the risk

of HIV acquisition by men (Auvert *et al.* 2005; Bailey *et al.* 2007; Gray *et al.* 2007), and while the effect on infection risks during sex with an HIV-positive partner remains somewhat controversial, MC has emerged as one of the core pillars of HIV prevention programs in SSA (Schwartländer *et al.* 2011; UNAIDS 2010). Recent estimates suggest population-level reductions in HIV infections for men and women as high as 28 percent in Zimbabwe (Hallett *et al.* 2011), where the reductions in infection risks for men result from the combined effect of a lower HIV prevalence among male partners and possible long-term direct reductions of male-to-female HIV transmission risks that are suggested by recent studies to result from circumcision after the wound healing is completed. Based on the recent evidence about the effectiveness of MC, Potts *et al.* (2008) argue that resources should be redirected from potentially ineffective interventions – including HIV testing, treatment of STIs, and abstinence programs – towards MC and selected other behavioral interventions that have been shown to effectively reduce HIV risks.

In addition to MC, new biomedical developments promise new approaches to substantially reducing the risk of transmitting HIV by offering anti-retroviral treatment (ART) to HIV-positive individuals as soon as they are infected (NIAID 2011; Smith *et al.* 2011). This test-and-treat strategy is based on the premise that reductions in viral load caused by ART will decrease an individual's infectiousness, and advocates regular, widespread HIV testing and immediate initiation of ART for infected people. Findings from the HPTN 052 study (NIAID 2011) for example attributed a 96 percent reduction of HIV transmission to the use of anti-retroviral drugs. Some studies have claimed that a comprehensive test-and-treat program could reduce HIV incidence and mortality to less than one case per 1,000 people per year by 2016 (Granich *et al.* 2009), and reduce the prevalence of HIV to less than 1 percent within 50 years. Based on this recent evidence, it is likely that ART will serve as a cornerstone of combination prevention of HIV-1 in the near future. Continued research will be essential to measure anticipated benefits and to detect implementation barriers and untoward consequences of such a program, especially increases in primary

Table 1.1 HIV prevalence, HIV incidence, and number of persons living with HIV in sub-Saharan Africa, 2009

	HIV prevalence (age 15–49)	HIV incidence (age 15–49)	Number of persons living with HIV (in '000)	Proportion of all HIV+ persons in SSA	Cumulative prop. of all HIV+ persons in SSA
Swaziland	25.9%	2.66	180	0.8%	0.8%
Botswana	24.8%	1.56	320	1.5%	2.3%
Lesotho	23.6%	2.58	290	1.3%	3.7%
South Africa	17.8%	1.49	5,600	25.9%	29.6%
Zimbabwe	14.3%	0.84	1,200	5.6%	35.2%
Zambia	13.5%	1.17	980	4.5%	39.7%
Namibia	13.1%	0.43	180	0.8%	40.5%
Mozambique	11.5%	1.19	1,400	6.5%	47.0%
Malawi	11.0%	0.95	920	4.3%	51.3%
Uganda	6.5%	0.74	1,200	5.6%	56.8%
Kenya	6.3%	0.53	1,500	6.9%	63.8%
Tanzania	5.6%	0.45	1,400	6.5%	70.3%
Cameroon	5.3%	0.53	610	2.8%	73.1%
Gabon	5.2%	0.43	46	0.2%	73.3%
Equatorial Guinea	5.0%	n.a.	20	0.1%	73.4%
Central African R.	4.7%	0.17	130	0.6%	74.0%
Nigeria	3.6%	0.38	3,300	15.3%	89.3%
Chad	3.4%	n.a.	210	1.0%	90.3%
Congo	3.4%	0.28	77	0.4%	90.6%
Cote d'Ivoire	3.4%	0.11	450	2.1%	92.7%
Burundi	3.3%	n.a.	180	0.8%	93.5%
Togo	3.2%	0.27	120	0.6%	94.1%
Rwanda	2.9%	0.18	170	0.8%	94.9%
Guinea-Bissau	2.5%	0.21	22	0.1%	95.0%
Angola	2.0%	0.21	200	0.9%	95.9%
Gambia, The	2.0%	n.a.	18	0.1%	96.0%
Ghana	1.8%	0.15	260	1.2%	97.2%
Sierra Leone	1.6%	0.14	49	0.2%	97.4%
Liberia	1.5%	n.a.	37	0.2%	97.6%
Guinea	1.3%	0.1	79	0.4%	98.0%
Benin	1.2%	0.1	60	0.3%	98.2%
Burkina Faso	1.2%	0.07	110	0.5%	98.8%
Mali	1.0%	0.06	76	0.4%	99.1%
Mauritius	1.0%	n.a.	9	0.0%	99.1%
Senegal	0.9%	0.08	59	0.3%	99.4%
Eritrea	0.8%	0.03	25	0.1%	99.5%
Niger	0.8%	0.08	61	0.3%	99.8%
Mauritania	0.7%	n.a.	14	0.1%	99.9%
Madagascar	0.2%	n.a.	24	0.1%	100.0%
Comoros	0.1%	n.a.	<1	<0.1%	100.0%

Source: AIDSinfo (www.aidsinfoonline.org), retrieved 8/4/2011
Note: HIV incidence = new HIV infections per 100 person years

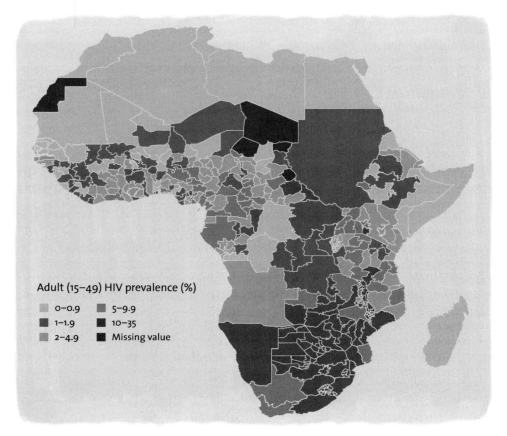

Figure 1.1 *Subnational estimates of HIV prevalence among adults (age 15–59) in sub-Saharan Africa, 2001–2010*
Note: *Subnational data not available for Angola, Eritrea, Gabon, the Gambia, Guinea-Bissau, Madagascar, Mauritania, Namibia, Somalia, Sudan, and Togo.*
Source: *UNAIDS (2011, page 74)*

ART resistance. Skeptics of this approach, however, point out the important role of recent HIV infections in propagating HIV – with studies claiming that up to 40 percent of HIV infections in urban Malawi are attributable to sexual contact with individuals with early infection (< 6 months) (Cohen and Corbett 2011; Powers *et al.* 2011), i.e., individuals who are highly infectious but unlikely to be covered by test-and-treat programs in resource-poor countries. Thus, without near-complete coverage, interventions during chronic infection will probably have incomplete effectiveness unless complemented by strategies targeting individuals with early HIV infection, or

by interventions that not only reduce HIV transmission risks but also result in behavioral changes and the adoption of risk-reduction strategies.

How do behavioral prevention programs fit into the policy mix? Behavioral strategies to prevent the sexual transmission of HIV include programs that aim to delay age of sexual debut, decrease the number of sexual partners and concurrent partnerships, increase the proportion of protected sexual acts, increase acceptance of HIV testing and counseling (HTC), and improve adherence to successful biomedical prevention strategies, such as condom use (Coates *et al.* 2008; McCoy *et al.* 2010). While biomedical interventions and their promise in reducing HIV infection risk have recently been dominating the headlines in both the scientific and policy-oriented discussion about alternative HIV prevention strategies, Halperin *et al.* (2011) and Coates *et al.* (2008) conclude, based on their analyses of declining HIV incidence in several SSA countries, that behavioral change must remain the core of prevention efforts. In particular, although there have been promising breakthroughs in biomedical interventions to reduce HIV infection risks (notably MC), given the limitations and challenges of biomedical interventions in terms of scaling-up, resource requirements, and potential reductions in effectiveness due to drug resistance, these biomedical programs cannot constitute the sole prevention efforts in resource-poor contexts such as SSA. Behavioral change programs and structural interventions facilitating behavior change are therefore widely recognized to be an important and essential – but not necessarily sufficient – part of comprehensive HIV prevention programs in SSA (Coates *et al.* 2008; Padian *et al.* 2011). The UNAIDS Strategy 2011–2015 concludes that evidence is mounting that comprehensive sexuality education empowers young people to make informed decisions regarding their sexual health and behavior while playing a part in combating damaging beliefs and misconceptions about HIV and sexual health (UNAIDS 2010).

While recognizing this important role of behavioral change programs, Schwartländer *et al.* (2011) argue that the policy mix needs to change from a "commodity approach" that encourages scaling-up of numerous strategies in parallel, irrespective of the evidence about the relative effects of these programs, towards a strategic "investment approach" that incorporates major efficiency gains through community mobilization, synergies among program elements, and benefits of the extension of ART for prevention of HIV transmission (Figure 1.2). This framework proposes three categories of investment, consisting of six basic programmatic activities, interventions that create a facilitating environment to achieve maximum effectiveness ("critical enablers"), and programmatic efforts in other health and development sectors related to HIV/AIDS. Four of the six program components focus on reducing the transmission of

HIV through sexual relationships, that is, prevention strategies that are within the scope of the analyses in this paper. The investment approach in Figure 1.2 also emphasizes the role of "critical enablers," i.e., the complementary program activities that are necessary to increase the effectiveness of prevention efforts. Social enablers include outreach for HIV/AIDS testing and HIV/AIDS treatment literacy, stigma reduction, advocacy to protect human rights, and monitoring of the equity and quality of program access and results and mass communication designed to raise awareness and support change in social norms. Program enablers include incentives for program participation, methods to improve retention of patients on anti-retroviral therapy, capacity-building for development of community-based organizations, strategic planning, communications infrastructure, information dissemination, and efforts to improve service integration and linkages from testing to care. As we will argue below, the cost of these enablers is often inadequately represented in studies assessing the costs of program interventions, despite the fact that they may constitute an important part of the overall program costs (e.g., up to 35 percent in the initial years of the investment approach in Figure 1.2). Based on their evaluation of this investment approach, Schwartländer *et al.* (2011) claim that at a yearly cost of achievement of universal access to HIV prevention, treatment, care, and support by 2015 of not less than $22 billion, this program can globally avert 12.2 million new HIV infections and 7.4 million deaths from AIDS between 2011 and 2020, compared with continuation of present approaches, and result in 29.4 million life-years gained.

In addition to emphasizing a multi-faceted approach to HIV prevention that combines biomedical, behavioral, and structural components, as for instance in the investment approach in Figure 1.2, there is also a broad recognition that the HIV/AIDS epidemic is heterogeneous – globally, but also within SSA – and that interventions need to be specific to local contexts (e.g., Wilson and Halperin 2008). The most important distinction is between the generalized epidemics in high-prevalence SSA countries, where interventions need to change behaviors and/or infection risks on the population level, versus the more concentrated or mixed

INVESTMENT FRAMEWORK

For whom? Explicitly identify and prioritize populations on the basis of the epidemic profile
How? Use the human rights approach to achieve dignity and security

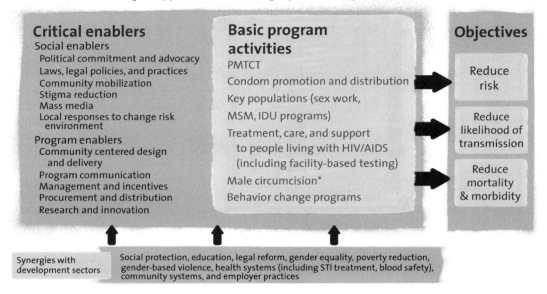

Figure 1.2 *"Investment approach" to HIV prevention that combines community mobilization, synergies between program elements, and benefits of the extension of anti-retroviral therapy for prevention of HIV transmission*
Notes: *Applicable in generalized epidemics with a low prevalence of male circumcision. MSM = men who have sex with men. IDU = injecting drug user. PMTCT = prevention of mother-to-child transmission. STI = sexually transmitted infection.*
Source: *Schwartländer et al. (2011)*

epidemics in much of the rest of the world and in low-prevalence SSA countries (note in Table 1.1 there are eight SSA countries with prevalence at 1 percent or less, and sixteen SSA countries with prevalences at 2 percent or less) where interventions can often be more targeted towards the highest risk groups. While programs clearly need to be adjusted to local contexts, even across different SSA countries, based on a nuanced understanding of the local social, economic, institutional, and epidemiological context, Coates *et al.* (2008) also warn of the dangers of extensive modifications to local contexts that are often based on weak empirical evidence about cross-country differences and that may undermine the synergies and scale effects that can be achieved if interventions are applied on a large scale. Evidence that this might be occurring

is provided in Figure 1.3 (Forsythe *et al.* 2009), which reports the allocation to HIV prevention in different SSA countries that are arranged from low prevalence (left) to high prevalence (right). While one would expect that the allocation of prevention effort varies by HIV prevalence, the pattern in Figure 1.3 appears quite random, with substantial variations across countries that seem to face relatively similar HIV epidemics. For example, focusing on the two highest prevalence countries, Botswana and Swaziland, the resources allocated to prevention efforts appear to be markedly different. In Botswana, most prevention resources are allocated to PMTCT, whereas in Swaziland, the majority of resources are spent on behavioral change communication (BCC), an intervention that is allocated a much smaller proportion of all resources

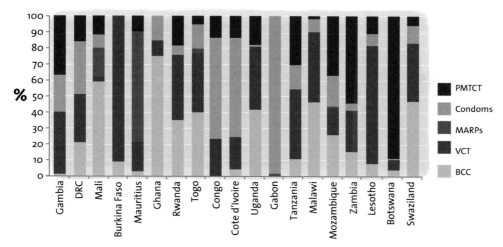

Figure 1.3 *Allocation of resources to HIV prevention in sub-Saharan Africa*
Notes: *BCC = behavior change communication. VCT = voluntary testing and counseling. MARPs =*
most at-risk populations. PMTCT = prevention of mother to child transmission.
Source: *Forsythe* et al. *(2009), with data from UNAIDS (2008)*

in Botswana. Of course there are other huge differences between markets, policies, and level of development between Botswana and Swaziland that may account for the variations in resource allocations to HIV prevention in the two countries. But if these factors account for the difference, the comparison between these two countries points to the importance of heterogeneities of other types even in countries with similar prevalences.

Assessing the evidence about the effectiveness and cost-effectiveness of interventions

Ideally, the interventions considered to reduce the sexual transmission of HIV would be based on solid empirical evidence about their effectiveness, and resources would be allocated efficiently to different programs. While there is a growing agreement that contemporary HIV prevention programs should adopt a multi-pronged approach combining biomedical, behavioral, and structural approaches, diverging advice exists in the current literature as to how to allocate resources to the different components. Forsythe *et al.* (2009) conclude, based on an analysis of how resources are allocated to

prevention efforts, that "there are clear indications that most countries are not allocating their HIV and AIDS resources in a way which is likely to achieve the greatest possible impact" (see also the discussion related to Figure 1.3). And while evidence is often far from conclusive, several criteria to improve allocation decisions exist: Schwartländer *et al.* (2011) argue that in their investment approach, "basic program activities [that] have a direct effect on reduction of transmission, morbidity, and mortality from HIV/AIDS...should be scaled up according to the size of the affected population." Potts *et al.* (2008), in agreement with other studies (e.g., Padian *et al.* 2011; Schwartländer *et al.* 2011), argue that intervention with established effectiveness in preventing HIV infection should be scaled up, while programs that have not been shown to reduce HIV should be faded out. Forsythe *et al.* (2009) propose an "evidence-based allocation strategy" as the overarching principle in which resources are spent in a way that is, based on the best currently available evidence, likely to achieve the greatest possible result in terms of preventing new infections, providing care and treatment, and mitigating impact. Basic economic theory (Behrman and Knowles 1998) suggests programs should be scaled up until their social marginal benefits equal their social marginal costs, while others have argued that programs with the largest cost-effectiveness (Drummond *et al*. 1997; Musgrove and Fox-Rushby 2006) or highest benefit to cost ratios (Brent 2010a) should receive priority. Equating social marginal benefits with social marginal costs, as suggested by Behrman and Knowles, implies that programs should be scaled up or scaled down to the point at which benefit to cost ratios are one. Political constraints on governmental budgets, high adjustment costs, and effective interest groups may preclude scaling up or scaling down all interventions so that all benefit to cost ratios are equal to one, so values different from one may be observed in real world programs. Tools such as the Resource Needs Model (RNM), which can provide policy-makers with a clearer idea of resource requirements, the Male Circumcision: Decision Makers' Program Planning Tool (DMPPT), or the Goals and Allocation by Cost-Effectiveness (ABCE) model can also provide decision-makers with a clearer vision of how they might reallocate funds. These different criteria and/or tools lead to different priorities in prevention efforts. The economic approaches, for example, may lead to much different allocations among interventions than some of the other "rules" for allocation suggested above because they focus on costs as well as impacts at the margin. Cost-effectiveness estimates, for another example, focus by definition on one objective rather than considering multiple objectives as in cost-benefit analysis.

In addition to possible disagreements about the general principles guiding the allocation of resources to different programs, there is considerable uncertainty about the efficacy and/or effectiveness of program interventions to reduce the sexual transmission of HIV. Ultimately, under any of the criteria stated above, only programs that reduce HIV risk behaviors, HIV infection risks, and/or HIV incidence should be considered. However, despite the substantial resources devoted to evaluating such interventions, the evidence remains weak (Padian *et al*. 2010; Ross 2010). For example, restricting studies to the "gold standard" of randomized controlled trials (RCTs) with biological outcome measures (HIV incidence), a systematic review of late phase RCTs evaluating interventions for the prevention of sexual transmission

of HIV by Padian *et al*. (2010) identified only thirty-seven HIV prevention RCTs reporting on thirty-nine unique interventions. Only six RCTs, all evaluating biomedical interventions, demonstrated definitive effects on HIV incidence. Five of the six RCTs significantly reduced HIV infection: all three male circumcision trials, one trial of sexually transmitted infection treatment and care, and one vaccine trial. Njeuhmeli *et al*. (2011) evaluate the potential population-level impacts of MC using the Male Circumcision: Decision Makers' Program Planning Tool to model the impact and cost of scaling up adult MC in Botswana, Lesotho, Malawi, Mozambique, Namibia, Rwanda, South Africa, Swaziland, Tanzania, Uganda, Zambia, Zimbabwe, and Nyanza province in Kenya. At a cost of about $80 per circumcision, scaling up adult MC to reach 80 percent coverage in these countries by 2015, and maintaining 80 percent coverage thereafter, would entail performing 20.33 million circumcisions between 2011 and 2015 and an additional 8.42 million between 2016 and 2025. Such a scale-up would result in averting 3.36 million new HIV infections and 386,000 AIDS deaths through 2025, and this scale-up would result in net savings (due to averted treatment and care costs) amounting to $16.55 billion. However, in contrast to the clear evidence documented for MC, almost 90 percent of HIV prevention trials reviewed in Padian *et al*. (2010) had "flat" results, i.e., the RCTs did not indicate statistically significant declines in HIV and/or STI incidence as a result of the intervention. In some cases, these flat results may be attributable to trial design and/or implementation, including for example inadequate sample sizes to detect changes in incidence, especially in light of the often lower-than-expected incidence in both arms of the RCTs, the requirement to provide "diluted" forms of the intervention to the control arm, or the "diffusion" of the intervention into the control group. An update of this review of RCTs (Padian *et al*. 2011) has further strengthened the evidence for biomedical interventions – MC and ART as prevention ("test-and-treat") – and also points to the potentials of structural interventions such as microfinance programs (Pronyk *et al*. 2006, 2008) or conditional cash transfers (Baird *et al*. 2010; Kohler and Thornton 2012) that are discussed in more detail below. Behavioral interventions that have been evaluated in RCTs

include some combination of risk reduction counseling, condom promotion, and referral and treatment for STIs that exceed the local standard of
care. But even the updated analyses in Padian
et al. (2011) fail to identify effective behavioral
interventions, and all seven RCTs reviewed in
the study found no statistically significant reductions in HIV incidence. In summary, therefore,
while for some biomedical interventions – and in
particular, male circumcision – strong evidence
about their efficacy and sometimes their effectiveness exists, outside of these biomedical interventions, the empirical evidence often needs to
be supported by circumstantial evidence, evidence
from observational studies – which generally do
not establish causal effects – or studies that use
behavioral outcomes rather than HIV incidence
itself in trying to establish the effectiveness of
interventions.

The aforementioned limited evidence from RCTs
about the effectiveness of behavioral strategies
to reduce the sexual transmission of HIV is in
sharp contrast with the important role that is often
attributed by others to behavioral changes in reducing HIV incidence in SSA (e.g., UNAIDS 2010).
Analyzing comprehensive data from Zimbabwe,
Gregson *et al.* (2010) and Halperin *et al.* (2011)
for example document that HIV incidence may
have peaked in the early 1990s, and fallen during
the 1990s. Household survey data shows that this
decline in HIV incidence in Zimbabwe is linked
to reductions in reported casual partners from the
late 1990s onwards, and in increases in condom
use in non-regular partnerships between 1998 and
2007. Gregson *et al.* (2010) claim that this study
provides the first convincing evidence of an HIV
decline accelerated by changes in sexual behavior in a southern African country. Declines in HIV
prevalence have been linked to behavioral changes
also in other SSA countries (Hallett *et al.* 2006;
the International Group on Analysis of Trends in
HIV Prevalence and Behaviors in Young People in
Countries most Affected by HIV 2010; UNAIDS
2010). Increases in AIDS mortality may have been
a key factor driving behavioral changes, and in
the specific case of Zimbabwe, another key factor may have been the adverse economic conditions that prevailed during this period. In terms of
interventions and behavioral change programs,

Halperin *et al.* identify condom distribution and
promotion programs, and community-based interventions, as plausibly making major contributions
to the HIV decline in Zimbabwe, while they
discount an important role related to HIV testing and counseling. Interpersonal communication
about HIV/AIDS and risk reduction strategy is
likely to have been an important facilitating factor (see also Behrman *et al.* 2009; Kohler *et al.*
2007). Potts *et al.* (2008) also argue that policies targeted at the reduction of multiple concurrent partnerships were one intervention that may
have contributed substantially to declines in HIV
in SSA, with potentially much greater effectiveness
if this prevention strategy had been adopted more
broadly.

In contrast, in a somewhat pessimistic summary about behavioral interventions to reduce HIV
infections in the context of generalized epidemics
such as HIV in SSA, Wilson and Halperin (2008)
observe that the most "trusted interventions" –
including HIV testing and counseling, condom promotion, and school and youth (including abstinence programs) – are "at best unproven, and
at worst disproven, for reducing HIV incidence."
Based on the mixed evidence that emerges from
the above review, no single behavioral HIV prevention approach has therefore emerged as the leading
behavioral intervention in SSA, and the claims that
these efforts contributed importantly to the recent
declines in HIV in some SSA countries are often
based on indirect – and sometimes weak – evidence.
While behavioral change programs continue to be
emphasized in most agendas aiming at reducing
HIV infections (Bertozzi *et al.* 2006; Schwartländer
et al. 2011; UNAIDS 2010), the evidence of dramatic behavioral changes as a response to these
programs in SSA remains controversial (McCoy
et al. 2010).

In reviewing the evidence about policy intervention, HIV testing and counseling (HTC) deserves
specific attention. HIV testing and counseling, and
in particular, the component of HTC formerly
referred to as voluntary counseling and testing
(VCT), has been a key component of AIDS control
programs for several years, predating the rise of
"test-and-treat" interventions in which HIV testing
is central for identifying HIV-positive individuals
and enrolling them in ART treatment. For example,

an op-ed piece in the *New York Times* several years ago declared that HTC is the "missing weapon" in the battle against AIDS (Holbrooke and Furman 2004), based on the argument that those who learn they are not infected will be more strongly motivated to avoid infection in the future, and those who learn that they are infected will be motivated to avoid infecting others. Yet, at least several RCT studies evaluating HTC programs have shown no consistent reduction for those who test HIV-negative, although risk reduction in some who test positive has occurred, and the studies found no population-level impact of HTC on HIV and/or STI incidence (Corbett *et al.* 2007; Denison *et al.* 2008; Metcalf *et al.* 2005; Sherr *et al.* 2007; the Voluntary HIV-1 Counseling and Testing Efficacy Study Group 2000). There is also little evidence, among HIV-negative individuals, of HTC impacts on behavioral risk reduction (e.g., condom use or reduction in the number of sexual partners) or even subjective risk assessments about being HIV-positive (Delavande and Kohler forthcoming; Matovu *et al.* 2006), and selectivity in HTC uptake and/or study participation may have affected the findings of existing studies (Glick 2005). Only one recent study by Cremin *et al.* (2010) documented that both HIV-positive and HIV-negative women receiving HTC have sustained significant reductions in the number of sexual partnerships (the reductions existed for males, but were not statistically significant). Based on the existing evidence, Ross (2010) speculates that HIV testing and counseling might be effective in persuading HIV-positive individuals to reduce their risk of onward transmission of HIV to their partners, but potentially leads to relative disinhibition among those who test HIV-negative, along the lines of "I have taken risks in the past and have not been infected, so maybe I can continue with my previous behaviors?"

It is important, however, to recognize that the contemporary context in which HIV testing and counseling is expanded is often substantially different from the context in which the above studies were conducted (Gersovitz 2011), as voluntary counseling is increasingly complemented by routine testing within health care settings, home-based testing and counseling, or even self-testing (Ganguli *et al.* 2009; Helleringer *et al.* 2009;

Weinreb and Stecklov 2009). New testing possibilities, including more frequent testing and home-based testing, a decreasing stigmatization of testing HIV-positive, and new incentives to get tested to gain access to ART for both treatment and prevention, may have changed the impact of HTC on behavioral risk reduction and behavioral change in SSA. Couple-based HIV testing and counseling (Painter 2001), incentives for getting tested (Thornton 2008), or programs facilitating the communications of HIV test results between spouses or with sexual partners (Anglewicz and Chitsanya 2011) may also enhance the effectiveness of HIV testing and counseling in reducing HIV infection risks, and community-based interventions using mobile technologies can be used to substantially increase the uptake of HIV testing services (Sweat *et al.* 2011). Despite the somewhat mixed evidence, therefore, UNAIDS Strategy 2011–2015 continues to emphasize the scaling-up of HIV testing and counseling as an essential component of prevention strategies, including particular foci for improving access to HIV testing and counseling among youths and HTC for couples. UNAIDS (2010) and Cremin *et al.* (2010) conclude that "[HTC in the form of] VCT arguably represents the best opportunity for encouraging sexual behavior[al] change, which is essential if the transmission of HIV is to be abated and the provision of treatment is to be sustainable." This conclusion is conditional on HTC leading to sustained risk reduction among both infected and uninfected individuals. This outcome is only likely if HTC is widespread, possibly relatively frequent, combined with high-quality counseling.

In addition to offering some revisionist perspectives on HIV testing and counseling, some recent studies also provide a more optimistic perspective within the otherwise generally inconclusive or controversial empirical evidence about the effectiveness of behavioral interventions. For example, cellphones and related technologies may offer new ways for delivering information campaigns, and for interacting with young adults in SSA, in ways that can reduce HIV risks (Swendeman and Rotheram-Borus 2010). A recent school-level randomized experiment has also provided information on the relative risk of HIV infection by partner's age, and documented that the sexual behaviors of teenagers are responsive to HIV risk information. In particular, this randomized study documented a 28 percent decrease in teen pregnancy, an objective proxy for the incidence of unprotected sex (Dupas 2011), among teenagers who received information about the local prevalence of HIV disaggregated by age and gender group, i.e., important – but generally not available – information that can affect partner selection and the adoption of condoms or other risk-reduction behaviors with a specific partner, while the official abstinence-only HIV curriculum had no impact on teen pregnancy. Besides offering HIV-related education and training in schools, some recent studies also suggest that encouraging school attendance by adolescents – and in particular girls – through monetary incentives can not only reduce school dropouts but can also reduce HIV infection risks by delaying sexual debut and/or other reducing risk factors associated with infection with human immunodeficiency virus (Baird *et al.* 2010; Cho *et al.* 2011; Hallfors *et al.* 2011). In addition, several other programs that deviate from the more conventional behavioral intervention programs that have been the focus of much of the above literature have emerged as potential HIV prevention approaches. For example, Pronyk *et al.* (2006, 2008) document with a large-scale RCT that the IMAGE Program in South Africa, which combines microfinance for women with gender training and community mobilization, resulted in increases in household economic well-being and women's empowerment, a 50 percent reduction in intimate partner violence, and reduced HIV risk behavior among young women participants. The program has scaled up to reach more than 12,000 women in South Africa. In addition, several studies have suggested the possibility that conditional cash transfers can effectively be implemented to reduce HIV infection risks, including a program that gave financial rewards for testing negative for non-HIV sexually transmitted diseases every few months in Tanzania (RESPECT) (de Walque *et al.* 2011; World Bank 2010b) and a program for adolescents in Mexico (Galarraga and Gertler 2010). Another program in Malawi found that conditional and unconditional cash transfers for adolescent girls were associated with lower rates of marriage (Baird *et al.* 2010) and HIV (World Bank 2010a). Recent press releases have heralded these conditional cash incentive programs as potentially promising and innovative approaches to HIV/AIDS prevention. The UC Berkeley news release about the RESPECT program for example begins: "Giving out cash can be an effective tool in combating sexually transmitted infections in rural Africa" (Yang 2010). Kohler and Thornton (2012), drawing on a program offering financial incentives for individuals to maintain their HIV status in Malawi, however, raise some concerns about the potential effectiveness of conditional cash transfer (CCT) programs for HIV prevention, and conclude that CCT programs that aim to motivate safe sexual behavior in Africa need to take into account that money given in the present may have much stronger effects than rewards in the future, and any effect of these programs may be fairly sensitive to the specific design of the program, the local and/or cultural context, and the degree of agency individuals have with respect to sexual behaviors.

In summary, current empirical evidence clearly points to MC as a promising intervention, with possible additional effective interventions being comprehensive testing and counseling, effective information and peer group campaigns, and possibly programs that encourage schooling or incentivize HIV risk reductions. Translating these findings into policy interventions, however, requires prioritization among different possible prevention approaches, as well as decisions about resource allocations to different components in multi-faceted approaches such as the "investment approach" in Figure 1.2. In choosing among these effective interventions, additional criteria are necessary to guide resource allocations and aid the prioritization of prevention strategies. Cost-effectiveness analyses and benefit-cost analyses can both fill this gap, and especially the former has been extensively applied to HIV prevention programs.

To provide guidance about the allocation of resources to prevention efforts, an extensive body of literature has emerged that studies the cost-effectiveness of interventions targeted towards reducing HIV infections through sexual relations. Cost-effectiveness is defined to yield the effectiveness in terms of some specific goal for the use of some specific amount of resources, often using summary measures of effectiveness such as the quality- or disability-adjusted life years (QALYs/DALYs) gained/averted through the same

Table 1.2 Cost per DALY and cost per infection averted for selected interventions in sub-Saharan Africa

| | Cost ($) per | | | |
	DALY	infection averted	Region/country	Source
HTC	82	1,315483*	SSA Kenya	Hogan *et al.* (2005) John *et al.* (2008)
Treatment of STIs	17–121	321–3,635	E. Africa	Oster (2005); Vickerman *et al.* (2006); White *et al.* (2008b)
School-based interventions	376–530	6,704–9,448	Africa	Hogan *et al.* (2005)
Male circumcision	–	176–3,554	SSA	Gray *et al.* (2007); Martin *et al.* (2007); White *et al.* (2008a)
Empowerment/social/peer-based programs/mass media	3	599	SSA	Hogan *et al.* (2005)

Sources: Adapted from Galarraga *et al.* (2009)
Note: *focuses on averting infant infections

resources used in different interventions (Drummond *et al.* 1997). Cost-effectiveness analysis (CEA) is then used to compare two or more alternatives in terms of their costs and effectiveness through a cost-effectiveness ratio that is computed as the difference in costs over the difference in effectiveness. In the context of HIV/AIDS, the costs per HIV infection averted and the costs per DALY/QALY are also often used as the outcome variables. A recent review by Galarraga *et al.* (2009), for example, conducted a systematic identification of publications through several methods: electronic databases, internet search of international organizations and major funding/implementing agencies, and journal browsing. Inclusion criteria included: HIV prevention intervention, publication in 2005–2008, setting in low- and middle-income countries, and cost-effectiveness estimation (empirical or modeling) using outcomes in terms of cost per HIV infection averted and/or cost per disability-adjusted life year (DALY) or quality-adjusted life year (QALY). The study found twenty-one studies analyzing the cost-effectiveness of HIV-prevention interventions published in 2005–2008. Seventeen cost-effectiveness studies analyzed biomedical interventions; only a few dealt with behavioral and environmental/structural interventions. Sixteen studies focused on SSA, and only a handful on Asia, Latin America, and Eastern Europe. They summarize the results of these studies to show that many HIV-prevention interventions are very cost-effective in absolute terms (using costs per DALY averted), and also in country-specific relative terms (in cost per DALY measured as percentage of GDP per capita). They also note that there are several types of interventions for which cost-effectiveness studies are still not available or insufficient, including surveillance, abstinence, school-based education, universal precautions, prevention for positives, and similar structural interventions. They further conclude that the sparse cost-effectiveness evidence is not easily comparable due to a lack of uniform reporting of costs and outcomes, and, thus, not very useful for decision making. There is still much work to be done both on costs and effectiveness to adequately inform HIV prevention planning. Some key findings of Galarraga *et al.*'s (2009) review, which are relevant for the discussions within the framework of *RethinkHIV* about the prevention of sexual infections, are reported in Table 1.2 (for a related study, see Uthman *et al.* 2010).

Based on their review of the literature, Galarraga *et al.* (2009) conclude that MC stands out as highly cost-effective, given the levels of efficacy suggested by recent RCTs, whereas no clear picture emerges for behavioral and structural interventions (see also Shepherd *et al.* 2010). For behavioral interventions, there is a lack of demonstrated efficacy in reducing HIV infections, and even where such evidence exists, careful cost-effectiveness data are often missing. A similar conclusion is obtained with respect to HTC, where cost-effectiveness results are strongly affected by the mixed findings about the extent to which HTC can reduce HIV. A possibly more optimistic perspective of the cost-effectiveness of HTC is suggested by a more recent study (Waters *et al.* 2011) that has cost-effectiveness of alternative HIV retesting frequencies, with testing frequencies ranging from three months to thirty years. The benefits of HTC occur as persons testing HIV-positive receive treatment, thereby reducing the further transmission probabilities (no behavioral change is assumed to result from HTC in this study). For example, accounting for secondary infections averted, the most cost-effective testing frequency was every 7.5 years for 0.8 percent incidence, every 5 years for 1.3 percent incidence, and every 2 years for 4.0 percent incidence. At a testing frequency of 7.5 years, the overall cost per QALY gained was $701, and the total cost per HIV-infected case identified was $2,030. Thus, even in low prevalence populations, regular HTC (re-)testing could be cost-effective – even if there are no behavioral changes resulting from HTC itself, as all the benefits in Waters *et al.* (2011) occur through ART treatment of HIV-positive individuals. In terms of structural interventions, Galarraga *et al.* (2009) primarily identify conditional cash transfer (CCT) programs as potentially cost-effective interventions, based on further studies confirming existing evidence about their effectiveness, while in many other structural interventions no clear conclusions about their cost-effectiveness could be established.

Beyond cost-effectiveness analyses, there is also a nascent literature on cost-benefit analyses for setting priorities for HIV/AIDS interventions (Brent 2010a). This cost-benefit approach considers benefits more broadly, including the subjective well-being of individuals, and tries to account for the fact that individuals make conscious choices with respect to sexual relations and other behaviors that affect their HIV infection risks (Philipson and Posner 1993). Brent (2010b), for example, evaluate the costs and benefits of scaling up HTC programs in Tanzania, formulating a welfare function based on an individual's, or in the case of couple-HTC, two individuals', expected utility functions and estimating the benefits the averted lives lost whenever discordant couples are revealed, while the costs also

include the utility costs of behavioral changes based on new information about one's (and possibly one's spouse's) HIV status. The study finds that the existing HTC program is only marginally worthwhile, while scaling up the program, and also scaling up couple-HTC, could increase the benefit to cost ratio to over three. A related study also finds that the benefits of education through delaying the onset of sexual activity outweigh the costs of the program and the possible positive effects of higher education on risk-taking behaviors (Brent 2009).

RethinkHIV: Possible solutions for the prevention of HIV infections through sexual relations

Our guidelines for selecting possible solutions for *RethinkHIV* that aim for the reduction of HIV infection through sexual relations are as follows: First, we focused on potential interventions for which there is reasonably strong empirical evidence from multiple SSA countries about the efficacy – and possibly even effectiveness – of the intervention. Second, we focused on interventions that are seen as important elements in the HIV/AIDS prevention efforts in SSA by international organizations and local governments. Third, we restricted ourselves to interventions for which reasonable estimates about both the benefits and costs of the intervention could be obtained. The later requirement, for example, ruled out the consideration of test-and-treat programs, as the efficacy of this possible intervention has just recently been established and the effectiveness of the intervention outside the context of randomized trials, as well as the challenges – and costs – of a scale-up of these interventions, are currently unknown.

Based on these guidelines, the three solutions for the prevention of HIV infections through sexual relations for which cost-benefit and cost-effectiveness estimates are presented in this assessment paper are male circumcision, HIV testing and counseling, and information campaigns through mass media and peer groups.

Male circumcision (MC)

Medical MC is currently the policy intervention with the strongest empirical evidence, based on

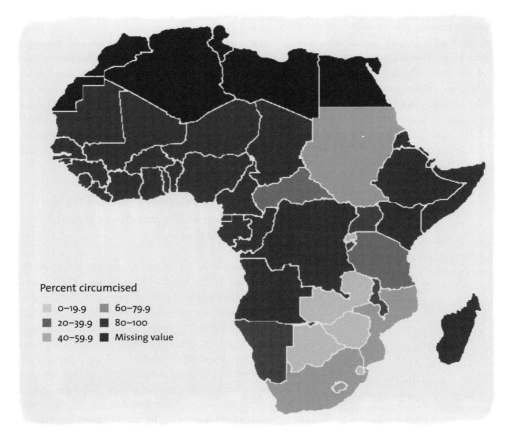

Figure 1.4 *Male circumcision prevalence in sub-Saharan Africa, 2010*
Source: *UNAIDS (2011, page 65)*

randomized controlled trials in SSA that have carefully assessed effectiveness in preventing sexually transmitted HIV. Extensive studies have also been conducted to assess the costs and challenges of implementing and scaling up MC. Multiple studies have suggested that this scale-up of MC is cost-effective. MC is also an important element of the prevention agenda promoted by UNAIDS as well as many governments or NGOs in SSA. The prevalence of MC continues to be relatively low in many countries most affected by the HIV/AIDS epidemic (Figure 1.4), and MC has been scaled-up in many SSA countries and seems to be accelerating rapidly. For example, UNAIDS (2011) reports that more than 100,000 men were circumcised in eight priority countries (Kenya, Malawi, Namibia, Rwanda,

South Africa, Swaziland, Zambia, Zimbabwe) in 2009, up from less than 50,000 in 2006, and more than 350,000 men were circumcised during 2010 in these eight countries. While some scholars have argued that behavioral disinhibition, that is, the adoption of riskier sexual behaviors among circumcised men, may reduce the effectiveness of MC for reducing HIV incidence, current empirical evidence suggests that behavioral disinhibition is unlikely to be a major factor that will substantially reduce the effectiveness of MC (for one of many related discussions on the validity of the evidence supporting MC and its potential for HIV reductions in SSA, see Geen *et al.* 2011, and Banerjee *et al.* 2011). For example, data from the three RCTs on MC (Auvert *et al.* 2008; Bailey *et al.* 2007;

Gray *et al.* 2007) and one prospective cohort study (Mattson *et al.* 2008) found no overall increases in risk behavior following circumcision. Among the Kenya RCT participants, Mattson *et al.* (2008) found that risk behavior actually decreased over the course of twelve months.

Most existing studies of MC have focused on circumcision of adolescents and young adults, and this focus is attractive because adolescents and young adults often represent the age groups most at risk of contracting HIV. It is clear, however, that MC can be performed at a variety of ages, including at very young ages. Evidence from Botswana suggests that infant MC may be very acceptable to mothers (Plank *et al.* 2010). Infant or neonatal circumcision is relatively easily performed in context where a large fraction of births occur within hospital contexts, or neonatal follow-ups in hospitals are common, and the marginal costs of performing a neonatal MC in the context of a hospital delivery might be small. Bollinger *et al.* (2009) for example estimate for Botswana that the costs of neonatal MC are about 20 percent lower than the costs of adult MC, due to lower complication rates and lower costs for commodities, and some studies – in the specific case for Rwanda – estimate costs for neonatal or infant circumcision that are only about 25 percent of the costs of adult MC (studies in the US suggest that the costs of neonatal/infant MC are only about 10 percent of the costs of adult MC, but the applicability of these estimates to SSA is questionable, given the generally less developed health systems). The primary disadvantage of neonatal/infant MC as compared to adult MC is that the benefits in terms of reduced HIV incidence will occur twenty to thirty years in the future, when individuals who were circumcised as infants reach their primary ages of sexual activity. We will discuss these pros and cons of neonatal/infant MC as compared to adult MC further in the context of our discussion of the benefit to cost ratios for MC. For example, White *et al.*'s (2008a) simulations suggest that circumcising neonates would begin to reduce HIV incidence in the general population after twenty to thirty years in men and thirty to forty years in women, whereas circumcising most men before sexual debut or in early adulthood would have much quicker impacts.

Although tens of millions of men remain uncircumcised in SSA, it is also important to recognize that the prevalence of MC is already fairly high in several countries and regions with high HIV prevalence (Figures 1.1 and 1.4), raising some doubts whether scale-ups in MC are a realistic effective scenario in all SSA contexts with severe epidemics.

HIV testing and counseling (HTC)

We consider HTC as a possible solution for the prevention of sexual transmission of HIV, even though the empirical evidence to date is mixed. HTC is likely to remain an important component of HIV prevention, especially given that it is a crucial element in providing HIV-positive individuals with ART for both treatment and possibly prevention. In addition, technological progress has changed the options for HTC substantially from the context in which earlier HTC programs were evaluated, thereby improving access to HTC as well as potential frequency and convenience of testing and the possible expansion of couple-based HTC. Relatively comprehensive repeated home-based HTC is therefore a realistic option in SSA, and recent studies suggest that such programs can lead to reductions in the sexual transmission of HIV. It is important to emphasize, however, that benefit-cost calculations for HTC are more speculative than those for MC, as both estimates of the program effects, and the costs of HTC programs to achieve these program effects, have great uncertainty.

Information campaigns through mass media and peer groups (IC)

Our consideration of information campaigns through mass media and peer groups (IC) is based on the fact that, despite the uncertain empirical evidence about their effectiveness, these programs continue to constitute an important component of HIV prevention strategies. While the alleged effectiveness of some of the "conventional" media and peer group campaigns are not generally backed by careful empirical evidence, more recent studies suggest that more innovative program designs – including for instance school-based interventions, information campaigns that provide specific local information relevant to risk reduction (e.g., the local HIV prevalence by age), or programs that rely on cellphones and related technologies – are effective in reducing HIV infections among young adults. As with HTC, it is important to emphasize that benefit-cost calculations for IC are more speculative than those for MC as both estimates of the program effects, and the costs of HTC programs to achieve these program effects, have great uncertainty.

The above policy options are attractive to consider in the context of *RethinkHIV* because the potential solutions cover a broad range of empirically and theoretically attractive interventions: first, our analyses include a biomedical intervention (male circumcision) that results in a long-term irreversible reduction in infection risk as a result of a one-time medical procedure; risk reductions are potentially stronger for female-to-male and male-to-male transmissions, but may also be important for male-to-female transmissions. The second option considers HTC campaigns that focus on information that individuals have about their own HIV status though HIV testing and counseling, where both theoretical and empirical arguments suggest that providing individuals with accurate information about their own – and possibly also their spouses' and/or other sexual partners' – HIV status should result in less risky decisions about sexual behaviors and sexual relationships. Finally, the third option focuses on information campaigns through mass media and peer groups that aim at reducing risk behaviors in populations affected by HIV by providing more information about HIV/AIDS and potential prevention strategies; information campaigns have also integrated peer groups and community mobilization for prevention efforts, and these aspects seem important for attaining program effectiveness.

Some readers may wonder why condom distribution is not an obvious solution to consider. The answer is that we have not been able to find systematic studies, such as RCTs, that provide persuasive evidence that interventions that focus primarily on condom distribution are likely to be high benefit-cost interventions.

Benefit-cost analyses for policy interventions: some general considerations

The remainder of this paper focuses on establishing benefit to cost ratios, as well as cost-effectiveness estimates, for the above interventions to reduce the sexual transmission of HIV in SSA. The approach that we pursue in this context combines several of the important themes discussed above: we focus on interventions for which there is reasonable evidence about their effectiveness. We adopt an explicit life-cycle perspective in which both the costs and benefits of the interventions occur throughout an individual's life, and we explicitly consider survival probabilities and levels of income and consumption as they occur across the life-cycle. We also consider how interventions are likely to affect the course of the HIV/AIDS epidemic, and how the benefits of an intervention may change as a result of the fact that the intervention affects the future HIV prevalence within which individuals will make decisions about sexual and related behaviors.

Within the scope of the present paper, however, it was also necessary to accept several limitations. First, some epidemiological models for cost-effectiveness analyses are based on fairly detailed models that derive the disease dynamics from assumptions about sexual behaviors, including mixing between different subpopulations, and model changes in prevalence as the combined effect of mortality, changes in infection risks, and behavioral change. But because of the scarcity of information our framework is more limited. We capture the effects of mortality, program interventions, and behavioral changes on prevalence by making reasonable assumptions about disease dynamics, rather than deriving the disease dynamics from micro-foundations. In addition, in order to estimate the benefits of interventions, we account for the additional DALYs lived by individuals in the presence of interventions to reduce the sexual transmission of HIV across the life-course, and we include the costs/benefits from losses in productivity and consumption through mortality and morbidity. Second, we do not derive individual behavior based on an explicit utility maximization model and a derived welfare function for individuals or couples, nor do we explicitly allow for behavioral changes in responses to interventions that would in part reduce the effectiveness of the intervention (e.g., increases in risky sex in response to the reduced HIV infection risks after circumcision are not explicitly modeled). We do, however, base our reductions of infection risks on empirical studies that have identified the net (or reduced form) consequences of different interventions, and these program effects tend to reflect the extent to which individuals have modified their risk-taking behaviors in response to interventions. Third, we also do not consider intergenerational perspectives, such as are relevant to account for the consequences of preventing a person's HIV infection on reduced mother-to-child transmission or the human capital investments of children in the person's household. Fourth, we also do not explicitly account for altruism. Several of these limitations can be addressed in future research. Despite these limitations, however, the benefit-cost approach utilized in this paper is an important contribution to the existing literature evaluating different interventions to reduce the sexual transmission of HIV because we ground our analysis in a systematic integration of the available evidence within a dynamic life-cycle perspective in which an individual faces evolving risks and ART prevalences, with age-specific survival probabilities, and with the incorporation of age-specific productivity and consumption effects in addition to DALYs.

Within the framework outlined above, benefit-cost analyses differ from studies of cost-effectiveness in several important dimensions, and benefit-cost analyses are likely to be preferable for guiding policy decisions about how to allocate scarce resources to different possible interventions. Benefit-cost analysis, or the equivalent in the present case of internal rates of returns, is the appropriate tool for prioritizing among solutions that have multiple impacts, such as those considered in this paper. The alternative of cost-effective analysis for only one impact is only partial and may be misleading if major impacts are ignored. For example the cost per life saved or per DALY saved may be quite misleading if there are impacts

on other outcomes such as productivity, as appears to be the case for HIV/AIDS. Therefore we focus in this paper on benefit-cost analysis, though we make some comparisons below with cost-effectiveness estimates to see whether or not the focus in cost-effectiveness analysis on single impacts leads to similar rankings of interventions.

Conceptually, benefit-cost analysis is straightforward. Simply compare the benefits with the costs – if the benefits exceed the costs, or equivalently the benefit to cost ratio exceeds one, then an intervention is warranted. The benefits are simply the sum of the present discounted values of the weighted impacts of the interventions. Likewise the costs are simply the sum of the present discounted values of the costs of the intervention. The devil – and the challenges – however, as usual are in the details. Some examples follow.[1]

Applying this general concept of benefit-cost analysis to the prevention of the sexual transmission of HIV requires the adoption of a life-cycle perspective in which both infection risks, as well as the costs and benefits of being HIV-negative or becoming infected with HIV, are dependent on an individual's life-cycle. Figure 1.5 illustrates some of the complexities with a representation of the dynamics of the process. The individual starts in year t unaffected when s/he is a given age and gender, say a twenty-year-old male, and in a particular context that reflects the prevalence of HIV at that time and his behaviors that put him at risk. The right-side of this figure gives the benefits for a twenty-year-old male of averting infection in terms of DALYs that would be lost, ART and other treatment costs, and losses of production minus consumption – all of which occur with lags due to the latency period

---

[1] Several of these issues are also relevant in the context of other mathematical models that are used to evaluate HIV prevention or treatment programs. For example, in a review of the key messages emerging from mathematical models of HIV/AIDS interventions, Johnson and White (2011) identify several themes and challenges that are common to these models: the positive (or possibly negative) effects of interventions beyond the groups in which they are introduced, the importance of intervening early, the potential for behavioral changes towards more risky behaviors to reverse gains made in HIV prevention, and the emerging threat of drug resistance.

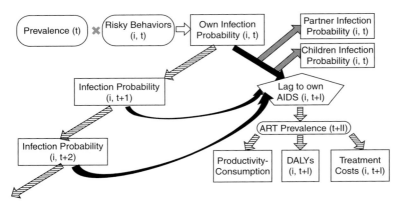

Figure 1.5 *Conceptual framework for the benefit-cost analyses of interventions to reduce the sexual transmission of HIV: Possible sequences for individual* i *starting at year* t

before HIV leads to AIDS and all of which depend on survival probabilities in the absence of AIDS and the prevalence and timing of ART among those infected with HIV. The left-side gives the dynamics over subsequent ages, depending on the nature of the intervention, including how it affects the HIV prevalence in the relevant population. In addition to the effects on the twenty-year-old male as he ages, as indicated in the upper right side of the figure there are effects on partners and possible intergenerational transmission of effects to children (for males, through infecting female partners prior to pregnancies). We elaborate on the particular assumptions that we make for our estimates, consistent with this figure, focusing on a particular age and gender for our estimates because, as discussed below, the probable costs and effects are age- and gender-specific. We consider interventions focused on twenty-year-olds because that age is likely to be an age in which the interventions have close to their maximum effectiveness. We focus on males because one of the leading possible solutions for reducing the sexual transmission of HIV/AIDS is MC.

The costs of an intervention are basically the real resource costs that are incurred to change the probability of infection through altering risky behaviors. The prevalence depends upon the rest of society and is likely to change over time, increasing during the spread of the epidemic and declining if there are effective means to reduce the epidemic that are adopted by others.[2] The prevalence that a

twenty-year-old male faces and his risky behaviors determine the probability of him becoming infected in the year when he is twenty. If he is not infected, then he faces infection probabilities the next year $(t + 1)$ when he is twenty-one, and if not infected that year, the infection probabilities of being infected in the subsequent year $(t + 2)$ when he is twenty-two, etc. The cross-hatched arrows to the left in Figure 1.5 illustrate this sequence.

Of course, in any year he may become infected. The solid black arrows in Figure 1.5 indicate what happens if he is infected. Once infected, there is increased probability of infecting sexual partners and (if the individual is a female) transferring the infection to new children, as indicated by the two stippled arrows. For our estimates in this assessment paper we assume that the impact on the individual's sexual partners' infection probabilities is captured on average by the changing prevalence. For the infected individual himself, there is a latency period (l) of on average of about ten years before he develops AIDS (Morgan *et al.* 2002). Once he develops AIDS (the large black arrows in the figure), the impact on average depends on the prevalence at that time (e.g., ten years after infection) of ART treatment, which also is likely

[2] Vernon Smith suggested in personal correspondence that the average HIV incidence within a period in a population (or subpopulation) can be viewed to depend on the interaction between the size of the infected and the size of the uninfected populations at the start of the period. Our simulations of individual behaviors are similar in spirit to this suggestion.

to change over time if, for example, coverage is extended by expanded efforts by governments or international organizations. The benefits of not being infected for those who would not receive ART include avoiding disability and mortality, as captured for example by DALYs, and losses of productivity above own consumption. Note that even if the value per year of premature disability and mortality as represented by DALYs is assumed to be independent of age, the loss (gain) to the rest of society because an individual would have produced more (less) than he consumed over the rest of his life is likely to be very dependent on age (see the next paragraph). The benefits of not being infected for those who would receive ART include the cost of ART for the rest of their lives. Based on *The Economist* (2011, 90), we assume that the cost of one year of ART is $500, the sum of $100 for a year's course of drugs plus around $400 for the cost of administration (for related estimates, see Galarraga *et al.* 2011; Schwartländer *et al.* 2011). We assume that the ART prevalence is initially 25 percent, and increases by 1 percentage point each year.

There are several important life-cycle patterns in these processes. (1) Risky behaviors are likely to increase in adolescence and reach a maximum in late adolescence and early adulthood and then decline. (2) Productivity is likely to be zero and then very low in childhood but increase during adolescence to reach a maximum in mature adulthood and then decline when the individual becomes elderly, in an inverted U-shaped pattern. (3) Own consumption is likely to also follow an inverted U-shaped pattern but with less sharp age patterns and positive consumption (in contrast to productivity) even when very young or very old, so that own consumption is likely to be greater than own productivity for the young and the elderly and own productivity is likely to be greater than own consumption for prime-age adults. (4) Survival probabilities affect all the forward-looking relevant outcomes such as future productivity, consumption, and ART costs. We incorporate all these life-cycle considerations into our estimates. We note here that they affect the estimated benefits and costs demonstrably, so estimates that ignored them might be quite misleading. We use the UN Population Division estimates of age-specific survival probabilities for SSA

uninfected populations to represent the relevant age patterns in mortality for uninfected populations (UN-ESA 2010).

Another factor is that some important dimensions of the costs and benefits are likely to vary importantly across societies depending inter alia on the average per capita income. For this reason we effectively consider two types of economies: lower per capital income economies for which $1,000 per year DALYs are assumed and somewhat higher per capita income economies for which $5,000 per year DALYs are assumed. These alternative DALYs are the alternatives being used by all the assessment papers in this project, so they assure consistency across the six assessment papers with regard to one important assumption. The values of DALYs used themselves are one important difference between these two types of economies, but hardly the only important difference. We also assume parallel differences in life-cycle paths of productivities and consumption and in the short-run costs beyond DALYs of the onslaught of AIDS for individuals not receiving ART in the form of other care by the health system or by their families. To investigate the sensitivity of the estimates to the assumption about the value of DALYs, we also simulate what happens if in an otherwise $1,000 per year DALY (i.e., relatively poor) economy the appropriate value of the DALYs themselves is $5,000 per year (and vice versa).

Further, as noted above, all the forward-looking costs and benefits from the time of an intervention that affects the probability of infection must be discounted to the same point of time in order to make sensible comparisons of benefits and costs for any particular intervention and across interventions, as well as with other uses of resources, ranging from increased schooling to improved environmental protection. We assume, as in the other five assessment papers that are part of this project, that alternative discount rates of interest are 3 percent and 5 percent.

Finally, an important factor is the initial HIV prevalence. For given risky behaviors, the probability of infection obviously depends on what the HIV prevalence is in the relevant pool of potential sexual partners. We assume two options: first, an initial high prevalence of 25 percent, which corresponds roughly to the prevalence level in Botswana, Lesotho, and Swaziland, i.e., the highest national adult HIV prevalence levels currently observed in SSA (Table 1.1). Second, a medium level of HIV prevalence of 11 percent. This level approximately evenly divides the number of HIV-positive persons in SSA, with about half living in countries above and half living in countries below that prevalence, and it broadly represents the cluster of countries that have an adult HIV prevalence rate of 10–15 percent in Table 1.1. We do not calculate benefit to cost ratios for low prevalence countries in SSA, say with an HIV prevalence of 5 percent or lower, because the prevention agenda in these countries arguably needs to have a different emphasis than in the high prevalence countries, and three-quarters of all HIV-positive persons in SSA currently live in countries with a prevalence of 5 percent or higher. We further assume that these prevalences will decline proportionally each year, depending on the assumed success of the intervention. Before we use this framework to evaluate the three possible solutions – MC, HIV testing and counseling, and information campaigns – for reducing sexual transmission of HIV/AIDS, we want to highlight some general considerations that are likely to have substantial impacts on the results of benefit-cost analyses and about which explicit and conscious assumptions need to be made. Uniformity in these assumptions across different studies is necessary for comparability.

(1) Range of impacts: averting HIV/AIDS for an individual has a number of impacts on that individual over his/her life cycle, depending on the life-cycle stage at which the individual is infected and the latency period between infection and development of HIV/AIDS. Averting HIV/AIDS results not only in later mortality, but less use of medical resources and increased productivity. Some interventions to lessen HIV/AIDS also may have important other impacts, such as increasing schooling of adolescents. And, in addition, averting HIV/AIDS has positive impacts through reducing the probability of HIV/AIDS for others, namely individuals' sexual partners and, for women of childbearing age, their subsequent children. Therefore estimating the benefits is

likely to be complicated not only because of the multiple impacts on a particular individual, but also the dependency on the life-cycle stage and the probable impacts on others.

(2) "Prices": impacts generally are multiple and measured in different units, but must be combined into the same units (normally monetary units with prices as weights) in order to sum them and in order to compare them with costs. For some impacts conceptually at least the measurements are relatively straightforward – for instance, market prices for the value of increased labor productivity or reduced use of medical goods and services under the assumption that such prices reflect the true social marginal value of the relevant good or service. But for other impacts, this evaluation is much more challenging. The key example for this project is the value of averting mortality. A range of methods have been proposed in the literature – for example, the lowest-cost alternative means of averting mortality (Summers 1992, 1994) and the revealed preference as reflected in wage-risk choices in labor markets (Aldy and Viscusi 2007; Hammitt 2007; Robinson 2007; Viscusi 1993, 2010). A related question is what prices should be used. For example, should prices (including wages) be used for a poor SSA developing country, or for a country like Denmark – under the argument that a life should be valued the same whether it be in a low- or a high-income country? How these questions are answered can make an enormous difference for the present project in which averted mortality is a major impact. For example, Summers (1992) reports that the cost of saving a life through measles immunization was of the order of magnitude of $800 per life saved in the early 1990s, or about $1,250 in 2004 (adjusting for inflation and the costs of raising resources; Behrman et al. 2004), while in a recent publication Bartick and Reinhold (2010) use $10.56 million per death in 2007 US dollars. For the present project, all of the assessment papers are using the same two alternatives – DALYs of $1,000 per year and $5,000 per year – to assure consistency within the project with regard to this critical assumption.

(3) Range of costs: what is of interest for the costs are the total true resource costs to society. These are not identical to governmental budgetary expenditures, though often analysts seem to assume that they are. On one hand governmental budgetary expenditures in some cases include substantial transfer components (e.g., in CCT programs), which typically involve some but much smaller resource costs than the amount of the fiscal expenditures. On the other hand, private costs and distortionary costs of raising funds for governmental programs may be considerable. Many programs, for example, may require time inputs from individuals that are not typically covered by governmental expenditures. Distortion costs of raising resources for governmental expenditures also have been estimated to be on the order of magnitude of 25 percent of those expenditures or more (e.g., Ballard *et al.* 1985; Devarajan *et al.* 1997; Feldstein 1995; Harberger 1997; Knowles and Behrman 2003, 2005). Because cost estimates vary considerably, it is important to present estimates that illustrate how robust the benefit to cost ratios are to different cost estimates.

(4) Discounting: the costs, and probably even more the benefits, may be distributed over a number of years. But the value to society of resources in the future is less than the value of the same resources now because they can be reinvested if they are available now. Therefore future costs and benefits should be discounted to the present for comparability, particularly for costs and benefits that are likely to occur some time into the future. And the discount rate makes a difference. For instance, the present discounted value (PDV) of $1,000 received in twenty years' time is $553 if the discount rate is 3 percent, $377 if the discount rate is 5 percent, and $149 if the discount rate is 10 percent (for forty years' time, the respective PDVs are $306, $142, and $22). However, there is a lack of agreement about what discount rates are appropriate, though rates in the 3–10 percent range are common for the social sectors. For the present project, all of the assessment papers are using the same two alternatives – discount rates of 3 percent per year and 5 percent per year –

to assure consistency within the project with regard to this critical assumption.

(5) Interaction among solutions: of necessity, we consider each solution in isolation, not only among those that we consider in this paper but also with regard to the other five categories considered in this project. It might be the case, for example, that "Research and Development" will come up with a cheap and widely applicable intervention that eliminates infection risks or cures HIV/AIDS. Were that to happen, the impacts of the solutions considered in this paper would change radically in a way that probably would mean that the solutions discussed in this assessment paper would become much lower priority. But our estimates are under the assumption that such developments are improbable. Of course, over time some of the solutions in the six categories, or other solutions, possibly will have widespread impacts – in which case it may be valuable to undertake again the current exercise in light of the very changed situation.

(6) Scale: scale can come into estimation of benefit to cost ratios in at least four ways. First, there may be high benefit-cost interventions that are effective for only a small select population, and therefore are not likely to be of interest for the present project with its broad perspective. Second, there may be interventions that have high benefit to cost ratios on a small scale but that are difficult to scale up because critical dimensions of the small-scale intervention (e.g., high-quality and particularly dedicated staff) cannot be maintained if the intervention is scaled up. Third, there may be important aggregate effects on markets if HIV/AIDS is averted on a large scale, such as increased demands on schooling systems and reduced wage rates along the lines in the opposite direction of Young's (2005) provocative article on "the gift of the dying" due to the HIV/AIDS epidemic in SSA. Fourth, the more an effective intervention is scaled up within a community, the lower the risk of infection, all else being equal.

(7) Estimation challenges: the estimation challenges for obtaining benefit to cost ratios are enormous not only for the reasons noted above,

but because of the difficulties in obtaining good response estimates due to endogenous behavioral choices, unobserved variables, selectivity of samples, and different market and policy contexts to which large numbers of academic studies have been devoted. Our above review of the literature reflects these uncertainties. For example, for many behavioral interventions and for the expansion of HTC, both program effects and the costs associated with potentially effective programs are difficult to pin down, and scaled-up programs may have different effects and be subject to different costs than programs that have been implemented as part of research studies. One could therefore conclude that the task of estimating benefit to cost ratios is so difficult that it would be better to abandon it. But that would leave society with little systematic guidance about policy choices in this important area. Therefore, in hopes of improving the basis for policy guidance, we swallow hard and proceed boldly and hopefully creatively (and hopefully not too foolhardily) to make the best estimates that we can given the present very imperfect information and strong assumptions necessary, with some efforts to explore the sensitivity of our estimates to important alternative assumptions.

Additional specific assumptions necessary for the estimates for the three solutions and benefit to cost ratios and cost-effectiveness estimates

Before turning to our estimates of benefit-cost and cost-effectiveness, we first summarize the critical elements in our benefit-cost estimates and then note several specific assumptions, in addition to the general considerations for benefit-cost calculations discussed above, that need to be made for the evaluation of the three possible solutions – male circumcision, HIV testing and counseling, and information campaigns through mass media and peer groups – for the reduction of sexual transmission of HIV.

Summary of procedures underlying our estimated benefit to cost ratios

Our general approach to estimating the benefit to cost ratios is the same for all three interventions. Consistent with the conceptual framework in Figure 1.5, we assumed that the benefits of averting an HIV infection has the following components, all of which are discounted to the time of the intervention to compare with costs of the intervention that are also discounted to the time of the intervention:

- DALYs saved from averting AIDS on average ten years after the infection given age-specific survival patterns in the absence of AIDS;
- differences in production minus consumption, both of which have life-cycle patterns (e.g., so that for prime-age adults production exceeds consumption, but not for those younger or older) and both of which reflect survival probabilities in the absence of AIDS and the prevalence of ART;
- treatment costs (other than ART) on average ten years after infection for those who develop AIDS and who do not receive ART until they die;
- ART costs that would have been expended on average ten years after the initial infection and continued over the remaining life of each infected individual who receives ART, again adjusted for survival probabilities in the absence of AIDS, that are saved due to reduced HIV infections; and
- infections averted through the reduction in the HIV prevalence in the broader population (see below for the specific assumptions for the alternative interventions).

These benefits are experienced for the year (male age twenty years) of the intervention and, if the individual is not affected, as he ages year by year, as indicated in the left side of Figure 1.5. For MC we assume that females benefit from the intervention similarly to males because of the dominance of heterosexual sexual transmissions, and for HTC and information campaigns we assume that females subjected to the intervention would benefit similarly to males. As noted above, there is considerable uncertainty in calculating all of these benefits, as well as the resource costs of the intervention, for which reason we present alternative estimates that illustrate the sensitivity of our estimates to alternative assumptions. But we note that we do not include some possible benefits, in particular the benefits from averting intergenerational transmission of the disease to children ("Children Infection Probability" on upper right side of Figure 1.5). For this reason, all else being equal, our estimates are lower-bound estimates of the true benefits. These benefits are compared to the real resource costs of interventions that vary across the interventions and are discussed below.

Additional specific assumptions for each of the three solutions

Male circumcision (MC): based on the literature review summarized above, we assume that MC reduces the probability of infection through sexual interaction by 30 percent. This is a permanent effect of a one-time intervention that lasts over the remaining lifetime of the circumcised male. We further assume that HIV prevalences will decline proportionally each year to 0.98 of the previous year value due to the changes induced by this proposed solution on the pool of potential sexual partners. That is, although we focus on one individual for our simulation, we assume that the same policy is applied broadly to others, not just for this one individual in isolation. We assume that the direct costs of circumcision are in the range of $40 to $70, based on estimates that have been reported for SSA (Gray *et al.* 2007; Martin *et al.* 2007; Schwartländer *et al.* 2011; White *et al.* 2008b). These are only the direct costs, and do not cover any cost of pain and suffering or possible infection risks or the costs of campaigns or programs to make men aware of the options and benefits of circumcision and to induce them to elect to do so, or additional capital costs that might be required to scale up the intervention beyond currently existing health clinics or other providers. Because some of the costs of circumcision are likely to depend on local costs and income levels, we assume a cost range of $30–52 for the low per capita economy, and $60–105 for the high per capita economy. Because the scale-up of

MC requires expansion of health services as well as information campaigns – and possibly explicit incentives – to achieve a high uptake of MC, we assume in our baseline calculations that the overall costs of one MC on average are twice the direct costs of the medical procedure. In lieu of detailed data on these costs, this assumption seems to be a more reasonable baseline scenario than calculations that focus on the direct costs of circumcision (as is often the case in existing studies). We comment below on the implications of such other costs for our benefit-cost estimates.

HIV testing and counseling (HTC): following recent studies about the population-level effect of HTC programs, we assume that a one-time large-scale HTC program that achieves a very comprehensive coverage can reduce HIV incidence by 20 percent (Waters *et al.* 2011), with the effect fading over a ten-year period. This effectiveness of a comprehensive HTC campaign is consistent with the literature reviewed above. This assumed reduction in incidence is the combined effect of behavioral changes in the HIV-positive partners who would be identified in a comprehensive HTC campaign as well as reductions in transmission risks that occur because HIV-positive individuals could identify treatment as a result of the HTC campaign. We further assume that during the initial ten-year period, the HIV prevalence will decline proportionally each year to 0.99 of the previous year value due to the changes induced by this proposed solution on the pool of potential sexual partners and higher mortality of HIV-positive persons; subsequently, HIV prevalence declines each year to .995 of the previous year, essentially as a result of higher mortality of HIV-positive persons. Schwartländer *et al.* (2011) estimate the costs of HTC in SSA at about $15, Hausler *et al.* (2006) report costs for clinic-based tests at $7–10, and Helleringer *et al.* (2010) estimate the cost of home-based HTC at around $15 in rural Malawi. In order to achieve the effectiveness in reducing HIV incidence that our calculations assume, it is important that the HTC campaign is comprehensive and reaches a majority of the population, and that it is accompanied by follow-up for persons who have not yet participated in HTC, a comprehensive counseling in connection with HTC, and potential referral to ART for those who are identified as HIV-positive. The direct costs of the HTC program are therefore likely to exceed the estimates that exist in the literature. We therefore assume direct HTC costs in the low per capita economy of $15–20 per HTC, and in the high per capita economy of $30–40. Moreover, because we anticipate that a comprehensive and effective HTC campaign requires some scaling-up of infrastructure as well as additional costs of associated information campaigns, we assume that the total costs of HTC exceed the direct costs by 50 percent.

Information campaigns through mass media and peer groups: the evidence on which to base these estimates is the weakest among the three possible solutions that we consider in this assessment paper. A skeptical reading of the literature reviewed above would suggest that the evidence about the effect of information campaigns on HIV incidence is weak, and that currently no proven strategies to reduce HIV incidence through such programs exist. A somewhat more optimistic reading of the literature suggests that some recent innovations in program design, and the possible combination with cellphones, provide new possibilities to design new information campaigns and peer group programs that might reduce incidence. Clearly, there is a considerable amount of speculation, and the existing literature is only of limited help. Similar uncertainty exists with respect to the costs of programs. For example, Hogan *et al.* (2005) provide some discussion, but it is difficult to figure out the costs per person for these interventions. If one looks at their estimates of costs per infection averted, and compares them to HTCs, then the costs per infection averted range from 0.1 to about 20 times of that of HTCs – a huge range. Schwartländer *et al.* (2011) estimate $3.38 for community mobilization programs in SSA, but it is unclear what activities are included in the types of programs that they are considering.

To provide at least some guidance about the benefit to cost ratios of information campaigns, we assume that a one-time program intervention can be designed that initially reduces HIV incidence by 15 percent, and that this effect declines linearly over ten years. Given the existing evidence, we assume that this effect can be achieved by a fairly intensive campaign that requires a fair amount of time

and effort in counseling/training young men and women. The required time substantially exceeds that of HTCs, and the extra time is not compensated by the fact that some of these are group sessions (e.g. many effective programs implement a curriculum that is based on repeated sessions with young adults to teach them about safe sex, etc.). Therefore we assume that the costs of information campaigns with the effectiveness noted above is from two to four times the costs of (the least expensive) HTC.

Benefit to cost ratios for interventions that reduce HIV infections through sexual interactions

Table 1.3 presents benefit-cost estimates for each of the three possible solutions based on the assumptions discussed above, in each case with alternative estimates for: $1,000 DALY economy and $5,000 DALY economy, 3 percent and 5 percent discount rates, 11 percent (medium) and 25 percent (high) initial HIV prevalence, and low and high costs for the interventions. By a "$1,000 DALY economy" we mean a relatively low-income economy in general, not only with respect to DALYs; likewise we mean a higher-income economy in general for a "$5,000 DALY economy." As noted, the "high" initial prevalence assumption of 25 percent is about the average prevalence rate for the three countries in SSA with the highest HIV prevalence in Table 1.1 – Swaziland, Botswana, and Lesotho. The "medium" initial prevalence rate of 11.0 percent is that of Malawi and slightly below Mozambique, Namibia, and Zambia. Though over a third of the SSA countries included in Table 1.1 have prevalence rates of less than 2 percent (and over half have prevalence rates of less than 3.5 percent), we do not consider a "low" prevalence case because it would double the number of estimates presented but not add much information. For all three solutions we assume that the target segments are all twenty-year-olds, not just some particular subpopulation such as prostitutes, or men having sex with men. As noted above, the benefit-cost calculations were performed for males, and it is assumed that females are identically

Table 1.3 Benefits, costs, and benefit to cost ratios for three possible solutions to reduce sexual HIV/AIDS infections in SSA

High prevalence (25% initially)

		Program costs										Benefit to cost ratios			
		Benefits				Direct costs		Total costs							
		3%, 1K	5%, 1K	3%, 5K	5%, 5K	1K	5K	1K	5K			3%, 1K	5%, 1K	3%, 5K	5%, 5K
Male circumcision	Low C	$1,989	$1,373	$9,945	$6,866	$30	$60	$60	$120			33.1	22.9	82.9	57.2
	High C	$1,989	$1,373	$9,945	$6,866	$52	$105	$104	$210			19.1	13.2	47.4	32.7
HTC	Low C	$322	$237	$1,612	$1,184	$15	$30	$23	$45			14.3	10.5	35.8	26.3
	High C	$322	$237	$1,612	$1,184	$20	$40	$30	$60			10.7	7.9	26.9	19.7
Info campaign	Low C	$244	$179	$1,219	$895	$30	$60	$30	$60			8.1	6.0	20.3	14.9
	High C	$244	$179	$1,219	$895	$80	$160	$80	$160			3.0	2.2	7.6	5.6

Medium prevalence (11% initially)

		Program costs										Benefit to cost ratios			
		Benefits				Direct costs		Total costs							
		3%, 1K	5%, 1K	3%, 5K	5%, 5K	1K	5K	1K	5K			3%, 1K	5%, 1K	3%, 5K	5%, 5K
Male circumcision	Low C	$972	$671	$4,862	$3,357	$30	$60	$60	$120			16.2	11.2	40.5	28.0
	High C	$972	$671	$4,862	$3,357	$52	$105	$104	$210			9.3	6.5	23.2	16.0
HTC	Low C	$142	$104	$709	$521	$15	$30	$23	$45			6.3	4.6	15.8	11.6
	High C	$142	$104	$709	$521	$20	$40	$30	$60			4.7	3.5	11.8	8.7
Info campaign	Low C	$107	$79	$536	$394	$30	$60	$30	$60			3.6	2.6	8.9	6.6
	High C	$107	$79	$536	$394	$80	$160	$80	$160			1.3	1.0	3.4	2.5

Notes: See text for details. 1K and 5K refer respectively to $1,000 and $5,000 DALY economies. 3% and 5% are discount rates. Low C and High C are the low and high cost assumptions.

affected by the intervention in the case of HTC and information campaigns; for male circumcision, we assume that females benefit symmetrically through the interaction with circumcised men. Because of this broad targeting to young adults (and young males, for male circumcision), there are assumed to be impacts on the overall prevalence rates over time, as noted. Examination of Table 1.3 suggests the following observations:

First, the estimated benefit to cost ratios are sensitive to some of the critical assumptions that are investigated in the table. The benefit to cost ratios are substantially higher:

- for a $5,000 DALY economy compared with a $1,000 DALY economy, they are about 2.5 times as large;
- for a 3 percent discount rate compared with a 5 percent discount rate, they are about 40 percent larger;
- for a high (25 percent) initial HIV prevalence compared with a medium (11 percent) initial HIV prevalence, they are a little more than twice as large;
- for our low-cost intervention estimates compared with our higher-cost intervention estimates, they are about 1.7, 1.3, and 2.7 times as large, respectively, for the three possible solutions.

Therefore it might be very misleading to assume away the heterogeneity in these various dimensions by considering, for example, only central values for DALYs, discount rates, HIV prevalence, and costs. Instead it is important to be sensitive to how the estimates vary, with plausible variations in all of these dimensions. Then it is desirable to try to pin down as much as possible which of these assumptions are appropriate for any particular situation being considered in order to inform the decision as to which benefit to cost ratios are most likely to be appropriate for that particular context. Of course in terms of prioritizing interventions, the patterns in our estimates suggest the higher the benefit to cost ratios the higher are DALYs, the lower are discount rates, the higher is HIV prevalence, and the lower are costs.

Second, nevertheless, overall these benefit-cost estimates tend to be high and all but one exceed one (the exception is the high-cost information cam-

paign in a $1,000 DALY economy with a 5 percent discount rate, in which case the benefit to cost ratio is 1.0), suggesting substantial possibilities for interventions that reduce the transmission of sexually transmitted HIV/AIDS. Note that in many cases the benefit to cost ratios would be relatively high even if the benefits are overestimated or the costs underestimated. For example, if the costs of MC were underestimated by a factor of 10 because of the exclusion of the costs of pain and suffering, the costs of informing and inducing men to participate, and the capital costs of scaling up beyond mere marginal additions to existing health clinics, the benefit to cost ratios still would be from 2.3 to 8.3 in high prevalence areas – though they would be around 2.0 or less for high-cost interventions in $1,000 DALY economies.

Third, MC of young adults emerges as the intervention with the highest benefit to cost ratios in both the high and medium prevalence context, for both 1K and 5K economies and independent of the discount rate. This dominance of MC over other interventions analyzed in this paper is due to the long-term sizable reduction in HIV infection risks resulting from a one-time procedure that can be performed at relatively moderate costs, and the fact that females benefit from the male-centered intervention through changes in the prevalence among their male partners and possible reductions in female to male transmission rates. While we do not analyze neonatal or infant MC in detail, the general tendency in the comparison of the benefit to cost ratios between adult and neonatal/infant MC can be easily established. At a discount rate of 3 percent, delaying the effect of reducing HIV infections two to three decades into the future would reduce benefits by about 45–60 percent. If the costs of neonatal/infant MC are less than 45–60 percent of the costs of adult circumcision, then the benefit to cost ratio for infant/neonatal MC would exceed that for adult MC; to the extent that the cost savings are less, adult MC would have higher benefit to cost ratios. Because there continues to be considerable uncertainty about the relative costs of neonatal/infant as compared to adult MC in SSA, and because most of the studies that point to very high cost savings by conducting infant/neonatal as compared to adult MC pertain to countries with contexts where a high fraction of births occur in hospitals and/or neonatal hospital follow-up is common, we conclude at this point that – at least broadly speaking – the benefit to cost ratios for infant/neonatal MC in a SSA context are likely to be relatively similar to that of adult MC (where young adults are the primary target).

Fourth, the benefit to cost ratios change some in predictable ways if a high value of DALYs is used for low-DALY economies and vice versa (estimates not presented), but basically give similar patterns. The benefits, and thus the benefit to cost ratios, increase if for the poorer economies DALYs are valued at $5,000 and decrease if for the better-off economies DALYs are valued at $1,000.

Cost-effectiveness estimates for interventions that reduce HIV infections through sexual interactions

Table 1.4 presents the costs per HIV infection averted (HIA) and the costs per DALY that are implied by our calculations of the benefit to cost ratios above. The first observation is that these costs per HIA and DALY are broadly consistent with other estimates in the literature (e.g., Galarraga *et al.* 2009; Table 1.2), and the broad conclusions obtained from the cost-effectiveness calculations in Table 1.4 are similar to those obtained from the benefit-cost analyses in Table 1.3. For example, MC is the most cost-effective intervention, both in terms of costs per infection averted and cost per DALY averted, in both the high- and medium-prevalence scenarios. HTC is also cost-effective if the program is sufficiently comprehensive and well-designed to result in the reductions of HIV infection risks that we have assumed in our calculations. Information campaigns are the least cost-effective intervention based on our calculations, with considerable uncertainty about the costs per DALY and HIA.

Comparing Tables 1.3 and 1.4, however, also reveals some important differences between the benefit-cost approach (Table 1.3) and the cost-effectiveness approach (Table 1.4). For example, based on cost-effectiveness calculations, MC

always dominates HTC, and MC is between three and four times more cost-effective than HTC (the costs per DALY and HIA for MC are between 25 and 33 percent of those for HTC). The ratio by which MC dominates HTC is somewhat less in the benefit-cost analyses. This results from the fact that the benefits are discounted, and while both programs result in sizable reduction in infection risks in the short term, they fade for HTC during ten years; for MC they remain throughout the life-course, but the additional DALYs and HIV occur further in the future, as well as potentially at stages of the life-course where consumption exceeds production, which reduces the benefits in the benefit-cost considerations but does not affect the cost-effectiveness considerations. Hence, benefit-cost considerations reflect the timing of the DALYs saved as a result of the interventions through discounting, and they reflect the stage of the life-cycle – and the consumption and production profiles corresponding to these stages of the life-cycle – at which DALYs are saved as a result of the intervention. These aspects, which can be important for prioritizing interventions, are not reflected in cost-effectiveness analyses. A further advantage of benefit-cost analyses is that they help to compare the costs of the intervention to the benefits on the same metric; for example, based on cost-effectiveness calculations one could wonder, assuming that more cost-effective interventions have already been exploited or are not available, if an intervention that can avert an HIV infection of costs of close to $10,000 or more is worthwhile. The benefit-cost considerations, which include an evaluation of life – combining both the valuation of DALYs and the patterns of production and consumption – reflect this valuation of life and show that even interventions that can avert an HIV infection of costs of close to $10,000 have benefit to cost ratios that exceed one. Moreover, benefit-cost calculations, but not the cost-effectiveness calculations in Table 1.4, reflect how different rates of intertemporal trade-offs (discount factors) affect the priority setting in HIV prevention and resource allocation to different programs.

Especially for biomedical interventions, for which substantial shares of program costs are spent on non-locally produced program inputs (e.g., drugs and medical technology), the costs of

Table 1.4 Costs per infection averted and costs per DALY for three possible solutions to reduce sexual HIV/AIDS infections in SAA

High prevalence (25% initially)

		Infections averted (per person)	DALYs saved (per person)	Costs of treatment		Total costs		Cost per infection averted		Cost per DALY	
				1K	5K	1K	5K	1K	5K	1K	5K
Male circumcision	Low C	0.277	6.72	$30	$60	$60	$120	$216	$433	$4	$9
	High C	0.277	6.72	$52	$105	$104	$210	$375	$758	$8	$16
HTC	Low C	0.025	0.85	$15	$30	$23	$45	$890	$1,779	$18	$35
	High C	0.025	0.85	$20	$40	$30	$60	$1,186	$2,372	$23	$47
Info campaign	Low C	0.019	0.65	$30	$60	$30	$60	$1,567	$3,133	$46	$93
	High C	0.019	0.65	$80	$160	$80	$160	$4,177	$8,355	$124	$247

Medium prevalence (11% initially)

		Infections averted (per person)	DALYs saved (per person)	Costs of treatment		Total costs		Cost per infection averted		Cost per DALY	
				1K	5K	1K	5K	1K	5K	1K	5K
Male circumcision	Low C	0.136	3.28	$30	$60	$60	$120	$443	$886	$9	$18
	High C	0.136	3.28	$52	$105	$104	$210	$768	$1,550	$16	$32
HTC	Low C	0.011	0.38	$15	$30	$23	$45	$2,022	$4,043	$40	$80
	High C	0.011	0.38	$20	$40	$30	$60	$2,696	$5,391	$53	$106
Info campaign	Low C	0.008	0.28	$30	$60	$30	$60	$3,560	$7,120	$105	$211
	High C	0.008	0.28	$80	$160	$80	$160	$9,494	$18,988	$281	$562

Notes: See text for details. 1K and 5K refer respectively to $1,000 and $5,000 DALY economies. 3% and 5% are discount rates.
Low C and High C are the low and high cost assumptions.

intervention are likely to vary less than proportionally with the income levels of the economy. Our assumptions about program costs reflect this. As a result, the benefit-cost calculations reflect generally strongly increasing benefit to cost ratios in comparing a $1,000 economy with a $5,000 economy, and for all interventions, the benefit to cost ratios are about 2.5 times as high in the latter as in the former. In cost-effectiveness calculations, however, higher income levels affect only the cost side – at least in our calculation as we use a uniform life table that reflects mortality in the absence of AIDS across all calculations. As a result, interventions become less cost-effective in higher income contexts as compared to lower income contexts, in sharp contrast to the benefit to cost ratios, that increase with income levels under our assumptions in our basic benefit-cost estimates that link DALYs to the overall income levels of the economies.

Application to selected high- and medium-prevalence countries

The interventions discussed in this paper focus on young adults. To provide an idea about the potential number of beneficiaries in SSA for these interventions, we observe that there are currently about 148 million individuals ("young adults") in their twenties in SSA, and about 215 million individuals will enter their twenties in the next decade. Considering current young adults, and individuals becoming young adults over the next decade, as the primary target of interventions to reduce the transmission of HIV therefore suggests that there are more than 350 million potential beneficiaries of such interventions over the next decade. About half of these individuals are male, of which a significant proportion – varying from less than 10 percent to more than 80 percent (Figure 1.4) – are circumcised based on existing cultural and/or religious norms and practices. Prevalence of circumcision tends to be lower in countries with high prevalence of HIV (Figures 1.1 and 1.4).

In the broadest sense, therefore, the potential pool of beneficiaries in SSA of such interventions targeted at young adults is very large. As is emphasized in our analyses, however, SSA countries vary importantly in their HIV prevalence, the prevalence of circumcision, the income levels, and other demographic and socioeconomic characteristics and trends. Policies are therefore likely to need to be prioritized differently to specific countries, policy mixes are likely to need to be adjusted to the specific contexts, and the feasibility, costs, and benefits of interventions will differ across different SSA countries.

Table 1.5 provides an illustrative example of the number of infections averted and the total benefits incurred if the three interventions – MC, HTC, and information campaigns – were implemented in selected high- and medium-prevalence countries. Based on the review of the literature, there is considerable uncertainty about the scale to which these interventions can be rolled out and implemented. Most clearly for MC, and to a lesser extent for HTC, the interventions require the expansion of health infrastructure for their implementation that may limit the short-term scale-up of these interventions. For MC, the implementation also requires overcoming possible cultural or normative inertias towards MC in countries where MC has not been widely practiced so far (see Figure 1.4). There is also considerable uncertainty about the scale of the intervention and the disease dynamics resulting from the intervention and other socioeconomic, demographic, and behavioral changes that occur parallel to the intervention. To illustrate the benefits resulting from the interventions in a comparable fashion, we therefore present summary calculations of the infections averted and the total benefits incurred assuming that a total amount of $10 million was devoted to each of these interventions as part of a broad HIV intervention across several years targeted at young adults. Because of the considerable heterogeneities among the high-prevalence countries and among the medium-prevalence countries in these and other relevant dimensions, we focus on the countries with the largest population corresponding to the high- and medium-prevalence levels for our calculations (see also Table 1.1 for a list of countries by HIV prevalence): Botswana for the high-prevalence scenario, and Mozambique for the medium-prevalence scenario (South Africa has a larger population, but is

Table 1.5 Application to selected high- and medium-prevalence countries – Botswana and Mozambique

	Scenario	
	High prevalence	Medium prevalence
Assumed initial HIV prevalence for benefit-cost calculations	25%	11%
Largest SSA country with HIV prevalence near scenario assumptions	Botswana	Mozambique
Total number of HIV+ persons aged 15–49 in above country (2009, in '000)	320	1,400
Total number of young adults aged 15–25 in above country (2010, in '000, males and females)	444	4,606
Fraction (already) circumcised	12%	51%
Intervention I: Male circumcision Number of beneficiaries, infections averted, and total benefits resulting from $10 million spent on intervention		
Total beneficiaries (= number of male circumcisions, in '000)	61	122
Number of infections avoided (in '000)	16.8	16.5
Total benefits of intervention (in million $)	603	119
Benefit to cost ratio	60.3	11.9
Intervention II: HTC Number of beneficiaries, infections averted, and total benefits resulting from $10 million spent on intervention		
Total beneficiaries (= number of HTCs (for males and females), in '000)	190	381
Number of infections avoided (in '000)	4.8	4.2
Total benefits of intervention (in million $)	307	54
Benefit to cost ratio	30.7	5.4
Intervention III: Information campaign Number of beneficiaries, infections averted, and total benefits resulting from $10 million spent on intervention		
Total beneficiaries (= number of persons reached by info campaign (males and females), in '000)	91	182
Number of infections avoided (in '000)	1.7	1.5
Total benefits of intervention (in million $)	111	19
Benefit to cost ratio	11.1	1.9

Notes:
Benefits are based on 3% discount rate.
Botswana is considered as a 5K economy, Mozambique as a 1K economy.
Costs of the intervention are the average of the low and high scenarios.
Number of infections avoided per person reached by intervention is obtained from Table 1.4.
Benefits per person reached by intervention is obtained from Table 1.3.
Total number of young adults is obtained from UN World Population Prospects 2010.
Number already circumcised is obtained from http://aidsinfoonline.org.

a combination of areas with different prevalences and an overall average between our high-prevalence and medium-prevalence country groups; see Figure 1.1). Reflecting the very different income levels, we consider Botswana as corresponding to a "5K economy" in our calculations, and Mozambique as a "1K economy." We use the average of the high- and low-cost scenario to represent costs and the benefits based on the calculations in Table 1.3 with a discount rate of 3 percent.

Based on our calculations, for example, $10 million devoted to MC of young males would result in approximately 61,000 male circumcisions in Botswana, resulting in approximately

17,000 averted HIV infections among both men and women and incurring about $600 million of benefits (benefit to cost ratio approximately 60) in terms of discounted DALYs saved, averted treatment costs, and net production. In contrast, the same amount devoted to MC in Mozambique would result in about 122,000 male circumcisions, more than in Botswana due to assumed lower costs in Mozambique as compared to Botswana. Because of the lower prevalence in Mozambique as compared to Botswana, fewer HIV infections would be averted in Mozambique as compared to Botswana (16,500 as compared to 16,800); combined with lower income levels in Mozambique, which affect the valuation of benefits, the total benefits are only about one-fifth of those in Botswana ($119 million as compared to $603 million). While MC continues to generate benefits that vastly exceed the costs, the benefit to cost ratio in Mozambique is "only" 11.9, as compared to more than 60 in Botswana.

Table 1.5 also reports analogous calculations for HTC and information campaigns. While $10 million allocated to these interventions would reach a larger number of individuals due to the lower costs of the intervention than of MC, the infections averted, the total benefits incurred, and the benefit to cost ratios would be lower for these interventions as compared to MC. Nevertheless, both of these interventions have benefit to cost ratios larger than one – and often substantially so – in both Botswana and Mozambique.

Conclusions

HIV/AIDS is primarily spread through sexual interactions in SSA. Therefore it is natural to ask what are the relative merits of possible solutions to the HIV/AIDS epidemic in SSA that work through reducing infections spread by sexual interactions. This assessment paper addresses three such possible solutions for which there is sufficient information to suggest that they might be quite promising:

- male circumcision (MC),
- HIV testing and counseling (HTC), and
- information campaigns through mass media and peer groups.

Even though there is more information on these possible solutions than on some other possibilities, the information is limited and the challenges of estimating benefits and costs within an appropriate dynamic life-cycle framework are considerable. This paper has proceeded, nevertheless, while trying to make as explicit as possible the various necessary assumptions. The estimated benefit to cost ratios obtained are shown to be sensitive to critical assumptions related to the value of averting mortality, the discount rate, the HIV prevalence rate, and the costs of interventions. Nevertheless the benefit-cost estimates suggest that under most plausible conditions the benefit to cost ratios for these interventions in high-prevalence and (somewhat less so) medium-prevalence countries are likely to be large, particularly for MC and probably for HTCs, though the smaller estimates for information campaigns in part reflect the greater fuzziness in the underlying information available for the estimates. Therefore interventions to reduce the spread of HIV/AIDS in SSA through reducing sexual infection rates indeed seem to have considerable promise – and greater promise where prevalence rates of DALYs are higher and resource costs of interventions and discount rates are lower. The estimates also show that cost-effectiveness estimates per HIV infection averted and per DALY in a broad general sense reveal similar patterns, but also differ importantly from benefit-cost estimates in specific respects because they do not incorporate some critical factors that are incorporated in the benefit-cost estimates such as intertemporal trade-offs that require discounting, life-cycle considerations, and impacts on production and consumption.

Because the benefits – including the values of DALYs and lives saved – in the benefit-cost calculations performed in this paper (and the *RethinkHIV* project more generally) increase more strongly with income levels than do the costs, benefit to cost ratios tend to be highest in relatively rich high-prevalence countries. Relatively rich high-prevalence countries would therefore receive priority if interventions were allocated based on benefit-cost criteria alone.

But, as generally is the case with public programs and policies, other criteria also may be important – most importantly poverty reduction and reductions in inequality. The utilization of such criteria in addition to benefit to cost ratios is likely to lead to increases in the relative priorities for investing in poorer countries.

References

Agot, K. E., Kiarie, J. N., Nguyen, H. Q., Odhiambo, J. O., Onyango, T. M. and Weiss, N. S. (2007). Male circumcision in Siaya and Bondo districts, Kenya: prospective cohort study to assess behavioral disinhibition following circumcision. *Journal of Acquired Immune Deficiency Syndromes* **44**(1): 66–70. doi:10.1097/01.qai. 0000242455.05274.20.

Aldy, J. E. and Viscusi, W. K. (2007). Age differences in the value of statistical life: revealed preference evidence. *Review of Environmental Economics and Policy* **1**: 241–60. doi:10.1093/reep/rem014.

Anglewicz, P. and Chitsanya, J. (2011). Disclosure of HIV status between spouses in Malawi. *AIDS Care* **23**(8), 998–1005.

Auvert, B., Taljaard, D., Lagarde, E., Sobngwi-Tambekou, J., Sitta, R. and Puren, A. (2005). Randomized, controlled intervention trial of male circumcision for reduction of HIV infection risk: the ANRS 1265 trial. *PLoS Medicine* **2**(11): 1112–22. doi:10.1371/journal. pmed.0020298.

Bailey, R. C., Moses, S., Parker, C. B., Agot, K., Maclean, I., Krieger, J. N., Williams, C. F. M., Campbell, R. T. and Ndinya-Achola, J. O. (2007). Male circumcision for HIV prevention in young men in Kisumu, Kenya: a randomised controlled trial. *The Lancet* **369**(9562): 643–56. doi:10.1016/S0140-6736(07)60312-2.

Baird, S., Chirwa, E., McIntosh, C. and Özler, B. (2010). The short-term impacts of a schooling conditional cash transfer program on the sexual behavior of young women. *Health Economics* **19**(S1): 55–68. doi:10.1002/hec.1569.

Ballard, C., Shoven, J. and Whalley, J. (1985). General equilibrium computations of the marginal welfare costs of taxes in the United States. *American Economic Review* **75**(1): 128–38.

Banerjee, J., Klausner, J. D., Halperin, D. T., Wamai, R., Schoen, E. J., Moses, S., Morris, B. J., Bailis, S. A., Venter, F., Martinson, N., Coates, T. J., Gray, G. and Bowa, K. (2011). Circumcision denialism unfounded and unscientific. *American Journal of Preventive Medicine* **40**(3): e11–e12.

Bartick, M. and Reinhold, A. (2010). The burden of suboptimal breastfeeding in the United States: a pediatric cost analysis. *Pediatrics* **125**(5): 1048–58.

Behrman, J. R., Alderman, H. and Hoddinott, J. (2004). Hunger and malnutrition. In: Lomborg, B. (ed.). *Global Crises, Global Solutions*. Cambridge University Press, 363–420. (See also www.copenhagenconsensus.com.)

Behrman, J. R. and Knowles, J. C. (1998). Population and reproductive health: an economic framework for policy evaluation. *Population and Development Review* **24**(4): 697–737.

Behrman, J. R., Kohler, H.-P. and Watkins, S. C. (2009). Lessons from empirical network analyses on matters of life and death in East Africa. In: Kleindorfer, P. R. and Wind, Y. (eds.). *The Network Challenge: Strategy, Profit, and Risk in an Interlinked World*. Upper Saddle River, NJ: Wharton School Publishing, chap. 28, 495–512. http://books.google.com/ books?id=gjq4mC3hW1QC.

Bertozzi, S., Padian, N. S., Wegbreit, J., DeMaria, L. M., Feldman, B., Gayle, H., Gold, J., Grant, R. and Isbell, M. T. (2006). HIV/AIDS prevention and treatment. In: Jamison, D. T., Breman, J. G., Measham, A. R., Alleyne, G., Claeson, M., Evans, D. B., Jha, P., Mills, A. and Musgrove, P. (eds.). *Disease Control Priorities in Developing Countries*, 2nd edn. Oxford University Press, 331–70. http://files.dcp2.org/pdf/DCP/DCP18. pdf.

Binagwaho, A., Pegurri, E., Muita, J. and Bertozzi, S. (2010). Male circumcision at different ages in Rwanda: a cost-effectiveness study. *PLoS Med* **7**(1): e1000211. doi:10.1371/journal.pmed. 1000211.

Bollinger, L., Stover, J., Musuka, G., Fidzani, B., Moeti, T. and Busang, L. (2009). The cost and impact of male circumcision on HIV/AIDS in Botswana. *Journal of the International AIDS Society* **12**(1): 7. doi:10.1186/1758-2652-12-7.

Brent, R. J. (2009). A cost-benefit analysis of female primary education as a means of reducing HIV/AIDS in Tanzania. *Applied Economics* **41**(14): 1731–43. doi:10.1080/ 00036840601032235.

Brent, R. J. (2010a). *Setting Priorities for HIV/AIDS Interventions: A Cost-Benefit Approach*. Cheltenham: Edward Elgar Publishing.

Brent, R. J. (2010b). A social cost-benefit criterion for evaluating voluntary counseling and testing with an application to Tanzania. *Health Economics* **19**(2): 154–72. doi:10.1002/hec.1457.

Cho, H., Hallfors, D. D., Mbai, I. I., Itindi, J., Milimo, B. W., Halpern, C. T. and Iritani, B. J. (2011). Keeping adolescent orphans in school to prevent human immunodeficiency virus infection: evidence from a randomized controlled trial in Kenya. *Journal of Adolescent Health* **48**(5): 523–6. doi:10.1016/j.jadohealth.2010.08.007.

Coates, T. J., Richter, L. and Caceres, C. (2008). Behavioral strategies to reduce HIV transmission: how to make them work better. *The Lancet* **372**(9639): 669–84. doi:10.1016/S0140-6736(08)60886-7.

Cohen, T. and Corbett, E. L. (2011). Test and treat in HIV: success could depend on rapid detection. *The Lancet* **378**(9787): 204–6. doi:S0140-6736(11)60896-9.

Corbett, E. L., Makamure, B., Cheung, Y. B., Dauya, E., Matambo, R., Bandason, T., Munyati, S. S., Mason, P. R., Butterworth, A. E. and Hayes, R. J. (2007). HIV incidence during a cluster-randomized trial of two strategies providing voluntary counselling and testing at the workplace, Zimbabwe. *AIDS* **21**(4): 483–9. doi:10.1097/QAD.0b013e3280115402.

Cremin, I., Nyamukapa, C., Sherr, L., Hallett, T., Chawira, G., Cauchemez, S., Lopman, B., Garnett, G. and Gregson, S. (2010). Patterns of self-reported behavior change associated with receiving voluntary counselling and testing in a longitudinal study from Manicaland, Zimbabwe. *AIDS and Behavior* **14**(3): 708–15. doi:10.1007/s10461-009-9592-4.

de Walque, D., Dow, W. H., Nathan, R., Medlin, C. A. and the RESPECT study team. (2011). Evaluating conditional cash transfers to prevent HIV and other sexually transmitted infections (STIs) in Tanzania. Paper presented at the Annual Meeting of the Population Association of America, Washington, DC, March 31–April 2, 2011, http://paa2011.princeton.edu/download.aspx?submissionId=112619.

Delavande, A. and Kohler, H.-P. (forthcoming). The impact of HIV testing on subjective expectations and risky behavior in Malawi. *Demography*.

Denison, J., O'Reilly, K., Schmid, G., Kennedy, C. and Sweat, M. (2008). HIV voluntary counseling and testing and behavioral risk reduction in developing countries: a meta-analysis, 1990–2005. *AIDS and Behavior* **12**(3): 363–73. doi:10.1007/s10461-007-9349-x.

Devarajan, S., Squire, L. and Suthiwart-Narueput, S. (1997). Beyond rate of return: reorienting project appraisal. *World Bank Research Observer* **12**(1): 35–46.

Drummond, M., O'Brien, B. J., Stoddart, G. L. and Torrance, G. (1997). *Methods for the Economic Evaluation of Health Care Programmes*. Oxford University Press.

Dupas, P. (2011). Do teenagers respond to HIV risk information? Evidence from a field experiment in Kenya. *American Economic Journal: Applied Economics* **3**(34): 1–34. doi:10.1257/app.3.1.1.

Feldstein, M. (1995). *Tax Avoidance and the Deadweight Loss of the Income Tax*. NBER Working Paper No. 5055, www.nber.org.

Forsythe, S., Stover, J. and Bollinger, L. (2009). The past, present and future of HIV, AIDS and resource allocation. *BMC Public Health* **9**.

Galarraga, O., Colchero, M. A., Wamai, R. and Bertozzi, S. (2009). HIV prevention cost-effectiveness: a systematic review. *BMC Public Health* **9**(Suppl 1): S5. doi:10.1186/1471-2458-9-S1-S5.

Galarraga, O. and Gertler, P. (2010). Cash and a brighter future: the effect of conditional transfers on adolescent risk behaviors: evidence from urban Mexico. Unpublished manuscript.

Galarraga, O., Wirtz, V. J., Figueroa-Lara, A., Santa-Ana-Tellez, Y., Coulibaly, I., Viisainen, K., Medina-Lara, A. and Korenromp, E. L. (2011). Unit costs for delivery of antiretroviral treatment and prevention of mother-to-child transmission of HIV: a systematic review for low- and middle-income countries. *PharmacoEconomics* **29**(7): 579–99.

Ganguli, I., Bassett, I., Dong, K. and Walensky, R. (2009). Home testing for HIV infection in resource-limited settings. *Current HIV/AIDS Reports* **6**(4): 217–23. doi:10.1007/s11904-009-0029-5.

Gersovitz, M. (2011). HIV testing: principles and practice. *The World Bank Research Observer* **26**(1): 1–41. doi:10.1093/wbro/lkp013.

Glick, P. (2005). Scaling up HIV voluntary counseling and testing in Africa. *Evaluation*

Review **29**(4): 331–57. doi:10.1177/
0193841X05276437.

Granich, R. M., Gilks, C. F., Dye, C., De Cock,
K. M. and Williams, B. G. (2009). Universal
voluntary HIV testing with immediate
antiretroviral therapy as a strategy for
elimination of HIV transmission: a
mathematical model. *The Lancet* **373**(9657):
48–57. doi:10.1016/S0140-6736(08)61697-9.

Gray, R. H., Kigozi, G., Serwadda, D., Makumbi, F.,
Watya, S., Nalugoda, F., Kiwanuka, N.,
Moulton, L. H., Chaudhary, M. A., Chen, M. Z.,
Sewankambo, N. K., Wabwire-Mangen, F.,
Bacon, M. C., Williams, C. F. M., Opendi, P.,
Reynolds, S. J., Laeyendecker, O., Quinn, T. C.
and Wawer, M. J. (2007). Male circumcision for
HIV prevention in men in Rakai, Uganda: a
randomised trial. *The Lancet* **369**(9562):
657–66. doi:10.1016/S0140-6736(07)
60313-4.

Green, L. W., Travis, J. W., McAllister, R. G.,
Peterson, K. W., Vardanyan, A. N. and Craig, A.
(2010). Male circumcision and HIV prevention:
insufficient evidence and neglected external
validity. *American Journal of Preventive
Medicine* **39**(5): 479–82. doi:S0749-
3797(10)00439-3.

Gregson, S., Gonese, E., Hallett, T. B., Taruberekera,
N., Hargrove, J. W., Lopman, B., Corbett, E. L.,
Dorrington, R., Dube, S., Dehne, K. and
Mugurungi, O. (2010). HIV decline in
Zimbabwe due to reductions in risky sex?
Evidence from a comprehensive
epidemiological review. *International Journal
of Epidemiology* **39**(5): 1311–23. doi:10.1093/
ije/dyq055.

Hallett, T. B., Aberle-Grasse, J., Bello, G., Boulos,
L.-M., Cayemittes, M. P. A., Cheluget, B.,
Chipeta, J., Dorrington, R., Dube, S., Ekra, A.
K., Garcia-Calleja, J. M., Garnett, G. P., Greby,
S., Gregson, S., Grove, J. T., Hader, S., Hanson,
J., Hladik, W., Ismail, S., Kassim, S., Kirungi,
W., Kouassi, L., Mahomva, A., Marum, L.,
Maurice, C., Nolan, M., Rehle, T., Stover, J. and
Walker, N. (2006). Declines in HIV prevalence
can be associated with changing sexual behavior
in Uganda, urban Kenya, Zimbabwe, and urban
Haiti. *Sexually Transmitted Infections* **82**(suppl
1): i1–i8. doi:10.1136/sti.2005.016014.

Hallett, T. B., Alsallaq, R. A., Baeten, J. M., Weiss,
H., Celum, C., Gray, R. and Abu-Raddad, L.
(2011). Will circumcision provide even more

protection from HIV to women and men? New
estimates of the population impact of
circumcision interventions. *Sexually
Transmitted Infections* **87**(2): 88–93. doi:10.
1136/sti.2010.043372.

Hallfors, D., Cho, H., Rusakaniko, S., Iritani, B.,
Mapfumo, J. and Halpern, C. (2011).
Supporting adolescent orphan girls to stay in
school as HIV risk prevention: evidence from a
randomized controlled trial in Zimbabwe.
American Journal of Public Health **101**(6):
1082–8.

Halperin, D. T., Mugurungi, O., Hallett, T. B.,
Muchini, B., Campbell, B., Magure, T.,
Benedikt, C. and Gregson, S. (2011). A
surprising prevention success: why did the HIV
epidemic decline in Zimbabwe? *PLoS Med* **8**(2):
e1000414. doi:10.1371/journal.pmed.1000414.

Hammitt, J. K. (2007). Valuing changes in mortality
risk: lives saved versus life years saved. *Review
of Environmental Economics and Policy* **1**:
228–40. doi:10.1093/reep/rem015.

Harberger, A. (1997). New frontiers in project
evaluation? A comment on Devarajan, Squire
and Suthiwart-Narueput. *The World Bank
Research Observer* **12**(1): 73–9.

Hausler, H. P., Sinanovic, E., Kumaranayake, L.,
Naidoo, P., Schoeman, H., Karpakis, B. and
Godfrey-Faussett, P. (2006). Costs of measures
to control tuberculosis/HIV in public primary
care facilities in Cape Town, South Africa.
Bulletin of the World Health Organization
84: 528–36. doi:10.1590/S0042-
96862006000700014.

Helleringer, S., Kohler, H.-P., Kalilani-Phiri, L.,
Mkandawire, J. and Armbruster, B. (2010).
Uptake and cost of repeated home-based HIV
testing and counseling campaigns in Likoma
(Malawi): a step closer to universal screening?
Philadelphia, PA: University of Pennsylvania,
unpublished manuscript.

Helleringer, S., Kohler, H.-P. and Mkandawire, J.
(2009). Increasing uptake of HIV testing and
counseling among the poorest in sub-Saharan
countries through home-based service
provision. *Journal of Acquired Immune
Deficiency Syndromes* **51**(2): 185–93.
doi:10.1097/QAI.0b013e31819c1726.

Hogan, D. R., Baltussen, R., Hayashi, C., Lauer, J. A.
and Salomon, J. A. (2005). Cost effectiveness
analysis of strategies to combat HIV/AIDS in
developing countries. *BMJ* **331**(7530):

1431–7. doi:10.1136/bmj.38643.
368692.68.

Holbrooke, R. and Furman, R. (2004). A global battle's missing weapon. *New York Times* Op-Ed, February 10, 2004.

John, F. N., Farquhar, C., Kiarie, J. N., Kabura, M. N. and John-Stewart, G. C. (2008). Cost effectiveness of couple counselling to enhance infant HIV-1 prevention. *Int J STD AIDS* **19**(6): 406–9. doi:10.1258/ijsa.2008.007234.

Johnson, L. F. and White, P. J. (2011). A review of mathematical models of HIV/AIDS interventions and their implications for policy. *Sexually Transmitted Infections*. doi:10.1136/sti.2010.045500.

Knowles, J. C. and Behrman, J. R. (2003). Assessing the economic returns to investing in youth in developing countries. The World Bank, Health, Nutrition and Population (HNP) Discussion Paper 2888, www.worldbank.org.

Knowles, J. C. and Behrman, J. R. (2005). Economic returns to investing in youth. In: *The Transition to Adulthood in Developing Countries: Selected Studies*. Washington, DC: National Academy of Science-National Research Council, 424–90.

Kohler, H.-P., Behrman, J. R. and Watkins, S. C. (2007). Social networks and HIV/AIDS risk perceptions. *Demography* **44**(1): 1–33. doi:10.1353/dem.2007.0006.

Kohler, H.-P. and Thornton, R. (2012). Conditional cash transfers and HIV/AIDS prevention: unconditionally promising? *World Bank Economic Review* **26**(2), 165–90.

Martin, G., Bollinger, L., Pandit-Rajani, T., Nkambula, R. and Stover, J. (2007). *Costing Male Circumcision in Swaziland and Implications for the Cost-Effectiveness of Circumcision as an HIV Intervention.* Washington, DC: USAID, Health Policy Initiative.

Matovu, J. K. B., Gray, R. H., Kiwanuka, N., Kigozi, G., Wabwire-Mangen, F., Nalugoda, F., Serwadda, D., Sewankambo, N. K. and Wawer, M. K. (2006). *Repeat Voluntary HIV Counseling and Testing (VCT), Sexual Risk Behavior and HIV Incidence in Rakai, Uganda.*

Mattson, C. L., Campbell, R. T., Bailey, R. C., Agot, K., Ndinya-Achola, J. O. and Moses, S. (2008). Risk compensation is not associated with male circumcision in Kisumu, Kenya: a multifaceted assessment of men enrolled in a randomized

controlled trial. *PLoS ONE* **3**(6): e2443. doi:10.1371/journal.pone.0002443.

McCoy, S., Kangwende, R. and Padian, N. (2010). Behavior change interventions to prevent HIV infection among women living in low and middle income countries: a systematic review. *AIDS and Behavior* **14**(3): 469–82. doi:10.1007/s10461-009-9644-9.

Metcalf, C. A., Douglas, J. M. J., Malotte, C. K., Cross, H., Dillon, B. A., Paul, S. M., Padilla, S. M., Brookes, L. C., Lindsey, C. A., Byers, R. H., Peterman, T. A. and the RESPECT-2 Study Group. (2005). Relative efficacy of prevention counseling with rapid and standard HIV testing: a randomized, controlled trial (respect-2). *Sexually Transmitted Diseases* **32**(2): 130–8.

Morgan, D., Mahe, C., Mayanja, B., Okongo, J. M., Lubega, R. and Whitworth, J. A. G. (2002). HIV-1 infection in rural Africa: is there a difference in median time to AIDS and survival compared with that in industrialized countries? *AIDS* **16**(4): 597–603.

Musgrove, P. and Fox-Rushby, J. (2006). Cost-effectiveness analysis for priority setting. In: Jamison, D. T., Breman, J. G., Measham, A. R., Alleyne, G., Claeson, M., Evans, D. B., Jha, P., Mills, A. and Musgrove, P. (eds.). *Disease Control Priorities in Developing Countries*, 2nd edn. Oxford University Press, 35–86. www.dcp2.org/pubs/DCP.

NIAID. (2011). Treating HIV-infected people with antiretrovirals protects partners from infection: findings result from NIH-funded international study. www.niaid.nih.gov/news/newsreleases/2011/pages/hptn052.aspx.

Njeuhmeli, E., Forsythe, S., Reed, J., Opuni, M., Bollinger, L., Heard, N., Castor, D., Stover, J., Farley, T., Menon, V. and Hankins, C. (2011). The impact and cost of expanding male circumcision for HIV prevention in eastern and southern Africa. Unpublished manuscript.

Oster, E. (2005). Sexually transmitted infections, sexual behavior, and the HIV/AIDS epidemic. *Quarterly Journal of Economics* **120**(2): 467–515.

Padian, N. S., McCoy, S. I., Abdool Karim, S. S., Hasen, N., Kim, J., Bartos, M., Katabira, E., Bertozzi, S. M., Schwartländer, B. and Cohen, M. S. (2011). HIV prevention transformed: the new prevention research agenda. *The Lancet* **378**(9787): 269–78. doi:10.1016/S0140-6736(11)60877-5.

Padian, N. S., McCoy, S. I., Balkus, J. E. and Wasserheit, J. N. (2010). Weighing the gold in the gold standard: challenges in HIV prevention research. *AIDS* **24**(5): 621–35. doi:10.1097/QAD.0b013e328337798a.

Painter, T. (2001). Voluntary counseling and testing for couples: a high-leverage intervention for HIV/AIDS prevention in sub-Saharan Africa. *Social Science and Medicine* **53**: 1397–1411.

Philipson, T. J. and Posner, R. A. (1993). *Private Choices and Public Health: The AIDS Epidemic in an Economic Perspective.* Cambridge, MA: Harvard University Press.

Plank, R. M., Makhema, J., Kebaabetswe, P., Hussein, F., Lesetedi, C., Halperin, D., Bassil, B., Shapiro, R. and Lockman, S. (2010). Acceptability of infant male circumcision as part of HIV prevention and male reproductive health efforts in Gaborone, Botswana, and surrounding areas. *AIDS and Behavior* **14**(5): 1198–202. doi:10.1007/s10461-009-9632-0.

Potts, M., Halperin, D. T., Kirby, D., Swidler, A., Marseille, E., Klausner, J. D., Hearst, N., Wamai, R. G., Kahn, J. G. and Walsh, J. (2008). Reassessing HIV prevention. *Science* **320**(5877): 749–50. doi:10.1126/science.1153843.

Powers, K. A., Ghani, A. C., Miller, W. C., Hoffman, I. F., Pettifor, A. E., Kamanga, G., Martinson, F. E. and Cohen, M. S. (2011). The role of acute and early HIV infection in the spread of HIV and implications for transmission prevention strategies in Lilongwe, Malawi: a modelling study. *The Lancet* **378**(9787): 256–68. doi:10.1016/S0140-6736(11)60842-8.

Pronyk, P. M., Hargreaves, J. R., Kim, J. C., Morison, L. A., Phetla, G., Watts, C., Busza, J. and Porter, J. D. H. (2006). Effect of a structural intervention for the prevention of intimate-partner violence and HIV in rural South Africa: a cluster randomised trial. *The Lancet* **368**(9551): 1973–83. doi:10.1016/S0140-6736(06)69744-4.

Pronyk, P. M., Kim, J. C., Abramsk, T., Phetla, G., Hargreaves, J. R., Morison, L. A., Watts, C., Busza, J. and Porter, J. D. H. (2008). A combined microfinance and training intervention can reduce HIV risk behavior in young female participants. *Aids* **22**(13): 1659–65.

Robinson, L. A. (2007). Policy monitor: how US government agencies value mortality risk reductions. *Review of Environmental Economics and Policy* **1**: 283–99. doi:10.1093/reep/rem018.

Ross, D. A. (2010). Behavioral interventions to reduce HIV risk: What works? *AIDS* **24**(Supplement 4): S4–S14. doi:10.1097/01.aids.0000390703.35642.89.

Schwartländer, B., Stover, J., Hallett, T., Atun, R., Avila, C., Gouws, E., Bartos, M., Ghys, P. D., Opuni, M., Barr, D., Alsallaq, R., Bollinger, L., de Freitas, M., Garnett, G., Holmes, C., Legins, K., Pillay, Y., Stanciole, A. E., McClure, C., Hirnschall, G., Laga, M. and Padian, N. (2011). Towards an improved investment approach for an effective response to HIV/AIDS. *The Lancet* –. doi:10.1016/S0140-6736(11)60702-2. Published online June 3, 2011.

Shepherd, J., Kavanagh, J., Picot, J., Cooper, K., Harden, A. and Barnett-Page, E. (2010). The effectiveness and cost-effectiveness of behavioral interventions for the prevention of sexually transmitted infections in young people aged 13–19: a systematic review and economic evaluation. *Health Technology Assessment* **14**(7): 1–230. doi:10.3310/hta14070. www.hta.ac.uk/project/1666.asp.

Sherr, L., Lopman, B., Kakowa, M., Dube, S., Chawira, G., Nyamukapa, C., Oberzaucher, N., Cremin, I. and Gregson, S. (2007). Voluntary counselling and testing: uptake, impact on sexual behavior, and HIV incidence in a rural Zimbabwean cohort. *AIDS* **21**(7): 851–60. doi:10.1097/QAD.0b013e32805e8711.

Smith, K., Powers, K. A., Kashuba, A. D. and Cohen, M. S. (2011). HIV-1 treatment as prevention: the good, the bad, and the challenges. *Current Opinion in HIV and AIDS* **6**(4): 315–25. doi:10.1097/COH.0b013e32834788e7.

Summers, L. H. (1992). Investing in all the people. *Pakistan Development Review* **31**(4): 367–406.

Summers, L. H. (1994). Investing in all the people: educating women in developing countries. World Bank, Economic Development Institute Seminar Paper No. 45, Washington, DC.

Sweat, M., Morin, S., Celentano, D., Mulawa, M., Singh, B., Mbwambo, J., Kawichai, S., Chingono, A., Khumalo-Sakutukwa, G., Gray, G., Richter, L., Kulich, M., Sadowski, A. and Coates, T. (2011). Community-based intervention to increase HIV testing and case detection in people aged 16–32 years in Tanzania, Zimbabwe, and Thailand (NIMH Project Accept, HPTN 043): a randomised study. *The Lancet Infectious Diseases* **11**(7): 525–32. doi:10.1016/S1473-3099(11)70060-3.

Swendeman, D. and Rotheram-Borus, M. J. (2010). Innovation in sexually transmitted disease and HIV prevention: internet and mobile phone delivery vehicles for global diffusion. *Current Opinion in Psychiatry* **23**(2): 139–44. doi:10.1097/YCO.0b013e328336656a.

The Economist. (2011). The end of AIDS? Thirty years on, it looks as though the plague can now be beaten, if the world has the will to do so. The Economist Print Edition, June 2, 2011.

The International Group on Analysis of Trends in HIV Prevalence and Behaviors in Young People in Countries most Affected by HIV. (2010). Trends in HIV prevalence and sexual behavior among young people aged 15–24 years in countries most affected by HIV. *Sexually Transmitted Infections* **86**(Suppl 2): ii72–ii83. doi:10.1136/sti.2010.044933.

The Voluntary HIV-1 Counseling and Testing Efficacy Study Group. (2000). Efficacy of voluntary HIV-1 counselling and testing in individuals and couples in Kenya, Tanzania, and Trinidad: a randomised trial. *The Lancet* **356**(9224): 103–12.

Thornton, R. L. (2008). The demand for learning HIV status and the impact on sexual behavior: evidence from a field experiment. *American Economic Review* **98**(5): 1829–63.

UN-ESA. (2010). World population prospects, the 2010 revision: AIDS and no-AIDS variants. United Nations, Department of Economic and Social Affairs, Population Division, http://esa. un.org/unpd/peps/EXCEL-Data_WPP2010/ aids_no-aids_variants.html.

UNAIDS. (2008). *Report on the Global HIV/AIDS Epidemic*. New York: World Health Organization and UNAIDS.

UNAIDS. (2010a). *2010 Global Report: Fact Sheet for Sub-Saharan Africa*. New York: World Health Organization and UNAIDS. www.unaids.org/globalreport/.

UNAIDS. (2010b). *Getting to Zero: 2011–2015 Strategy*. Joint United Nations Programme on HIV/AIDS (UNAIDS). www.unaids.org.

UNAIDS. (2010c). *Global Report: UNAIDS Report on the Global AIDS Epidemic 2010*. New York: World Health Organization and UNAIDS. www.unaids.org/globalreport/.

UNAIDS. (2011a). *AIDS at 30: Nations at the Crossroads*. New York, NY: United Nations

Joint Program on AIDS (UNAIDS). www.unaids.org/unaids_resources/aidsat30/ aids-at-30.pdf.

UNAIDS. (2011b). UNAIDS webpage on "sexual transmission of HIV." Accessed August 2, 2011, www.unaids.org/en/strategygoalsby2015/ sexualtransmissionofhiv/.

Uthman, O. A., Popoola, T. A., Uthman, M. M. B. and Aremu, O. (2010). Economic evaluations of adult male circumcision for prevention of heterosexual acquisition of HIV in men in sub-Saharan Africa: a systematic review. *PLoS ONE* **5**(3): e9628. doi:10.1371/journal.pone. 0009628.

Vickerman, P., Terris-Prestholt, F., Delany, S., Kumaranayake, L., Rees, H. and Watts, C. (2006). Are targeted HIV prevention activities cost-effective in high prevalence settings? Results from a sexually transmitted infection treatment project for sex workers in Johannesburg, South Africa. *Sexually Transmitted Diseases* **33**(10): S122–S132. doi:10.1097/01.olq.0000221351.55097.36.

Viscusi, W. K. (1993). The value of risks to life and health. *Journal of Economic Literature* **31**: 1912–46.

Viscusi, W. K. (2010). The heterogeneity of the value of statistical life: introduction and overview. *Journal of Risk and Uncertainty* **40**(1): 1–13.

Waters, R. C., Ostermann, J., Reeves, T. D., Masnick, M. F., Thielman, N. M., Bartlett, J. A. and Crump, J. A. (2011). A cost-effectiveness analysis of alternative HIV retesting strategies in sub-Saharan Africa. *JAIDS–Journal of Acquired Immune Deficiency Syndromes* **56**(5): 443–52.

Weinreb, A. A. and Stecklov, G. (2009). Social inequality and HIV-testing: comparing home- and clinic-based testing in rural Malawi. *Demographic Research* **21**(21): 627–46. doi:10.4054/DemRes.2009.21.21.

White, R. G., Glynn, J. R., Orroth, K. K., Freeman, E. E., Bakker, R., Weiss, H. A., Kumaranayake, L., Habbema, J. D. F., Buve, A. and Hayes, R. J. (2008a). Male circumcision for HIV prevention in sub-Saharan Africa: who, what and when? *AIDS* **22**(14): 1841–50. doi:10.1097/QAD. 0b013e32830e0137.

White, R. G., Orroth, K. K., Glynn, J. R., Freeman, E. E., Bakker, R., Habbema, J. D. F., Terris-Prestholt, F., Kumaranayake, L., Buve, A. and Hayes, R. J. (2008b). Treating curable sexually transmitted infections to prevent HIV in Africa: still an effective control strategy? *Journal of Acquired Immune Deficiency Syndromes* **47**(3): 346–53. doi:10.1097/QAI. 0b013e318160d56a.

Wilson, D. and Halperin, D. T. (2008). Know your epidemic, know your response: a useful approach, if we get it right. *The Lancet* **372**(9637): 423–6. doi:10.1016/S0140-6736(08)60883-1.

World Bank. (2010a). Malawi and Tanzania research shows promise in preventing HIV and sexually-transmitted infections. World Bank News & Broadcast, July 18, 2010. The World Bank, Washington, DC, http://go.worldbank. org/XDHE04P2G0.

World Bank. (2010b). The RESPECT study: evaluating conditional cash transfers for HIV/STI prevention in Tanzania. Washington, DC: World Bank, *Results Brief*, http:// siteresources.worldbank.org/DEC/Resources/ HIVExeSummarypercent28Tanzaniapercent29. pdf.

Yang, S. (2010). Cash rewards and counseling could help prevent STIs in rural Africa. University of California at Berkeley Press Release, July 18, 2010, http://berkeley.edu/news/media/releases/ 2010/07/18_sti-africa.shtml.

Young, A. (2005). The gift of the dying: the tragedy of AIDS and the welfare of future African generations. *Quarterly Journal of Economics* **120**(2): 423–66.

Sexual transmission of HIV

Perspective paper

DAMIEN DE WALQUE

In their assessment paper, Jere R. Behrman and Hans-Peter Kohler (2011) have identified three possible interventions for the prevention of sexual transmission of HIV: 1) medical male circumcision, 2) voluntary counseling and testing, and 3) information campaigns through mass media and peer groups. They identified those solutions based on an extensive and updated literature review building on the review of cost effectiveness of HIV prevention interventions performed by Galárraga *et al.* (2009).

They selected those three solutions based on their assessment that the current empirical evidence clearly points to medical male circumcision as a promising intervention, with possible additional effective interventions being comprehensive testing and counseling and effective information and peer group campaigns. They stress that the information about the effectiveness of those HIV prevention interventions and others is limited and that the challenges of estimating benefits and costs within an appropriate dynamic life-cycle framework are considerable. They show that the benefit to cost ratios they obtained are sensitive to critical assumptions related to the value of life, the discount rate, the HIV prevalence rate, and the costs of interventions. Nevertheless their benefit-cost estimates suggest that under most plausible conditions the benefit-cost ratios for these interventions in high-prevalence and medium-prevalence countries are likely to be large, particularly for male circumcision and probably for HIV testing and counseling (HTC). They obtain smaller estimates for information campaigns which in part reflect the greater uncertainty in the underlying information available for the estimates. They conclude that interventions to reduce the spread of

HIV/AIDS in sub-Saharan Africa through reducing sexual infection rates seem to have considerable promise – and greater promise where prevalence rates and DALYs are higher and resource costs of interventions and discount rates are lower. Their estimates also show that cost-effectiveness estimates per HIV infection averted and per DALY in a broad general sense reveal similar patterns, but also differ importantly from benefit-cost estimates in specific respects because they do not incorporate some critical factors that are incorporated in the benefit-cost estimates such as intertemporal trade-offs that require discounting, life-cycle considerations, and impacts on production and consumption.

The assessment paper by Behrman and Kohler (2011) is comprehensive, clear, and supported by a strong analysis. Their selection of three interventions makes sense, based on the current evidence. Using the assessment paper as a starting point, the role of this perspective paper is to propose a discussion of the assessment paper findings and offer further perspectives on the topics, possibly on the basis of more recent or more tentative evidence. This perspective paper will start by stressing the need for more and better impact evaluations of HIV/AIDS prevention interventions. Next, it will argue that cost-effectiveness calculations should better integrate potential behavioral responses to prevention interventions. Further, it will discuss implications

I thank Sinith Mehtsun for excellent research assistance. The findings, interpretations, and conclusions in this paper are those of the author and do not necessarily represent the views of the World Bank, its Executive Directors, or the governments they represent.

for cost-effectiveness of scaling-up interventions, especially male circumcision. It will also argue in favor of more targeted approaches. Finally, it will review three other possible solutions mentioned but not thoroughly analyzed in the assessment paper because they have been proposed and tested only recently and the evidence about their efficacy and effectiveness remains very limited: a) treatment as prevention, b) pre-exposure chemoprophylaxis for HIV prevention, and c) conditional cash transfers.

The need for more and better impact evaluations of HIV/AIDS prevention interventions

Behrman and Kohler (2011) make clear that the evidence on the efficacy and cost-effectiveness of prevention intervention is limited. First, too few impact evaluations have been conducted and too few have been conducted rigorously. As pointed out by Bertozzi (2009), "we need to stop spending billions implementing large-scale interventions without measuring effectiveness." Bertozzi follows by giving as an example the billions spent on abstinence campaigns without any measure of whether these campaigns held any value in preventing HIV.[1] As pointed out by Behrman and Kohler (2011), it also seems that there is very limited evidence available about the effectiveness of condom distribution.

When impact evaluations have been conducted, they are often not rigorous enough. HIV/AIDS prevention is a field where impact evaluation is challenging because evaluators are confronted with endogenous behavioral choices, unobserved variables, selectivity of samples, and response bias, in particular when measuring self-reported sexual behaviors. Only few of the studies presented as evaluating the impact of HIV prevention information have research designs that allow them to overcome those challenges.

Even when rigorous impact evaluations have been used, the results are not always clear evidence of the efficacy and cost-effectiveness of the intervention. Padian et al. (2010) review thirty-seven randomized controlled trials of HIV prevention interventions and find only six demonstrating effects in reducing HIV incidence. The review suggests that lack of statistical power, poor adherence,

and diluted versions of the intervention in comparison groups may have been important issues in some of the trials that did not show any results.

An example of such uncertainty in the impact evaluation results for an HIV prevention intervention is the treatment of other sexually transmitted infections (STIs). As summarized in Galárraga et al. (2009), the earliest study of the efficacy of treating other STIs on HIV incidence conducted in Mwanza, Tanzania suggested that when STIs are treated, HIV infection declined by almost 40 percent over a two-year period (Grosskurth et al. 1995). Following this result, STI treatment was included in the catalogue of HIV prevention measures endorsed by the WHO and UNAIDS. However, another randomized control trial in Rakai Uganda showed contradictory results (Wawer et al. 1998) and other studies have not replicated the Mwanza level of efficacy. The treatment of other STIs is not included in the solutions identified in the assessment paper probably because of the divergence in the results from those impact evaluations.

With the current amount and level of evidence, as acknowledged by Behrman and Kohler (2011), identifying the most cost-effective interventions for preventing sexual infections is already a challenge. With, as discussed further in this perspective paper, new solutions for HIV prevention being currently advocated and tested, it is crucial that the development of these new solutions goes hand-in-hand with rigorous impact evaluations having enough statistical power and using biomarkers as endpoints.

Considering potential behavioral responses to prevention interventions

Part of the economics literature on HIV/AIDS has investigated disinhibition – or risk compensation – behaviors. The main proposition of this literature is that people may alter their behavior in response to perceived changes in risk.[2] In the specific case of HIV/AIDS, the focus has been mainly related to

---

[1] Zikusooka (2010) provides very useful information about the cost of abstinence and faithfulness interventions in Uganda, but without providing any evidence of impact on HIV prevention.

[2] See Peltzman (1975) for an early study on the introduction of mandatory car seat belts in the US.

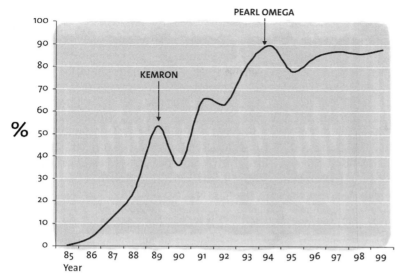

Figure 1.1.1 *Percent condom use in a cohort of sex workers: Nairobi 1985–99*
Source: *Jha* et al. *(2001)*

the increased access to ART. The concern is that increased access to ART may lead to a decrease in the perceived risk and costs of contracting HIV and, as a consequence, may lead to an increase of risky sexual behaviors (e.g., Eaton and Kalichman 2007). Such disinhibition behaviors, if large enough, may (at least partially) offset the benefits of scaling up access to ART. This conjecture is supported by several studies in the United States and Europe which have identified an upward trend in risky sexual behaviors since the introduction of ART in 1996 (e.g., Gremy and Beltzer 2004; Lakdawalla, Sood and Goldman 2006). More specifically, an association has been identified between decreased concern about HIV due to ART availability and unprotected sex, and in particular among men who have sex with men (e.g., Dukers *et al.* 2001; Kalichman 1998; Lakdawalla, Sood and Goldman 2006; Mechoulan 2007).

Investigations of disinhibition behaviors in sub-Saharan Africa are limited. One of the earliest studies looked at change in the use of condom by sex workers in Nairobi, Kenya (Jha *et al.* 2001). The findings are summarized in Figure 1.1.1 above.

This figure provides at least some suggestive evidence that condom use by sex workers decreased when "fake" cures of AIDS ("Kemron" and "Pearl Omega") were announced. Such a pattern is consistent with disinhibition behaviors, although the result may not be generalizable to the general population since it uses a very selected segment of the population. Cohen *et al.* (2009) is one of the few studies which use population-based surveys to test risk compensation behavior in a sub-Saharan African context. The authors found that in Kisimu (Kenya), ART-related risk compensation, and the belief that ART cures HIV, were associated with an increased HIV sero-prevalence in men, but not in women.

Behrman and Kohler's (2011) analysis does not explicitly allow for behavioral changes in responses to interventions that would in part reduce the effectiveness of the intervention (e.g., increases in risky sex in response to the reduced HIV infection risks after circumcision are not explicitly modeled) even though they consider such compensating behaviors when looking at the evidence on the efficacy of HIV/AIDS testing and counseling, referring to the analysis conducted by Ross (2010), who advances that HIV testing and counseling might be effective in persuading HIV-positive individuals to reduce their risky behaviors and the risk of transmission of HIV to their partners, but potentially leads to disinhibition among those who receive an HIV-negative test result.

This perspective paper is not focused on HIV/AIDS treatment, but disinhibition behaviors could also be present as a consequence of HIV prevention interventions for HIV testing, as suggested by Ross (2010). I would also think it should be considered and investigated especially in the case of male circumcision. It is possible that as a consequence of male circumcision – which is protective, but only to a certain extent – male individuals and their partners opt for less safe sexual practices and for example become less likely to use condoms, or more likely to engage in concurrent partnerships. Such a compensatory behavior would tend to diminish the benefits from male circumcision. Behrman and Kohler (2011) also discuss compensating behaviors related to male circumcision, but their assessment is that the current empirical evidence does suggest that disinhibition is unlikely to substantially reduce the effectiveness of medical male circumcision. This assessment is based on the evidence from self-reported sexual behaviors of study participants in the randomized control trials that have established the efficacy of medical male circumcision. As discussed in the next section, it would be important to assess the possibility of disinhibition from male circumcision interventions at scale.

An additional and related problem might be caused by so-called "bush" circumcisions, i.e. circumcisions performed outside health care settings, for example during traditional initiation ceremonies. For example, Corno and de Walque (2007) report that a particular type of traditional circumcision is performed in Lesotho. In the Basotho culture, many young males are sent by their parents to so-called "initiation schools" that represent a passage from adolescence to adulthood. Traditionally, initiation schools are places where young people are given information about sexual relations and reproductive health. During their stay at the initiation school, these boys are circumcised. This circumcision has a symbolic meaning and the procedure is very different from the circumcision adopted in most other African countries, especially by those in the Muslim tradition. It is not a complete removal of the foreskin but rather a more symbolic incision. It is also likely to be performed in unhygienic conditions. Moreover, after the initiation school, boys consider themselves adults and may engage more readily in sexual intercourse. It is also possible that their recent "circumcision" makes them more vulnerable to infection. These traditional practices combined with the dissemination of the message that male circumcision is proven to be protective might lead to disinhibition behavior even among males who are not properly circumcised, unless information campaigns clearly identify the type of circumcision which is actually protective and efforts are made to scale-up circumcision in health care settings.

Behrman and Kohler (2011) also compare neonatal or infant male circumcision to circumcision among adults and adolescents. They make the valid point that the benefits of infant male circumcision will be heavily discounted. Further, it has been suggested that disinhibition behaviors are less likely to occur in the case of infant circumcision, presumably because circumcision would have taken place well before the onset of sexual activity. While this seems plausible, this remains to be demonstrated empirically.

Overall, it is fair to conclude that the evidence on disinhibition behaviors is limited and inconclusive. Crepaz, Hart and Marks (2004) have provided a comprehensive review, with studies finding evidence of disinhibition and others not. The evidence is even more limited in sub-Saharan Africa. This is probably a good reason for not modeling it explicitly in the assessment paper as chosen by Behrman and Kohler (2011). But the potential risks associated with disinhibition on a large scale are important enough to be taken into consideration. As much as possible, future impact evaluations of HIV prevention interventions should consider and measure possible risk compensating behaviors, in particular in the case of male circumcision.

The importance of measuring efficiency of prevention intervention at scale

In the current literature, most interventions have been evaluated in randomized controlled trials or other type of pilot projects. As *RethinkHIV* is aiming at identifying the most promising prevention interventions, it is important to stress the difference between efficacy and efficiency studies (Gertler *et al.* 2010) and note that interventions which have demonstrated impact under closely managed conditions may not necessarily be as successful under normal, at scale, conditions. In other words, the external validity of efficacy studies needs to be investigated.

This is especially true for male circumcision, as advocated in Over (2010). Currently, the evidence showing the protective effect of male circumcision relies on three closely managed randomized control trials (Auvert *et al.* 2005; Bailey *et al.* 2007; Gray *et al.* 2007) showing a strong protective effect. But to date, to the best of my knowledge, there is no rigorous impact evaluation of male circumcision at scale. Those would be important studies to carry out, not only to confirm the external validity of the randomized control trials, but also to learn, for example, what are the most effective delivery mechanisms for scaling-up male circumcision. Obviously, such impact evaluations at scale could also help in investigating the issue of disinhibition behaviors discussed in the previous section.

The two other interventions identified by Behrman and Kohler (2011), HIV testing and counseling, and information campaigns through mass media and peer groups, have been scaled up to a larger extent than male circumcision, although it is not always obvious that the limited evidence available on their impact comes from efficiency rather than efficacy studies. Given the fragmentary and sometimes contradictory evidence about the impact of those interventions, it would also be beneficial to conduct impact evaluations of those interventions at scale. It must be said, however, that evaluating the impact of information campaigns through mass media is particularly difficult precisely because most media campaigns are conducted on a large scale and it is therefore difficult to identify control groups and estimate the counterfactual.

Considering more targeted approaches

Behrman and Kohler (2011) have mainly considered approaches that can be scaled up to the general population as they consider those as more likely to have a broad impact in reducing the overall sexual transmission of HIV. While this is a valid point, it is also true that interventions targeted at high-risk groups, such as men who have sex with men (MSM), or sex workers, can be very effective and have a significant impact on HIV transmission. Thailand's success in stemming its HIV epidemic has generally been attributed to a vigorous prevention strategy aimed at high risk groups. Such targeted interventions might be more adequate in countries with moderate to low HIV epidemics, but as evidenced in Table 1.1 and Figure 1.1 of Behrman and Kohler (2011), many African countries fall in that category. Ainsworth, Vaillancourt and Gaubatz (2005) among others have argued that the limited efficacy of interventions such as information campaigns through peer groups might be due, in part, to the fact that they were not targeted well enough to people really at risk of being infected by or of transmitting the HIV virus.

New solutions for the prevention of sexual transmission of HIV might offer new perspectives

Behrman and Kohler (2011) explicitly analyze the cost effectiveness of three existing prevention interventions but they also briefly discuss other more recent approaches without analyzing their cost-effectiveness. In this perspective paper, I will devote more attention to these new approaches which at this stage appear promising and might – or might not – play an important role for the prevention of sexual transmission of HIV in the future. Those three approaches are "treatment for prevention" (or "test-and-treat"), pre-exposure chemoprophylaxis for HIV prevention, and conditional cash transfers.

Treatment for prevention

The "treatment for prevention" approach proposes to test regularly a large fraction of the population and treat immediately with anti-retroviral therapies those who have tested positive without waiting for the AIDS symptoms to develop. By treating HIV-positives immediately after they have tested, the objective is to reduce the viral load of HIV-positives, and therefore their infectiousness. While earlier studies advocating this approach were based on modeling (Granich *et al.* 2009), recent results from the HPTN 052 study (NIAID 2011) indicate that treatment for prevention is efficacious (Padian *et al.* 2011). The treatment for prevention approach, however, needs further efficacy and efficiency trials, and the implications and obstacles to bringing it up to scale need to be further investigated and tested. This approach is discussed in more detail in the assessment paper of AIDS treatment and I will therefore not comment further on it.

Pre-exposure chemoprophylaxis for HIV prevention

Padian *et al.* (2011) also report on recent trials evaluating pre-exposure chemoprophylaxis for HIV prevention. In the Caprisa Study in South Africa, high-risk women used an applicator that delivered 1 percent tenofovir gel into the vaginal vault up to 12 hours before, and within 12 hours after intercourse. Investigators reported a 39 percent reduction in overall acquisition of HIV, and maximum reduction was 54 percent among the most adherent women (Abdool Karim *et al.* 2010). In the iPrEx study in 2010 (Grant *et al.* 2010), HIV-negative men who have sex with men were given daily an anti-retroviral combination, emtricitabine and tenofovir disoproxil fumarate (TDF plus FTC), for up to 2.8 years. The study recorded a 44 percent reduction in HIV acquisition and, as with the CAPRISA study, efficacy was strongly associated with concentrations of anti-retroviral drugs, a direct marker of adherence. By contrast, the FEM-PrEP trial of TDF plus FTC offered to high-risk women was discontinued because an equal number of infections occurred in both the placebo and treatment groups. As with treatment for prevention, the efficacy and efficiency of pre-exposure chemoprophylaxis for HIV patients needs to be further established and confirmed, but if they are confirmed it would open very promising perspectives for the prevention of sexual transmission. Compared to treatment as prevention, pre-exposure chemoprophylaxis offers two advantages. First, there is no need for frequent and widespread testing in order to identify HIV-positive individuals. This is logistically challenging in most settings in sub-Saharan Africa, especially if one of the objectives is to detect individuals with recent HIV infections which are more infectious, but more difficult to detect with accuracy. Second, pre-exposure chemoprophylaxis for HIV prevention can be self-targeted by individuals who feel they are most at risk. However, both approaches require a high level of adherence in the absence of symptoms, and both have the potential to trigger risk compensating or disinhibition behaviors described earlier.

Conditional cash transfers

I will focus more extensively, among the potentially promising new solutions, on conditional cash transfers as I have more experience in that field. I will first lay out the rationale for applying the conditional cash transfer logic to the prevention of the sexual transmission of HIV, summarizing the argument in Medlin and de Walque (2008). Then, I will briefly present the current evidence which has also been discussed by Behrman and Kohler (2011).

Rationale for applying conditional cash transfers to HIV prevention

Conditional cash transfer (CCT) programs which provide cash to poor households in exchange for their active participation in educational and health care services have proven very popular among developing country governments, sweeping the globe from Mexico to other parts of Latin America and, much more recently, to Africa. The principle of conditionality – which may be applied differently in practice, but generally requires families to send their children to school or to receive a range of health care services, such as nutritional counseling, childhood vaccination programs, etc. – distinguishes CCT programs from more traditional social assistance programs which provide cash or vouchers directly to poor or otherwise distressed families, with no conditions attached. The CCT programs that emphasize the use of market-oriented "demand-side" interventions provide incentives for longer-term human capital investments (Rawlings and Rubio 2005; Fiszbein and Schady 2008).

The CCT programs that have received the most attention are those having an explicit orientation toward poverty alleviation, involving both education and health components as part of a broader, long-term strategy of human capital investments. Such programs have been rigorously evaluated, and, on the whole, have been found to be effective at increasing levels of household consumption and improving uptake rates of a wide range of education and preventive health care services. Specifically with regard to health outcomes, several studies have shown an impact on anthropometric outcomes, such as improvement in the nutritional status of newborns and infants (Colombia), height gains among children aged 12 to 36 months (Mexico), and decreases in stunting and the proportion of underweight children aged 0 to 5 years (Nicaragua).

The substantial evidence demonstrating positive effects on the uptake of health care services and a range of critical health outcomes in different countries and socioeconomic settings has triggered significant interest in exploring potential applications of CCTs to other areas of health, including HIV prevention. This is certainly the case in sub-Saharan Africa, where interest in replicating the results of such programs has led to pilot projects to support the care of AIDS orphans, and the uptake of HIV testing services (Thornton 2008). These experiments, observed in combination with programs in other countries seeking to use CCTs to increase contraceptive use and to discourage pregnancies, particularly among adolescent girls, raise the question of whether CCTs may be usefully applied to improve outcomes in sexual and reproductive health, generally, and in particular as a tool to prevent STI/HIV transmission.

Existing CCT programs provide powerful evidence into the linkages between financial incentives and behavior change. In addition, they provide compelling evidence that such programs can have a direct impact on selected health outcomes at a large scale, and over an extended period of many

years. However, there remain questions about the importance of the conditionality to the effectiveness of such programs. For a richer exploration of this issue, it is also useful to turn to the contingency management (CM) literature which addresses risky health behaviors such as substance abuse, smoking, and over-eating.

In a similar manner as for the CCT poverty alleviation programs, CM relies on the mechanism of conditionality to elicit behaviors that are viewed to be in one's long-term interest (or those of society), and to discourage those behaviors that may ultimately be detrimental to one's own health and well-being but that may not be easily perceived or experienced as such in the short term. However, while traditional CCT programs, or those focused on improving uptake rates, require a "simple" behavioral response (e.g. involving a single finite action, such as attending a health clinic), the latter require a "complex" change (e.g. abstaining from a behavior that may be desirable, and habit-forming, in the short run, but in the long run is detrimental to one's health) (Kane et al. 2004). Thus, with regard to the importance of the conditionality and in the domain of sexual and reproductive health, per se, more might be gleaned from an examination of the evidence from contingency management rather than the CCTs.

The essential principles of CM, as outlined by Petry et al. (2000), are to reinforce the treatment goals by 1) closely monitoring the target behavior; 2) providing tangible, positive reinforcement of the target behavior; and 3) removing the positive reinforcement when the target behavior does not occur. CM techniques have been developed and tested in the context of clinical trials and settings, but have rarely, if ever, been implemented on a large scale in the manner of CCT programs. However, studies of the behavioral and health impacts of CM are valuable for their focus on different aspects of the conditionality that is expected to bring about the required behavioral changes in the domain of preventing the sexual transmission of HIV.

As with CCTs, CM interventions have been tied to participation and the uptake of services in several domains, although risk behaviors are the important determinant for participant selection, rather than income constraints. CM has been shown to increase uptake rates of counseling sessions for drug abuse; attendance at weight loss sessions; and attendance in smoking cessation clinics.[3] Of particular interest, however, is the use of CM to trigger a complex behavioral change – usually, to discourage an unhealthy behavior by positively reinforcing the cessation of that activity (e.g. drug or alcohol abuse, smoking, or over-eating). The conceptual basis of CM and CCTs is thus largely similar, although advocates of CM impose no *a priori* assumptions about the effectiveness of the use of cash as the incentive or reinforcement device, and have experimented with a variety of reward mechanisms, including vouchers and prizes.[4] In addition, many CM studies are designed to explore effect differences due to variations in the value of the incentives (known as the "dose-response" curve), the frequency of monitoring and payments, and the length of time that the elicited behavior change is sustained after the program has ended.

Conditional cash transfers and contingency management offer an innovative alternative to traditional behavioral strategies, and therefore may have important applications to sexual and reproductive health, and HIV prevention, in particular.

The conceptual foundations of conditional cash transfers are rooted in traditional economic theory, which is based on the assumption that individuals make rational decisions that maximize their own individual well-being or utility. The theory acknowledges that individuals face risky choices with benefits (e.g. personal enjoyment) and costs (e.g. health risks), and assumes that individuals will make sensible choices after taking these costs and benefits into careful consideration. The modeling of individual decision making in this manner has led to major new insights into apparently "irrational" risk-taking behavior, and has been used to explain risky occupational choices such as formal and informal sex work. For example, Gertler *et al.* (2005) found in a study of Mexican sex workers that "risky sex," i.e. unprotected sex, carries a 23 percent higher price tag than sex with condoms. In a study of informal sex workers in Western Kenya, Robinson and Yeh (2011) found that sex workers charge more for anal sex, and that risky sexual activity fluctuates in response to consump-

tion expenditures and income shocks experienced within the household.

Another promising area of research in behavioral economics and decision theory offers an understanding of risk-taking behavior that may be radically and irreconcilably inconsistent with rational decision-making, such as the decision to engage in risky sex in a setting with high HIV prevalence. For example, O'Donoghue and Rabin (2001) have developed a behavioral model in which young people are assumed to make decisions by weighing costs and benefits, but they may also choose to act compulsively in certain instances. In this model, the benefits and costs incurred in the future are discounted in the same way that they would be in rational choice models, except that youth may place higher value on rewards received instantaneously. Behavioral economics refers to this as "hyperbolic time discounting" and it is a similar concept to that of "immediate gratification" used in developmental psychology.

The conceptual foundations of CCTs rest easily within either economic framework of decision-making, since cash payments can be used either to alter the cost-benefit parameters of the decision calculus of the rational individual, or it can be used to counter impulsive tendencies by rewarding, in the short term, behaviors that are likely to bring longer-term health benefits. Applied to poverty alleviation, the goal is to compensate individuals in the short term for the "costs" associated with investments in health and education that have a longer-term pay-off. Applied to risky behavior, the goal is to shift potential future costs of weight gain, smoking, and substance abuse higher to the present, so they can be more immediately perceived. Clearly, some behavioral changes may be more "costly" than others. For example, the uptake of health and educational services likely places fewer demands on the individual than, for example, the decision to refrain from specific behaviors, particularly those

---

[3] See, for example, Higgins *et al.* (1994); Petry (2000); and Emont and Cummings (1992).
[4] The findings of studies reviewed for this study suggested that cash is typically preferred by research subjects, and in some studies it has been shown to have a greater behavioral effect than the equivalent non-cash reward (Kamb *et al.* 1998), although the findings are hardly conclusive.

that afford pleasurable short-term benefits. This has been described as a difference between "simple" behavioral change and "complex" change, and the latter may require a larger incentive to bring about the desired change (Kane *et al.* 2004).

The same framework is useful in regards to sexual and reproductive health. As O'Donoghue and Rabin (2001) remind us, the decision to have sex involves a trade-off between the short-term benefit of sexual pleasure and intimacy, and the long-term (probabilistic) cost of getting pregnant, acquiring an STI, or contracting AIDS. Thus, risky decisions – such as whether or not to have unprotected sex – may be the result of a realistic assessment of trade-offs and probabilities, or may result from problems associated with undervaluing the future (or excessive discounting, in economic parlance). Of course, this is a stylized view of the decision-making process that may be conditioned and constrained by the cultural, social, and economic context. In fact, many studies have highlighted how poverty, lack of economic opportunity, and powerlessness close off options to the point that individuals (and especially, young girls) do not experience their engagement in risky sexual behavior as the outcome of a deliberate decision (Krishnan *et al.* 2008).

With regards to preventing HIV transmission, an added difficulty is that the "costs" of engaging in risky sexual behavior may not be perceived for many years, due to the lag between infectivity and presentation of acute and/or chronic symptoms of AIDS. Thus, one goal of the CCT intervention would be to shorten the horizon of the future by offering cash rewards at regular but more importantly frequent intervals. The premise is that a system of rapid feedback and positive reinforcement using cash as an incentive to shape behavior can effectively discourage risky sexual activity and therefore contribute to reduced rates of HIV transmission.

Current evidence on applying conditional cash transfers to HIV prevention

The evidence on the efficacy of conditional cash transfers for STI or HIV prevention is still unfolding and remains limited. In Malawi, small financial incentives have been shown to increase the uptake of HIV testing and counseling (Thornton 2008). Another study in Malawi conducted a conditional cash transfer program for adolescents in which the cash transfer was conditional on school attendance but which, in addition to increased enrollment and attendance, also caused a reduction in HIV and HSV-2 incidence (Baird *et al.* 2012). The same program also led to a modification of self-reported sexual behaviors, with adolescent girls having younger partners (Baird *et al.* 2010).

To date, two studies evaluated conditional cash transfers in which the condition is attached to negative test results for sexually transmitted infections. In Malawi, Kohler and Thornton (2012) tested an intervention promising a single cash reward in one year's time for individuals who remained HIV-negative. This design had no measurable effect on HIV status, but the number of sero-conversions in the sample was very small, and statistical power was therefore low. The RESPECT study (de Walque *et al.* 2010) evaluated a randomized intervention that used economic incentives to reduce risky sexual behavior among young people aged eighteen to thirty and their spouses in rural Tanzania. The goal was to prevent HIV and other sexually-transmitted infections (STIs) by linking cash rewards to negative STI test results assessed every four months. The study tested the hypothesis that a system of rapid feedback and positive reinforcement using cash as a primary incentive to reduce risky sexual behavior could be used to promote safer sexual activity among young people who are at high risk of HIV infection. Initial results of the randomized controlled trial after one year showed a significant reduction in STI incidence in the group that was eligible for the $20 quarterly payments, but no such reduction was found for the group receiving the $10 quarterly payments. Further, while the impact of the CCTs did not differ between males and females, the impact was larger among poorer households and in rural areas. While the RESPECT study results are important in showing that the idea of using financial incentives can be a useful tool for preventing HIV/STI transmission, this approach would need to be replicated elsewhere and implemented on a larger scale before it could be concluded that such conditional cash transfer

programs (for which administrative and laboratory capacity requirements are significant) offer an
efficient, scalable, and sustainable HIV prevention
strategy.

Conclusions

Using the assessment paper as a starting point,
this perspective paper on the prevention of sexual transmission of HIV offers further perspectives on the basis of more recent or more tentative evidence. It stresses the need for more and
better impact evaluations of HIV/AIDS prevention
interventions. It also argues that cost-effectiveness
calculations should better integrate potential behavioral responses to prevention interventions known
as disinhibition behaviors. Further, it recommends
considering the implications for cost-effectiveness
of scaling-up interventions, especially in the case of
medical male circumcision. It also argues in favor
of not neglecting approaches more targeted towards
vulnerable groups such as sex workers or men who
have sex with men. Finally, it reviews three other
possible solutions mentioned but not thoroughly
analyzed in the assessment paper because they have
been proposed and tested only recently and the evidence about their efficacy and effectiveness remains
very limited: a) treatment as prevention, b) pre-
exposure chemoprophylaxis for HIV prevention,
and c) conditional cash transfers.

References

Abdool Karim, Q., Abdool Karim, S. S., Frohlich,
J. A. *et al.* for the CAPRISA 004 Trial Group.
(2010). Effectiveness and safety of tenofovir
gel, an antiretroviral microbicide, for the
prevention of HIV infection in women. *Science*
329: 1168–74.

Ainsworth, M., Vaillancourt, D. and Gaubatz, J. H.
(2005). *Committing to Results: Improving the
Effectiveness of HIV/AIDS Assistance. An OED
Evaluation of the World Bank's Assistance for
HIV/AIDS Control.* Washington DC, The World
Bank.

Auvert, B., Taljaard, D., Lagarde, E., Sobngwi-
Tambekou, J., Sitta, R. and Puren, A. (2005).
Randomized, controlled intervention trial of

male circumcision for reduction of HIV
infection risk: the ANRS 1265 Trial. *PLoS
Medicine* **2**(11): 1112–22. doi:10.1371/
journal.pmed.0020298.

Bailey, R. C., Moses, S., Parker, C. B., Agot, K.,
Maclean, I., Krieger, J. N., Williams, C. F. M.,
Campbell, R. T. and Ndinya-Achola, J. O.
(2007). Male circumcision for HIV prevention
in young men in Kisumu, Kenya: a randomised
controlled trial. *The Lancet* **369**(9562): 643–56.
doi:10.1016/S0140-6736(07)60312-2.

Baird, S., Chirwa, E., McIntosh, C. and Özler, B.
(2010). The short-term impacts of a schooling
conditional cash transfer program on the sexual
behavior of young women. *Health Economics*
19(S1): 55–68. doi:10.1002/hec.1569.

Baird, S., Garfein, R., McIntosh, C. and Özler, B.
(2012). Effect of a cash transfer programme for
schooling on prevalence of HIV and herpes
simplex type 2 in Malawi: a cluster randomised
trial. *The Lancet* **379**(9823): 1320–9.

Behrman, J. R. and Kohler, H. P. (2011). *RethinkHIV*:
Assessment Paper on the Prevention of Sexual
Transmission of HIV. Forthcoming.

Bertozzi, S. M. (2009). Financing the Long Term
Solution. Fifth International AIDS Society
Conference on HIV Pathogenesis, Treatment
and Prevention, Cape Town, South Africa,
abstract TUPL103.

Cohen, C., Montandon, M., Carrico, A., Shiboski, S.,
Bostrom, A., Obure, A., Kwena, Z., Bailey, R.,
Nguti, R. and Bukusi, E. (2009). Association of
attitudes and beliefs towards antiretroviral
therapy with HIV-seroprevalence in the general
population of Kisumu, Kenya. *PLoS ONE* **4**(3).

Corno, L. and de Walque, D. (2007). *The
Determinants of HIV Infection and Related
Sexual Behaviors: Evidence from Lesotho.*
World Bank Policy Research Working Paper
No. 4421, Washington DC, The World Bank.

Crepaz, N., Hart, T. A. and Marks, G. (2004). Highly
active antiretroviral therapy and sexual risk
behavior. *JAMA* **292**(2): 224–36. doi:10.1001/
jama.292.2.224.

de Walque, D., Dow, W., Nathan, R., Abdul, F.,
Abilahi, E., Gong, Z., Isdahl, J., Jamison, B.,
Jullu, S., Krishnan, A., Majura, E., Miguel, J.,
Moncada, S., Mtenga, M. A., Mwanyangala, L.,
Packel, J., Schachter, K., Shirima and Medlin,
C. A. (2012). Incentivising safe sex: a
randomised trial of conditional cash transfers
for HIV and sexually transmitted infection

prevention in rural Tanzania. *BMJ Open* 2012;2:e000747. doi:10.1136/bmjopen-2011-000747.

Dukers, N., Goudsmit, J., de Wit, J., Prins, M., Weverling, G. and Coutinho, R. (2001). Sexual risk behavior relates to the virological and immunological improvements during highly active antiretroviral therapy in HIV-1 infection. *AIDS* **15**(3): 369.

Eaton, L. and Kalichman, S. (2007). Risk compensation in HIV prevention: implications for vaccines, microbicides, and other biomedical HIV prevention technologies. *Current HIV/AIDS Reports* **4**(4): 165–72.

Emont, S. and Cummings, K. (1992). Using a low-cost, prize-drawing incentive to improve recruitment rate at a work-site smoking cessation clinic. *Journal of Occupational Medicine* **34**: 771–4.

Family Health International. (2010). FHI Statement on the FEM-PrEP HIV Prevention Study. April 18, 2011. www.fhi.org/en/AboutFHI/Media/Releases/FEM-PrEP_statement041811.htm (accessed September 13, 2011).

Fiszbein, A. and Schady, N. (2009). *Conditional Cash Transfers: Reducing Present and Future Poverty*. Washington DC, The World Bank.

Galarraga, O., Colchero, M. A., Wamai, R. and Bertozzi, S. (2009). HIV prevention cost-effectiveness: a systematic review. *BMC Public Health* **9**(Suppl 1): S5. doi:10.1186/1471-2458-9-S1-S5.

Gertler, P., Shah, M. and Bertozzi, S. M. (2005). Risky business: the market for unprotected sex. *Journal of Political Economy* **113**: 518–50.

Gertler, P. J., Martinez, S., Premand, P., Rawlings, L.B. and Vermeersch, C. M. J. (2010). *Impact Evaluation in Practice*. Washington DC, The World Bank.

Granich, R. M., Gilks, C. F., Dye, C., De Cock, K. M. and Williams, B. G. (2009). Universal voluntary HIV testing with immediate antiretroviral therapy as a strategy for elimination of HIV transmission: a mathematical model. *The Lancet* **373**(9657): 48–57. doi:10.1016/S0140-6736(08)61697-9.

Grant, R. M., Lama, J. R., Anderson, P. L. *et al.* for the iPrEx. (2010). Preexposure chemoprophylaxis for HIV prevention in men who have sex with men. *N Engl J Med* **363**: 2587–99.

Gray, R. H., Kigozi, G., Serwadda, D., Makumbi, F., Watya, S., Nalugoda, F., Kiwanuka, N., Moulton, L. H., Chaudhary, M. A., Chen, M. Z., Sewankambo, N. K., Wabwire-Mangen, F., Bacon, M. C., Williams, C. F. M., Opendi, P., Reynolds, S. J., Laeyendecker, O., Quinn, T. C. and Wawer, M. J. (2007). Male circumcision for HIV prevention in men in Rakai, Uganda: a randomised trial. *The Lancet* **369**(9562): 657–66. doi:10.1016/S0140-6736(07)60313-4.

Gremy, I. and Beltzer, N. (2004). HIV risk and condom use in the adult heterosexual population in France between 1992 and 2001: return to the starting point? *AIDS* **18**(5): 805.

Grosskurth, H., Mosha, F., Todd, J., Mwijarubi, E., Klokke, A., Senkoro, K., Mayaud, P., Changalucha, J., Nicoll, A., ka-Gina, G. *et al.* (1995). Impact of improved treatment of sexually transmitted diseases on HIV infection in rural Tanzania: randomised controlled trial. *The Lancet* **346**(8974): 530–6.

Higgins *et al.* (1994). Incentives improve outcomes in outpatient behavioral treatment of cocaine dependence. *Archives of General Psychiatry* **51**: 568–76.

Jha, P., Vaz, L., Plummer, F., Nagelkerke, N., Willbond, B., Ngugi, E., Moses, S., John, G., Nduati, R., MacDonald, K. *et al.* (2001). *The Evidence Base for Interventions to Prevent HIV Infection in Low and Middle-Income Countries*. Geneva: Commission on Macroeconomics and Health Working Paper Series WG 5.

Kalichman, S. (1998). Post-exposure prophylaxis for HIV infection in gay and bisexual men: implications for the future of HIV prevention. *American Journal of Preventive Medicine* **15**(2): 120–7.

Kamb, M. L. *et al.* (1998). What about money? Effect of small monetary incentives on enrollment, retention, and motivation to change behavior in an HIV/STD prevention counseling intervention. The Project RESPECT Study Group. *Sexually Transmitted Infections* **74**: 253–5.

Kane, R. *et al.* (2004). A structured review of the effect of economic incentives on consumers' preventive behavior. *American Journal of Preventive Medicine* **27**(4): 327–52.

Kohler, H.-P. and Thornton, R. (2012). Conditional cash transfers and HIV/AIDS prevention: unconditionally promising? *World Bank Economic Review* **26**(2), 165–90.

Krishnan, S., Dunbar, M. S., Minnis, A. M., Medlin, C. A., Gerdts, C. E. and Padian, N. S. (2008). Poverty, gender inequities and women's risk of human immunodeficiency virus/AIDS. *Annals of the New York Academy of Sciences* **1136**: 101–10.

Krishnan-Sarin, S. *et al.* (2006). Contingency management for smoking cessation in adolescent smokers. *Experimental Clinical Psychopharmacology* **14**(3): 306–10.

Lakdawalla, D., Sood, N. and Goldman, D. (2006). HIV breakthroughs and risky sexual behavior. *The Quarterly Journal of Economics* **121**(3): 1063–102.

Mechoulan, S. (2007). Risky sexual behavior, testing, and HIV treatments. *Forum for Health Economics & Policy* **10**(2).

Medlin, C. and de Walque, D. (2008). *Potential Applications of Conditional Cash Transfers for Prevention of Sexually Transmitted Infections and HIV in Sub-Saharan Africa.* Policy Research Working Paper 4673, The World Bank.

NIAID (2011). Treating HIV-infected people with anti-retrovirals protects partners from infection: findings result from NIH-funded international study. www.niaid.nih.gov/news/newsreleases/2011/pages/hptn052.aspx (accessed September 13, 2011).

O'Donoghue, T. and Rabin, M. (2001). Risky behavior among youths: some issues from behavioral economics. In Gruber, J. (ed.) *Risky Behavior Among Youths.* University of Chicago Press, 29–68.

Over, M. (2010). Adult male circumcision as an HIV prevention tool: should the scale up of an efficacious intervention be evaluated? Blog Post. January 26, 2010. Center for Global Development. http://blogs.cgdev.org/globalhealth/2010/01/adult-male-circumcision-as-an-hiv-prevention-tool-should-the-scale-up-of-an-efficacious-intervention-be-evaluated.php (accessed September 12, 2011).

Padian, N. S., McCoy, S. I., Abdool Karim, S. S., Hasen, N., Kim, J., Bartos, M., Katabira, E., Bertozzi, S. M., Schwartländer, B. and Cohen, M. S. (2011). HIV prevention transformed: the new prevention research agenda. *The Lancet* **378**(9787): 269–78. doi:10.1016/S0140-6736(11)60877-5.

Padian, N. S., McCoy, S. I., Balkus, J. E. and Wasserheit, J. N. (2010). Weighing the gold in the gold standard: challenges in HIV prevention research. *AIDS* **24**(5): 621–35. doi:10.1097/QAD.0b013e328337798a.

Peltzman, S. (1975). The effects of automobile safety regulation. *Journal of Political Economy* **83**(4): 677–726.

Petry, N. (2000). A comprehensive guide to the application of contingency management procedures in clinical settings. *Drug and Alcohol Dependence* **58**: 9–25.

Petry, N. *et al.* (2001). Contingency management interventions: from research to practice. *American Journal of Psychiatry* **158**(5): 694–702.

Rawlings, L. and Rubio, G. (2005). Evaluating the impact of conditional cash transfer programs. *The World Bank Research Observer* **20**(1): 29–55.

Robinson, J. and Yeh, E. (2011). Transactional sex as a response to risk in Western Kenya. *American Economic Journal: Applied Economics* **3**: 35–64.

Ross, D. A. (2010). Behavioral interventions to reduce HIV risk: what works? *AIDS* **24**(Supplement 4): S4–S14. doi:10.1097/01.aids.0000390703.35642.89.

Thornton, R. (2008). The demand for and impact of learning HIV status. *American Economic Review* **98**: 1829–63.

Wawer, M. J., Gray, R. H., Sewankambo, N. K., Serwadda, D., Paxton, L., Berkley, S., McNairn, D., Wabwire-Mangen, F., Li, C., Nalugoda, F. *et al.* (1998). A randomized, community trial of intensive sexually transmitted disease control for AIDS prevention, Rakai, Uganda. *AIDS* **12**(10): 1211–25.

Zikusooka, C. M. (2010). Cost of PEPFAR-funded interventions: case study of abstinence and be faithful and community mobilization strategies in Uganda. Presentation made at the International AIDS Economics Network Pre-Conference Meeting, July 16–17, 2010, Vienna, Austria.

Sexual transmission of HIV

Perspective paper

ALAN WHITESIDE

This project sets out to answer the question: if we raised an additional $10 billion over the next five years to combat HIV and AIDS in sub-Saharan Africa, how could it best be spent? What are the benefits and costs of the interventions? This perspective paper comments on the assessment paper focusing on prevention of sexual infections, taking into account the comments made at the Washington meeting and the subsequent revisions. The assessment paper identifed three of the most promising solutions and provided cost benefit analysis; the perspective paper provides an analysis of the assumptions and calculations used in the assessment paper as well as other viewpoints.

The work should be seen in the context of how HIV and AIDS are perceived and funded. The disease was first reported in 1981. The cause, a retrovirus, identified in 1983. By the early 1990s the epidemic was under control in the West, but prevalence was rising rapidly across much of sub-Saharan Africa (SSA). In 1996, the year UNAIDS was established, there was $3 million available globally for HIV and AIDS. There was then an almost exponential increase in funding until, by 2008, there was $15.6 billion. The early years of the century saw the establishment of the Global Fund to Fight AIDS, TB, and Malaria (GFATM) and the US Presidential Emergency Plan for AIDS Relief (PEPFAR): both bringing significant additional resources to the table (Smith and Whiteside 2010).

Since 2008 the situation has changed. AIDS is no longer at the top of the global health agenda, and indeed for most of the world this makes sense: it is not *the* priority. The amount of money available rose slightly to $15.9 billion in 2009 and dropped to $15.3 billion in 2010. At best, resources will be stable; at worst they may fall. The pledges made at the October 2010 replenishment conference for the GFATM were below expectations. PEPFAR has indicated that its funding is unlikely to rise. A number of other donors have either not fulfilled their commitments or have cut back. The UN Non-Communicable Disease Summit in New York in September 2011 has the potential to further shift AIDS out of the spotlight. Unfortunately the nature of the disease (the long period between infection and illness) means needs are growing as more people become eligible for (comparatively) expensive treatment.

RethinkHIV comes at a critical juncture in the response to the epidemic. It is not enough to simply invest $10 billion; the key is to get the best returns. This issue is increasingly important in the light of flat-lining of resources. Unfortunately, the question we may ultimately be faced with is not how to invest additional money, but rather how to make best use of what we have. This paper looks at prevention. There is a Ugandan saying that "we should not keep mopping the floor while the tap is running." Prevention must be at the heart of the AIDS response.

The assessment paper

Behrman and Kohler (2011) describe how they arrive at possible solutions for prevention of sexual transmission of HIV infections in SSA. There are initially three criteria for interventions:

- those for which there is reasonably strong empirical evidence from multiple countries about the efficacy – and possibly even effectiveness – of the intervention;
- ones seen as important elements in HIV/AIDS prevention efforts by international organizations and local governments; and
- interventions where reasonable estimates of benefits and costs could be obtained.

The question is, what works? Behrman and Kohler recognize "considerable uncertainty about the efficacy and/or effectiveness of program interventions to reduce the sexual transmission of HIV. Ultimately, under any of the criteria stated above, only programs that reduce HIV risk behaviors, HIV infection risks, and/or HIV incidence should be considered." The evidence – as to which interventions make a difference – is weak.

Three interventions are identified for further analysis. First, biomedical: male circumcision (MC), which results in a long-term irreversible reduction in infection risk for men. Second: those HIV testing and counseling (HTC) campaigns which focus on an individual's information about their HIV status. According to Behrman and Kohler, theoretical and empirical arguments suggest that if individuals know their HIV status (and that of their spouses and other sexual partners), they will make less risky decisions about sexual behaviors and relationships. The third intervention is information campaigns (IC) through mass media and peer groups, aiming to reduce risk behaviors by providing information about the disease and prevention. The commissioning brief to the authors was to pick "at least three of the most promising interventions" – it is troubling that they struggled to come up with just these three, but this is a criticism of HIV responses, not their work.

The limitations and assumptions are clearly stated by Behrman and Kohler. The analysis is grounded in "a systematic integration of the available evidence within a *dynamic life-cycle perspective* in which an individual faces evolving risks and ART prevalences, with age-specific survival probabilities and with the incorporation of age-specific productivity and consumption effects in addition to DALYs" (emphasis mine). They say, somewhat

touchingly: "One could therefore conclude that the task of estimating benefit to cost ratios is so difficult that it would be better to abandon it. But that would leave society with little systematic guidance about policy choices in this important area. Therefore, in hopes of improving the basis for policy guidance, we swallow hard and proceed boldly and hopefully creatively (and hopefully not too foolhardily) to make the best estimates that we can." The three solutions are summarized below.

Male circumcision (MC)

Medical male circumcision programs are in place in many African countries. Behrman and Kohler (2011) view MC as the policy intervention with the strongest empirical evidence. This is based on randomized controlled trials in SSA, with extensive studies to assess the costs and challenges of implementing and scaling up. These suggest scale-up is cost-effective. MC has the added advantage of being high on the UNAIDS agenda as well as that of many governments, donors, and NGOs. Early work (pre-1990) showed that high HIV prevalence coincided with low rates of circumcision (ecological evidence). It should be noted that the campaign is for *medical* male circumcision. In settings where this is done as part of coming of age rituals, the circumcision may be effective, but only if enough of the foreskin is removed. Following the meeting in Washington Behrman and Kohler added neonatal or male circumcision as a possible intervention.

HIV testing and counseling (HTC)

HTC is considered, although empirical evidence is mixed. The reason for its continued inclusion is that it remains "an important component of HIV prevention, especially given that it is a crucial element in providing HIV-positive individuals with ART for both treatment and possibly prevention. In addition, technological progress has changed the options for HTC substantially from the context in which earlier VCT programs were evaluated, thereby improving access to HTC as well as potential frequency and convenience of testing and the possible expansion of couple-based HTC." This inclusion of HTC is partly based on the recent finding on the role of treatment in reducing infection; this is critiqued below. The authors note benefit-cost calculations for HTC are more speculative than those for MC because program effects and costs are uncertain. It is not clear from the paper as to exactly what we should be funding in HTCs, as they are many and varied.

Information campaigns through mass media and peer groups (IC)

The third solution is information campaigns through mass media and peer groups. It is included because, although there is little clear evidence on their effects, they "constitute an important component of HIV prevention strategies." Behrman and Kohler (2011) state: "While the alleged effectiveness of some of the 'conventional' media and peer group campaigns are not generally backed by careful empirical evidence, more recent studies suggest that more innovative program designs – including for instance school-based interventions, information campaigns that provide specific local information relevant to risk reduction (e.g., the local HIV prevalence by age), or programs that rely on cell phones and related technologies – are effective in reducing HIV infections among young adults." The benefit-cost calculations for IC are speculative, and even more uncertain than for HTC programs.

Findings

The conclusions of the paper are presented in two tables. Both look at the three solutions with alternative estimates for: a $1,000 DALY economy and a $5,000 DALY economy; 3 percent and 5 percent discount rates; 11 percent (medium) and 25 percent (high) initial HIV prevalence; and low and high costs for the interventions. The authors correctly exclude low-prevalence countries from the analysis. This is a good decision because the HIV epidemic is not high on the agenda, nor should it be, in these settings.

The first table presents benefit-cost estimates. Overall these are high. The lowest ratio is in the case of the high-cost information campaign in a $1,000 DALY economy with a 5 percent discount rate where the benefit to cost ratio is 1.0. In all other

scenarios it is above this; at the peak it is 82.9 for low-cost circumcision at a 3 percent discount rate in a $5,000 DALY, high-prevalence economy.

This means there are "substantial possibilities for interventions that reduce the transmission of sexually transmitted HIV/AIDS." Benefit to cost ratios remain high even if benefits are overestimated or costs underestimated. These ratios are about 2.5 times as large for the $5,000 DALY economy than the $1,000 DALY economy; they are 40 percent larger for the 3 percent discount rate than for a 5 percent discount rate; are twice as large for a high (25 percent) initial HIV prevalence than for a medium (11 percent) initial HIV prevalence; and low-cost intervention estimates are higher for each solution than the higher-cost intervention estimates.

A plain language conclusion is: the less the intervention costs, the higher the prevalence, and the higher the value of a life, the greater the benefits against the cost. For the low-cost alternatives, MC has the highest benefit to cost ratios, with HTCs second, and IC third. But for the high-cost intervention assumptions, HTCs tend to have the highest benefit to cost ratios with MC second and IC third.

The second table presents the costs per HIV infection averted (HIA) and the costs per DALY that are implied by calculations of the benefit to cost ratios. MC is the most cost-effective intervention, both in terms of costs per infection averted and cost per DALY averted, in high- and medium-prevalence scenarios. HTC is cost-effective if the program is sufficiently comprehensive and well designed to result in the reductions of HIV infection risks that are assumed in the authors' calculations. Information campaigns are the least cost-effective intervention with considerable uncertainty about the costs per DALY and HIA.

There are important differences between the benefit-cost approach and the cost-effectiveness approach. Based on cost-effectiveness calculations, MC always dominates HTC, and MC is between 1.5 and 2 times more cost-effective than HTC (the costs per DALY and HIA for MC are 50–66 percent those for HTC). In the benefit-cost analyses for the high-cost scenario and high initial prevalence, HTC is the intervention with the higher benefit to cost ratio than MC. This is because benefits are discounted, and circumcision is for life, while the other interventions fade over time.

The plain language conclusion is benefit-cost analysis is more relevant for policy analysis. On this basis if we had an extra $10 billion and the cost of the intervention is high we should invest in HTC, otherwise MC will produce the best return. This is interesting but not terribly helpful to policy- and decision-makers, as will be discussed. It illustrates the complexity of the epidemic and the limitations of this approach.

How should we assess success: the role of RCTs

Behrman and Kohler (p. 18) write:

> despite the substantial resources devoted to evaluating such interventions, the evidence remains weak (Padian *et al.* 2010; Ross 2010). For example, restricting studies to the "gold standard" of randomized controlled trials (RCTs) with biological outcome measures (HIV incidence), a systematic review of late phase RCTs evaluating interventions for the prevention of sexual transmission of HIV by Padian *et al.* (2010) identified only 37 HIV prevention RCTs reporting on 39 unique interventions. Only six RCTs, all evaluating biomedical interventions, demonstrated definitive effects on HIV incidence. Five of the six RCTs significantly reduced HIV infection: all three male circumcision trials, one trial of sexually transmitted infection treatment and care, and one vaccine trial.

It is on the basis of this analysis that they put forward their three solutions for the prevention of sexually transmitted HIV infections (with cost-benefit and cost-effectiveness estimates). It is worth noting we have not found any other work at the time of completing this paper.

In science the gold standard to assess if something works is a randomized controlled trial (RCT). This is a scientific experiment where subjects are randomly allocated to receive one or other of alternative treatments. Usually one group is the intervention arm, the other the control. Ideally the trial is blind – the participants do not know which intervention they are receiving. There may be additional levels of "blinding": those administering the intervention, collecting results, and carrying out first stage of analysis should not know what the partici-

pants are getting – double and triple blinding. What is crucial is if the outcome of the intervention can be measured. In the case of HIV prevention the outcome should be biologically measurable: reduced HIV incidence is the best result, but proxies such as pregnancy rates may be used.

There are concerns with using RCTs as a measure of effectiveness of HIV prevention – they are better suited to assessing treatment. They are complex, expensive, and take time. An example is the microbicide trials, a prevention method not prioritized here, for good reason, as it is not yet available. The idea of a female controlled prevention method was first mooted in 1990 by Professor Zena Stein (Stein 1990). The Centre for the AIDS Programme of Research in South Africa (CAPRISA), based in Durban, completed the most recent study on microbicides. They looked at whether a gel containing the anti-retroviral drug tenofovir, applied vaginally by women, would reduce the risk of infection. Following years of design work and preparation, the trial began in May 2007 in an area outside Pietermaritzburg in South Africa. It finished in December 2009, and data were first published in March 2010. The trial had 1,800 participants; half the women were given the gel with tenofovir and others the gel with no drug. They were asked to use the first dose 12 hours prior to and 12 hours after having sex. All were given HIV risk reduction counseling, and received condoms.

The headline result was: a microbicide containing 1 percent tenofovir was 39 percent effective in reducing risk of contracting HIV during sex, and 51 percent effective in preventing genital herpes infections (Mbadi and CAPRISA 2010; Fox 2010). Further trials will need to be done (and are in process) before the gel is approved by the regulatory agencies – the Food and Drug Administration in the USA and Medicines Control Council in South Africa. This probably won't happen before 2015 – twenty-five years after the idea was first mooted.

The situation is further complicated because a number of prevention RCTs have been halted early, as they were shown to be effective and it was considered unethical to withhold the intervention. It is worth noting that this unfortunately does not mean that the interventions are either sustained or scaled-up.

Some interventions do not lend themselves to RCTs. For example, how can a national media program be tested in a control population? All and sundry would be exposed to billboards, and radio messages are available to everyone with a receiver.

Finally while results from a RCT are considered the gold standard, they can be wrong. Again an HIV prevention intervention illustrates this. It was thought in the 1990s that the presence of sexually transmitted infections (STIs) was an important cofactor for HIV infection, and that pre-emptive treatment of STIs might be a way of bringing down HIV incidence. Indeed the belief was so strong that trials went into the field to find out what impact STI prevention and control might have on HIV infection rates. The two landmark trials were in Mwanza, Tanzania and across the border in Rakai in Uganda.

In 1995, the first results of the Mwanza study showed 40 percent of HIV infections had been prevented in the communities receiving the intervention. At this point there was nothing else with such promising outcomes, and it was greeted with great excitement by the AIDS community. The Rakai study, which reported in 1999, showed no HIV infections were prevented in the intervention communities. Subsequent studies have not been able to replicate the Mwanza work (Hitchcock and Fransen 1999; Grosskurth *et al.* 2000).

The gold standard is to have a number of RCTs which can then be subjected to a systematic review. A systematic review is usually regarded as a literature review focused on a research question. It tries to identify, appraise, select, and synthesize all high-quality research evidence relevant to the question. Systematic reviews of high-quality randomized controlled trials are considered crucial to evidence-based medicine. The best way to do such reviews in medicine is by using the well-known Cochrane methodology.[1]

Returning to the example of STI control, there is a current Cochrane review on the impact of population-based biomedical STI interventions on the incidence of HIV infection. This states:

> We failed to confirm the hypothesis that STI control is an effective HIV prevention strategy. Improved STI treatment services were shown in one study

to reduce HIV incidence in an environment characterized by an emerging HIV epidemic (low and slowly rising prevalence), where STI treatment services were poor and where STIs were highly prevalent; Incidence was not reduced in two other settings. There is no evidence for substantial benefit from a presumptive treatment intervention for all community members. There are, however, other compelling reasons why STI treatment services should be strengthened, and the available evidence suggests that when an intervention is accepted it can substantially improve quality of services provided. (Ng *et al.* 2011.)

Social science has its own systematic review body, the Campbell Collaboration, which "helps people make well-informed decisions by preparing, maintaining and disseminating systematic reviews in education, crime and justice, and social welfare" (Campbell Collaboration 2011). This may be of help moving forward but it is still in its early stages.

Differences in philosophy between social sciences, natural science, and humanities are beyond the scope of this paper but are nonetheless important. Kagan (2009) puts forward three components to intellectual efforts: the unquestioned premises that create preferences for particular questions and hence particular answers – in the case of this project that economic analysis works; the analytical tools used – here, monetary costs and benefits; and a preferred set of concepts that are the core of explanations – for *RethinkHIV* that is cost benefit analysis.

The underlying assumptions for critiquing the paper

The scale of the epidemic

There are three major epidemics in the subcontinent. This is well illustrated on the map in Behrman and Kohler's paper (2011). First and easiest to deal with are those areas where prevalence is low. This predominantly encompasses the Muslim countries of North and West Africa. The main modes of transmission are probably drug use, men having sex with men, and commercial sex work. The drug use is the topic of the non-sexual transmission paper. One

[1] See www.cochrane.org/cochrane-reviews.

question that is relevant but beyond the scope of this paper is: why are infection rates so low? Levels of male circumcision may be a critical reason. The Behrman and Kohler (2011) assessment paper correctly does not consider these countries further.

The second cohort consists of countries where HIV rates are stable or falling, yet high – 5–15 percent among adults. These include East African nations where the epidemic first emerged: Kenya, Tanzania, and Uganda, and some West African countries. It should be noted that the big unknown in terms of prevalence is Nigeria; both because the data are unreliable and the size of the population means the numbers could be huge. These countries are dealt with as medium prevalence in the paper.

Worst affected are the hyper-endemic countries of Southern Africa: Zambia, Malawi, Zimbabwe, Mozambique, South Africa, Swaziland, Botswana, and Lesotho (but not, interestingly, Angola, a country where males are circumcised early). Here prevalence is shockingly high. There are two important points about prevalence. The first is the rate and the second is the numbers. It is appalling that 50 percent of women aged between twenty-five and twenty-nine in Swaziland are infected; this translates into a lifetime risk of probably close to 80 percent. It is also worth noting that while South Africa does not appear to have the same infection rates as Botswana, Lesotho, and Swaziland, this is because some provinces have diluted overall prevalence. It is estimated that over five million South Africans are infected. There are more people with HIV in the province of KwaZulu-Natal than in Botswana, Lesotho, Namibia, and Swaziland combined. In these situations HIV has to be an overriding priority. These countries are identified as high prevalence in the paper.

Modes of transmission

The main modes of transmission among adults are sex, injecting drug use, blood transfusions, and contaminated medical equipment (nosocomial infection). In sub-Saharan Africa, sexual contact accounts for the largest proportion of infections, although other modes of transmission are present and important in some settings. It must be remembered that sexual contact can be sex between men

and women (heterosexual sex), and sex between men, known as men who have sex with men (MSM).

The probability of sexual transmission can be expressed as

$$I = S\,[1 - \{pB[1 - \beta']\alpha(1 - v)$$
$$+ p(1 - B)[1 - \beta]\alpha(1 - v) + (1 - p)\}n]$$

S = number susceptible
p = HIV prevalence in partners
B = prevalence of sexually transmitted infections (STIs) in partners
β = probability of transmission (with STI (β'), without STI (β))
α = contacts per partner
v = proportion of acts protected by condom use
n = number of partners (UNAIDS 2011a)

There are a number of important studies from UNAIDS on modes of transmission. These are well described on the UNAIDS website, which also has tools, guidelines and gives access to country reports (UNAIDS 2011b). The chance of infection for heterosexual intercourse is 0.006 per risky exposure act with an STI present, and 0.002 with no STI, no matter whether the person is a sex worker or in a long-term relationship. It is higher for men who have sex with men: the probability per risky act is 0.030 if there is an STI and 0.010 with no STI. If, in a population, many men (S) visit commercial sex workers (CSW) frequently (α), who in turn have high levels of infections and STIs (p and B), and these sex acts are unprotected (v), then the chance of transmission increases. It is perhaps worth noting that people do not think rationally about probability; indeed, to coin a phrase, good or bad luck is simply probability personalized.

What therefore drives the epidemic (in the absence of interventions) is the underlying prevalence, frequency of sex, multiple partners, levels of STIs, and condom usage. These determine the chance of exposure and the number of exposures. The very different epidemics in Africa are illustrated in Figure 1.2.1.

In Swaziland and Lesotho over 60 percent of infections are between people engaged in so-called "long term cohabiting monogamous heterosexual sex." Of considerable significance are those

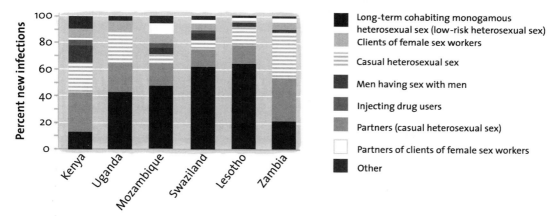

Figure 1.2.1 *Incidence by modes of HIV transmission (sexual)*
Source: *Results from Know your Epidemic project in Southern and Eastern Africa.*
Reports available from www.unaidsrstesa.org/hiv-prevention-modes-of-transmission.

having "casual heterosexual sex" and their part-ners. The figure is also telling because it shows a small but significant contribution from MSM in Kenya, Mozambique, and Swaziland; numbers are smaller in Lesotho and Zambia. There appear to be no transmissions via this route in Uganda, but MSM activities are illegal and highly stigmatized there. Indeed MSM is illegal in a number of countries and stigmatized in most – in Malawi, two gay men were jailed in mid-2011. This impacts on reporting and makes interventions problematic. Also significant are infections between commercial sex workers and their clients. Again in some settings this may be illegal, which causes problems for identifying and addressing the problem.

Basics of sexually transmitted HIV prevention

Preventing HIV transmission through sexual inter-course is not rocket science. There are behavioral interventions: abstinence, delaying sexual debut, sticking to one partner, having fewer partners, and not having concurrent partners. In the equation above, this is intervening in the α (contacts per partner) and n (number of partners) to reduce the S (number susceptible) and hence the incidence. In terms of the Schwartländer *et al.* (2011) invest-ment approach, this is reducing risk. The second set of options are about making the chance of trans-mission in an act of sexual intercourse less likely.

Interventions available at the moment focus on the B (prevalence of STIs in partners) and the ν = pro-portion of acts protected by condom use. Not in the equation is circumcision, which is a biomedi-cal intervention. When microbicides and vaccines become available they will fall into the category of interventions that make sex less risky.

Of course in getting prevention programs that work, the devil is in the detail (as with benefit-cost analysis). Obviously, not engaging in sex is a sure way to avoid infection. The abstinence option was pushed in the PEPFAR funding, where one-third of prevention money was earmarked for this. There is little evidence that this type of interven-tion works. My unit undertook an evaluation of a project in Durban, where a faith-based organization was providing an intervention in schools. We found the project had mixed results. Qualitative analysis showed the community valued the intervention and it created a safe space for adolescents to discuss HIV and abstinence, life skills, and socio-economic challenges. Quantitative analyses showed that par-ticipation was associated with higher scores on a number of resilience dimensions, including hope, mastery, and optimism. Participation was statis-tically related to a lower likelihood of report-ing ever having had sex (42.1 percent of learners reported having had sex, compared to 52.8 percent of those who had not received the intervention). This effect was stronger in boys: 20 percent of male learners exposed to the intervention reported having had sex in the past year, compared to 35.3 percent of those who were not. However, those exposed to this intervention had less favourable attitudes towards using condoms as the most reliable form of HIV prevention (Casale *et al.* 2010; Nixon *et al.* 2009). The good news is that participants delayed sexual debut; the bad news was that they were less likely to use condoms. I think the problem with faith-based abstinence programs is that to have sex is a "sin"; but to use a condom is a worse "sin," because it implies premeditation and a willingness to "sin." Therefore to have sex and use a condom is not a "sin + sin = 2 sins" equation, but rather "sin + sin + premeditation = sin^3."

If a person cannot abstain, they can avoid infection by not being exposed to infected partners. Having one uninfected lifetime partner will achieve this. Other ways of decreasing risk include delaying sexual debut – this is particularly important for younger women, for physiological reasons; having fewer partners; not having concurrent partners; and choosing partners from pools where infection levels are lower. This last option is cited by Behrman and Kohler (2011) who cite a study showing that sexual behaviors of female teenagers are responsive to HIV risk information. When girls were informed of the HIV prevalence rates in men of various ages, they chose their sexual partners from those with lower infection rates. This randomized study documented a 28 percent decrease in teen pregnancy (Dupas 2011). These are the HTC and IC options. They are social interventions.

If a person is exposed through sex to someone who is infected, then the likelihood of transmission can be reduced. If they do not have STIs (B = prevalence of STIs in partners), then transmission is reduced, but as the RCTs show that STI interventions as currently designed do not work, Behrman and Kohler (2011) correctly do not pursue this option. To repeat the quote, "There is no evidence for substantial benefit from a presumptive treatment intervention for all community members. *There are, however, other compelling reasons why STI treatment services should be strengthened*" (emphasis mine). For both men and women, using condoms – male or female – will reduce the chance of exposure; and men who are engaged in heterosexual sex are at lower risk if they are circumcised.

The assessment paper critique

The assessment paper identifies three possible solutions for lessening sexual transmission of HIV: male circumcision; HIV counseling and testing; and information campaigns. This is essentially one biomedical intervention and two social interventions. Before commenting on these solutions it is worth noting that in all cases the assessment paper discusses this as a decrease in infection among young men. This is of concern, as the bulk of infections are in young women.

The paper assumes that male circumcision will reduce the probability of infection by 30 percent. The data suggests that the reduction is about 60 percent, so this is a conservative estimate. Voluntary counseling and testing is assumed to reduce infection by 25 percent. Information through mass media and peer groups is assumed to reduce the rate of infection by 25 percent. The data for these interventions are rather a guesstimate.

Male circumcision

Medical male circumcision is the prevention intervention for which there is the most evidence and there are RCTs. It is a straightforward binary option: circumcised/not circumcised, and works for life. However, it is protective for uninfected men, not women. If enough men in a population are circumcised, then it will impact transmission in the population.

There can be no doubt that this is a good option. In 2006, following the publication of the second edition of *AIDS in the Twenty-first Century: Disease and Globalization* (Barnett and Whiteside 2006), my co-author Tony Barnett and I felt that we lacked solutions and convened a meeting of senior people from a range of organizations to talk about what was needed. All were invited in their personal capacity. The meeting was attended by the AIDS ambassadors, senior donor agency staff, a representative of a pharmaceutical company, and people from hyper-endemic countries. The conversation, which took place over two days on a sailing boat in the IJsselmeer, was private, but at the end we agreed an *Informal Aide Memoire of the Silos to Windmill Meeting*, which was to be realistic, advocating and discussing limited issues to see if they were feasible.

We agreed on four key issues. In order of priority they were:

1. We advocated routine opt-out male infant circumcision. Evidence so far is substantial enough to make this case. Opt-in circumcision should be available for older males.
2. We perceived a disconnect between those who (desperately) need funding and their potential donors, due to communication problems, bureaucracy, and different perceptions and expectations. The donor community needs to get to know its "customers" better.
3. We argued for investigating the need for and possibilities of establishing health insurance funds.
4. We felt the need to find a system for accountability on all levels.

Medical male infant circumcision was included following the Washington meeting. It will take a long time to become effective. Boys become sexually active in their late teens or early twenties so, at worst, it would take twenty-five years to show an impact. This is the same period from conceptualization to delivery of the microbicide! Reworking their paper Behrman and Kohler note that there is uncertainty about the relative costs of infant and adult circumcision but conclude that the benefit to cost ratios for infant circumcision are likely to be much the same as for adults.

In general, HIV/AIDS scholars and activists are reactive and have tended to focus on immediate quick fixes and to conceptualize "impacts" as sequential and short-term effects resulting from the virus, rather than considering the complexities and inter-generational dimensions of epidemics and their consequences. I worked with colleagues in thinking about key conceptual limitations through a novel, comparative analysis of historical trends and contemporary debates within HIV/AIDS and

climate change scholarship. These share certain similarities. Scholars in both areas are struggling to understand phenomena that are unprecedented, complex, highly dynamic, and that have different impacts on different people and places. However, whereas in climate change people look forward, in AIDS we don't (Chazan, Brklacich, and Whiteside 2009).

Ignored in this paper is the issue of MSM. Is medical male circumcision effective at reducing transmission between men who have sex with men? These numbers may be significant. A recently published Cochrane systematic review (Wiysonge *et al.* 2011) designed to answer this question found there to be no conclusive evidence suggesting a protective role of medical male circumcision (MMC) between men who have sex with men, although there may be some protection for men who practice primarily insertive anal sex. At present there is no completed randomized controlled trial (RCT) that has assessed the effects of male circumcision on acquisition of HIV and other sexually transmitted infections among MSM. It will be important to watch for the results of an RCT currently being conducted in China among MSM (Wiysonge *et al.* 2011).

HIV counseling and testing and treatment as prevention

The HTC solution is conditional on it "leading to sustained risk reduction among both infected and uninfected individuals. This outcome is only likely if HTC is widespread, possibly relatively frequent, combined with high-quality counseling" (Behrman and Kohler 2011). It is not entirely clear what these solutions will look like, but they do advocate for early treatment of those found to be infected, and the critique needs to devote a few paragraphs to this.

The idea of AIDS treatment as prevention has been around for some time. Montaner of the British Columbia Center for Excellence on HIV/AIDS suggested that, by getting many of the small cohort of HIV-infected people on treatment in his province, HIV transmission would be greatly reduced (Montaner *et al.* 2006). He further argued, albeit on the basis of very poor data, that this was cost effective. The publication of a model by Ruben Granich and others in 2009 (Granich *et al.* 2009) suggested that if people were tested regularly and those infected were immediately put on therapy, this would, over time, eliminate HIV transmission. This was a mathematical model. Nonetheless there was a great deal of interest in operationalizing it. Swiss authorities released guidance in which discordant couples, on anti-retroviral therapy, were advised they had no need for other prevention techniques. Most recently a study, HPTN-052, showed that there were 96 percent fewer HIV transmission events in couples who began treatment immediately, than in couples who started later.

There are a number of important questions that need to be raised before this is adopted as a gold standard policy, with the expectation that it will bring an end to the HIV epidemic. These are particularly important in resource-poor settings:

What is the meaning of immediately? Recent work shows a significant number of HIV transmissions take place in the early stages of a person being infected (Powers *et al.* 2011). A comment in the *Lancet* (Cohen and Corbett 2011) notes: "if individuals within the first 6 months of their HIV infection are indeed responsible for a high proportion of all transmission events, a substantial proportion needs to be rapidly identified and treated during this stage to have any prospect of the large decreases in HIV prevalence." This adds to logistical challenges and costs, especially since HIV is still stigmatizing. It also means that the idea of a limited period of population-wide safe sex could work, in conjunction with treatment (Parkhurst and Whiteside 2010).

What will the costs be? The early detection needs more expensive kits. People will be on treatment for longer, adding to the price of therapy. Cost benefit analysis from the treatment papers of *RethinkHIV* may be of value in addressing these questions.

What are the population effects? Will this accelerate the emergence of antiviral resistance?

What are the individual effects? Will there be risk compensation (more risky sexual behav-

iors when an individual feels protected)? Does it make sense for an individual to go on early treatment in resource-constrained environments where, should they develop resistance and side-effects, they have a shorter period of access to ART, and earlier death?

Information campaigns and mass media

This is the third and weakest part of the proposal. There are numerous such programs, but trying to evaluate them is extremely difficult and there are no RCTs or robust cost analyses. Two examples spring to mind: LoveLife and Swaziland's *Makhwapheni* Campaign, both from hyperendemic Southern Africa.

LoveLife was a campaign in South Africa supported primarily by the Kaiser Family Foundation.[2] Millions of dollars were mobilized in support of its programs from 1999. I, along with many other South Africans, found the messaging impenetrable. The most visible were billboards that left us confused. One giant lime-green billboard featured the words, "Score" and "Red Card," with corresponding check boxes beside them. Other posters featured cryptic word pairs: "Your Body/Anybody," "Climax/Anticlimax," or "Drop Dead Gorgeous/ The Drop."

There was an evaluation planned. It began successfully, but as the research began to suggest that this program was not having the impact claimed, the two researchers found their work blocked. So with regard to the biggest IC campaign we have no clear data on its impact (Halperin and Williams 2001).

In Swaziland a bold initiative was instigated, the *Makhwapheni* Campaign. Literally this means something "hidden in the armpit," but in Swaziland it was known to mean "secret lover." It was bold and explicit. In Swaziland most people have cellphones and they were at the center of the campaign. This began in July 2006 and lasted just a few weeks. It was based on billboards showing the screen of a cellphone with invitations in cellphone talk. One said, "i'm all alone. cum 4 a quicky." Another said, "she's working late, cum work on me." Beside these

---

[2] See www.lovelife.org.za/.

invitations were strong punch lines, in siSwati. One example, "why kill your family?"; another, "and more orphans were left behind." The slogan for the entire campaign was "*makhwapheni uyabulala*": "your secret lover can kill you."

The campaign got the country talking, but it resulted in a backlash from some AIDS activists. They felt they were singled out, accused of spreading HIV and being stigmatized. Others read it as focusing on women's sexuality. There were demonstrations, the billboards came down, and one of the most successful campaigns (at least in terms of getting people to talk) ended.

On the basis of available evidence, IC campaigns cannot be evaluated. However, they are important, and to understand this we should look at the Schwartländer *et al.* (2011) paper. Many interventions fall into the category of critical enablers. Necessary but not sufficient!

What is missing and what might come in the future

The assessment paper identifies the interventions for which there is cost and benefit information. We are left asking, with Behrman and Kohler, is that all? Microbicides are not available, but may be important in the future. Condoms seem not to be evaluated. It would, on the basis of this work, seem that resource allocation decisions are not being made on good data and analysis.

One wild idea is to explore the concept of a "sexual abstinence month" to reduce HIV incidence, a behavioral intervention where a population-wide "safe sex/no sex" effort for a set period of time could make a significant contribution to global prevention efforts. This is based on the idea that people have higher viral loads immediately after they are infected, and if they could avoid infecting others then the population viral load and infectivity would be reduced. This idea is a hypothesis which requires further exploration and testing. A month of "safe sex/no sex" would produce easily verifiable data with regards to adherence, evidenced in the number of births occurring nine months after the campaign (Parkhurst and Whiteside 2010).

What policy recommendations can come out of this work?

The Copenhagen Consensus Center is known for taking difficult issues and applying rigorous analysis to them. For those of us working in the field of AIDS, and especially coming from Southern Africa, where the epidemic is at its worst, this project offered the opportunity to grapple with critical issues. From an economic point of view it suggests where resources should be allocated. At this stage I have to say it does not yet provide the answers.

On the basis of the paper I have critiqued, male circumcision takes priority, but note that this is something available only for young men, while the worst epidemic is located among women. If we do succeed in circumcising enough young men, it will make a difference to the epidemic, but not for years to come. Beyond circumcision the answers remain unclear. It may be that the investment framework put forward by Schwartländer *et al.* (2011) needs to be looked at in conjunction with this process. Ultimately it may also be that it is only through equitable development that is gender sensitive, or through restrictive regimes and religions, that we can hope to bring the epidemic under control. This is all rather depressing.

References

Barnett, T. and Whiteside, A. (2006). *AIDS in the Twenty-first Century: Disease and Globalization*, 2nd edn. Basingstoke: Palgrave.

Behrman, J. R. and Kohler, H.-P. (2011). RethinkHIV: assessment paper on the prevention of sexual transmission of HIV.

Campbell Collaboration. (2011). www. campbellcollaboration.org/about_us/index.php.

Casale, M., Dawad, S., Flicker, S., Hynie, M., Jenney, A., Jobson, G., Nixon, S., O'Brien, K., Rogan, M., Rubincam, C., Cele, P., Magadlela, O., Mhlongo, W., Phakathi, P., Radebe, S. and Zwane, T. (2010). They made us who we are today: a retrospective evaluation of the 1st 5-year cohort of the iThembaLethu HIV Prevention Programme (2002–2006). Final evaluation report available on the HEARD website at: www.heard.org.za/heard-resources/2010#reports.

Chazan, M., Brklacich, M. and Whiteside, A. (2009). Rethinking the conceptual terrain of AIDS scholarship: lessons from comparing 27 years of AIDS and climate change research. *Globalization and Health* **5**: 12. doi:10.1186/1744-8603-5-12.

Cohen, T. and Corbett, E. L. (2011). Test and treat in HIV: success could depend on rapid detection. *The Lancet* **378**(9787): 204–6. doi:S0140-6736(11)60896-9.

Dupas, P. (2011). Do teenagers respond to HIV risk information? Evidence from a field experiment in Kenya. *American Economic Journal: Applied Economics* **3**(34): 1–34. doi:10.1257/app.3.1.1.

Fox, M. (2010). AIDS gel with Gilead drug protects women in study. 19 July. Reuters. www.reuters.com/article/2010/07/19/aids-gel-idUSN1920562920100719, retrieved March 28, 2011.

Granich, R. M., Gilks, C. F., Dye, C., De Cock, K. M. and Williams, B. G. (2009). Universal voluntary HIV testing with immediate antiretroviral therapy as a strategy for elimination of HIV transmission: a mathematical model. *The Lancet* **373**: 48–57.

Grosskurth, H., Gray, R., Hayes, R., Mabey, D. and Wawer, M. (2000). Control of sexually transmitted diseases for HIV-1 prevention: understanding the implications of the Mwanza and Rakai trials. *The Lancet* **355**(9219): 1981–7.

Halperin, D. and Williams, B. (2001). This is no way to fight AIDS in Africa. *Washington Post*, August 26.

Hitchcock, P. and Fransen, L. (1999). Preventing HIV infection: lessons from Mwanza and Rakai. *The Lancet*, **353**(9152): 513–15.

Kagan, J. (2009). *The Three Cultures: Natural Sciences, Social Sciences and the Humanities in the 21st Century*. New York: Cambridge University Press.

Mbadi, N. and CAPRISA. (2010). Study of microbicide gel shows reduced risk of HIV and herpes infections in women, 2011. www.caprisa.org/joomla/Micro/CAPRISA%20004%20Press%20Release%20for%2020%20July%202010, retrieved January 23, 2011.

Montaner, J. S. G., Hogg, R., Wood, E., Kerr, T., Tyndall, M., Levy, A. R. and Harrigan, R. (2006). The case for expanding access to highly active antiretroviral therapy to curb the growth of the HIV epidemic. *The Lancet* August 5; **368**: 531–6.

Ng, B. E., Butler, L. M., Horvath, T. and Rutherford, G. W. (2011). Population-based biomedical sexually transmitted infection control interventions for reducing HIV infection. *Cochrane Database of Systematic Reviews 2011*, Issue 3. Art. No.: CD001220. DOI: 10.1002/14651858.CD001220.pub3.

Nixon, S., Flicker, S., Hynie, M., Casale, M., Rogan, M., Rubincam, C., O'Brien, K. and Jenney, A. (2009). Destiny, disease and desire: unpacking the results of a school-faith-based HIV intervention. Fourth Southern African AIDS Conference, March 31 to April 3, 2009.

Padian, N. S., McCoy, S. I., Balkus, J. E. and Wasserheit, J. N. (2010). Weighing the gold in the gold standard: challenges in HIV prevention research. *AIDS* **24**(5): 621–35. doi:10.1097/QAD.0b013e328337798a.

Parkhurst, J. O. and Whiteside, A. (2010). Innovative responses for preventing HIV transmission: the protective value of population-wide interruptions of risk activity. *South African Journal of HIV Medicine* **3**, April.

Powers, K. A., Ghani, A. C., Miller, W. C., Hoffman, I. F., Pettifor, A. E., Kamanga, G., Martinson, F. E. and Cohen, M. S. (2011). The role of acute and early HIV infection in the spread of HIV and implications for transmission prevention strategies in Lilongwe, Malawi: a modelling study. *The Lancet* **378**(9787): 256–68. doi:10.1016/S0140-6736(11)60842-8.

Ross, D. A. (2010). Behavioral interventions to reduce HIV risk: what works? *AIDS* **24**(Supplement 4): S4–S14. doi:10.1097/01.aids.0000390703.35642.89.

Schwartländer, B., Stover, J., Hallett, T., Atun, R., Avila, C., Gouws, E., Bartos, M., Ghys, P. D., Opuni, M., Barr, D., Alsallaq, R., Bollinger, L., de Freitas, M., Garnett, G., Holmes, C., Legins, K., Pillay, Y., Stanciole, A. E., McClure, C., Hirnschall, G., Laga, M. and Padian, N. (2011). Towards an improved investment approach for an effective response to HIV/AIDS. *The Lancet* –. doi:10.1016/S0140-6736(11)60702-2. Published online June 3.

Smith, J. and Whiteside, A. (2010). The history of AIDS exceptionalism. *Journal of the International AIDS Society* **13**: 47.

Stein, Z. A. (1990). HIV prevention: the need for methods women can use. *American Journal of Public Health* **80**(4): 460–2.

UNAIDS. (2011a). Modelling the expected distribution of new HIV infections by exposure group. Slide presentation from UNAIDS, accessed July 11, 2011 at www.unaids.org/en/media/unaids/contentassets/restore/mot_gen_2007_pres_en.pdf.

UNAIDS. (2011b). Know your epidemic and modes of transmission. www.unaidsrstesa.org/thematic-areas/hiv-prevention/know-your-epidemic-modes-transmission, accessed July 11, 2011.

Wikipedia. (2011). http://en.wikipedia.org/wiki/Systematic_review#Cochrane_Collaboration, accessed August 31, 2011.

Wiysonge, C. S., Kongnyuy, E. J., Shey, M., Muula, A. S., Navti, O. B., Akl, E. A. and Lo, Y. R. (2011). Male circumcision for prevention of homosexual acquisition of HIV in men. *Cochrane Database of Systematic Reviews*, Issue **6**.

Prevention of non-sexual transmission of HIV

LORI A. BOLLINGER

Although much progress against the HIV/AIDS epidemic has been made, the level of new HIV infections remains substantial, and the majority of these new infections continue to occur in sub-Saharan Africa. In 2009, an estimated 2.6 million new HIV infections were recorded worldwide, with nearly 70 percent of these occurring in sub-Saharan Africa. The pace of the epidemic in sub-Saharan Africa has slowed, however: between 2001 and 2009, the number of new infections in sub-Saharan Africa decreased from 2.2 million to 1.8 million. The recent Political Declaration on HIV/AIDS adopted by the United Nations program on AIDS (UNAIDS) General Assembly on 10 June 2011 renewed member countries' commitment to avert new HIV infections through focused prevention efforts, including eliminating HIV infections transmitted vertically, and to increase the number of people on anti-retroviral therapy to 15 million by 2015 (UNAIDS 2011).

The continued need for both prevention and treatment funding for HIV/AIDS is combined with stagnant or even diminishing financial resources. Although funding has increased substantially in the last decade, spending remained approximately the same between 2008 and 2009, only increasing from $15.6 billion to $15.9 billion. Because the funding need increased over that year, the funding gap increased from $7.7 billion in 2008 to $10 billion in 2009 (UNAIDS 2010). The question asked by *RethinkHIV* is thus particularly relevant at this juncture: how can an additional $10 billion be spent over the next five years to fight HIV/AIDS in sub-Saharan Africa?

A recent series of studies modeling the modes of transmission for five Eastern and Southern Africa countries estimated that the majority of new HIV infections are transmitted via sexual behavior. The studies found, however, that some new infections did occur via non-sexual transmission, including unsafe medical injections, unsafe blood transfusions, and needle-sharing behavior among injecting drug users (IDUs) (UNAIDS 2009; see Figure 2.1).

The average percentage of new HIV infections (excluding those transmitted vertically) from unsafe medical injections was 1 percent across the five countries summarized in the study, ranging from 0.2 percent in Swaziland to 2.21 percent in Kenya. The average percentage due to blood transfusions was even lower, at 0.16 percent, ranging from zero percent in Lesotho and Uganda to 0.4 percent in Swaziland. Finally, the average percentage of new HIV infections that was attributed to IDU needle-sharing behavior averaged 1.8 percent for the five countries, ranging from zero percent in Lesotho to almost 4 percent in Kenya. Note that, although these modes of transmission modeling studies did not examine the proportion of new infections due to vertical transmission, a significant number of new infections do continue to occur via transmission from mother to child throughout sub-Saharan Africa; approximately 350,000 new HIV infections occurred in children due to vertical transmission in 2008, or 18 percent of the total number of new HIV infections that occurred in sub-Saharan Africa in 2008 (UNAIDS 2010).

For most HIV infections caused by non-sexual transmission there are proven cost-effective solutions to reduce and virtually eliminate transmission of new infections. Transmission of HIV through unsafe medical injections can be eliminated through the use of automatic disposable syringes, a relatively inexpensive intervention, along with appropriate waste disposal methods. Screening blood that is to be used in blood transfusions for HIV has been shown to be extremely cost-effective in a wide variety of settings. Preventing mother-to-child transmission of HIV by

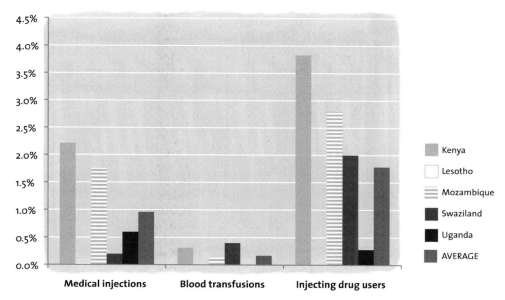

Figure 2.1 *HIV transmission by selected modes in five sub-Saharan African countries*

providing anti-retroviral drugs to both mother and child is also a cost-effective intervention, even when continued throughout the breastfeeding period in order to reduce transmission via breastfeeding. Finally, some interventions preventing transmission through needle-sharing behavior among injecting drug users may be cost-effective, such as outreach programs including information and education campaigns, as well as needle and syringe exchange programs, although other programs such as opioid substitution therapy (OST) may not be cost-effective.

This paper will examine the cost-effectiveness of each of these proposed solutions for sub-Saharan Africa, using a variety of models across all of the relevant countries, described in the Methodology section below.

Methodology

The purpose of economic evaluation is to assist policy-makers in making decisions among various program alternatives. Several different approaches can be taken: cost-effectiveness analysis, which evaluates the cost of an intervention relative to a nonmonetary outcome, such as number of cases averted for a particular disease or number of life years saved; cost-utility analysis, which evaluates the cost of an intervention relative to an outcome expressed in utility terms, such as quality-adjusted life years (QALYs); or benefit-cost analysis, which evaluates the cost of an intervention relative to a monetized outcome, calculated as the monetary benefits that accrue from implementing the intervention. In this paper, both cost-effectiveness and benefit-cost analyses are performed for the four sets of interventions described above.

Within HIV/AIDS, the cost-effectiveness of prevention interventions is analyzed by examining the incremental cost of averting one HIV infection. Two different sets of assumptions must be made in order to perform this analysis: the incremental costs associated with implementing the prevention intervention, and the number of HIV infections averted, usually derived from modeling exercises. The incremental cost effectiveness ratio (ICER) can then be calculated by dividing the incremental cost associated with the intervention by the number of DALYs saved through implementing the intervention, following recent literature in multiplying HIV infections averted by 20 for adults and 25 for children to calculate DALYs (Bertozzi *et al.* 2006; Murray *et al.* 1996). The incremental costs are calculated by multiplying a unit cost specific to the intervention and country by the increase in the number of people reached by the intervention. Using the standardized definitions developed by the Commission on Macroeconomics and Health and utilized by the World Health Organization (WHO) CHOICE (CHOosing Interventions that are Cost-Effective) network, we define an intervention as highly cost-effective if the ICER is less than the country's annual gross national income (GNI) per capita, cost-effective if the ICER is between one and three times the country's annual GNI per capita, and not cost-effective if the ICER is greater than three times the country's annual GNI per capita (Commission on Macroeconomics and Health 2001; WHO 2011). Note that the GNI per capita using the Atlas method across sub-Saharan Africa in 2009 was $1,125, while the GNI per capita adjusted for purchasing power parity in sub-Saharan Africa in 2009 was $2,051 (World Bank 2011).

Details of specific costs, coverage rates, and target populations are described for each of the four sets of interventions in their specific sections below. The general methodology used in modeling HIV infections averted is described further below.

Calculating benefits

In order to calculate the benefit to cost ratio (B/C ratio), an additional set of assumptions must be made regarding the benefits associated with averting one HIV infection. In this paper, following guidelines provided by *RethinkHIV*, benefits are assumed to be the sum of the treatment savings associated with an averted HIV infection, as well as the value of the number of lives saved with the valuation performed at two different levels: $1,000 per life year gained, and $5,000 per life year gained.

The savings that accrue because an HIV infection does not have to be treated consist of two parts: the lifetime discounted cost of providing someone with anti-retroviral therapy (ART), including assumptions about the costs of ART, survival on ART, as well as the appropriate discount rate, and the lifetime discounted cost of treating opportunistic infections, again with assumptions about costs

and discount rates. Following the recommendation of *RethinkHIV*, in order to ensure consistency of results across papers, we assume that the cost of ART is either $500 or $1,000 per year for twenty years, with the discount rate varying between 3 percent and 5 percent. The ART cost consists of all costs associated with delivering ART, including the cost of anti-retroviral drugs, laboratory monitoring tests, and service delivery costs.

Note that the assumption of a twenty-year time horizon for providing ART assumes that the continuation rate is 97 percent throughout the duration of treatment. This twenty-year time horizon aligns with recent findings from a cohort study in Uganda that found an average life expectancy of between 26.7 and 27.9 years for over 22,315 ART patients (Mills *et al.* 2011). This study assumes a 30 percent mortality rate for those lost to follow-up, a rate which was found to be 6.4 percent of the total patient population. Note that another study finds a slightly higher mortality rate of 47 percent to those lost to follow-up (Mahy *et al.* 2010); applying this higher mortality rate to the Uganda data would result in a decrease of the overall life expectancy calculated in the Uganda study, aligning it even more closely with the life expectancy of twenty years assumed here.

In addition to the benefits that accrue from savings associated with not providing ART because of the averted HIV infection, savings are realized because opportunistic infections (OIs) do not have to be treated, either. Here, we assume that one averted HIV infection results in three years of savings regarding OIs, with the first year occurring at the beginning of the time of infection, and the second and third years occurring at the end of life discounted appropriately. The OI savings consist of two parts: the drug and laboratory test costs used in treating opportunistic infections, and the associated service delivery cost. Because different opportunistic infections occur with varying frequency across patients and countries, we use a cost of $47.94 for drugs and laboratory tests, which is calculated from the annual median cost for drugs and laboratory tests across four recent studies in sub-Saharan Africa: Cote d'Ivoire (Goldie *et al.* 2006); Rwanda (Vinard *et al.* 2005); Uganda (Chandler and Musau 2005); and Zambia (Kombe *et al.* 2003). This unit

Table 2.1 Value of lifetime discounted ART and opportunistic infection treatment, $

Treatment cost per year	Discount rate of 3%	Discount rate of 5%
ART: 500 per year	7,052	6,044
ART: 1,000 per year	14,068	12,056
Opportunistic infections	424	355

cost for drugs and laboratory tests is combined with the cost of delivering the treatment, which in turn consists of two parts. The first part is the cost of treating opportunistic infections in the hospital, and is calculated as the product of the annual median number of inpatient days for patients being treated for opportunistic infections, calculated from the same literature cited above, and an average cost for sub-Saharan Africa for one bed day at a primary-level hospital, available from the WHO-CHOICE database for sub-Saharan Africa (WHO 2011). The second part of the service delivery cost for OIs is the cost of treating opportunistic infections in a health center setting, and is calculated as the annual median number of outpatient visits for patients being treated for opportunistic infections, calculated using the literature cited above, and an average cost for sub-Saharan Africa per twenty-minute outpatient visit at a health center, at the mid-range of capacity utilization, again from the WHO-CHOICE database for sub-Saharan Africa. Overall, the service delivery portion of the unit cost for treating opportunistic infections equals $145.48, which implies a total annual cost saving of $193.42 due to each averted HIV infection.

Combining all of the assumptions above results in the lifetime discounted value of ART varying from $6,044 to $14,068, depending on both the assumption of ART cost per year and the discount rate, while the lifetime discounted cost of treating opportunistic infections varies between $355 and $424, depending on the discount rate (see Table 2.1). Note, however, that not all people who became infected with HIV would have received ART, as coverage is less than 100 percent in sub-Saharan Africa; thus we apply the 2009 estimated ART coverage for sub-Saharan Africa of 37 percent to calculate the averted ART costs associated with one HIV infection averted. We assume, however,

that all HIV-infected people would receive treatment for opportunistic infections.

In addition to the benefits that accrue from an averted HIV infection because of the averted treatment costs, both for anti-retroviral therapy and for opportunistic infections, *RethinkHIV* requested that the value of life years gained be included in the calculation of benefits associated with an averted HIV infection, valuing each life year gained at both $1,000 and $5,000, discounted at both 3 percent and 5 percent. We assume further that the 63 percent of HIV-infected people not receiving ART survive on average an additional eleven years, and that ART provision begins on average seven years after someone becomes infected. We assume an average life expectancy for sub-Saharan Africa of sixty-five years for adults (United Nations 2011), while further assumptions are made below regarding the age at which an adult infection is averted for each of the sets of interventions.

The exception to this is the set of assumptions regarding the age at which an infection is averted for interventions preventing mother-to-child transmission (pMTCT), as these interventions avert infant HIV infections. First, we assume that the 72 percent of HIV-infected children not receiving ART survive on average five years, and that children begin receiving ART at age one year. Second, we assume a life expectancy at birth of 52.5 years (United Nations 2011). Finally, note that some controversy surrounds the valuation of an infant's life; some economists argue that high rates of infant and child mortality in developing countries imply that the value of an infant's life that is saved should not receive full weight for every year of life expectancy (Jamison 2010). Because this assumption is crucial here in the evaluation of the benefits associated with pMTCT programs, we calculate the number of life years gained by an averted infant HIV infection in two ways: assuming that the averted infection receives the full credit of 52.5 years for life expectancy, and receiving half of the credit of life expectancy.

Combining all of these assumptions regarding the valuation of a saved life from averting one HIV infection results in benefits varying from about $4,900 to $91,000 (see Table 2.2). The values in this table will be used in calculating the benefits in

Table 2.2 Value of life saved, by age, value of life year, and discount rate ($000)

	Value of life year saved = $1,000, discounted 3%	Value of life year saved = $5,000, discounted 3%	Value of life year saved = $1,000, discounted 5%	Value of life year saved = $5,000, discounted 5%
Life saved as infant	$18.2	$91.0	$13.3	$66.3
Life-year of infant = 0.5 adult life-year	$9.1	$45.5	$6.6	$33.1
Life saved at 22	$11.4	$56.9	$6.9	$34.5
Life saved at 27	$8.5	$42.6	$4.9	$24.4

each of the sections below, along with the benefits associated with averted treatment costs.

Modeling HIV infections averted

Here, two different models are used to calculate the number of HIV infections averted due to implementing the four different sets of prevention interventions: the AIDS Impact Model in Spectrum is used to model the impact of pMTCT programs, and the Goals model along with a minor adaptation of it called Goals Express is used to estimate the impact of the other three prevention interventions. Each of the models is described in detail below.

AIDS Impact Model in Spectrum

Spectrum is a suite of easy-to-use policy models which provide policy-makers with an analytical tool to support the decision-making process. Spectrum consists of several software models, including a demographic projection module (DemProj), a module for family planning (FamPlan), the AIDS Impact Model which examines the demographic and social impact of the HIV/AIDS epidemic, the Goals module which examines the cost and impact of HIV interventions, the Lives Saved Tool (LiST), and the RAPID model (Resources for the Awareness of Population Impacts on Development), among others.

The AIDS Impact Model (AIM) projects the consequences of the HIV epidemic, including the number of people living with HIV, new infections for both adults and children, and AIDS deaths by age and sex, as well as the new cases of tuberculosis and AIDS orphans. AIM requires an input assumption about the past and future course of adult HIV

incidence, usually calculated by using the Estimation and Projection Package (EPP),[1] as well as assumptions about current programmatic statistics regarding treatment coverage of both ART and pMTCT programs. Note that both EPP and AIM are reviewed by the UNAIDS Reference Group on Estimates, Models and Projections, a group established to provide advice on estimating national HIV prevalence patterns.

After adult HIV incidence and treatment coverage are entered into the Spectrum/AIM model, assumptions about other HIV/AIDS characteristics can also be entered for variables such as the survival period from HIV infection to AIDS death, the age and sex distribution of new HIV infections, and the perinatal transmission rate. Before AIM can be used, a demographic projection must be prepared using DemProj, one of the Spectrum systems of policy models. The demographic projection is modified by AIM through AIDS deaths and the impact of HIV infection on fertility. The Epidemiology section of AIM calculates the number of HIV infections, AIDS cases, and AIDS deaths. This information is then used in the Treatment Costs section to calculate the costs of treatment for pMTCT, HIV/AIDS, and AIDS-associated tuberculosis and opportunistic infections; the Impacts section to calculate various indicators of demographic and social impact; and the Orphans section to calculate the number of orphans. The manuals associated with the various modules describe the underlying equations and assumptions for all of the components of each module.[2]

---

[1] Available at www.unaids.org/en/dataanalysis/tools/estimationandprojectionpackageepp/.
[2] Modules and manuals are available at http://futuresinstitute.org/.

AIM is used by UNAIDS in collaboration with their national partners to make the national and regional estimates it releases every two years (Stover *et al.* 2010). In this exercise, national HIV/AIDS programs collaborate with UNAIDS to estimate the HIV/AIDS incidence and prevalence in their country, including providing programmatic statistics on coverage of anti-retroviral therapy and programs preventing mother-to-child transmission (pMTCT). Default data files are available with the public release of Spectrum for all low- and middle-income developing countries; these files contain the approved national-level HIV estimates and programmatic statistics.

We use these default data files in the AIM module to calculate new HIV infections due to vertical transmission. The mother-to-child transmission rate is the percentage of babies born to HIV-infected mothers who will be infected themselves. Studies have found that this percentage varies substantially depending on whether anti-retrovirals (ARV) are used and whether breastfeeding occurs, ranging from a low level of transmission around 2 percent when women receive triple preventive therapy and do not breastfeed, to 35 percent or more when women receive no preventive ARV drugs and continue breastfeeding for more than 18 months. We describe further below in the pMTCT section the scenarios utilized in this analysis, including the treatment options selected with their associated HIV vertical transmission rates, costs assumed, and scale-up patterns utilized.

Goals model (and Goals Express)

The Goals model is intended to support strategic planning at the national level by providing a tool to link program goals and funding. The model has been used by many countries to assist in the national planning process (Forsythe *et al.* 2009).

The model can help answer several key questions in the fight against HIV/AIDS, including:

- Which goals can be achieved?
- How much funding is required to achieve these goals?
- How does funding allocation influence achieving strategic program goals?

The Goals model links budget line items to coverage of services, behavior change, and prevention of new infections. The model starts with budget line items. These are mapped to the major categories of prevention (e.g., voluntary counseling and testing (VCT), school-based programs, condom promotion), care and treatment (e.g., palliative care, treatment of opportunistic infections, provision of ART), and program operation (e.g., policy, advocacy, management). For each of the prevention, care, and support categories the model calculates coverage, that is, the percentage of the population in need of the service that is exposed to the information or utilizes the service, by dividing the budget amount by the target population. This calculation uses unit costs that are either based on local cost studies, if available, or on international experience.

Coverage of prevention activities is then linked to behavior change (see Figure 2.2). The model contains an impact matrix developed from almost 200 studies of prevention interventions (Bollinger 2008). This matrix describes how coverage of various prevention activities (such as VCT, school-based programs, and community mobilization) affects four key behaviors (condom use, number of partners, age at first sex, and sharing needles) among five risk groups (high-risk heterosexual, medium-risk heterosexual, low-risk heterosexual, men who have sex with men, and injecting drug users (IDUs)). In a typical application, high-risk refers to sex workers and their clients, medium-risk refers to men and women who have multiple partners, and low-risk refers to men and women who have a single partner. People who are in more than one risk group are classified according to their highest-risk group.

An HIV transmission model calculates how changes in sexual behavior reduce the number of new infections. The model also calculates the impact of needle-sharing on new infections in the IDU population. The results are displayed in terms of HIV prevalence or incidence among all adults (15–49) in the five risk groups. The model also calculates the incremental cost per infection averted.

The probability of infection is calculated using an equation implemented in the AVERT model (Weinstein *et al.* 1989; Bouey *et al.* 1998). This equation calculates the probability of infection as a function of HIV prevalence in the partner population, the

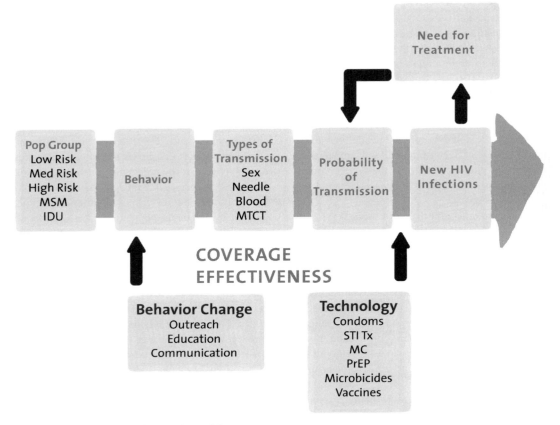

Figure 2.2 *Schematic of the Goals model*

transmissibility of HIV, the impact of a sexually transmitted infection on HIV transmissibility, the proportion of the population with sexually transmitted infections, condom use or needle-sharing use, number of partners per year, and number of sexual or needle-sharing contacts with each partner. The general equation is:

$$\text{ProbInf}_{r,s} = 1 - \left\{ p_p \sum_s w_s[1 - r_{gs}(1 - f_r e)]^{n_r} + (1 - p_{r,p}) \right\}^{m_r}$$

Where:

$\text{ProbInf}_{r,s}$ = probability of a person in the target population of risk group r becoming infected with HIV

p_p = HIV prevalence in the partner population

w_s = proportion of the target population in one of four possible states (has no sexually transmitted infection, has an ulcerative STI, has an inflammatory STI, has both an ulcerative and inflammatory STI)

r_{gs} = the transmissibility of HIV given STI state s and partner combination g, where g has three possible states (male to female, female to male, and male to male)

f_r = proportion of sexual contacts involving condom use/needle-sharing use

e = efficacy of condom use in preventing HIV transmission

n_r = number of sexual/injecting contacts per partner per year in risk group r

m_r = number of partners per year in risk group r

The prevention interventions are intended to reduce the transmission of new HIV infections. Except for safe blood and safe medical injections, all the prevention interventions operate by changing behaviors that are linked to HIV transmission. Four types of behavior are affected by the prevention interventions in the model:

- condom use;
- number of sexual partners;
- age at first sex;
- injecting drug user behavior.

Each prevention intervention can affect any or all of the four key behaviors. The effects may be different depending on the risk group. Thus a sex worker intervention may affect condom use and number of partners among high-risk women or men, but would not be expected to affect age at first sex or other behaviors among low-risk men or women. School-based interventions may affect age at first sex, condom use, and number of partners among the medium-risk population, but would not be expected to affect high-risk populations.

Several prevention interventions may affect the same behaviors in the same risk groups. Therefore, the impact of interventions on condom use is calculated as the percentage reduction in non-use. Impacts on the other behaviors are calculated as percentage reductions in the number of partners per year and reduction in percentage of IDU sharing needles, as well as percentage increases in age at first sex.

Goals Express adapts the general methodology of the fully articulated Goals model by utilizing the framework of the UNAIDS Modes of Transmission (MOT) model (UNAIDS 2007; Futures Institute 2011). Because the MOT model includes consideration of the two medical interventions examined here (safe medical injection, blood safety), while the full Goals model does not, we use a combination of the Goals Express and MOT models to model the number of infections averted by each of these two interventions. Basically, the same HIV transmission equation is used, but is adapted to the context of medical injections and blood transfusions and utilized in this transformed state in the MOT model, where:

- partner HIV prevalence is assumed to be the HIV prevalence rate for the general population, which varies by country;

- the number of partners is assumed to be one, as the analogous risk here is one syringe in the case of safe medical injections, and one unit of blood in the case of blood safety;
- the number of acts of exposure per year is the number of unsafe medical injections adults receive on average during a year and the probability that a blood transfusion is received;
- the percentage of acts protected is the coverage rate of those injections that occur following safe injection practices and the percentage of donated blood units that are tested for HIV, which varies by country.

Results

Safe medical injections

Unsafe injection practices exist throughout the developing world; research has found that up to 40 percent of injections across the developing world follow the practice of reusing syringes (Hutin *et al.* 2003). There are many reasons for these practices, among them a lack of awareness of the possible dangers in reusing syringes, a limited supply of syringes, and a lack of training of medical staff in safe disposal of medical waste. In addition, people tend to receive more injections per capita as part of standard medical treatment protocols, partly because of the belief that the injections are medically necessary, and partly because injection-based treatments sometimes receive higher fees (AIDSTAR-One 2011). One recent study in Uganda found that HIV prevalence was significantly higher among those people who received five or more medical injections in the previous year relative to those who did not receive a medical injection at all (Mishra *et al.* 2008).

A complete program to make medical injections safer has a number of different components (MMIS 2011):

- adequate supply of auto-disposable (AD) syringes;
- training for staff to utilize syringes;
- safe disposal of medical waste;
- information for the public regarding the program.

Although not all medical injections are unsafe for HIV transmission, as even those injections that

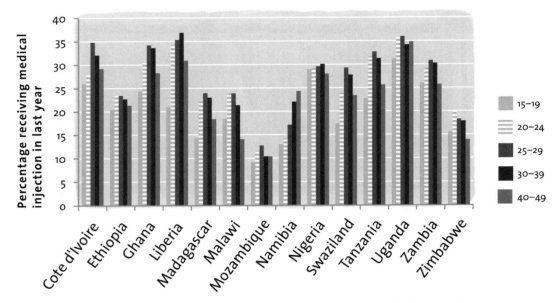

Figure 2.3 *Percentage of men and women receiving a medical injection in the last year, by age group, various demographic and health surveys*

reuse syringes must be contaminated with HIV in order to transmit the virus, *all* injections must be made safe in order to ensure safe medical injections. We calculate here the costs, the benefits, and the infections averted from making all medical injections safe, based on assumptions regarding target population, coverage rates for safe medical injections (both baseline and target coverage rates), unit costs, and the transmission probability for each of the sub-Saharan African countries. Note that in this paper we only examine implications for the HIV infections that would be averted; other infections would also be averted, such as hepatitis B and hepatitis C, the benefits of which are not calculated here.[3]

Target population

We begin by following the MOT model methodology in assuming that the adult population is the main source of new HIV infections occurring via unsafe medical injections. We assume that the HIV prevalence rate faced by uninfected adults is the general HIV prevalence rate for that population throughout the time period; the implicit assumption here is that the number of new HIV infections

resulting from any unsafe medical injections will be small enough that the general population HIV prevalence rate is not affected. We use the adult population and relevant HIV prevalence rate (ages fifteen and above) from the most recent publicly available Spectrum demographic projection files, which use projections from the United Nations Population Division, for the forty-four sub-Saharan countries listed in Appendix A. In addition, we follow assumptions used in calculating previous Global Burden of Disease statistics that adults in sub-Saharan Africa receive an average of 2.1 injections per year, and that 18 percent of those injections are unsafe (Hauri *et al.* 2004).

In order to ascertain the average age to use to calculate the value of life years gained with an HIV infection averted through safe medical injections, we examined the frequency of medical injections by

[3] The benefits would be extremely small, as the protocol for hepatitis B exposure is to receive the vaccination for hepatitis B, which the person may already have had, while no prophylaxis at all is recommended for hepatitis C exposure (Centers for Disease Control 2001). Note that the cost for a single vial dose of the hepatitis B vaccine is $0.40 (UNICEF 2011).

age group for several sub-Saharan African Demographic and Health Surveys. Figure 2.3 shows that the highest frequency of injections generally occurs in the age group 25–29; hence an average age of 27 is used here in order to calculate the number of life years gained.

Coverage

Where available, we use initial baseline coverage rates for safe medical injections from country-level workbooks developed by national teams in a series of workshops sponsored by UNAIDS. These workshops estimated the resources required to address the HIV/AIDS epidemic in their country, and contain country-validated data for a large number of interventions (Stover and Forsythe 2010). Where no country-level workbook exists, we use a regional median calculated based on these data, which in this case is about 5 percent. We assume that coverage levels reach 95 percent of all those receiving a medical injection with an AD syringe and appropriate waste disposal by 2015, using a linear scale-up pattern.

Unit cost

The cost of each of the four different prevention interventions varies both by intervention and by country, except in the case of safe medical injections. For safe medical injections, we use two different assumptions regarding unit cost. First, we assume that the incremental cost of using an AD syringe is equal to the international price achieved by UNICEF in their immunization programs, based on the assumption that sub-Saharan Africa would be able to achieve this same low price, and that there are no non-traded goods or services associated with the intervention. The incremental cost of an AD syringe used here for all countries is the difference between the UNICEF price for a regular syringe ($0.04) and the UNICEF price for an AD syringe ($0.06), or $0.02 (UNICEF 2009 and 2010a). In addition, we include costs for training, waste disposal, and public education programs related to safe medical injections. One recent estimate calculated the cost for these three components to be less than $0.01 per injection (WHO SIGN 2007). Adding this to the unit cost of an AD syringe would result

in a total unit cost per injection of $0.03, or total annual cost per person of $0.062.

We vary this unit cost assumption by utilizing data from a South African intervention which reported a cost of $0.036 for the AD syringe and a disposal cost of $0.024, for a total cost per injection of $0.06 (PATH 2007), which is double the first unit cost. Note that these unit costs are for AD syringes; the cost of retractable syringes is significantly higher.

Transmission probability

We follow the methodology in the MOT and Goals Express models in using an HIV transmission probability of 0.45 percent per injection, which is calculated as the average of the HIV transmission risk for accidental needle sticks of 0.24 percent and the risk of HIV transmission in IDU needle-sharing behavior of 0.65 percent (Lopman *et al.* 2006).

Based on the above assumptions, the modeling exercise indicates that a total of approximately 68,000 HIV infections could be averted across sub-Saharan Africa between 2011 and 2015 as a result of making 95 percent of all medical injections safe. Assuming a 3 percent discount rate and a unit cost of $0.03 per injection, the ICER for safe medical injections across sub-Saharan Africa is $136, which is significantly lower than the PPP-adjusted GNI per capita value of $2,051 for sub-Saharan Africa, making this a highly cost-effective intervention.

We then proceed to calculate the benefits associated with implementing this intervention. Table 2.3 presents eight different scenarios, which vary depending on the values for the three different sets of parameters requested by *RethinkHIV* regarding calculating benefits, that is, the discount rate, the value of life year saved, and the annual cost of ART. These scenarios are:

Scenario I: Discount rate of 3 percent, value of one life year saved equal to $1,000, annual cost of ART $500.

Scenario II: Discount rate of 5 percent, value of one life year saved equal to $1,000, annual cost of ART $500.

Scenario III: Discount rate of 3 percent, value of one life year saved equal to $5,000, annual cost of ART $500.

Table 2.3 Benefits associated with safe medical injections by discount rate, value of life year gained, and ART cost ($ million)

	Scenario I (3%, $1,000, $500)	Scenario II (5%, $1,000, $500)	Scenario III (3%, $5,000, $500)	Scenario IV (5%, $5,000, $500)	Scenario V (3%, $1,000, $1,000)	Scenario VI (5%, $1,000, $1,000)	Scenario VII (3%, $5,000, $1,000)	Scenario VIII (5%, $5,000, $1,000)
Years of life gained (undiscounted)	1.4							
Value of years gained	$581	$332	$2,907	$1,661	$581	$332	$2,907	$1,661
OI treatment costs averted	$29	$24	$29	$24	$29	$24	$29	$24
ARV treatment costs averted	$178	$153	$178	$153	$355	$304	$355	$304
Total	$788	$509	$3,114	$1,838	$965	$661	$3,291	$1,989

Scenario IV: Discount rate of 5 percent, value of one life year saved equal to $5,000, annual cost of ART $500.

Scenario V: Discount rate of 3 percent, value of one life year saved equal to $1,000, annual cost of ART $1,000.

Scenario VI: Discount rate of 5 percent, value of one life year saved equal to $1,000, annual cost of ART $1,000.

Scenario VII: Discount rate of 3 percent, value of one life year saved equal to $5,000, annual cost of ART $1,000.

Scenario VIII: Discount rate of 5 percent, value of one life year saved equal to $5,000, annual cost of ART $1,000.

Assuming that the average age of an averted HIV infection for safe medical injections is twenty-seven, the number of HIV infections averted translates into 2.6 million life years gained (undiscounted – see Table 2.3).

To give an initial example of calculating the value of life years gained, we examine Scenario I, assuming that the discount rate is 3 percent, the value of each life year gained is $1,000, and the annual cost of ART is $500. We then calculate the value of life years gained by multiplying the number of HIV infections averted (about 68,000) by the value of a life saved at age twenty-seven (about $8,500 – see Table 2.2). The OI treatment costs averted are calculated by multiplying the number of HIV infections averted by the discounted lifetime cost of

treating OIs, discounted at 3 percent ($424 – see Table 2.1). Finally, we calculate the averted ARV treatment costs by multiplying the number of HIV infections averted assuming that the annual cost of delivering ART is $500 and the discount rate is 3 percent ($7,052 – see Table 2.1), and then multiplying this by the ART coverage rate of 37 percent. The three components are then summed, to reach the total benefits associated with Scenario I.

If a value of $1,000 per life year gained is assumed, the table indicates that the value of the total number of life years gained varies between $332 million and $581 million, depending on whether a 3 percent or a 5 percent discount rate is used. If the value of each life year gained is increased to $5,000 instead of $1,000, the value of the total number of life years gained also increases, varying from $1.7 billion to $2.9 billion, again depending on the discount rate used.

The first two scenarios in Table 2.3 display the results for averted costs relative to treating opportunistic infections (OI) that vary depending on whether a 5 percent discount rate or 3 percent discount rate is assumed, varying between $24 million and $29 million, respectively. Since the only parameter that varies with respect to treating OIs is the discount rate, these two results are repeated three times across the columns of the results table.

Scenarios I and II also display the results of the ARV treatment costs that are averted, assuming that the cost of providing ART is $500 per year for twenty years, discounted by 3 and 5 percent

Table 2.4 Benefit/cost ratios for safe medical injections by value of life year gained, discount rate, costs of ART, and unit cost of injection ($ million)

Value of life year	Discount rate	Benefits		Costs		B/C ratio (A)/(A)	B/C ratio (A)/(B)	B/C ratio (B)/(A)	B/C ratio (B)/(B)
		$500 ART (A)	$1,000 ART (B)	$0.03 (A)	$0.06 (B)				
$1,000	3%	$788	$965	$166	$333	4.7	2.4	5.8	2.9
$1,000	5%	$509	$661	$155	$311	3.3	1.6	4.3	2.1
$5,000	3%	$3,114	$3,291	$166	$333	18.7	9.4	19.8	9.9
$5,000	5%	$1,838	$1,989	$155	$311	11.8	5.9	12.8	6.4

respectively. In the first scenario, $178 million is saved in averted ART costs by scaling up safe medical injections to cover 95 percent of the population in sub-Saharan Africa. In the second scenario, where a 5 percent discount rate is used instead of a 3 percent discount rate, the total ART costs averted amount to over $150 million. When the cost of providing ART is assumed to increase to $1,000 per year for twenty years, using a discount rate of 3 percent results in total savings associated with averted ARV treatment costs of approximately $304 million (see Scenarios V and VII). Using a discount rate of 5 percent results in a slight decrease in these overall ARV treatment cost savings, reducing the total amount saved to slightly less than $355 million (see Scenarios VI and VIII).

When all three components of the benefits associated with averting an HIV infection through a safe medical injection are summed, the total amount saved varies from a low of $509 million, which results from assuming a 5 percent discount rate, a value per life year gained of $1,000, and an annual cost of $500 to deliver ART, to a high of $3.3 billion, which results from assuming a 3 percent discount rate, a value per life year gained of $5,000, and an annual cost of $1,000 to deliver ART. Thus the savings associated with scaling up safe medical injections to cover 95 percent of all injections delivered in sub-Saharan Africa by 2015 will result in substantial savings.

Once the benefits of this intervention are calculated and aggregated, we can compare the total sum of benefits with the associated costs by calculating the various benefit-cost (B/C) ratios associated with the eight different scenarios. We add one more parameter to the mix in calculating the

various B/C ratios by varying the unit costs associated with performing a safe medical injection, in order to provide a range of estimates. We double the cost here in order to provide an upper bound on the possible costs associated with the intervention, which then becomes a lower bound on the B/C ratio (see Table 2.4).

We present four different sets of B/C ratios, which are based on different combinations of benefits associated with a $500 annual cost of ART (Benefits (A)) and benefits associated with a $1,000 annual cost of ART (Benefits (B)), as well as with costs associated with a unit cost of $0.03 per injection (Costs (A)) and costs associated with a unit cost of $0.06 per injection (Costs (B)). The scenarios for parameters that vary for the benefits calculated, described in detail in Table 2.3 opposite, are displayed in the rows of Table 2.4 above, with the value per life year gained varying between $1,000 and $5,000 and the value of the discount rate varying between 3 and 5 percent.

Results shown in the table indicate that the B/C ratio for covering 95 percent of all medical injections safely in sub-Saharan Africa by 2015 varies from a low of 1.6, that is $1.60 of benefits are gained for every dollar of expenditure, to a high value of 19.8, that is $19.80 of benefits are gained for every dollar expended. The lowest B/C ratio is attained when the value of a life year is $1,000, ART costs are only $500 per year, the cost per AD syringe used is $0.06, and the discount rate is 5 percent. The highest B/C ratio calculated is based on a value per life year gained of $5,000, ART costs of $1,000 per year, the lower cost per AD syringe of $0.03, and a discount rate of 3 percent. In all cases, providing safe medical injections results in B/C ratios significantly greater than one, the break-even point.

Safe blood transfusions

Due to the presence of anemia and other factors, blood transfusions are more common in sub-Saharan Africa than in developed countries. Studies have found that up to 70 percent of all admitted hospital patients are anemic, a condition that can be caused either by poor nutrition (i.e., a lack of iron in the diet) or by infection with malaria, particularly in the case of pregnant women (Soares and Clements 2011; Kasili 1990). Safe blood transfusions are reported to exist in sub-Saharan Africa, although rigorous quality control standards are still lacking to some degree (Harries *et al.* 2010). South Africa in particular has had success in providing safe blood transfusions; by 2008, the South African government reported that since the introduction of nucleic acid amplification testing (NAT) for HIV in 2005, no HIV transmission had been linked to blood transfusions in the country (Flanagan 2008).

Testing donated blood for possible contamination with HIV in a quality-assured manner is one of the required indicators for country-level reporting for UNGASS. Many of the countries report that 100 percent of their blood supply meets this requirement, while there are still some countries reporting less than 100 percent coverage of their blood supply (UNAIDS 2010, Annex 2). While some sub-Saharan African countries with less than universal coverage report rates close to 100 percent (Benin, Togo), other countries report rates substantially lower (Angola, Niger, United Republic of Tanzania) (see Figure 2.4). We calculate below the costs and benefits of increasing coverage so that all sub-Saharan African countries have 100 percent coverage rates of blood tested in a quality-assured manner by 2015.

Target population

We assume that anybody in the general population may require a blood transfusion throughout the year, with one central blood supply used for both adults and children. We calculate the number of blood units required using the information reported

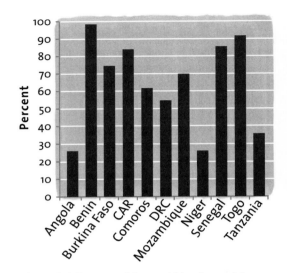

Figure 2.4 *Percent of donated blood tested for HIV contamination in a quality-assured manner: countries with less than 100 percent coverage*

by countries in the 2010 series of workshops sponsored by UNAIDS described above (Stover and Forsythe 2010). The number of blood units required per 1,000 population reported by the countries is shown in Figure 2.5; for those countries that did not attend a workshop, we use the median value calculated from the countries below of 3.3 units required per 1,000 population.

Based on the assumption that donated blood will be almost entirely donated by the adult population, we assume that the HIV prevalence rate faced by the uninfected population throughout the time period is the adult HIV prevalence rate; again the implicit assumption here is that unsafe blood transfusions will result in a small number of new HIV infections, such that the HIV prevalence rate will not change substantially. We use the total population and relevant HIV prevalence rate (ages fifteen and above) from the same Spectrum files described above in the section on unsafe medical injections. Because women are more likely than men to receive blood transfusions (Mishra and Khan 2008), as transfusions occur due to anemia associated with pregnancy (Zucker *et al.* 1994), we assume that the averted HIV infections occur on average at the peak childbearing age of twenty-seven.

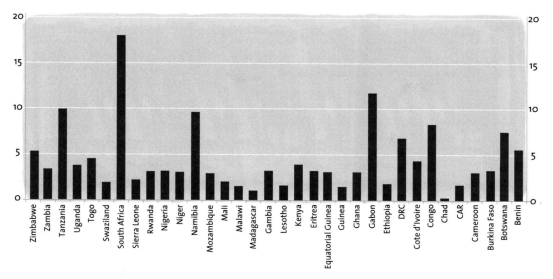

Figure 2.5 *Number of blood units required per 1,000 population; data from countries attending 2010 UNAIDS-sponsored workshops*

Coverage

For baseline coverage, we use the coverage rates reported for 2009 in the country-specific 2010 UNGASS reports, available publicly on the UNAIDS website. For those countries that report less than 100 percent coverage of testing donated blood for HIV, we assume that 100 percent of the blood supply will be tested by 2015, scaling up coverage in a linear fashion.

Unit cost

The unit costs used here are taken from the same resource needs estimates developed by national experts in the series of workshops in 2010 sponsored by UNAIDS (Stover and Forsythe 2010). In the case where a country did not attend a workshop, the median cost across the available countries is used.

Note that the unit cost of this intervention is defined as the marginal cost to test one unit of donated blood for HIV in a quality-assured manner. Since donated blood is tested for a number of different viruses in sub-Saharan Africa, including hepatitis B and hepatitis C, countries are instructed to include only the cost relevant to testing for HIV in the calculations, rather than the full cost of testing one unit of donated blood. Since only the marginal

cost of testing blood for HIV is included here, we include only HIV infections averted in calculating the benefits associated with this cost.

Transmission probability

We assume an HIV transmission probability of 90 percent per unit of contaminated blood that is transfused (Donegan *et al.* 1990).

Ensuring that 100 percent of all blood transfusions in sub-Saharan Africa is safe from HIV contamination by 2015 results in averting slightly more than 131,000 HIV infections. Relatively more infections are averted through this intervention than through safe medical injections because, although initial baseline coverage is greater here, the transmission probability is so much higher via blood transfusions than with medical injections that more HIV infections occur. Using a 3 percent discount rate results in an ICER of $3, a figure substantially lower than the PPP-adjusted GNI per capita figure of $2,051 for sub-Saharan Africa, making this a highly cost-effective intervention.

Turning to the benefit-cost analysis, we again present results based on the eight different scenarios described above, as requested by *RethinkHIV*, varying the scenarios by value of life year gained, cost of ART, and discount rate (see Table 2.5).

Table 2.5 Benefits associated with safe blood transfusions by discount rate, value of life year gained, and ART cost ($ million)

	Scenario I (3%, $1,000, $500)	Scenario II (5%, $1,000, $500)	Scenario III (3%, $5,000, $500)	Scenario IV (5%, $5,000, $500)	Scenario V (3%, $1,000, $1,000)	Scenario VI (5%, $1,000, $1,000)	Scenario VII (3%, $5,000, $1,000)	Scenario VIII (5%, $5,000, $1,000)
Years of life gained (undiscounted)	2.8							
Value of years gained	$1,119	$639	$5,595	$3,197	$1,119	$639	$5,595	$3,197
OI treatment costs averted	$56	$47	$56	$47	$56	$47	$56	$47
ARV treatment costs averted	$343	$294	$343	$294	$683	$586	$683	$586
Total	$1,517	$980	$5,993	$3,537	$1,858	$1,272	$6,334	$3,829

Assuming that the average age at an averted HIV infection is twenty-seven, the number of life years gained overall is 2.8 million, undiscounted. If the value of each life year gained is assumed to be $1,000, then the total value of life years gained varies between $639 million and $1.1 billion, as the discount rate varies between 3 and 5 percent (see Scenarios I and II). If instead the value of one life year gained is changed so that it is equal to $5,000, then the value of life years gained varies from $3.2 billion with a discount rate of 5 percent to $5.6 billion with a discount rate of 3 percent (see Scenarios III and IV).

The benefits associated with averted treatment costs of OIs due to averting HIV infections range from $47 million using a 5 percent discount rate to $56 million using a 3 percent discount rate (see Scenarios I and II). Since the only parameter that varies for OI treatment costs is the discount rate, this number is repeated across the remaining scenarios.

Finally, we examine the total benefits associated with averted ARV treatment costs. Assuming that the annual cost of ARV treatment is $500, then the total amount of cost savings from providing a safe blood supply varies between $294 million and $343 million for 5 percent and 3 percent discount rates, respectively. If we change the assumption regarding the cost of delivering ART so that the annual cost becomes equal to $1,000, then the treatment savings vary between $586 million and $683 million for 5 percent and 3 percent discount rates.

Overall, the total benefits that accrue from scaling-up testing of the donated blood supply for HIV to reach 100 percent coverage of all countries in sub-Saharan Africa range from a low of $980 million, when the value of one life-year gained is $1,000, the annual cost of ART is assumed to be $500, and a 5 percent discount rate is used, to a high of $6.3 billion, when the value of one life-year gained is $5,000, the annual cost of ART is assumed to be $1,000, and a 3 percent discount rate is used.

These calculated benefits can then be associated with the relevant costs to calculate eight different benefit to cost ratios (see Table 2.6). The B/C ratio ranges from a low of 146 to a high of 882, making this a highly beneficial intervention at any level.

Preventing mother-to-child transmission

Although the number of new infant infections declined by 26 percent between 2001 and 2009, vertical transmission still accounts for a significant proportion of new HIV infections in the developing world, inspiring a call by UNAIDS for a virtual elimination of new vertical infections (UNAIDS 2011). In the twenty-five largest countries in sub-Saharan Africa, the number of new infant infections declined by 24 percent between 2001 and 2009, with one-third of that decline occurring in 2009 alone (Mahy *et al.* 2010), although 350,000

Table 2.6 Benefit to cost ratios of providing safe blood supply, by value of life year gained, discount rate, and cost of ART ($ million)

Value of life year	Discount rate	Benefits		Costs	B/C ratio (A)	B/C ratio (B)
		$500 ART (A)	$1,000 ART (B)			
$1,000	3%	$1,517	$1,858	$7.18	211	259
$1,000	5%	$980	$1,272	$6.70	146	190
$5,000	3%	$5,993	$6,334	$7.18	834	882
$5,000	5%	$3,537	$3,829	$6.70	528	572

new vertical transmissions occurred in 2008 in the region as a whole, as described above. Programs that prevent mother-to-child transmission (pMTCT) of HIV are among the most cost-effective interventions available in the HIV/AIDS arsenal; two factors that have limited the uptake of pMTCT programs, however, are low levels of antenatal clinic attendance and/or deliveries at a facility, and high levels of stigma associated with an HIV-positive diagnosis, particularly when treatment is not available (Ekouevi *et al.* 2004).

In 2010, the World Health Organization released new guidelines for treating pregnant women and infants in order to prevent HIV vertical transmission (WHO 2010a). For those pregnant women in need of ART for their own health (currently those with CD4 counts under 350 cells/mm^3), the guidelines recommend lifelong ART. For those pregnant women who are not in need of ART based on current guidelines, the guidelines for treating pregnant women recommend one of two options:

- *Option A*: the pregnant woman receives zidovudine beginning as early as fourteen weeks' gestation, followed by a single dose of nevirapine when labor begins and zidovudine/lamivudine during delivery. This is followed by zidovudine/lamivudine for seven days postpartum if zidovudine began at less than four weeks before delivery. Breastfeeding infants receive nevirapine daily until one week beyond the cessation of breastfeeding; non-breastfeeding infants receive either nevirapine or zidovudine for six weeks after birth.
- *Option B*: the pregnant woman receives triple ART beginning as early as fourteen weeks' ges-

tation through the period of breastfeeding (one week beyond cessation of breastfeeding), while the infant receives nevirapine or zidovudine for four to six weeks after birth.

Since a panel of experts found that transmission rates are reduced by the same percentage for both Options A and B (WHO 2010b), and Option B is substantially more expensive to provide than Option A, for the most part countries are preferring Option A in their pMTCT programs. We calculate here the costs and benefits of scaling up Option A in pMTCT programs from current levels to 90 percent coverage of all pregnant women by 2015, using a linear scale-up pattern. We use the publicly available Spectrum/AIM projections and model, described above, to calculate the number of HIV infant infections averted by scaling-up Option A in the forty-four sub-Saharan African countries, as well as the associated costs. The specific assumptions used for the projections are described in more detail below.

Target population

As described above, Spectrum is a fully articulated demographic model with sub-modules focusing on different topics, including family planning, child and maternal mortality, and the demographic and social impacts of HIV/AIDS. We use the publicly available projection files for both the demographic (DemProj) and HIV/AIDS (AIDS Impact Model, or AIM) modules to calculate the number of infant infections averted through implementing Option A, as well as the associated costs. The target population for the pMTCT programs is all pregnant women, along with their subsequent live births, in the forty-four sub-Saharan African countries listed in Appendix A. As described above, we perform two sets of benefit calculations, the first assuming that each life year saved via an averted infant infection receives a weight of one, and the second assuming that each life year saved via an averted infant infection receives a weight of 0.5.

Coverage

Baseline coverage rates for each country are available in the publicly available Spectrum/AIM files; these are program statistics regarding the number of women served in each country's pMTCT program that were provided and validated by each country's government. We follow the recent UNAIDS call to virtually eliminate all new infant HIV infections by scaling-up coverage to reach 90 percent of all pregnant women and their infants by 2015, using a linear scale-up pattern.

Unit cost

We adapt the unit costs used in the recent UNAIDS Global Plan (UNAIDS 2011). For that plan, the cost of screening women and the cost of Option A were calculated as normalized using an index of an average purchasing power parity (PPP) adjusted GNI per capita for twenty-one representative sub-Saharan African countries. In that study, the cost of screening HIV-negative women was assumed to be $3.90, including testing costs, while the cost of screening HIV-positive women was assumed to be $13, including testing and post-test counseling costs. The cost of Option A was assumed in the study to be on average $237, consisting of $30 for the average amount of zidovudine/lamivudine used, $63 for nevirapine, $54 for laboratory costs, and $90 for service delivery costs.[4] The representative costs used in that study are adjusted here for each of the forty-four countries individually by multiplying each cost by the country-specific PPP-adjusted GNI per capita divided by the average PPP-adjusted GNI per capita for the twenty-one representative countries used above. We follow the recent UNAIDS Investment Framework analysis (Schwartländer *et al.* 2011) in assuming that scaling-up delivery of treatment will occur to a large extent through community health care workers, which does not require construction of additional antenatal clinic facilities.

Transmission probability

We follow the methodology approved for use in the Spectrum/AIM model (WHO 2010b) and assume that Option A reduces perinatal vertical transmission to 2 percent, while breastfeeding has a monthly transmission probability of 0.2 percent.

Given the above assumptions, over 265,000 new infant HIV infections could be averted by 2015 by increasing the coverage of pMTCT programs to 90 percent, using a linear scale-up rate. The calculated ICER across all forty-four countries using an initial discount rate of 3 percent is about $30, well below the average GNI per capita in 2009 of $2,051, making this a highly cost-effective intervention.

We turn to calculating the benefits associated with saving over 265,000 infants through this intervention. We calculate two sets of the eight scenarios displayed above for the benefits associated with safe medical injections and a safe blood supply, as recommended by *RethinkHIV*; the first panel, Panel A, assumes that each life year saved from an averted infant infection receives a weight of one, that is it equals one full life year gained, while the second panel, Panel B, assumes that each infant life year gained receives a weight of 0.5 (see Table 2.7).

Examining the results in Panel A first, where each life year gained receives a full weight of one, it can be seen that averting 265,000 infant infections results in a gain of 13.9 million (undiscounted) life years. Assuming that the value of each life year gained is $1,000, the total value of life years gained ranges from $3.5 billion to $4.8 billion for discount rates of 5 and 3 percent, respectively. If the value of each life year gained is $5,000, then total value increases to range from $17.6 billion to $24.1 billion for the two different discount rates. If instead each life year gained receives a weight of 0.5, or half of one year, the total value of life years gained is reduced by approximately 50 percent, ranging from a low of $1.8 billion when the value of each year equals $1,000 and a discount rate of 5 percent is used, to a high of $12.1 billion when the value of each year is $5,000 and a 3 percent discount rate is used.

---

[4] Note that these costs are nearly identical to the costs calculated independently by Brent (2011) for one of the perspective papers written for this same project, *RethinkHIV*.

Table 2.7 Benefits associated with pMTCT programs, by discount rate, value of life year gained, cost of ART, and different weights for life years gained ($ million)

	Scenario I (3%, $1,000, $500)	Scenario II (5%, $1,000, $500)	Scenario III (3%, $5,000, $500)	Scenario IV (5%, $5,000, $500)	Scenario V (3%, $1,000, $1,000)	Scenario VI (5%, $1,000, $1,000)	Scenario VII (3%, $5,000, $1,000)	Scenario VIII (5%, $5,000, $1,000)
Panel A (life year weighted at 1.0)								
Years of life gained (undiscounted)	13.9							
Value of years gained	$4,825	$3,511	$24,125	$17,557	$4,825	$3,511	$24,125	$17,557
OI treatment costs averted	$112	$94	$112	$94	$112	$94	$112	$94
ARV treatment costs averted	$691	$593	$691	$593	$1,379	$1,182	$1,379	$1,182
Total	$5,629	$4,198	$24,929	$18,243	$6,317	$4,788	$25,617	$18,833
Panel B (life year weighted at 0.5)								
Years of life gained (undiscounted)	7.0							
Value of years gained	$2,412	$1,756	$12,062	$8,778	$2,412	$1,756	$12,062	$8,778
OI treatment costs averted	$112	$94	$112	$94	$112	$94	$112	$94
ARV treatment costs averted	$691	$593	$691	$593	$1,379	$1,182	$1,379	$1,182
Total	$3,216	$2,442	$12,866	$9,465	$3,904	$3,032	$13,554	$10,054

Because treatment costs are not dependent on the number of life years gained, but instead are based on the number of HIV infections averted, the calculation of treatment costs averted are the same in the two panels, Panels A and B. The total amount saved by not treating OIs associated with averting one HIV infection varies between $94 million and $112 million for 5 and 3 percent discount rates, respectively. The total amount saved by avoiding treating an HIV-infected person with ARVs ranges from $593 million to $691 million when the annual cost of ARV treatment is $500, depending on the discount rate, and ranges from $1.2 billion to $1.4 billion when the annual cost of ARV treatment is $1,000, again depending on the discount rate.

By aggregating all three factors in Table 2.7, we see that the total benefits associated with scaling up pMTCT programs to reach 90 percent of all pregnant women by 2015 in sub-Saharan Africa ranges by a factor of ten, from a low value of $2.4 billion (life year weighted at 0.5, discount rate of 5 percent, value of life year gained of $1,000, and annual ARV treatment cost of $500), to a high value of $25.6 billion (life year weighted at 1.0, discount rate of 3 percent, value of life year gained of $5,000, and annual ARV treatment cost of $1,000).

The total benefits above are used to calculate the benefit to cost ratios associated with scaling up pMTCT programs (see Table 2.8). All of the benefit to cost ratios are significantly greater than one, ranging from a low value of 15 to a high value of 146, implying that spending one dollar on a pMTCT program results in a benefit of between $15 and $146, an excellent return on investment examining any of the scenarios.

As countries debate which pMTCT protocol to use, one possibility (known as "Option B+") is to test and then treat all HIV-positive pregnant women with triple ART. Although arguably the marginal cost of Option B+ relative to Option A should be attributed to the overall treatment budget rather than the pMTCT budget, we perform a sensitivity analysis here by calculating the cost of Option B+, assuming that treatment begins at fourteen weeks' gestation and continues for six months. We use the ART unit costs from the UNAIDS Investment

Table 2.8 Benefit to cost ratios of providing pMTCT programs, by discount rate, value of life year gained, cost of ART, and different life year weights ($ million)

	Discount rate	Benefits		Costs	B/C ratio (A)	B/C ratio (B)
Panel A (life year weighted at 1.0)		$500 ART (A)	$1,000 ART (B)			
$1,000	3%	$5,629	$6,317	$175	32	36
$1,000	5%	$4,198	$4,788	$163	26	29
$5,000	3%	$24,929	$25,617	$175	142	146
$5,000	5%	$18,243	$18,833	$163	112	115
Panel B (life year weighted at 0.5)						
$1,000	3%	$3,216	$3,904	$175	18	22
$1,000	5%	$2,442	$3,032	$163	15	19
$5,000	3%	$12,866	$13,554	$175	73	77
$5,000	5%	$9,465	$10,054	$163	58	62

Framework between 2011 and 2015. As expected, the incremental costs for pMTCT increase significantly, from about $196 million to over $333 million between 2011 and 2015. This also has an impact on the benefit to cost ratios, which now range from 9 to 84; note, however, that the ratios are still significantly greater than one.

Prevention interventions for injecting drug users

Although the source of the vast majority of new HIV infections in sub-Saharan Africa has been heterosexual transmission, recently new HIV infections have begun to be transmitted via injecting drug use (IDU) behavior. There are only a few countries in sub-Saharan Africa for which this appears to be an issue, including Kenya, South Africa, the United Republic of Tanzania, and Mauritius (UNAIDS 2010a). Reported rates of HIV infection are quite high in the IDU population in some of these countries, reaching 36 percent in Nairobi, Kenya (Odek-Ogunde *et al.* 2004), 26 percent in Zanzibar (Dahoma *et al.* 2006), and about 12 percent in South Africa (Mathers *et al.* 2010). Even with high levels of HIV infection, however, the number of new infections associated with IDU and partners, including sexual behavior, is usually

relatively low (e.g., 3.8 percent in Kenya (Kenya National AIDS Control Council 2009)).

Both the United Nations and the guidance provided by PEPFAR (PEPFAR 2010) recommend a comprehensive package of interventions for IDU, including:

- outreach and information, education, and communication (IEC) programs;
- needle and syringe exchange programs (NSEP);
- opioid substitution therapy (OST);
- HIV counseling and testing, along with ART for HIV-positive IDU;
- counseling and treatment for sexual behavior, including providing condoms and STI treatment;
- vaccination, diagnosis, and treatment of viral hepatitis.

In this paper, we examine the impact of interventions targeting IDU in Kenya, South Africa, the United Republic of Tanzania, but not Mauritius, as the overall burden of HIV/AIDS disease is substantially greater in the first three countries than in Mauritius. We explore the set of harm reduction interventions targeting IDU which includes three of the key interventions listed above: outreach/information and education campaigns, needle and syringe exchange programs, and opioid substitution therapy. Since condom distribution affects the sexual transmission portion of the HIV/AIDS epidemic, and this paper examines non-sexual HIV transmission, its impact is not included here.

We use the Spectrum/Goals model, described in detail in the Methodology section above, to calculate the impact of increasing coverage of IDU-targeted interventions on injecting behavior in Kenya, South Africa, and the United Republic of Tanzania. We use the country-specific Goals models developed by the aids2031 Consortium for each of the three countries (Hecht *et al.* 2009, 2010); note that the epidemiological fits of the model were performed by the aids2031 Modelling Working Group. Complete details of the specifications are available upon request.

Target population

We target the injecting behavior of the IDU population in each of the three countries. We assume here that, because the IDU population is generally a younger population, an HIV infection among the IDU population is averted on average at age twenty-two.

Coverage

We use the baseline coverage rates provided by the three countries in the resource needs workshops sponsored by UNAIDS referred to above (Stover and Forsythe 2010). Each of the three countries examined here attended a workshop and validated their initial results upon return to their home country. Note that baseline coverage rates are quite low for the three interventions in each of the countries, with zero percent coverage reported for OST programs from all three countries, zero percent coverage reported for NSEP in Tanzania and South Africa, 5 percent coverage reported for NSEP in Kenya, and outreach/IEC intervention baseline coverage rates reported to be 5 percent in South Africa, 10 percent in Kenya, and 29 percent in Tanzania.

A crucial question here is what the target coverage rates should be for each of the three IDU interventions. Although it is reasonable to assume that some HIV prevention interventions can reach very high levels of coverage, e.g., 100 percent for a safe blood supply and for school-based programs, it is unlikely that similarly high coverage levels can be reached for interventions targeting marginalized populations such as IDUs. We adopt the practice followed by UNAIDS where universal access targets for most-at-risk populations, such as IDU, sex workers, and men who have sex with men, assume that the maximum feasible coverage rate is 60 percent for outreach/IEC programs and NSEP, while the maximum feasible coverage rate is 40 percent for OST programs (Schwartländer *et al.* 2011). Note that the assumption regarding maximum achievable coverage for OST programs is based on the maximum coverage achieved in existing OST programs (Mathers *et al.* 2010; Needle and Zhao 2010; Verster *et al.* 2009).

Unit cost

Again we utilize the information provided by the three countries in the UNAIDS-sponsored resource needs workshops to estimate the annual unit costs for each of the three interventions. Note in turn that the values were validated after the countries received default values in the workshops, discussed in detail in Verster *et al.* (2009).

Transmission probability

Although HIV transmission for IDU in the Goals model can occur either via injecting or sexual behavior, we focus here on the impact of increasing coverage of interventions targeting injecting behavior. We perform a sensitivity analysis regarding the impact of these interventions by varying the number of HIV infections averted by two times a standard deviation of 20 percent in both directions.

Assuming that the coverage of the first two IDU interventions (IEC and NSEP) reaches 60 percent by 2015, and that coverage of OST programs reaches 40 percent by 2015, by 2015 approximately 570 new HIV infections could be averted among the IDU population. Using an initial discount rate of 3 percent, the ICER across the three countries is $758, implying that this set of interventions is highly cost-effective.

The monetary benefits associated with scaling up interventions to reduce injecting behavior are displayed in Table 2.9. Assuming that each infection averted occurs at an average age of twenty-two, as injecting drug users tend to be quite young (Dolan and Niven 2005), in total approximately 15,000 life years are gained when interventions targeting IDU are scaled up to reach the universal access coverage

Table 2.9 Benefits associated with IDU interventions, by discount rate, value of life year gained, and cost of ART ($ million)

	Scenario I (3%, $1,000, $500)	Scenario II (5%, $1,000, $500)	Scenario III (3%, $5,000, $500)	Scenario IV (5%, $5,000, $500)	Scenario V (3%, $1,000, $1,000)	Scenario VI (5%, $1,000, $1,000)	Scenario VII (3%, $5,000, $1,000)	Scenario VIII (5%, $5,000, $1,000)
Years of life gained (undiscounted)	0.015							
Value of years gained	$6.5	$3.9	$32.4	$19.7	$6.5	$3.9	$32.4	$19.7
OI treatment costs averted	$0.24	$0.20	$0.24	$0.20	$0.24	$0.20	$0.24	$0.20
ARV treatment costs averted	$1.5	$1.3	$1.5	$1.3	$3.0	$2.5	$3.0	$2.5
Total	$8.2	$5.4	$34.1	$21.1	$9.7	$6.7	$35.6	$22.4

targets described above. If the value of one life year gained is assumed to be $1,000, then the total value of life years gained ranges from $3.9 million to $6.5 million when the discount rate varies between 5 and 3 percent. If the value of one life year gained is set at $5,000, then the total value of life years gained ranges from $19.7 million to $32.4 million, depending on the discount rate.

In addition to the benefits associated with the value of life years gained, savings will also be realized in averted treatment costs for both OIs as well as ARV treatment costs. Savings from averted OI treatment costs range from $0.2 million to $0.24 million as the discount rate varies between 5 and 3 percent. If the annual cost of providing ART is assumed to be $500, then the ARV treatment costs averted range from $1.3 million to $1.5 million, depending on the value of the discount rate, while if the annual cost of providing ART is assumed to be $1,000, then the ARV treatment cost savings range from $2.5 million to $3.0 million.

Overall, the benefits associated with scaling up the three different interventions – outreach/IEC interventions, NSEP and OST programs – that reach IDU in Kenya, South Africa, and the United Republic of Tanzania range from $5.4 million, which occurs when the discount rate is 5 percent, the value of one life year gained is $1,000, and the annual ART cost is $500, to $35.6 million, which occurs when the discount rate is 3 percent, the value of one life year gained is $5,000, and the annual ART cost is $1,000.

In order to perform a sensitivity analysis on the HIV transmission rate used in the model, we calculate the monetary benefits associated with increasing the coverage of interventions to reduce risky injecting behavior when the number of HIV infections averted changes by two times the standard deviation in both directions (see Table 2.10).

Varying the number of HIV infections averted by 40 percent in both directions results in a similar change in the calculation of the associated monetary benefits. When the number of HIV infections averted is decreased by 40 percent, the number of life years gained decreases to 9,000, while the decrease in total monetary benefits resulting ranges from a new low figure of $3.2 million to a new high figure of $21.4 million. When the number of HIV infections averted is increased by 40 percent, there is an increase in the number of life years gained of 21,000, while the associated monetary benefits increase from a low of $10.6 million to a high of $56.9 million.

Applying the results from the initial analysis of benefits presented in Table 2.9, we calculate the benefit to cost ratios associated with providing interventions to change needle-sharing behavior among IDU (see Table 2.11).

The benefit to cost ratios of this set of interventions are not as high as the B/C ratios derived in the other interventions targeting non-sexual transmission of HIV in this paper, and in fact the B/C ratios drop under one for certain scenarios, that is, the

Table 2.10 Sensitivity analysis of the benefits associated with IDU interventions, by discount rate, value of life year gained, cost of ART, and infections averted ($ million)

		Scenario I (3%, $1,000, $500)	Scenario II (5%, $1,000, $500)	Scenario III (3%, $5,000, $500)	Scenario IV (5%, $5,000, $500)	Scenario V (3%, $1,000, $1,000)	Scenario VI (5%, $1,000, $1,000)	Scenario VII (3%, $5,000, $1,000)	Scenario VIII (5%, $5,000, $1,000)
Panel A: Infections averted 40% lower									
Years of life gained (undiscounted)	0.009								
Value of years gained		$3.9	$2.4	$19.4	$11.8	$3.9	$2.4	$19.4	$11.8
OI treatment costs averted		$0.15	$0.12	$0.15	$0.12	$0.15	$0.12	$0.15	$0.12
ARV treatment costs averted		$0.9	$0.8	$0.9	$0.8	$1.8	$1.5	$1.8	$1.5
Total		$4.9	$3.2	$20.5	$12.7	$5.8	$4.0	$21.4	$13.4
Panel B: Infections averted 40% higher									
Years of life gained (undiscounted)	0.021								
Value of years gained		$9.1	$5.5	$45.4	$27.5	$9.1	$5.5	$45.4	$27.5
OI treatment costs averted		$0.34	$0.28	$0.34	$0.28	$0.34	$0.28	$0.34	$0.28
ARV treatment costs averted		$2.1	$1.8	$2.1	$1.8	$4.2	$3.6	$4.2	$3.6
Total		$15.0	$10.6	$51.3	$32.6	$20.6	$15.4	$56.9	$37.4

Table 2.11 Benefit to cost ratios of providing IDU interventions, by discount rate, value of life year gained, and cost of ART ($ million)

		Benefits				
Value of life year	Discount rate	$500 ART (A)	$1,000 ART (B)	Costs	B/C ratio (A)	B/C ratio (B)
$1,000	3%	$8.2	$9.7	$7.6	1.1	1.3
$1,000	5%	$5.4	$6.7	$7.0	0.8	0.9
$5,000	3%	$34.1	$35.6	$7.6	4.5	4.7
$5,000	5%	$21.1	$22.4	$7.0	3.0	3.2

amount of benefits that accrue are lower than the amount that is spent in delivering the interventions. The B/C ratio varies from a low of 0.8 when the discount rate is 5 percent, the value of one life year gained is $1,000, and the annual cost of the averted ART is $500, to a high of 4.7, which occurs when the discount rate is 3 percent, the value of one life year gained is $5,000, and the annual cost of the averted ARV treatment is $1,000. When the sensitivity analysis regarding the number of HIV infections averted is repeated in calculating the benefit

to cost ratios, the B/C ratio drops well below one (see Table 2.12). The B/C ratios resulting from the sensitivity analysis range from a low of 0.5, when infections averted are 40 percent lower, the discount rate is 5 percent, the value of one life year gained is $1,000, and the annual cost of averted ART is $500, to a high of 7.5, which occurs when the number of infections averted is 40 percent higher, the discount rate is 3 percent, the value of one life year gained is $5,000, and the annual cost of averted ARV treatment is $1,000.

Table 2.12 Sensitivity analysis of the benefit to cost ratios of providing IDU interventions, by discount rate, value of life year gained, cost of ART, and number of infections averted ($ million)

	Discount rate	Benefits		Costs	B/C ratio (A)	B/C ratio (B)
Panel A: Infections averted 40% lower						
Value of life year		$500 ART (A)	$1,000 ART (B)			
$1,000	3%	$4.9	$5.8	$7.6	0.7	0.8
$1,000	5%	$3.2	$4.0	$7.0	0.5	0.6
$5,000	3%	$20.5	$21.4	$7.6	2.7	2.8
$5,000	5%	$12.7	$13.4	$7.0	1.8	1.9
Panel B: Infections averted 40% higher						
Value of life year		$500 ART (A)	$1,000 ART (B)			
$1,000	3%	$15.0	$20.6	$7.6	2.0	2.7
$1,000	5%	$10.6	$15.4	$7.0	1.5	2.2
$5,000	3%	$51.3	$56.9	$7.6	6.8	7.5
$5,000	5%	$32.6	$37.4	$7.0	4.6	5.3

Table 2.13 Summary of benefits and costs associated with interventions to reduce non-sexual HIV transmission

Proposed solution	Cumulative increase in beneficiaries by 2015 (millions)	Cumulative incremental costs ($ million)	Number of HIV infections averted	Range of benefits ($ million)	Range of costs ($ million)	Range of B/C ratio
Safe medical injections	1,223	$184.98	68,000	$509 to $3,291	$155 to $333	1.6 to 19.8
Safe blood supply	489	$2.19	131,000	$980 to $6,334	$6.7 to $7.2	146 to 882
Preventing mother-to-child transmission	1.21	$195.90	265,000	$2,442 to $25,617	$163 to $175	15 to 146
Interventions to reduce risky IDU behavior (Kenya, South Africa, United Republic of Tanzania)	0.020	$8.43	570	$3.2 to $56.9	$7.0 to $7.6	0.5 to 7.5
Grand total	1,713	$391.48	464,570			

Conclusion and recommendations

Although progress has been made in both reducing the number of new HIV infections and providing anti-retroviral treatment to those who are HIV-positive, HIV/AIDS is still the leading cause of death for adults in sub-Saharan Africa. This paper examined four possible solutions to the non-sexual transmission of HIV that can be undertaken to further reduce the burden of HIV/AIDS in the continent.

We used both the AIM/Spectrum and Goals models to examine ICERs and B/C ratios for 44 sub-Saharan African countries, except in the case of

interventions targeting IDU behavior, where we examined three countries: Kenya, South Africa, and the United Republic of Tanzania. Overall, the first three interventions result in very high benefit to cost ratios, ranging from 1.6 to 19.8 for safe medical injections, 146 to 882 for safe blood supplies, and 15 to 146 for programs preventing mother-to-child transmission (see Table 2.13). The benefit to cost ratios for interventions to reduce risky injecting behavior are not as high as the other B/C ratios, and drop below one in some scenarios, ranging from 0.5 to 7.5. In some scenarios, however, interventions to reduce risky injecting behavior are still cost-saving, that is, the benefits are higher than the costs.

In addition, it is important to note that the overall resources required to achieve these target coverage rates is not large. Over the course of the five-year scale-up period 2011 to 2015, the cumulative incremental costs to make medical injections safer is $185 million and benefits 1.2 billion people cumulatively who receive injections over that time period. The cumulative incremental costs to ensure a safe blood supply is only $2 million, and that intervention benefits almost 500 million people cumulatively over the five-year time period. The cumulative incremental cost to finish scaling up pMTCT programs is $196 million, with over 1.2 million HIV-positive pregnant women receiving ARV prophylaxis between 2011 and 2015, while the cumulative incremental cost to institute interventions targeting IDU is $8.5 million, serving 20,000 IDU over five years. The grand total required for all four sets of interventions to reduce non-sexual transmission of HIV is $391 million.

Some caveats should be attached to these results, some of which will be addressed by other papers in this series. For example, although pMTCT programs are extremely cost-effective, the challenge is to increase uptake so that full benefits can be experienced, and virtual elimination of vertical transmission is achieved. As noted above, two impediments to achieving full coverage of pMTCT interventions are access to care, both through antenatal clinic facilities and community health care workers, and reducing stigma associated with an HIV diagnosis. Since the cost of increasing antenatal care access is a cost to the health system in general, this is being addressed by the health systems paper. Reducing stigma is integrally linked with an increase in availability of ART; this topic will be addressed in the paper on anti-retroviral treatment. In addition, reducing unnecessary medical injections via interventions elsewhere in the health system, such as treating anemia, are not costed here.

Finally, there are other possible non-sexual transmission interventions with less well-defined benefits, including family planning and treating neglected tropical diseases such as schistosomiasis. For example, a recent paper found that increasing the availability of family planning could avert a substantial number of new infant HIV infections through reducing unmet need for family planning in HIV-positive women (Mahy *et al.* 2010). In addition, some argue that a minimal investment in treating certain tropical diseases would result in averting HIV infections as well (Hotez *et al.* 2011; Stillwaggon 2009), while a recent study found that delivering an integrated package of treatment for both HIV and some neglected tropical diseases would increase the cost-effectiveness for both sets of diseases (Noblick *et al.* 2011).

Appendix A: List of countries in analysis

Angola
Benin
Botswana
Burkina Faso
Burundi
Cameroon
Central African Republic
Chad
Comoros
Congo
Cote d'Ivoire
Democratic Republic of the Congo
Djibouti
Equatorial Guinea
Eritrea
Ethiopia
Gabon
Gambia
Ghana
Guinea
Guinea-Bissau
Kenya
Lesotho
Liberia
Madagascar
Malawi
Mali
Mauritania
Mauritius
Mozambique
Namibia
Niger
Nigeria
Rwanda
Senegal

Sierra Leone
Somalia
South Africa
Swaziland
Togo
Uganda
United Republic of Tanzania
Zambia
Zimbabwe

References

AIDSTAR-One. (2011). Injection Safety. Available at: www.AIDSTAR-One.com, accessed July 20, 2011.

Bertozzi, S. M., Padian, N. S., Wegbreit, J., DeMaria, L. M., Feldman, B., Gayle, H., Gold, J., Grant, R. and Isbell, M. T. (2006). HIV/AIDS prevention and treatment. In Jamison, D. T., *et al.* (eds.) *Disease Control Priorities in Developing Countries*, Vol. 2. New York and Washington, DC: Oxford University Press/World Bank, 331–70.

Bollinger, L. (2008). How can we calculate the "E" in "CEA"? *AIDS*. Jul; **22** Suppl 1: S51–7.

Bouey, P., Saidel, T. and Rehle, T. (1998) *AVERT: A Tool for Estimating Intervention Effects on the Reduction of HIV Transmission*. Arlington, VA: Family Health International.

Brent, R. J. (2011). Perspective Paper for Rethink-HIV: Treatment. Available at: www.rethinkhiv.com/, accessed October 18, 2011.

CEGAA and Results for Development. (2010). The Long Run Costs and Financing of HIV/AIDS in South Africa. Available at: www.resultsfordevelopment.org/sites/resultsfordevelopment.org/files/aids2031_South-Africa_Report_FINAL2.pdf, accessed June 20, 2011.

Centers for Disease Control. (2001). Updated U.S. Public Health Service Guidelines for the Management of Occupational Exposures to HBV, HCV, and HIV and Recommendations for Postexposure Prophylaxis. Available at: www.cdc.gov/mmwr/PDF/rr/rr5011.pdf, accessed August 20, 2011.

Chandler, R. and Musau, R. (2005). Estimating Resource Requirements for Scaling Up Anti-retroviral Therapy in Uganda. PHRPlus paper, October 2005. Available at: www.

healthsystems2020.org/files/1629_file_Tech078_fin.pdf, accessed July 20, 2011.

Commission on Macroeconomics and Health. (2001). Report of the Commission on Macroeconomics and Health, presented to World Health Organization. Available at: http://whqlibdoc.who.int/publications/2001/924154550x.pdf, accessed July 20, 2011.

Dahoma, M. J. U. *et al.* (2006). HIV and substance abuse: the dual epidemics challenging Zanzibar. *African Journal of Drug and Alcohol Studies*, 2006, **5**: 129–38.

Demographic and Health Surveys, various years, various countries. Available at: www.measuredhs.com, accessed August 20, 2011.

Dolan, K. A. and Niven, H. (2005). A review of HIV prevention among young injecting drug users: a guide for researchers. *Harm Reduct J*. 2005 Mar 17; **2**(1): 5.

Donegan, E., Stuart, M., Niland, J. C. *et al.* (1990). Infection with human immunodeficiency virus type 1 (HIV-1) among recipients of antibody-positive blood donations. *Ann. Intern. Med.* **113**(10): 733–9.

Ekouevi, D. K., Leroy, V., Viho, A., Bequet, L., Horo, A., Rouet, F., Sakarovitch, C., Welffens-Ekra, C., Dabis, F.; ANRS 1201/1202 Ditrame Plus Study Group. (2004). Acceptability and uptake of a package to prevent mother-to-child transmission using rapid HIV testing in Abidjan, Côte d'Ivoire. *AIDS*. Mar 5; **18**(4): 697–700.

Flanagan, L. (2008). Transfusion of Blood Safer from HIV than Ever, *The Star* (Johannesburg); July 15, 2008.

Forsythe, S., Stover, J. and Bollinger, L. (2009). The past, present and future of HIV/AIDS and resource allocation. *BMC Public Health*. 2009 Nov 18; **9** Suppl 1: S4.

Futures Institute. (2011). See http://policytools.futuresinstitute.org/goals.html.

Goldie, S. J., Yazdanpanah, Y., Losina, E. *et al.* (2006). Cost-effectiveness of HIV treatment in resource-poor settings – the case of Cote d'Ivoire. *NEJM* **355**; 11(1141–53).

Harries, A. D., Zachariah, R., Tayler-Smith, K., Schouten, E. J., Chimbwandira, F., Van Damme, W. and El-Sadr, W. M. (2010). Keeping health facilities safe: one way of strengthening the interaction between disease-specific programmes and health systems. *Trop Med Int Health*. Dec; **15**(12): 1407–12.

Hauri, A. M., Armstrong, G. L. and Hutin, Y. J. F. (2004). The global burden of disease attributable to contaminated injections given in health care settings. *International Journal of STDs & AIDS* **15**: 7–16.

Hecht, R., Bollinger, L., Stover, J., McGreevey, W., Muhib, F., Madavo, C. E. and de Ferranti, D. (2009). Critical choices in financing the response to the global HIV/AIDS pandemic. *Health Affair* **28**: 6; 1–15. doi:10.1377/HlthAff28.61.

Hecht, R., Stover, J., Bollinger, L., Muhib, F., Case, K. and de Ferranti, D. (2010). Financing of HIV/AIDS programme scale-up in low-income and middle-income countries, 2009–2031. *Lancet* Oct 9; **376**(9748): 1254–60.

Hotez, P. J., Mistry, N., Rubinstein, J. and Sachs, J. D. (2011). Integrating neglected tropical diseases into AIDS, tuberculosis, and malaria control. *N Engl J Med.* Jun 2; **364**(22): 2086–9.

Hutin, Y. J., Hauri, A. M. and Armstrong, G. L. (2003). Use of injections in healthcare settings worldwide, 2000: literature review and regional estimates. *BMJ.* Nov 8; **327**(7423): 1075.

Jamison, D. (2010). Disease control. In Lomborg, B. (ed.) *Smart Solutions to Climate Change: Comparing Costs and Benefits*. Cambridge University Press.

Kasili, E. G. (1990). Malnutrition and infections as causes of childhood anemia in tropical Africa. *Am J Pediatr Hematol Oncol.* Fall; **12**(3): 375–7.

Kenya National AIDS Control Council. (2009). HIV Prevention Response and Modes of Transmission Analysis. Republic of Kenya. Available at: http://siteresources.worldbank.org/INTHIVAIDS/Resources/375798-1103037153392/KenyaMOT22March09Final.pdf, accessed July 22, 2011.

Kombe, G. and Smith, O. (2003). *The Costs of Anti-Retroviral Treatment in Zambia*. Technical Report No. 029. Bethesda, MD: The Partners for Health Reform*plus* Project, Abt Associates Inc. www.who.int/hiv/amds/countries/zmb_CostsARVTreatment.pdf, accessed July 20, 2011.

Lopman, B. A., French, K. M., Baggaley, R., Gregson, S. and Garnett, G. P. (2006). HIV-contaminated syringes are not evidence of transmission. *AIDS.* Sep 11; **20**(14): 1905.

Mahy, M., Lewden, C., Brinkhof, M. W., Dabis, F., Tassie, J. M., Souteyrand, Y. and Stover, J. (2010). Derivation of parameters used in Spectrum for eligibility for anti-retroviral therapy and survival on anti-retroviral therapy. *Sex Transm Infect.* Dec; **86** Suppl 2: ii28–34.

Mahy, M., Stover, J., Kiragu, K., Hayashi, C., Akwara, P., Luo, C., Stanecki, K., Ekpini, R. and Shaffer, N. (2010). What will it take to achieve virtual elimination of mother-to-child transmission of HIV? An assessment of current progress and future needs. *Sex Transm Infect.* Dec; **86** Suppl 2: ii48–55.

Mathers, B. M., Degenhardt, L., Ali, H., Wiessing, L., Hickman, M., Mattick, R. P., Myers, B., Ambekar, A. and Strathdee, S. A. (2010). 2009 Reference Group to the UN on HIV and Injecting Drug Use. HIV prevention, treatment, and care services for people who inject drugs: a systematic review of global, regional, and national coverage. *Lancet.* Mar 20; **375**(9719): 1014–28. Epub 2010 Feb 26.

Mills, E., Bakanda, C., Birungi, J., Chan, K., Ford, N., Cooper, C., Nachega, J. B., Dybul, M. and Hogg, R. (2011). Life expectancy of persons receiving combination antiretroviral therapy in low-income countries: a cohort analysis from Uganda. *Ann Intern Med.* **155**: 209–16.

Mishra, V. and Khan, S. (2008). Medical Injection Use and HIV in Sub-Saharan Africa. Demographic and Health Surveys Comparative Reports 21, USAID.

Mishra, V., Kottiri, B. and Liu, L. (2008). The Association between Medical Injections and Prevalent HIV Infection: Evidence from a National Sero-Survey in Uganda. Demographic and Health Surveys Working Papers, USAID.

MMIS. (2011). Available at: http://portalprd1.jsi.com/portal/page/portal/MMIS_WEBSITE_PGG/MMIS_HOMEPAGE_PG/MMIS_HOME_TAB:MMIS_OVRVW_TAB, accessed June 16, 2001.

Murray, C. J. L. and Lopez, A. D. (1996) *The Global Burden of Disease: A Comprehensive Assessment of Mortality and Disability from Diseases, Injuries, and Risk Factors in 1990 and Projected to 2020*. Boston, MA: Harvard University Press.

Needle, R. H. and Zhao, L. (2010). HIV prevention among injection drug users. Strengthening U.S. support for core interventions. A Report of the CSIS Global Health Policy Center. Washington DC: Center for Strategic and International Studies, 2010. Available at: http://csis.org/files/

publication/100408_Needle_HIVPrevention_web.pdf, accessed July 21, 2011.

Noblick, J., Skolnik, R. and Hotez, P. J. (2011). Linking global HIV/AIDS treatments with national programs for the control and elimination of the neglected tropical diseases. *PLoS Negl Trop Dis* **5**(7): e1022. doi:10.1371/journal.pntd.0001022.

Odek-Ogunde, M. *et al.* (2004). Seroprevalence of HIV, HBC and HCV in injecting drug users in Nairobi, Kenya: World Health Organization Drug Injecting Study Phase II findings. XV International Conference on AIDS, Bangkok, Thailand, 11–16 July (Abstract WePeC6001); http://gateway.nlmnih.gov/MeetingAbstracts/ma?f=102283927.html, accessed July 21, 2011.

PATH. (2007). Evaluation of a Retractable Syringe in South Africa. Available at: www.path.org/files/TS_eval_rtr_syr_sa.pdf, accessed October 19, 2011.

PEPFAR. (2010). Comprehensive HIV Prevention for People Who Inject Drugs, Revised Guidance. July 2010. Available at: www.pepfar.gov/documents/organization/144970.pdf, accessed July 22, 2011.

Schwartländer, B., Stover, J., Hallett, T., Atun, R., Avila, C., Gouws, E., Bartos, M., Ghys, P. D., Opuni, M., Barr, D., Alsallaq, R., Bollinger, L., de Freitas, M., Garnett, G., Holmes, C., Legins, K., Pillay, Y., Stanciole, A. E., McClure, C., Hirnschall, G., Laga, M. and Padian, N. (2011). Investment Framework Study Group. Towards an improved investment approach for an effective response to HIV/AIDS. *Lancet.* Jun 11; **377**(9782): 2031–41.

Soares Magalhães, R. J. and Clements, A. C. (2011). Mapping the risk of anaemia in preschool-age children: the contribution of malnutrition, malaria, and helminth infections in west Africa. *PLoS Med.* Jun; **8**(6): e1000438. Epub 2011 Jun 7.

Stillwaggon, E. (2009). Complexity, cofactors, and the failure of AIDS policy in Africa. *J Int AIDS Soc.* Jul 10; **12**(1): 12.

Stover, J. and Forsythe, S. (2010). *Financial Resources Required to Achieve National Goals for HIV Prevention, Treatment, Care and Support.* Glastonbury, CT: Futures Institute.

Stover, J., Johnson, P., Hallett, T., Marston, M., Becquet, R. and Timaeus, I. M. (2010). The Spectrum projection package: improvements in estimating incidence by age and sex, mother-to-child transmission, HIV progression in children and double orphans. *Sex Trans Infect*; **86**(Suppl 2): ii16–ii21. doi:10.1136/sti.2010.044222.

UNAIDS. (2007). www.unaids.org/en/dataanalysis/tools, accessed June 16, 2011.

UNAIDS. (2009). www.unaidsrstesa.org/thematic-areas/hiv-prevention/know-your-epidemic-modes-transmission, accessed June 16, 2011.

UNAIDS. (2010). UNAIDS Global Report for 2010. Available at: www.unaids.org, accessed June 16, 2011.

UNAIDS. (2011). AIDS at 30: Nations at the Crossroads. Available at: www.unaids.org/en/resources/unaidspublications/2011/#c_60139, accessed July 21, 2011.

UNICEF. (2009). 2009 AD Syringes Projections: Quantities and Prices.

UNICEF. (2010a). Interview with Dr Edward Hoekstra, Senior Health Advisor, Health Section, UNICEF. Available at: www.unicef.org/immunization/23244_safety.html, accessed June 10, 2011.

UNICEF. (2010b). Children and AIDS Fifth Stocktaking Report. Available at: www.unicef.org/publications/files/Children_and_AIDS-Fifth_Stocktaking_Report_2010_EN.pdf, accessed June 10, 2011.

UNICEF. (2011). UNICEF Supply Catalog, online at: https://supply.unicef.org/unicef_b2c/app/displayApp/(cpgsize=0&layout=7.0-12_1_66_68_115_2&uiarea=2&carea=4D69FD959FD33516E10000009E710FC1&cpgnum=1)/.do?rf=y, HepB Vaccine, Single dose. Accessed August 22, 2011.

United Nations, Department of Economic and Social Affairs, Population Division. (2011). World Population Prospects: The 2010 Revision, CD-ROM Edition.

Verster, A. D., Clark, N. C., Ball, A. L. and Donoghoe, M. C. (2009). *Interventions for HIV Prevention, Treatment and Care Among People Who Inject Drugs: Methods and Assumptions Recommended by the Working Group. Methodological Annex – IX. Financial resources required to achieve universal access to HIV prevention, treatment, care and support.* Geneva: WHO and UNAIDS.

Vinard, P., Nzigiye, B. and Rugabirwa, S. (2005). Etude sur le cout de la prise en charge des PVVIH. Prejet Int/107 – Initiative ESTHER en collaboration avec la CNLS. Dec 04–Mar 05.

Weinstein, M. C., Graham, J. D., Siegel, J. E. and
    Fineberg, H. V. (1989). Cost-effectiveness
    analysis of AIDS prevention programs:
    concepts, complications, and illustrations.
    In Turner, C. F., Miller, H. G. and Moses, L. E.
    (eds.) *Confronting AIDS: Sexual Behavior
    and Intravenous Drug Use*. Washington,
    DC: National Academy Press, 471–
    99.
WHO. (2010a). Anti-retroviral drugs for treating
    pregnant women and preventing HIV infection
    in infants. Available at: www.who.int/hiv/pub/
    mtct/anti-retroviral2010/en/index.html,
    accessed July 21, 2011.
WHO. (2010b). Consultative meeting on updating
    estimates of mother-to-child transmission rates
    of HIV. Available at: www.epidem.org/
    Publications/UpdatingMTCTratesReport.pdf,
    accessed July 22, 2011.

WHO. (2011). www.who.int/choice/costs/
    CER_thresholds/en/index.html, accessed
    June 16, 2011.
WHO Safe Injection Global Network (SIGN).
    (2007). Cited in Koska, M. and Baker, L. Smart
    Injection Programme. Available at:
    www.safepointtrust.org/smartinjections_files/
    Smart_Injection_Programme_Nov07.pdf,
    accessed July 21, 2011.
World Bank. (2011). World Development Indicators
    database. Available at: http://data.worldbank.
    org/region/SSA.
Zucker, J. R., Lackritz, E. M., Ruebush, T. K.,
    Hightower, A. W., Adungosi, J. E., Were, J. B.
    and Campbell, C. C. (1994). Anaemia, blood
    transfusion practices, HIV and mortality among
    women of reproductive age in western Kenya.
    Trans R Soc Trop Med Hyg. 1994 Mar–Apr;
    88(2): 173–6.

Prevention of non-sexual transmission of HIV

Perspective paper

ROB BALTUSSEN AND JAN HONTELEZ

The contribution by Bollinger (Bollinger 2011) on the costs, effect, and cost-effectiveness of prevention of non-sexual HIV infections in sub-Saharan Africa is an ambitious undertaking. This perspective paper qualifies the merits of the analysis, and puts forward a number of important issues to consider when interpreting its results. We first reflect on the options and limitations of detailed continent-wide analysis in the absence of comprehensive data and then identify a number of analytical shortcomings. We proceed by presenting results from other studies based on country-level analysis, and finally draw a number of conclusions.

Options and limitations of multi-country analyses

The study provides cost, effect, and cost-effectiveness estimates at the continent level, on the basis of individual analyses for each of forty-four countries in sub-Saharan Africa. Compared to previous similar analysis by e.g. Floyd *et al.* (Creese *et al.* 2002) that provided single cost-effectiveness estimates for sub-Saharan Africa as a whole, and Hogan *et al.* (Hogan *et al.* 2005) that provided estimates for several African sub-regions, the study has the potential to bring more detail and therefore credibility to its estimates. At the same time, the question is whether the study can actually live up to these standards – does it really provide estimates that are sufficiently transparent, valid, and reliable at the country level? Unfortunately, we do have doubts on this, and we identify four key issues.

First, at the analytical level, the study relies on a range of models under the name of SPECTRUM to make country-specific models and subsequently projections of the HIV/AIDS epidemic – it is not clear to what extent these models reflect the actual epidemiology in the country of analysis. Estimates are said to be based on a number of country-level workshops, but no indication is given as to the goodness of fit of the resulting models. Second, in these kinds of analyses, where subgroups of the HIV epidemic are investigated, it is important to have adequate estimates of the relative contribution of each transmission route to the overall epidemic. Although the Modes of Transmission (MoT) initiative (Colvin *et al.* 2011) aims at mapping the attributable fraction of different transmission routes in individual countries, the methodology is questionable and ultimately depends on local data, which is often unreliable or missing. The assumed number of infections caused by unsafe medical injections, IDU use, or blood transfusions is therefore subject to high levels of uncertainty. Third, and closely related, the impact of the interventions is estimated on the basis of an impact matrix, that reflects the reported evidence of almost 200 preventive interventions – however, it is not known to what extent these reflect the intervention effectiveness of the countries under study. Average effectiveness estimates are not necessarily locally meaningful, as they are subject to a wide range of local practices (e.g. needle exchange programs are culturally very sensitive). Fourth, the study often relies on costing data that is extrapolated from a small number of other countries, or are based on international prices (e.g. that of ARV drugs) and its accuracy can only be guessed. Having said this, it should be noted that the above limitations are inherent to the task at hand and therefore virtually inevitable – any detailed country analysis in the absence of comprehensive data is fraught with difficulties. At the same time, this places question marks on the usefulness of studies of this nature, and whether series of high-quality country-level studies may not be more relevant.

Methods of analysis

The study also suffers from a number of shortcomings related to (analytical) choices made by the author. First, the study falls short in its presentation – most importantly, it only presents summary information for sub-Saharan Africa as a whole, and not for the individual countries. A more detailed documentation of the analysis, country by country, would add the necessary transparency to the study. Also, sources of data are not always presented, or are presented without argumentation. For example, the HIV transmission probability of contaminated blood is assumed to be 90 percent, but the reader cannot make a judgement on the strength of the evidence behind this assumption. Tables listing all variables and their values, including sources and strengths of evidence, would have been most useful. More generally, the author presents some overview of the cost-effectiveness of preventive interventions to reduce non-sexual transmission – it is not clear whether this is a literature review (if so, what are the sources?) or a summary of the present study (if so, how did the author come to the conclusion that opioid substitution therapy may not be cost-effective?).

Second, cost estimates are not optimal. For example, the author assumes linear cost function whereas evidence is available that, with increasing coverage, costs increase or diminish depending on the program under study (Johns and Torres 2005). Detailed estimates are also available (WHO-CHOICE 2011). Also, in estimating costs of averted infections, the author assumes all patients receive anti-retroviral treatment – this is of course a gross overestimate and not realistic. Furthermore, in extrapolating cost estimates

from country to country, proper analysis distinguishes prices and quantities and adapts the former to price levels of the country under study, and where possible the latter to local resource utilization patterns. The author follows this methodology to calculate unit costs of the prevention of mother-to-child transmission (pMTCT) but fails to do this for safe medical injections and safe blood transfusions – the unit costs of the latter are based on median costs as reported in a limited number of studies, and one can only guess whether this reflects real costs.

Third, effectiveness and benefit estimates have important shortcomings resulting in a gross overestimation of the number of life years gained and net financial gains of the evaluated prevention interventions. The direct effectiveness outcomes – that result from the modeling exercise – are the number of infections prevented, which are then used to calculate the number of life years saved by multiplying the number with a certain standard. This approach ignores the dynamics of an HIV infection and antiretroviral therapy such as the natural history, time till treatment eligibility (i.e., when CD4 cell counts drop below 350 cells/μL), health-seeking behavior of individuals, treatment coverage, etc. This introduces important biases into the analysis. Most importantly, it seems like the author simply subtracts the age of infection from the life expectancy at birth to calculate the number of life years gained per averted infection (e.g., an averted infection due to reduced unsafe drug injections at, on average, age twenty-two would lead to $65 - 22 = 43$ life years gained). This implies that a person with an HIV infection dies at age twenty-two, which is an unrealistic assumption, resulting in a gross overestimation of the number of life years gained of preventing an infection. The average survival of an untreated HIV infection is about eleven years, while ART will further increase life expectancy by about twenty years. Thus, a person would not die at age twenty-two (age of infection), but at age fifty, resulting in fifteen life years gained, almost three times lower compared to the forty-two years calculated by the author. This overestimation becomes especially apparent in the calculations regarding pMTCT, where the number of life years gained of one prevented infection is sixty-five. Also, estimates of life years gained are based on a standardized average African life expectancy of sixty-five years – the rationale must be that the use of realistic but lower life expectancies in some countries (as in Sierra Leone, where life expectancy is thirty-seven years) would render interventions in these countries less cost-effective. However, this rationale is only valid where countries can be compared in terms of economic attractiveness of interventions, which is not the purpose in the present study. Hence, the use of an artificial life expectancy of sixty-five years is misleading, and overestimates the economic attractiveness.

Fourth, the author presents cost-effectiveness estimates in terms of cost per infection averted, and compares these to international benchmarks as put forward by the Commission of Macroeconomics and Health (CMH). CMH states that interventions that cost, per DALY averted, less than one time gross national income (GNI) per capita can be considered cost-effective. The author makes a clear mistake by comparing *cost per infection* averted to the CMH benchmark, that is – as said – expressed as *cost per DALY* averted. Since the number of DALYs saved from (preventive) interventions is 10–15 times higher than the number of averted infections, the resulting conclusions are seriously flawed, and the economic attractiveness of intervention – when compared to CMH benchmarks – is much better than presented. Also, the author used the PPP-adjusted GNI in the calculations, whereas the cost estimates are in ordinary dollars: the result is that the benchmark – already wrongly interpreted – is also wrongly valued. In addition, it is rather confusing and theoretically incorrect to employ two different monetary benchmarks for a life year saved, i.e., that of the CMH ($1,125) and the value as put forward by *RethinkHIV* ($1,000–5,000). These values have the same conceptual underpinning, and either one of them should be used throughout the analysis.

Fifth, and more specifically, in the analysis on IDU-related infections, the author combines costs and effectiveness of three different interventions – (i) outreach/information and education campaigns; (ii) needle and syringe exchange programs; and (iii) opioid substitution therapy. This very much limits the interpretation of results. Together, the interventions are said to be moderately economically attractive – but it is not clear whether there is large variation in the cost-effectiveness of the individual interventions and e.g. one, highly cost-ineffective, intervention that dominates the others.

Preventive versus treatment interventions

A more general observation relates to the role of this study in the broader *RethinkHIV* project. We applaud the use of a fairly consistent methodological approach in the present paper to evaluate sets of interventions. This is definitely a virtue, and allows a direct comparison of the relative economic attractiveness of these interventions and the identification of "best buys." The "science" of cost-effectiveness analyses typically focuses on a single intervention only and employs different methodological approaches, and as a consequence their results are difficult to compare. The present study design overcomes this problem. However, an important caveat is that present results may be difficult to compare to other studies in the same series of *RethinkHIV*. Most important is the choice to express health effects of interventions in terms of infections averted – this provides an uneven playing level for the comparison of economic attractiveness of preventive and treatment interventions as it is not the sole aim of the latter to prevent infections. In other words, by defining outcomes in averted infections, preventive interventions are advantaged over treatment interventions. The use of life years gained as a common outcome measure would have provided a more equal playing ground.

Given the above-mentioned important limitations, the added value of the presented analyses should be considered carefully. The cost-effectiveness of preventing non-sexually transmitted HIV – especially mother-to-child transmission – in sub-Saharan Africa has been extensively studied by others (Wilkinson, Floyd *et al.* 2000; Sweat, O'Reilly *et al.* 2004; Maclean and Stringer 2005; Soorapanth, Sansom *et al.* 2006; Robberstad and Evjen-Olsen 2010; van Hulst, Smit Sibinga *et al.* 2010; Alistar, Owens *et al.* 2011; Johri and Ako-Arrey 2011; Shah, Johns *et al.* 2011). Although these studies are usually country-based rather than continent-based, they do provide more comprehensive data and analyses on the likely impact of interventions that prevent the non-sexual transmission of HIV. Robberstad *et al.* found that the incremental cost of preventing one child infection of HIV in Tanzania is $4,062, while the cost per DALY averted is $162 (Robberstad and Evjen-Olsen 2010). These results are in line with Shah *et al.* who modeled the cost-effectiveness of the new WHO recommendations on pMTCT in Nigeria, showing that new WHO treatment guidelines cost $113 per DALY averted (Shah, Johns *et al.* 2011). Although the comparison with the results of Bollinger is difficult, since the author only presents continent-wide results and gives costs per averted infection, the cost estimates and thus cost-effectiveness ratios in the analyses by Robberstad *et al.* and Shah *et al.* are considerably higher than the $520 per infection averted calculated by Bollinger (nearly eight times lower than estimated by Robberstad *et al.*), indicating that the results presented by Bollinger might be overly optimistic.

In addition, others have shown that needle exchange programs and opiate substitute therapies can be highly cost-effective (Alistar, Owens *et al.* 2011), which is in contrast to Bollinger, who concludes that these interventions are not cost-effective. However, the cost-effectiveness of HIV prevention interventions in IDUs is largely determined by the HIV prevalence in the IDU population (Cohen, Wu *et al.* 2004). Here, Bollinger highlights an important gap in knowledge: some information regarding injecting drug use was available in only four of the forty-four countries in the analyses. For most sub-Saharan African countries, data on the size of the injecting drug use population and HIV prevalence among these drug users are absent (Strathdee and Stockman 2010), leaving us guessing as to the real size of the problem and the likely cost-effectiveness of interventions. Finally, current knowledge regarding the cost-effectiveness of preventing HIV through providing safe medical injections or screening of donor blood is considerably less. Nevertheless, these interventions are relatively cheap and easy to implement, and are therefore likely to be highly economically attractive (van Hulst, Smit Sibinga *et al.* 2010).

Equity in resource allocation

A general critique on cost-effectiveness and cost-benefit analysis is that it ignores the question of *who benefits* from interventions. For purposes of equity, policy-makers may well want to give priority to certain disadvantaged groups in society to give them as much of a fair chance to live a healthy life. However, interventions that target disadvantaged groups in society may well be more costly and/or yield less health effects, and will not necessarily be most cost-effective or cost-beneficial. For example, mobile clinics are more costly than central distribution of ARVs but greatly improve service coverage among remote areas. Policy-makers thus need to strike a balance between efficiency and equity objectives in health when setting priorities. Unfortunately, as in the present study, these equity aspects are seldom reported, and it is not clear at what (extra) costs disadvantaged groups can be reached.

Conclusion

To conclude, the effort of the author to conduct an economic analysis of the prevention of non-sexual infection of HIV in not less than forty-four sub-Saharan African countries is an ambitious undertaking. The study suffers from the inherent limitations of such a continent-wide analysis, and a number of other, avoidable, methodological shortcomings which hamper the interpretation of the results. On the other hand, the results from this and other studies regarding the cost-effectiveness of the presented interventions – either because the intervention is easy and cheap (providing clean needles for medical injections and screening donated blood) or because a large number of infections can be prevented (prevention of mother-to-child transmission) – are so overwhelming that we tend to agree with the author's conclusions that interventions to reduce non-sexual transmission of HIV are generally economically attractive.

References

Alistar, S. S., Owens, D. K. *et al.* (2011). Effectiveness and cost effectiveness of expanding harm reduction and antiretroviral therapy in a mixed HIV epidemic: a modeling analysis for Ukraine. *PLoS Med* **8**(3): e1000423.

Bollinger, L. (2011 forthcoming). Prevention of non-sexual transmission of HIV. Assessment paper for *RethinkHIV*.

Cohen, D. A., Wu, S. Y. *et al*. (2004). Comparing the cost-effectiveness of HIV prevention interventions. *J Acquir Immune Defic Syndr* **37**(3): 1404–14.

Colvin, M., Gorgens-Albino, M. and Kasedde, S. Analysis of HIV Prevention Response and Modes of HIV Transmission: The UNAIDS-GAMET Supported Synthesis Process. Available at www.unaidsrstesa.org/sites/default/files/modesoftransmission/analysis_hiv_prevention_response_and_mot.pdf, accessed August 15, 2011.

Creese, A., Floyd, K., Alban, A. and Guinness, L. (2002). Cost-effectiveness of HIV/AIDS interventions in Africa: a systematic review of the evidence. *Lancet*. May 11; **359**(9318): 1635–43.

Hogan, D. R., Baltussen, R., Hayashi, C., Lauer, J. A. and Salomon, J. A. (2005). Cost effectiveness analysis of strategies to combat HIV/AIDS in developing countries. *BMJ*. Dec 17; **331**(7530): 1431–7. Epub 2005 Nov 10.

Johns, B. and Torres, T. T. (2005). Costs of scaling up health interventions: a systematic review. *Health Policy Plan*. Jan; **20**(1): 1–13.

Johri, M. and Ako-Arrey, D. (2011). The cost-effectiveness of preventing mother-to-child transmission of HIV in low- and middle-income countries: systematic review. *Cost Eff Resour Alloc* **9**: 3.

Maclean, C. C. and Stringer, J. S. (2005). Potential cost-effectiveness of maternal and infant antiretroviral interventions to prevent mother-to-child transmission during breast-feeding. *J Acquir Immune Defic Syndr* **38**(5): 570–7.

Robberstad, B. and Evjen-Olsen, B. (2010). Preventing mother to child transmission of HIV with highly active antiretroviral treatment in Tanzania – a prospective cost-effectiveness study. *J Acquir Immune Defic Syndr* **55**(3): 397–403.

Shah, M., Johns, B. *et al*. (2011). Cost-effectiveness of new WHO recommendations for prevention of mother-to-child transmission of HIV in a resource-limited setting. *AIDS* **25**(8): 1093–102.

Soorapanth, S., Sansom, S. *et al*. (2006). Cost-effectiveness of HIV rescreening during late pregnancy to prevent mother-to-child HIV transmission in South Africa and other resource-limited settings. *J Acquir Immune Defic Syndr* **42**(2): 213–21.

Strathdee, S. A. and Stockman, J. K. (2010). Epidemiology of HIV among injecting and non-injecting drug users: current trends and implications for interventions. *Curr HIV/AIDS Rep* **7**(2): 99–106.

Sweat, M. D., O'Reilly, K. R. *et al*. (2004). Cost-effectiveness of nevirapine to prevent mother-to-child HIV transmission in eight African countries. *AIDS* **18**(12): 1661–71.

van Hulst, M., Smit Sibinga, C. T. *et al*. (2010). Health economics of blood transfusion safety – focus on sub-Saharan Africa. *Biologicals* **38**(1): 53–8.

WHO-CHOICE website, available at www.who.int/choice. Accessed August 15, 2011.

Wilkinson, D., Floyd, K. *et al*. (2000). National and provincial estimated costs and cost effectiveness of a programme to reduce mother-to-child HIV transmission in South Africa. *S Afr Med J* **90**(8): 794–8.

2.2 Prevention of non-sexual transmission of HIV

Mother-to-child transmission

Perspective paper

MIRA JOHRI

This perspective paper focuses on a single mode of non-sexual HIV transmission, mother-to-child transmission (MTCT), currently responsible for about 20 percent of new HIV infections annually in sub-Saharan Africa. Specifically, it examines the assessment paper (AP) proposal to evaluate the costs and benefits of a single strategy to prevent MTCT, consisting of WHO Option A delivered to over 90 percent of pregnant women by 2015 via a pattern of linear scale-up from current levels (Bollinger 2011). After some general comments on the methods and findings of the AP, a critical assessment is developed in three steps:

(1) The first section reviews the reasoning surrounding the choice of WHO Option A as the key MTCT strategy. It assesses representation of Option A in the analysis and finds that it fails fully to capture costs. It also demonstrates that methodological and modeling choices lead to a truncated assessment of benefits, such that potentially relevant differences among therapeutic options A, B, and B+ are not considered. The section concludes that analysis of a more comprehensive range of MTCT intervention options is required, including family planning, reproductive counseling, cotrimoxazole prophylaxis, early infant diagnosis, maternal ART for women requiring therapy for their own health, and WHO Options A, B, and B+.
(2) The second section examines the assumption of linear program scale-up. The production function for an intervention is rarely described in economic evaluations and results are usually given without regard to program scale. The costs and cost-effectiveness of preventing

mother-to-child transmission (pMTCT) programs are substantially affected by variations in HIV prevalence and health system infrastructure. Within countries, existing MTCT programs are generally located in settings of higher HIV prevalence and better health infrastructure, with the result that the costs of scale-up are likely to be importantly non-linear. The term pMTCT "cascade" has been used to describe the sequence of steps required to deliver antiretroviral-based MTCT interventions to HIV-positive mothers and their infants. It is argued that, at the population level, health system performance at each step of the cascade is likely to be the single most important factor for determining the number of infections in children.

(3) The final section sketches four additional MTCT intervention strategies that are likely to offer good value for money in some contexts and have received less attention to date. These include interventions to improve health system performance, HIV screening in the labor ward, and interventions to interrupt MTCT for HIV-positive women not delivering in a health facility. Most importantly, this section highlights the potential of an emerging "leapfrog" technology, multiplex point-of-care diagnostics, to overcome the problems outlined above. This technology could play a decisive role in increasing access to the pMTCT cascade while providing good value for money and thus, in synergy with health system improvements, in

My sincere thanks to Dr. Nigel Rollins, World Health Organization, for very insightful comments. All errors remain my own.

elimination of new infant HIV infections. Prevention of HIV transmission from mother-to-child is a high leverage intervention with implications for health and development. It is an opportunity too important to miss.

General comments

Methods of the assessment

The main purpose of an economic evaluation is to inform judgments about the relative worth or "value for money" of two or more alternative interventions or strategies. *RethinkHIV* requires that interventions be assessed through cost-benefit analysis (CBA). The measure of net benefit calculated in the assessment paper considers the costs of providing the intervention, and the benefits in monetary terms associated with an HIV infection averted. Benefits accrue from two sources. First, HIV infections averted are translated into an estimate of life years gained, and these life years are valued at levels recommended by *RethinkHIV*. Second, the analysis considers savings in treatment costs associated with HIV infections averted; specifically, expenditure averted for provision of anti-retroviral therapy and treatment of opportunistic infections.

Although not commonly used in health care settings, CBA is the only form of economic evaluation that directly addresses allocative efficiency (efficiency between sectors), and it can consider dimensions not included in standard cost-effectiveness analyses. However, the assessment paper analysis does not take up the opportunity to address the broader economic and social benefits of the interventions studied, such as productivity gains, impact on household poverty, orphaned children, catastrophic expenditure, impact on epidemic spread, educational attainment, fertility patterns, and macroeconomic impact. Data on these broader impacts may be difficult to assemble in a convincing way, and the complexity of the causal chains introduces additional difficulties for modeling of consequences. Nonetheless, it is important to note that the CBA analysis of benefits in the assessment paper is driven entirely by the outcome of an HIV infection averted. I will return to the

issue of comprehensiveness of the CBA below, in the context of pMTCT.

Prevention of mother-to-child transmission of HIV

Access to services to prevent MTCT has increased worldwide, leading to a steep drop in the number of children newly infected with HIV. Incident cases of pediatric HIV are 24 percent lower in 2009 as compared to five years earlier (United Nations Joint Programme on HIV/AIDS (UNAIDS) 2010), an unprecedented achievement that has led to calls for virtual elimination of HIV transmission from mother-to-child (United Nations Joint Programme on HIV/AIDS (UNAIDS) 2011). Despite these successes, an estimated 370,000 (95 percent CI: 230,000 to 510,000) children were newly infected in 2009 (United Nations Joint Programme on HIV/AIDS (UNAIDS) 2010). Twenty-two countries have the highest burden of HIV-positive pregnant women and therefore account for almost 90 percent of all new infant HIV infections. Twenty-one are in sub-Saharan Africa (SSA) (United Nations Joint Programme on HIV/AIDS (UNAIDS) 2010).

Comprehensive versus narrow approaches to pMTCT

Earlier this year, UNAIDS released a global plan to eliminate new HIV infections among children and to keep their mothers alive (United Nations Joint Programme on HIV/AIDS (UNAIDS) 2011). The plan is based on two targets: (1) reducing the number of new HIV infections among children by 90 percent; and (2) reducing the number of AIDS-related maternal deaths by 50 percent (United Nations Joint Programme on HIV/AIDS (UNAIDS) 2011). The strategy is multifaceted, consistent with the UN comprehensive approach to prevent MTCT based on four components: (1) primary prevention of HIV infection among women of childbearing age; (2) preventing unintended pregnancies among women living with HIV; (3) preventing HIV transmission from a woman living with HIV to her infant; and (4) providing appropriate treatment, care, and support to mothers living with HIV and their children and families. With respect to component 3, the virtual elimination goal specifies that MTCT be reduced to below 5 percent in breastfeeding populations, and 2 percent in non-breastfeeding populations (Mahy, Stover *et al.* 2010; United Nations Joint Programme on HIV/AIDS (UNAIDS) 2011).

Like virtually all cost-effectiveness analyses to date, the AP focuses only on "component 3" of the recommended four-prong MTCT strategy; that is, prevention of HIV transmission from a woman living with HIV to her infant (Johri and Ako-Arrey 2011). In policy terms, this focus appears too narrow, as prongs 1, 2, and 3 are synergistic and necessary to achieve the targeted 90 percent reduction in child HIV infections, and prongs 1 and 2 have received less support and success to date (Reynolds, Janowitz *et al.* 2006; Halperin, Stover *et al.* 2009; Mahy, Stover *et al.* 2010). Although this focus is to some extent encouraged by the division of topics mandated by *RethinkHIV* for this assessment of HIV/AIDS, it is important to take note of this choice from the outset and to trace its implications for the analysis. Noting that family planning is required to achieve the targeted 90 percent reduction in child HIV infections, a recent investment case analysis included a cost of $20 per woman screened per year (Schwartländer, Stover *et al.* 2011). Inclusion of a similar program component in the AP would add a minimum of one hundred million dollars to the costs of the strategy,[1] as well as appreciable additional benefits due to a reduction in non-HIV deaths among children and mothers.

Prevention of HIV transmission from mother to child: intervention options

Virtually all HIV-infected children acquire the infection through mother-to-child transmission (MTCT), which can occur during pregnancy, labor, and delivery, or through breastfeeding. In the absence of any intervention an estimated 15–30 percent of mothers with HIV infection will transmit the infection during pregnancy and delivery, and breastfeeding by an infected mother increases

the risk by a further 5–20 percent, to 20–45 percent overall (World Health Organization 2010; UNAIDS Reference Group on Estimates Modelling and Projections 2011).

Interventions to prevent transmission from an HIV-positive mother to her child (component 3 of the comprehensive pMTCT strategy) can dramatically reduce this risk, and have succeeded in virtually eliminating MTCT in high-income countries (HICs).[2] A number of intervention options exist, each with different resource requirements and levels of associated clinical benefit. All involve administration of anti-retroviral drugs to mother and infant. For low- and middle-income countries (LMICs), new WHO guidelines introduced in 2010 depart from previous approaches in emphasizing the importance of treating eligible pregnant women living with HIV requiring treatment for their own health (the suggested criterion is a CD4 cell count of less than 350 cells/μl) with triple combination anti-retroviral therapy (ART)[3] (World Health Organization 2010). The guidelines also recommend two equivalent options of anti-retroviral prophylaxis to prevent MTCT for women with CD4 cell counts greater than 350 cells/μl, and for the first time make provision for prophylaxis to the mother or child during breastfeeding (World Health Organization 2010). "Option A" is based on a less intensive

---

[1] The AP projects 265,000 infant infections averted. Multiplying by 20 gives the number of women screened, under the approximation that HIV prevalence among adults 15–49 years in sub-Saharan Africa is 5% (UNAIDS 2010). These 5.3 million women screened would incur costs of $20 each for a twelve-month family planning intervention = $106 million. This constitutes a minimum cost estimate. Assuming that roughly one million women are screened in each of the five years of the strategy, and that women receive family planning in each subsequent program year, the family planning intervention would cost roughly $300 million (or $270 million with 3% discounting).

[2] Country income classifications are taken from the World Bank (World Bank 2009).

[3] Following emerging practice, this paper uses "ARV" to refer to any single or dual anti-retroviral drug regimen used for pMTCT, and "ART" to refer to three-drug combination therapy (whether used for pMTCT or treatment of maternal HIV disease). "Prophylaxis" refers to the situation where ARV or ART is administered for purposes of pMTCT and is contrasted with "treatment" which refers to the situation where ART is administered for a woman's health.

medications anti-retroviral prophylaxis regimen (ARV) during pregnancy and breastfeeding, while "Option B" is based on triple drug prophylaxis (ART) during pregnancy and breastfeeding (World Health Organization 2010). An additional strategy now under discussion, "Option B+," proposes that all HIV-positive women be given lifelong ART, regardless of CD4 count or disease stage (National Institutes of Health: IMPAACT Trial Network 2010; Schouten, Jahn et al. 2011).

Of these therapeutic options, Option A has the lowest medication costs. Moreover, the effectiveness of these strategies in preventing MTCT in the perinatal period and during breastfeeding is considered equivalent (World Health Organization 2010; UNAIDS Reference Group on Estimates Modelling and Projections 2011). The AP therefore chooses to evaluate the costs and benefits of a single strategy, consisting of Option A delivered to over 90 percent of pregnant women by 2015. The analysis of costs associated with Option A includes counseling and testing, medication and service delivery, and a laboratory component, drawn from a recent investment framework analysis by Schwartländer and colleagues (Schwartländer, Stover et al. 2011).

The AP analysis of costs associated with Option A is importantly underestimated. Since CD4 cell counts are unknown at the time of screening, Option A offers the medication regimens costed in the AP for women with CD4 cell counts above 350, and also includes the provision that women detected as HIV-positive with CD4 <350 should receive ART for their own health. At the point of screening, approximately 48 percent of HIV-positive women are expected to have a CD4 cell count <350 (2010), and should therefore receive ART. The costs associated with provision of ART from week 14 (start of therapy) to 12 months (recommended cessation of breastfeeding according to WHO guidelines) should hence be included in the costs for Option A, for the 48 percent of women expected to have CD4 counts below 350 cells/μl. This was the practice followed in the investment framework analysis from which unit costs for this section were otherwise directly drawn (Schwartländer, Stover et al. 2011). Concretely, this means that base case costs for Option A should increase by almost $100 million.[4]

Second, laboratory facilities are often lacking and the investment framework analysis explicitly does not include the costs of laboratory start-up and infrastructure (Schwartländer, Stover et al. 2011). Implications of the linear scale-up assumption for laboratory and other infrastructure costs are considered below.

A corollary of this correction is that the difference in cost between intervention options is considerably less than portrayed in the AP.[5] A number of additional elements enter into selection of an appropriate MTCT intervention option, as countries must make decisions that balance a wide range of factors and in the face of considerable uncertainty. In terms of effectiveness in preventing infant infections, the current estimates should be viewed as provisional, as no studies report specifically on all components of the ARV interventions recommended in either Options A or B in the population for whom the option is recommended (UNAIDS Reference Group on Estimates Modelling and Projections 2011). Furthermore, no empirical study has as yet provided a comparison of Options A and B (UNAIDS Reference Group on Estimates Modelling and Projections 2011). Option B+ has not yet been directly studied, although a number of studies now in the field are soon expected to contribute new information (Mofenson 2010). Operationally,

---

[4] The AP presents 265,000 infant infections averted, which is roughly 265,000 women treated. If 48% have CD4 <350 at the point of screening and therefore require ART for their own health, and ART costs an additional $363 per patient ($600 ART – $237 medication costs already included in the analysis), the revised costs should be: 265,000*0.48*363 = $96.2 million.

[5] The AP assesses the cost of Option A as $196 million. Correcting for the omitted costs for women with CD4 counts below 350 during the period of pregnancy and breastfeeding yields a revised cost for Option A of (196 + 96) $292 million. The strategy presented in the AP as Option B+ considers costs from fourteen weeks' gestation to six months. Option B thus costs at least $333 million. The difference between Options B and B+ is impossible to capture within the timeframe of the analysis, and we agree with Dr. Bollinger that costs outside the period of pregnancy and breastfeeding may not be properly attributable to the pMTCT program. All unit costs here and in the AP are from the UNAIDS investment framework (Schwartländer, Stover et al. 2011); the AP considers a six- rather than a twelve-month breastfeeding period.

Option A requires a CD4 cell count reading to initiate therapy; however, the laboratory infrastructure required to provide a CD4 cell count is often lacking. Provision of Option A to breastfeeding mothers with CD4 counts of 200–350 is not recommended; yet this situation may arise where the infrastructure needed to perform CD4 counts is not in place (UNAIDS Reference Group on Estimates Modelling and Projections 2011). Option B requires a CD4 reading only to stop therapy, leaving time for travel or transport of specimens to be arranged. Option B+ proposes to guide therapy with minimal laboratory monitoring. In terms of safety to mothers, there are concerns about nevirapine-induced rash associated with Option A, provision of ART to healthy women associated with Options B and B+, and the impact on maternal health of the ART initiation and discontinuation strategies required by Option B (Mofenson 2010). In terms of safety to infants, Options B and B+ also raise unanswered questions about potential adverse pregnancy outcomes associated with receipt of ART, and potential teratogenicity associated with unintentional use of Efavirenz during the first trimester (Mofenson 2010). All three options are likely to stimulate resistance in infants who are infected during breastfeeding, making it necessary to foresee the use of second-line therapies (Mofenson 2010). Despite these concerns, there are important factors favoring Options B and B+.

Study conclusions can be importantly influenced by methodological and modeling choices (Brisson and Edmunds 2006). The AP uses a static natural history model to depict the process of HIV transmission from mother to child, focusing on the outcome of averting an infant HIV infection. The analysis is potentially truncated in several ways, such that potentially relevant differences among options are not captured.

- Maternal health and child survival: the WHO (2010) guidelines for pMTCT introduce new therapeutic strategies that promote the use of ART for a woman's own health and antiviral regimens during the breastfeeding period to prevent HIV transmission from mother to child (World Health Organization 2010). The most important gains of the new strategy are likely to be through impact on maternal health and child survival, which are not considered in the AP nor in any cost-effectiveness models of pMTCT published to date (Johri and Ako-Arrey 2011). With respect to child survival, the proposed interventions (Options A or B, including ART as required for a woman's health) are designed to make breastfeeding a good option for HIV-infected mothers as opposed to formula feeding. This is one of the greatest benefits of the new strategy, as it substantially reduces infection of HIV-exposed infants during the breastfeeding period. In addition, infants who are able to breastfeed safely are thereby protected against other major causes of mortality such as diarrhoea, pneumonia, and malnutrition (World Health Organization 2010). Also of relevance to assessment of the 2010 pMTCT strategies is the effect of ART on maternal survival and the downstream effect of maternal survival on child survival. Cost-effectiveness estimates that fail to capture these dimensions are likely to be inaccurate and to underestimate the full benefits of pMTCT interventions.

- In addition, focus on an infant HIV infection averted may fail to capture potentially relevant differences among specific intervention options. For example, therapeutic options may have different impacts on maternal health. A model-based comparison of the effectiveness of Options A, B, and B+ contextualized to Zimbabwe found that projected maternal and infant life expectancy was highest for Option B+ (Ciaranello, Perez *et al.* 2011). This finding is limited by lack of data and cannot be considered conclusive at this juncture. However, it illustrates the importance of capturing differences in the survival of mothers and infants in the analysis.

- Analytic timeframe: published cost-effectiveness studies of pMTCT have been based on a cohort perspective and consider a short timeframe bounded by the initiation of antenatal care (ANC) and cessation of breastfeeding (Johri and Ako-Arrey 2011). Fertility is very high in SSA and it is of relevance that a woman who is detected as HIV-positive during pregnancy is likely to have children in future. MTCT rates are substantially lower for women taking ART prior to pregnancy, such that Option B+ may

Table 2.2.1 Comparison of recommended therapeutic options in women with CD4 >350 who do not require therapy for their own health[1]

Criterion	Option A: Maternal AZT and Infant daily NVP	Option B: Maternal Triple ARV Prophylaxis	Option B+: Lifelong Maternal Triple ARV Prophylaxis
Efficacy in preventing MTCT[2]	Peripartum 2% Postpartum 0.2% per month	Peripartum 2% Postpartum 0.2% per month	Peripartum 2% Postpartum 0.2% per month
Feasibility	CD4 monitoring required to initiate therapy	ART initiated for all HIV-infected pregnant women CD4 monitoring needed to determine when to stop ART	ART for all HIV-infected pregnant women
Protection against forward (adult-to-adult) transmission of the HIV virus?	No	Yes, during pregnancy and breastfeeding	Yes
Optimal protection against HIV transmission for future pregnancies?[3]	No	No	Yes Pre-pregnancy ART Tx rates Peripartum 0.5% Postpartum 0.16% per month

[1] This table does not consider clinical criteria relating to the possible differential impact of therapeutic options on maternal and child health, as the key issues are as yet unresolved.
[2] All three strategies are viewed as identical in efficacy at the present time. These are estimates for MTCT transmission rates peripartum, and per month of postpartum HIV exposure through breastfeeding. Estimates are based on expert consensus synthesizing data from studies using similar regimens. There are no studies that report specifically on all components of the ARV interventions recommended in either Options A or B in the population for whom the option is recommended (UNAIDS Reference Group on Estimates Modelling and Projections 2011). Option B+ has not yet been studied.
[3] These are expert consensus estimates for MTCT transmission rates in women taking ART prior to pregnancy. Rates are given separately for the peripartum period, and per month of postpartum HIV exposure through breastfeeding (UNAIDS Reference Group on Estimates Modelling and Projections 2011).

be of substantial benefit to future children of an HIV-infected mother (Schouten, Jahn *et al.* 2011). Consideration of a longitudinal perspective would clarify this point and likely suggest a different ranking of strategies.

- Impact on forward transmission: receipt of ART by an HIV-positive person reduces HIV viral load, which has been demonstrated to provide protection against transmission of the virus to non-HIV-infected partners (Anglemyer, Rutherford *et al.* 2011). Option B+, which offers lifelong ART, may therefore have a positive impact on epidemic transmission (Schouten, Jahn *et al.* 2011). However, the dynamics of infection and transmission in the general population are not considered the assessment paper.

A broader comparison of therapeutic options A, B, and B+ is presented in Table 2.2.1. Questions remain about the comparative efficacy and safety of the three options; however, from a population health perspective, the "test and treat" approach reflected in Option B+ has the potential to offer substantially higher health benefits. The advantages it offers are likely to be particularly important when HIV prevalence is high, fertility rates are high, and health system infrastructure limited. Medication costs associated with Option B+ are higher, but potentially offset by lower laboratory costs and enhanced feasibility leading to greater uptake. In some contexts, Option B+ may thus have a more favorable cost-benefit profile.

In sum, the AP's focus on Option A as the intervention of choice seems to be shaped importantly by modeling decisions, as many relevant factors cannot be captured in a static natural history model with a short timeframe. All three options are of live policy importance. Of the seventeen sub-Saharan African high-burden countries that have chosen a policy option, ten (Cameroon, Kenya, Lesotho, Mozambique, Namibia, South Africa, Swaziland, Uganda, Zambia, and Zimbabwe) have chosen

Option A, five (Botswana, Burundi, Chad, Côte d'Ivoire, and Ghana) have chosen Option B, one (Nigeria) has chosen a combination of Options A (rural) and B (urban), and one (Malawi) has chosen Option B+ (UNICEF 2011). Both Options A and B were considered in a recent analysis of investment needs for HIV, as well as family planning, reproductive counseling, cotrimoxazole prophylaxis, and early infant diagnosis (Schwartländer, Stover et al. 2011). These interventions are similar to those considered in the UNAIDS global plan to eliminate new infant HIV infections (United Nations Joint Programme on HIV/AIDS (UNAIDS) 2011). I have argued above that Option B+ should also be given serious consideration. A more comprehensive range of MTCT intervention options is required.

Scale-up of interventions to prevent transmission from HIV-positive mother to child: key challenges

Interventions to prevent transmission from a woman living with HIV to her infant (component 3 of the comprehensive pMTCT strategy) are simple, modest in cost, and highly effective interventions backed by strong technical guidance, and as such, ideal candidates for widespread scale-up (Yamey 2011). While acknowledging the importance of additional investment in infrastructure for reproductive and child health (considered in a separate paper for this HIV/AIDS exercise), the AP models a linear scale-up pattern for the proposed pMTCT strategy, starting from contemporary levels and increasing linearly until 90 percent coverage is reached in 2015. It is useful to examine factors likely to affect the linearity of scale-up, particularly with respect to costs.

The costs of preventing transmission from a woman living with HIV to her child can be divided into two categories: the cost of detecting a case of HIV in a pregnant woman, and the cost of administering appropriate interventions to prevent MTCT once detected. These costs depend on two factors:

- HIV prevalence: currently recommended interventions to prevent pediatric infections have been found to be cost-effective in a variety of LMIC

settings as measured against accepted international benchmarks (Orlando, Marazzi et al. 2010; Robberstad and Evjen-Olsen 2010; Johri and Ako-Arrey 2011; Shah, Johns et al. 2011); however, there are challenges for efficient delivery of these interventions in low HIV prevalence settings (Rely, Bertozzi et al. 2003; Kumar, Birch et al. 2006; Johri and Ako-Arrey 2011). In settings of low HIV prevalence, the costs of case findings may be high relative to health benefits obtained. Collectively, the published literature suggests that, in settings where HIV prevalence in the general population is low, MTCT strategies based on universal or targeted testing of pregnant women may not compare well against cost-effectiveness benchmarks, or may satisfy formal criteria for cost-effectiveness but offer a low relative value in relation to competing interventions to improve population health (Johri and Ako-Arrey 2011).

- Health system infrastructure: published evaluations of pMTCT cost-effectiveness in LMICs have been based on decision models of hypothetical patient cohorts, with the exception of two studies, which used modeling in conjunction with data drawn from specific patient cohorts in Malawi (Orlando, Marazzi et al. 2010) and Tanzania (Robberstad and Evjen-Olsen 2010). With rare exceptions (Sweat, O'Reilly et al. 2004; Reynolds, Janowitz et al. 2006), modeling studies have generally assumed that the infrastructure required to provide the interventions under consideration is currently in place. The two studies using data from specific patient cohorts (Orlando, Marazzi et al. 2010; Robberstad and Evjen-Olsen 2010) take place in fully functioning centers, such that operational costs are considered, but infrastructure investments to create new facilities are not.

The production function for the intervention is rarely known in economic evaluations, and CEA estimates are usually given without specifying the degree of program scale (Moatti, Marlink et al. 2008). Some populations are more difficult to reach or to help. Variations in HIV prevalence principally affect the costs of case findings, while variations in infrastructure increase the costs of case

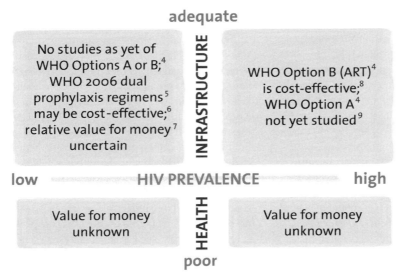

Figure 2.2.1 *Value for money of "component 3" pMTCT interventions in LMICs[1,2,3]*
[1] *Updated summary of a systematic review of HIV pMTCT cost-effectiveness in low- and middle-income countries (LMICs) (Johri and Ako-Arrey 2011).*
[2] *These are interventions to prevent transmission from a woman living with HIV to her infant (World Health Organization 2010c).*
[3] *For empirical studies, we refer to the infrastructure of the study location, not necessarily of the country. Modeling studies generally take infrastructure as given or linearly scalable.*
[4] *Currently recommended WHO pMTCT regimens (World Health Organization 2010b). Option B+ has not yet been studied.*
[5] *Formerly recommended WHO pMTCT anti-retroviral prophylaxis regimens focusing on the last trimester of pregnancy (World Health Organization 2006).*
[6] *Associated studies (Rely et al. 2003; Kumar et al. 2006).*
[7] *This is relative value as compared to competing interventions to improve population health.*
[8] *Associated studies (Orlando et al. 2010; Robberstad and Evjen-Olsen 2010; Shah et al. 2011).*
[9] *Option A should be at least as cost-effective as Option B for models considering only impact on infant HIV transmission, as Option A is considered to be lower in cost and equal in effectiveness to Option B in terms of preventing infant HIV transmission.*

findings and potentially also treatment. The costs and cost-effectiveness of HIV pMTCT is likely to be non-linear in these dimensions. These factors should be considered in interpreting CEA results (Figure 2.2.1).

To guide strategic planning and programming for HIV prevention, UNAIDS and other agencies advocate the use of data on disease burden and programmatic response to match resources to need, reflected in the principle "know your epidemic; know your response" (United Nations Joint Programme on HIV/AIDS (UNAIDS) 2007; The

Global Fund to Fight HIV 2011; UNICEF 2011). Table 2.2.2 presents key indicators for the forty-four sub-Saharan African countries included in the analysis.

Several points are worth noting:

- HIV prevalence varies substantially. Eight countries (Senegal, Niger, Mauritania, Madagascar, Eritrea, Comoros, Mauritius, and Mali) have HIV prevalence of less than 1 percent, and in an additional six countries HIV prevalence lies between 1 and 2 percent (Benin, Guinea, Burkina Faso,

Table 2.2.2 Key indicators[1]

Country	High burden?[2]	HIV prevalence (adult)[3]	2010 HDI[4]	Total fertility rate[5]	< 5 mortality (per 1,000)	Maternal mortality (per 100,000)	Unmet need for family planning	1 ANC visit (%)	Skilled birth attendance (%)	% ANC with pMTCT services	HIV testing in pregnant women (%)	ARV coverage for pMTCT (mothers, %)[6]	ARV coverage for pMTCT (infants, %)[7]
Angola	1	2	146	5.79	161	610	30	80	8	23	26	19	15
Benin	0	1.2	134	5.49				84	78		49	46	
Botswana	1	24.8	98	2.90	57	190		94.5	97	100	93	>95	>95
Burkina Faso	0	1.2	161	5.95			29	85	54		42	32	
Burundi	1	3.3	166	4.66	166	970	29	92	34	41	40	12	9
Cameroon	1	5.3	131	4.67	154	600	20	80	63	79	41	27	25
CAR	0	4.7	159	4.85				69	53		28	34	
Chad	1	3.4	163	6.20	209	1,200	23.3	39	14	8	6	6	4
Comoros	0	0.1	140	5.08				94			5		
Congo	0	3.4	126	4.64			16	86	86		23	12	
Cote d'Ivoire	1	3.4		4.65	119	470		85	57	44	47	54	33
Djibouti			147	3.95				92	93		39	10	
DRC	1	1.2–1.6	168	6.07	199	670	24	85	74	8	9	6	6
Equatorial Guinea	0	5	117	5.36							63	26	
Eritrea	0	0.8		4.68							25	34	
Ethiopia	1	1.5	157	4.60	104	470	22	28	6	86	16	18	15
Gabon	0	5.2	93	3.35							23	30	
Gambia	0	2	151	5.10				98	57		50		
Ghana	1	1.8	130	4.34	69	350	35	90	57	19	51	27	13
Guinea	0	1.3	156	5.45			21	88	46		10	17	
Guinea-Bissau	0	2.5	164	5.27				78	39		21	24	
Kenya	1	6.3	128	4.80		530	26	92	44	58	63	73	49
Lesotho	1	23.6	141	3.37	84	530	31	92	62	86	50	64	33
Liberia	0	1.5	162	5.42			36	79	46		22	16	
Madagascar	0	0.2	135	4.83			19	86	44		20		
Malawi	1	11	153	6.00	100	510	28	92	54	95	52	58	41
Mali	0	1	160	6.46			31	70	49		16		
Mauritania	0	0.7	136	4.71				81	61		6		
Mauritius	0	1	72	1.67					99.5		83		
Mozambique	1	11.5	165	5.11	142	550	18	89	55	78	77	70	43
Namibia	1	13.1	105	3.40	48	180	7	95	81	86	90	93	88

(cont.)

Table 2.2.2 (cont.)

Country	High burden?[2]	HIV prevalence (adult)[3]	2010 HDI[4]	Total fertility rate[5]	< 5 mortality (per 1,000)	Maternal mortality (per 100,000)	Unmet need for family planning	1 ANC visit (%)	Skilled birth attendance (%)	% ANC with pMTCT services	HIV testing in pregnant women (%)	ARV coverage for pMTCT (mothers, %)[6]	ARV coverage for pMTCT (infants, %)[7]
Niger	0	0.8	167	7.19			16	46	33		19		
Nigeria	1	3.6	142	5.61	138	840	20.2	58	39		13	22	8
Rwanda	0	2.9	152	5.43			38	96	52		71	65	
Senegal	0	0.9	144	5.03			32	87	52		35		
Sierra Leone	0	1.6	158	5.22			28	87	42		74	19	
Somalia	0			6.40				26	33		<1		
South Africa	1	17.8	110	2.55	62	410	14	92	91	95	95	88	56
Swaziland	1	25.9	121	3.57	73	420	24	85	69	79	73	88	82
Tanzania	1	5.6	148	5.58	108	790	21.8	76	43	72	66	70	51
Togo	0	3.2	139	4.30				84	62		20	26	
Uganda	1	6.5	143	6.38	128	430	41	94	42	51	64	53	28
Zambia	1	13.5	150	6.20	141	470	27	94	47	64	>95	69	39
Zimbabwe	1	14.3	169	3.47	90	790	13	93	60	55	46	56	35

[1] For the 21 high-burden countries (note 2), all data are taken from UNICEF unless otherwise specified (UNICEF 2011). For other countries, data comes from the WHO Global Health Observatory unless otherwise specified (World Health Organization 2010a). Data may be from different years, leading to some inconsistencies. Empty cells reflect missing information.

[2] These are the 22 countries (21 in sub-Saharan Africa) that have the highest burden of HIV-positive pregnant women and therefore account for almost 90 percent of all new infant HIV infections (United Nations Joint Programme on HIV/AIDS (UNAIDS) 2011).

[3] HIV prevalence in adults aged 15–49, as reported in the 2010 UNAIDS Epidemic Update (United Nations Joint Programme on HIV/AIDS (UNAIDS) 2010).

[4] The Human Development Index (HDI) provides a composite measure of three basic dimensions of human development: health, education, and income. This is the country rank for 2010 out of 169 countries with comparable data (United Nations Development Programme (UNDP) 2011).

[5] The average number of children a hypothetical cohort of women would have at the end of their reproductive period if they were subject during their whole lives to the fertility rates of a given period and if they were not subject to mortality. It is expressed here as children per woman for the period 2005–2010 (United Nations Department of Economic and Social Affairs 2010).

[6] The percentage of HIV-infected pregnant women who received anti-retroviral medicines to reduce the risk of mother-to-child transmission, among the estimated number of HIV-infected pregnant women.

[7] The percentage of HIV-exposed infants who received anti-retroviral medicines to reduce the risk of mother-to-child transmission, among the estimated number of HIV-exposed infants.

Ghana, Ethiopia, and Democratic Republic of the Congo). Even in the twenty-one high-burden countries, HIV prevalence ranges from just 1–2 percent in Ghana and the Democratic Republic of the Congo, to almost 26 percent in Swaziland. HIV prevalence also varies widely within coun-

tries. In Ethiopia, for example, HIV prevalence is estimated at 8 percent in the urban population and 1 percent in the rural population. The efficiency of interventions can be improved by targeting resources according to need. However, even in areas with very high need, HIV prevalence varies

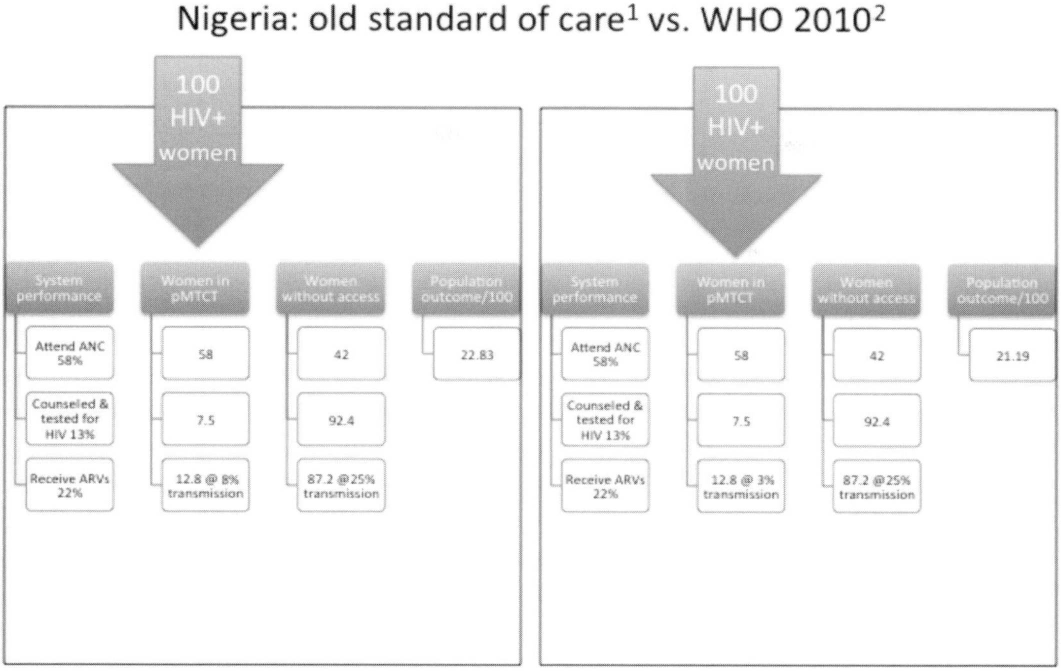

Nigeria: old standard of care[1] vs. WHO 2010[2]

Figure 2.2.2 *Impact of health system performance on childhood HIV infections[3]*
[1] *Currently recommended WHO pMTCT regimens (World Health Organization 2010b) are estimated to reduce infant transmission from the natural history rate of 25 percent to 3 percent and are shown on the right. Under this scenario, we expect 21 infant infections per 100 HIV-positive women.*
[2] *Adapted from Barker et al. (2011). System performance data are taken from Table 2.2.2. Due to inconsistencies in the data, the percent of HIV-positive women attending ANC is multiplied directly by the percent of HIV-positive women receiving to obtain the number of women benefiting from pMTCT. All transmission rates in this figure are for illustration only.*
[3] *Older anti-retroviral prophylaxis regimens focusing on the last trimester of pregnancy (World Health Organization 2006) are estimated to reduce infant transmission from the natural history rate of 25 percent to 8 percent and are shown on the left. Under this scenario, we expect almost 23 infant infections per 100 HIV-positive women.*

markedly. Moreover, targeting resources only to areas of high prevalence is insufficient to meet the elimination goal for infant HIV infections.

- Family planning is an important entry point to reducing infant HIV infections. Fertility rates are very high in SSA and unmet needs for family planning considerable, demonstrating the strategic importance of family planning, reproductive counseling, and potentially Option B+ for reducing infant infections.
- Health system infrastructure is often lacking. The term pMTCT "cascade" has been used to describe the sequence of steps required to

deliver anti-retroviral-based MTCT interventions to HIV-positive mothers and their infants (Barker, Mphatswe et al. 2011). A simplified three-step version is used for illustrative purposes (Barker, Mphatswe et al. 2011). The first step in the pathway involves access to antenatal care (ANC). As Table 2.2.2 demonstrates, access to ANC is highly variable in the countries in the analysis, ranging from 26 to 98 percent. Moreover, populations arrive in ANC at twenty-two weeks on average, while anti-retroviral regimens are to start at fourteen weeks. Timing is an important determinant of therapeutic effectiveness. The second step in the pathway involves access to HIV (and CD4) testing, to enable a woman to know her HIV status. The percentage of pregnant women receiving an HIV test was also highly variable, ranging from 6 percent to over 95 percent. The third step is provision of anti-retroviral treatment to women living with HIV and their infants. This also ranged from 6 percent to over 95 percent among the countries in our analysis.

At the population level, access to the pMTCT "cascade" is likely to be the single most important factor for determining the number of infections in children (Mahy, Stover *et al.* 2010; Mofenson 2010; Barker, Mphatswe *et al.* 2011). The vast majority of MTCT occurs in women who receive no treatment. Triple regimens will be important in reducing transmission in mother–infant dyads but, at a population level, will not have a large impact on MTCT rates. A study modeling the impact of the WHO Option B regime in Nigeria as compared to WHO 2006 dual prophylaxis found that at current coverage rates (10 percent of HIV-infected mothers) expected values for mother-to-child HIV transmission were 24.3 percent with WHO 2006 and 23.7 percent with Option B – a difference of 0.6 percent (Shah, Johns *et al.* 2011). Introduction of more effective combination ARV regimens will yield only marginal reductions in childhood HIV infections and mortality unless health systems achieve high performance at each step of the pMTCT pathway (Barker, Mphatswe *et al.* 2011). What is required is to ensure high coverage at each step of the cascade, and to avoid losses to follow-up occurring at each linkage point (Mahy, Stover *et al.* 2010; Mofenson 2010; Barker, Mphatswe *et al.* 2011).

A final insight emerging from this situational analysis relates to concerns for fair distribution of health benefits. Efficiency and equity are widely recognized as vital, independent goals for health systems (World Health Organization 2000). Almost all countries in the analysis document substantial inequities in access by wealth quintile and area of residence, with poor and rural populations having less access (UNICEF 2011). Achieving an equitable distribution of the benefits of enhanced pMTCT services will require substantial improvements to infrastructure and enhancements to access.

Within countries, existing MTCT programs are generally located in settings of higher HIV prevalence and better health infrastructure. Scale-up of pMTCT initiatives is likely to be highly non-linear in terms of costs, and resolution of health system issues will be of paramount importance in achieving elimination goals for new infant HIV infections. We should anticipate that future scale-up might require new means to provide access for more difficult to reach populations.

Scale-up of interventions to prevent transmission from HIV-positive mother to child: solutions

I next sketch four additional "solutions" not as yet discussed in the AP, the UNAIDS investment framework (Schwartländer, Stover *et al.* 2011), or the UNAIDS global plan to eliminate new infant HIV infections (United Nations Joint Programme on HIV/AIDS (UNAIDS) 2011):

- Interventions to improve health system performance: interventions to improve uptake at each step in the pMTCT cascade have the potential to confer substantial improvements in maternal and child survival (Youngleson, Nkurunziza *et al.* 2010; Barker, Mphatswe *et al.* 2011). Moreover, efforts to reduce losses to follow-up help to counter stigma and promote equity, since those who are lost to care are often among the most vulnerable. Health system improvements are feasible and can be achieved at reasonable cost (Youngleson, Nkurunziza *et al.* 2010).
- Screening in the labor ward: rapid point of care HIV screening in the labor ward can serve as an alternative pMTCT entry point. It is important for at least three reasons:
  (1) Many women in sub-Saharan Africa do not receive an HIV test during ANC, and present at labor with undocumented HIV status.
  (2) The highest rates of HIV transmission from mother to child are associated with new infections acquired during pregnancy and breastfeeding. Rates have been estimated at 30 percent (13–30 percent) for peripartum transmission, and 28 percent (14.3–56

percent) during the postnatal period (UNAIDS Reference Group on Estimates Modelling and Projections 2011).

(3) Male partners are more frequently present at the time of delivery than at ANC.

- Findings from clinical trials show that ARV prophylaxis given to mother during labor and neonate immediately after birth can reduce HIV MTCT by as much as 50 percent (UNAIDS Reference Group on Estimates Modelling and Projections 2011). Although the effectiveness of this strategy is lower than for interventions delivered in ANC, in settings of high HIV prevalence and weak maternal-child health infrastructure, HIV screening in the labor ward has been demonstrated to be feasible and effective in capturing a large number of cases for which effective intervention is possible (Temmerman, Quaghebeur et al. 2003; Homsy, Kalamya et al. 2006; Sagay, Musa et al. 2006; Beltman, Fitzgerald et al. 2010; Bello, Ogunbode et al. 2011), and in encouraging couple counseling (Homsy, Kalamya et al. 2006). Moreover, enabling a woman to have knowledge of her diagnosis provides her with an opportunity to improve her own health and to promote more favorable outcomes in future pregnancies. It is hence plausible that this strategy represents good value for money in some settings.

- Innovations to deliver care to women not delivering in a health facility: in developing countries, most poor women deliver at home (Montagu, Yamey et al. 2011). HIV-infected pregnant women living far from a clinic may be unable to afford long, repeated trips for treatment. In addition, many clinics in SSA suffer from stockouts, further endangering continuity of care. For women who know their HIV-positive status and are likely to deliver at home, innovative strategies have been developed to increase the uptake of more efficacious ARV prophylactic regimens for pMTCT in line with the most recent WHO guidelines (World Health Organization 2010). For example, the Mother-Baby Pack developed by WHO and UNICEF gives pregnant women living with HIV a complete, pre-packaged set of drugs to prevent transmission of the virus to their children.

My final suggestion highlights the potential of an intervention currently under development and not yet discussed in the context of HIV pMTCT:

- Multiplex point-of-care (POC) diagnostic tests: through its Grand Challenges program, the Bill and Melinda Gates Foundation has recently focused attention on the need to develop POC diagnostics that are easy to use, low-cost, and suitable to assess conditions and pathogens at the point-of-care in a variety of settings (The Bill and Melinda Gates Foundation 2011). Some initiatives involve multiplex tests, which provide diagnostic information on several conditions simultaneously. This is potentially a "leapfrog technology" for pMTCT as multiplex tests provide a means to circumvent both the health infrastructure problem and the HIV prevalence problem outlined above.

(1) As we have seen, structural factors in country health systems, in particular lack of access to ANC and HIV testing, are a critical factor in impeding pMTCT scale-up. Our ability to affect MTCT transmission rates at the population level depends crucially on improving access to the pMTCT cascade. HIV POC tests can be implemented even in rural and remote areas and require less highly trained personnel, making them a vital tool to improve access and potentially appropriate timing of administration.

(2) The ratio of costs to health benefits of single condition HIV POC tests depends on testing costs, and HIV prevalence. In settings where HIV prevalence in the general population is low, or costs of outreach are high, MTCT strategies based on universal or targeted testing of pregnant women may offer low value for money as compared to competing interventions to improve population health (Johri and Ako-Arrey 2011). Multiplex tests can be engineered to the epidemiology of the local context. Provided that testing costs can be kept low, it should therefore be possible to guarantee that diagnostic testing will detect a sufficient number of (HIV or non-HIV) cases to improve the value-to-money profile of universal antenatal screening. Multiplex

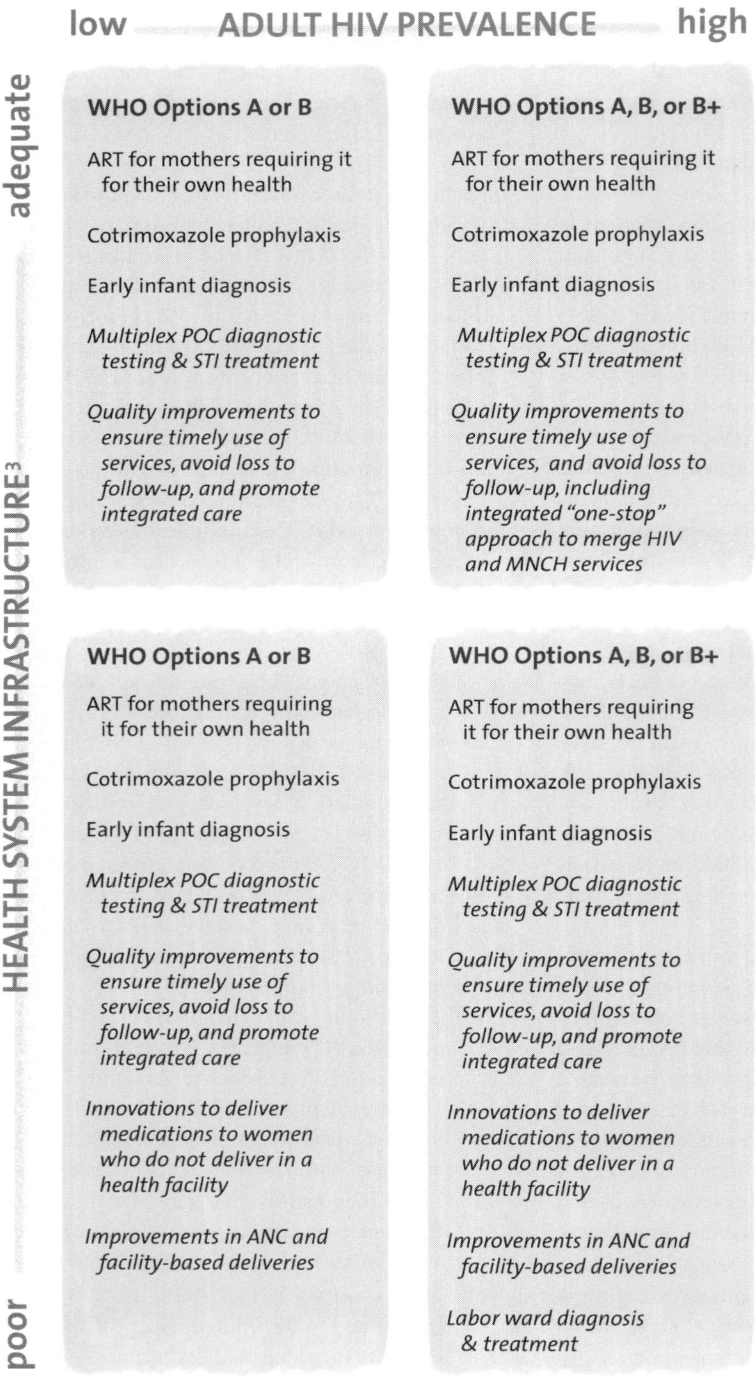

HEALTH SYSTEM INFRASTRUCTURE[3] (adequate → poor)

WHO Options A or B

ART for mothers requiring it for their own health

Cotrimoxazole prophylaxis

Early infant diagnosis

Multiplex POC diagnostic testing & STI treatment

Quality improvements to ensure timely use of services, avoid loss to follow-up, and promote integrated care

---

WHO Options A, B, or B+

ART for mothers requiring it for their own health

Cotrimoxazole prophylaxis

Early infant diagnosis

Multiplex POC diagnostic testing & STI treatment

Quality improvements to ensure timely use of services, and avoid loss to follow-up, including integrated "one-stop" approach to merge HIV and MNCH services

---

WHO Options A or B

ART for mothers requiring it for their own health

Cotrimoxazole prophylaxis

Early infant diagnosis

Multiplex POC diagnostic testing & STI treatment

Quality improvements to ensure timely use of services, avoid loss to follow-up, and promote integrated care

Innovations to deliver medications to women who do not deliver in a health facility

Improvements in ANC and facility-based deliveries

WHO Options A, B, or B+

ART for mothers requiring it for their own health

Cotrimoxazole prophylaxis

Early infant diagnosis

Multiplex POC diagnostic testing & STI treatment

Quality improvements to ensure timely use of services, avoid loss to follow-up, and promote integrated care

Innovations to deliver medications to women who do not deliver in a health facility

Improvements in ANC and facility-based deliveries

Labor ward diagnosis & treatment

Figure 2.2.3 *Innovative "component 3" strategies to prevent mother-to-child transmission*[1,2]
[1] *These are interventions to prevent transmission from a woman living with HIV to her infant (World Health Organization 2010c).*
[2] *This figure highlights strategies likely to offer good value for money in different epidemic and health system contexts. Strategies in italics highlight dimensions that have received less attention to date (Bollinger 2011; Schwartländer et al. 2011; United Nations Joint Programme on HIV/AIDS (UNAIDS) 2011).*

POC diagnostic tests combining detection of HIV with several other conditions are being developed for antenatal care populations in India (Pai, Joseph et al. 2010).

Concluding remarks

I have argued that increasing coverage of prevention of mother-to-child transmission services to 90 percent for all childbearing women living with HIV to reach elimination of new child infections by 2015 will require a substantially more comprehensive set of options than that presented in the AP, and for that reason find the cost estimate of $196 million to scale up pMTCT in SSA by 2015 (Bollinger 2011) implausibly low.[6] Two recent assessments may serve as useful comparisons. In its global plan towards virtual elimination of new HIV infections among children, UNAIDS evaluates resources required to increase coverage of a comprehensive set of pMTCT interventions to 90 percent of pregnant women in the twenty-two high-burden countries that are home to nearly 90 percent of pregnant women living with HIV who need services. For these priority countries (twenty-one of which lie in SSA and also figure in the AP analysis), UNAIDS evaluated the shortfall for pMTCT scale-up at $2.5 billion for the period 2011–2015 (United Nations Joint Programme on HIV/AIDS (UNAIDS) 2011). This resource needs estimate is of a similar order of magnitude to that identified in the investment framework by Schwartländer and colleagues, which also took a more comprehensive approach to MTCT and considered savings due to treatment costs offset (Schwartländer, Stover et al. 2011). Like the CCC HIV/AIDS exercise, the analysis by Schwartländer and colleagues studies investments in health infrastructure and HIV treatment separately (Schwartländer, Stover et al. 2011). All three analyses assess similar health benefits (90 percent coverage of pMTCT for all pregnant women) over a similar time period (2011–2015).[7]

The analysis also fails to capture some of the important benefits associated with pMTCT scale-up. The new therapeutic strategies for pMTCT introduced in the WHO 2010 guidelines (World Health Organization 2010) yield important benefits for maternal survival via use of ART for a woman's own health. They also confer important benefits for child survival, as anti-retroviral interventions can interrupt mother-to-child transmission, enable HIV-exposed infants to benefit from the protection against competing sources of child mortality afforded by safe breastfeeding, and contribute indirectly to child survival through enhanced maternal survival. Cost-effectiveness estimates that fail to capture these dimensions are likely to be inaccurate and to underestimate the full benefits of pMTCT interventions on HIV-related morbidity and mortality. A unique feature of pMTCT programs is that the same interventions required to achieve virtual elimination of new infant HIV infections will also necessarily transform health for non-HIV-infected mothers and children. For example, improved access to maternal and child health services (including family planning) through strengthened antenatal care infrastructure can be expected to make a definitive improvement to general maternal and child health.

The key question posed by *RethinkHIV* is: "If we successfully raised an additional $10 billion over the next five years to combat HIV/AIDS in sub-Saharan Africa, how could it best be spent?" Prevention of HIV transmission from mother-to-child is a high leverage intervention with implications for health and development. Even at substantially higher cost, a comprehensive approach to pMTCT has the potential to make a decisive contribution to achievement of Millennium Development Goal (MDG) 6 (combat HIV/AIDS, malaria, and other diseases), MDG 4 (reduce child mortality), and MDG 5 (improve maternal health), thereby yielding high value for money and return on investment.

---

[6] Even the corrected estimate of $292 million for Option A is implausibly low as an estimate of the costs of pMTCT scale-up.

[7] Schwartländer and colleagues evaluate resource requirements for a broader set of countries, but data are available by region. Similar to *RethinkHIV*, their investment framework does not include infrastructure costs nor primary prevention of HIV in the pMTCT component, but considers these elements separately (Schwartländer, Stover et al. 2011).

Simply put, scale-up of pMTCT is an opportunity too important to miss.

Currently recommended anti-retroviral-based options for pMTCT provide excellent value for money under certain conditions. However, the costs and cost-effectiveness of pMTCT programs are substantially affected by variations in HIV prevalence and health system infrastructure. Within countries, existing MTCT programs are generally located in settings of higher HIV prevalence and better health infrastructure, with the result that scale-up of interventions is likely to pose challenges in terms of feasibility and efficiency. Since most transmission occurs in women who do not receive treatment, at the population level, access to the pMTCT "cascade" may be the single most important factor for determining the number of new HIV infections in children.

While many of the most important interventions to reduce MTCT rates lie at the level of health systems, leapfrog technologies can help to change the rules of the game. An innovative way of increasing access to the pMTCT cascade may come by means of an emerging technology, multiplex point-of-care diagnostics. POC diagnostics allow one to partially bypass weak maternal and child health infrastructure, ensuring that diagnostic testing in pregnancy can be conducted without advanced laboratory facilities or highly skilled technicians, and thereby facilitating entry to the initial phase of the pMTCT cascade. While POC HIV tests have been in the field for several years, multiplex POC tests that provide results for several conditions simultaneously are still in the development pipeline. The additional and essential contribution of multiplex tests lies in their potential to increase the value for money associated with antenatal screening, by offering on average more health benefits per test due to detection and treatment of a wider range of health conditions. This will be particularly important in contexts where HIV prevalence is low, or costs of outreach are high. This technology could play a decisive role in increasing access to an HIV diagnosis during pregnancy and thus, in synergy with interventions to improve health system performance throughout the pMTCT cascade, in elimination of new infant HIV infections.

References

(2010). Report from the Consultative Meeting on Updating Estimates of Mother-to-Child Transmission Rates of HIV. Washington DC.

Anglemyer, A., Rutherford, G. W. *et al.* (2011). Anti-retroviral therapy for prevention of HIV transmission in HIV-discordant couples. *Cochrane Database Syst Rev*(8): CD009153.

Barker, P. M., Mphatswe, W. *et al.* (2011). Anti-retroviral drugs in the cupboard are not enough: the impact of health systems' performance on mother-to-child transmission of HIV. *J Acquir Immune Defic Syndr* **56**(2): e45–48.

Battersby, A., Feilden, R. *et al.* (1999). Sterilizable syringes: excessive risk or cost-effective option? *Bull World Health Organ* **77**(10): 812–19.

Bello, F. A., Ogunbode, O. O. *et al.* (2011). Acceptability of counselling and testing for HIV infection in women in labour at the University College Hospital, Ibadan, Nigeria. *Afr Health Sci* **11**(1): 30–5.

Beltman, J. J., Fitzgerald, M. *et al.* (2010). Accelerated HIV testing for PMTCT in maternity and labour wards is vital to capture mothers at a critical point in the programme at district level in Malawi. *AIDS Care* **22**(11): 1367–72.

Bollinger, L. (2011). Prevention of non-sexual transmission of HIV. Assessment paper for *RethinkHIV*.

Brisson, M. and Edmunds, W. J. (2006). Impact of model, methodological, and parameter uncertainty in the economic analysis of vaccination programs. *Med Decis Making* **26**(5): 434–46.

Canadian Agency for Drugs and Technologies in Health (CADTH). (2006). Guidelines for the Economic Evaluation of Health Technologies: Canada.

Ciaranello, A. L., Perez, F. *et al.* (2011). WHO 2010 guidelines for prevention of mother-to-child HIV transmission in Zimbabwe: modeling clinical outcomes in infants and mothers. *PLoS One* **6**(6): e20224.

Drain, P. K., Nelson, C. M. *et al.* (2003). Single-dose versus multi-dose vaccine vials for immunization programmes in developing countries. *Bull World Health Organ* **81**(10): 726–31.

Drummond, M. F., Sculpher, M. J. *et al.* (2005). *Methods for the Economic Evaluation of Health Care Programmes*. New York: Oxford University Press.

Halperin, D. T., Stover, J. *et al.* (2009). Benefits and costs of expanding access to family planning programs to women living with HIV. *AIDS* **23** Suppl 1: S123–130.

Homsy, J., Kalamya, J. N. *et al.* (2006). Routine intrapartum HIV counseling and testing for prevention of mother-to-child transmission of HIV in a rural Ugandan hospital. *Journal of Acquired Immune Deficiency Syndromes: JAIDS* **42**(2): 149–54.

Johri, M. and Ako-Arrey, D. (2011). The cost-effectiveness of preventing mother-to-child transmission of HIV in low- and middle-income countries: systematic review. *Cost Eff Resour Alloc* **9**: 3.

Koska, M. and Baker, L. (2007). Smart Injection Programme Proposed by Safepoint Trust.

Kumar, M., Birch, S. *et al.* (2006). Economic evaluation of HIV screening in pregnant women attending antenatal clinics in India. *Health Policy* **77**(2): 233–43.

Mahy, M., Stover, J. *et al.* (2010). What will it take to achieve virtual elimination of mother-to-child transmission of HIV? An assessment of current progress and future needs. *Sex Transm Infect* **86** Suppl 2: ii48–55.

Moatti, J. P., Marlink, R. *et al.* (2008). Universal access to HIV treatment in developing countries: going beyond the misinterpretations of the cost-effectiveness algorithm. *AIDS* **22** Suppl 1: S59–66.

Mofenson, L. M. (2010). Prevention in neglected subpopulations: prevention of mother-to-child transmission of HIV infection. *Clin Infect Dis* **50** Suppl 3: S130–48.

Montagu, D., Yamey, G. *et al.* (2011). Where do poor women in developing countries give birth? A multi-country analysis of demographic and health survey data. *PLoS One* **6**(2): e17155.

National Institutes of Health: IMPAACT Trial Network. (2010). p1077 The PROMISE Study (Promoting Maternal and Infant Survival Everywhere).

Orlando, S., Marazzi, M. C. *et al.* (2010). Cost-effectiveness of using HAART in prevention of mother-to-child transmission in the DREAM-Project Malawi. *J Acquir Immune Defic Syndr* **55**(5): 631–4.

Pai, N. P., Joseph, L. *et al.* (2010). Multiplex screening assays for HIV and co-infections: will they benefit patients, providers and health systems?, Canadian Institutes for Health Research (CIHR).

Program for Appropriate Technology in Health (PATH). (2011). An Overview of PATH's Injection Safety Work: 1999–2009. Retrieved August 25, 2011.

Rely, K., Bertozzi, S. M. *et al.* (2003). Cost-effectiveness of strategies to reduce mother-to-child HIV transmission in Mexico, a low-prevalence setting. *Health Policy and Planning* **18**(3): 290–8.

Reynolds, H. W., Janowitz, B. *et al.* (2006). The value of contraception to prevent perinatal HIV transmission. *Sex Transm Dis* **33**(6): 350–6.

Robberstad, B. and Evjen-Olsen, B. (2010). Preventing mother to child transmission of HIV with highly active antiretroviral treatment in Tanzania – a prospective cost-effectiveness study. *J Acquir Immune Defic Syndr* **55**(3): 397–403.

Sagay, A. S., Musa, J. *et al.* (2006). Rapid HIV testing and counselling in labour in a northern Nigerian setting. *Afr J Reprod Health* **10**(1): 76–80.

Schouten, E. J., Jahn, A. *et al.* (2011). Prevention of mother-to-child transmission of HIV and the health-related Millennium Development Goals: time for a public health approach. *Lancet* **378**(9787): 282–4.

Schwartländer, B., Stover, J. *et al.* (2011). Towards an improved investment approach for an effective response to HIV/AIDS. *Lancet* **377**(9782): 2031–41.

Shah, M., Johns, B. *et al.* (2011). Cost-effectiveness of new WHO recommendations for prevention of mother-to-child transmission of HIV in a resource-limited setting. *AIDS* **25**(8): 1093–102.

Sweat, M. D., O'Reilly, K. R. *et al.* (2004). Cost-effectiveness of nevirapine to prevent mother-to-child HIV transmission in eight African countries. *AIDS* **18**(12): 1661–71.

Tamplin, S. A., Davidson, D. *et al.* (2005). Issues and options for the safe destruction and disposal of used injection materials. *Waste Manag* **25**(6): 655–65.

Tan-Torres Edeger, T., Baltussen, R. *et al.* (2003). *Making Choices in Health: WHO Guide to Cost-Effectiveness Analysis*. Geneva: World Health Organization, 1–250.

Temmerman, M., Quaghebeur, A. *et al.* (2003). Mother-to-child HIV transmission in resource poor settings: how to improve coverage? *AIDS* **17**(8): 1239–42.

The Bill and Melinda Gates Foundation. (2011). Grand Challenges: Point-of-Care Diagnostics Grant Opportunity. Retrieved August 29, 2011, from www.grandchallenges.org/diagnostics/Pages/POCDiagnosticsInformation.aspx.

The Global Fund to Fight HIV, T. a. M. (2011). *Global Fund Information Note: Matching Resources to Need Opportunities to Promote Equity*. Geneva, 10.

UNAIDS Reference Group on Estimates Modelling and Projections. (2011). Working Paper on Mother-to-Child HIV Transmission Rates for Use in Spectrum, Geneva.

UNICEF. (2011). Preventing Mother-to-Child Transmission (PMTCT) of HIV. Retrieved August 28, 2011, from www.unicef.org/aids/index_preventionyoung.html.

United Nations Joint Programme on HIV/AIDS (UNAIDS). (2007). *Practical Guidelines for Intensifying HIV Prevention: Towards Universal Access*. Geneva: UNAIDS.

United Nations Joint Programme on HIV/AIDS (UNAIDS). (2010). UNAIDS Report on the Global AIDS Epidemic 2010. www.unaids.org/globalreport/default.htm.

United Nations Joint Programme on HIV/AIDS (UNAIDS). (2011). *Global Plan Towards the Elimination of New HIV Infections Among Children by 2015 and Keeping their Mothers Alive: 2011–2015*. Geneva: UNAIDS.

World Bank. (2009). 2008 Country Classification Tables. Data & Statistics: Country Classification. Retrieved September 25, 2009, from http://go.worldbank.org/K2CKM78CC0.

World Health Organization. (2000). *Health Systems: Improving Performance. World Health Report*. Geneva: World Health Organization, i–141.

World Health Organization. (2001). *Macroeconomics and Health: Investing in Health for Economic Development*. Canada: World Health Organization, 1–200.

World Health Organization. (2010). *Anti-Retroviral Drugs for Treating Pregnant Women and Preventing HIV Infection in Infants: Recommendations for a Public Health Approach – 2010 Version*. Geneva: World Health Organization.

World Health Organization. (2010). *PMTCT Strategic Vision 2010–2015: Preventing Mother-to-Child Transmission of HIV to Reach the UNGASS and Millennium Development Goals*. Geneva: World Health Organization.

Yamey, G. (2011). Scaling up global health interventions: a proposed framework for success. *PLoS Med* **8**(6): e1001049.

Youngleson, M. S., Nkurunziza, P. *et al.* (2010). Improving a mother to child HIV transmission programme through health system redesign: quality improvement, protocol adjustment and resource addition. *PLoS One* **5**(11): e13891.

Treatment

Assessment paper

MEAD OVER AND GEOFFREY P. GARNETT

Anti-retroviral treatment has changed the nature of the HIV pandemic and has been a major driver of an increase in resources devoted to health care in low-income countries (Walensky and Kuritzkes 2010), but there are questions about whether treatment has been adequately expanded, and about how to maintain the gains that have been achieved (Bertozzi, Martz *et al.* 2009). The global pandemic of human immunodeficiency virus (HIV) and the associated acquired immune deficiency syndrome (AIDS), emerging in 1981, was initially characterized by an exceptionally high fatality rate, where almost everyone infected would die, after a long and variable incubation period (Hendriks, Medley *et al.* 1993). Successful combination treatment, which uses three drugs to suppress the virus to levels where the immune system ceased to be damaged and where the virus could not easily evolve into a resistant genotype, dramatically changed the outcome of HIV infection, turning it into a manageable chronic disease (Palella, Delaney *et al.* 1998). However, this introduction of successful treatment in 1996 quickly highlighted the gross inequities in access to health care and treatments globally, with a declining mortality seen in North America and Western Europe that was not possible in lower income settings. A remarkable advocacy campaign led to reduced costs per person per year of anti-retroviral medication, along with increasing resources globally (UNAIDS 2009, 2010). The goal of universal access to anti-retrovirals was embraced by politicians at the Gleneagles summit in 2006, and again endorsed in June 2011 by the UN General Assembly (World Health Organization 2010). Currently there are over six million people on effective anti-retroviral treatment globally, a great tribute to the efforts of many (UNAIDS 2010). However, this is less than half of those in current "need" of treatment, and the growth in resources, which for

nearly a decade was 28 percent per year, has ceased. Would more resources be a good investment to stop deaths from HIV and stop the spread of HIV? In what follows, we model the spread of HIV, the impact of anti-retroviral treatment, and show how the trade-offs necessary in decisions about who to treat and how to treat them influence the benefits derived from treatment programs.

The stage of HIV infection at which it is best to treat someone has been a source of uncertainty, with changing perspectives, which have in part reflected evidence of clinical benefit, but for some also reflect resource allocation decisions. CD4 positive T-cells are so called as they are the helper cells of the immune system which have CD4 receptor molecules via which HIV enters the cell over their surface. These are the cells that are depleted by HIV infection, their loss leading to an inability to control opportunistic diseases. The CD4 count is a marker of disease progression, with AIDS in part being defined by a CD4 count of less than 200 cells per microliter of blood. Following HIV infection, there is a short (two- to three-month) acute period with a peak in viremia and dip in CD4 count which recovers somewhat. Thereafter, when the host's immune system reasserts itself, viral load more or less stabilizes and a steady decline in CD4 count ensues, until direct and indirect damage undermines the health of the infected person. Early thinking in HIV treatment was that hitting the virus hard and early might eradicate the infection in the individual. This proved unfounded, and because of the toxicity of drugs and the evolution of resistance and treatment failure, clinical fashions changed to reserve treatment till late in infection. Unfortunately, cohort studies showed that those treated late had already suffered much damage and had a higher risk of mortality (May, Boulle *et al.* 2010; Sabin and Phillips 2009). Concomitantly, drugs were developed that were less toxic and more effective, removing some reasons for delay. Treatment guidelines moved from a threshold of 200 CD4 cells, to 250 CD4 cells (so as not to allow measurement error and progression between tests to undermine treatment), to 350 CD4 cells in the 2009 WHO treatment guidelines (Bendavid, Grant *et al.* 2011; Walensky, Wood *et al.* 2010). This greatly increased global treatment need, when universal coverage of those with CD4 counts less than 200 was still a long way off (UNAIDS 2010).

The advantage of earlier treatment has been further highlighted by both observational studies and a clinical trial showing that the risk of HIV transmission is related to viral load and that treatment which reduces the viral load also reduces the risk of HIV transmission (Cohen, Chen *et al.* 2011; Donnell, Baeten *et al.* 2010). A retrospective analysis of HIV transmission in couples in Rakai, Uganda found a clear relationship between the serum viral load of the untreated infectious individual and the risk of HIV transmission (Quinn, Wawer *et al.* 2000). This observational evidence suggested that antiviral treatment, which reduces viral load, would also reduce transmission. Further evidence emerged from couples, where transmission was observed in those not yet on treatment but not for those successfully treated (Donnell, Baeten *et al.* 2010). Finally, evidence from a randomized control trial of early versus late treatment showed 96 percent efficacy in reducing transmission from the successfully treated partner to his or her uninfected partner in discordant couples (Cohen, Chen *et al.* 2011).[1] Modeling work based on the reduced transmissibility of those treated has argued that elimination of HIV is possible (Granich, Gilks *et al.* 2009). However, further studies suggest this would depend on who is treated, how early they can be diagnosed and started on treatment, and whether they maintain their adherence and do not fail treatment (Dodd, Garnett *et al.* 2010).

The improvements in our HIV treatment regimens and our understanding of the clinical and prevention benefits to be derived from treatment have paralleled improvements in the cost of antiviral drugs in resource-poor settings (Waning, Kyle *et al.* 2010; Waning, Kaplan *et al.* 2009; Wirtz, Forsythe *et al.* 2009) and an improved understanding of what drives costs. There is a range of first-line treatments, with different costs, and these costs have been driven down by donations, access agreements, tiered pricing, and generic manufacture. If the first-line regimen fails, second-line drugs are used which are more expensive (by about twofold in developing countries) (Keiser, Tweya *et al.* 2009; Waning, Kaplan *et al.* 2009). Thus, a program with a fixed drug budget that uses second-line drugs will have fewer resources for first-line drugs. To date, few patients in low- and middle-income countries receive second-line treatments (UNAIDS 2010). This is in part because the tests used to determine whether treatment is failing are expensive or in short supply (Keiser, Tweya *et al.* 2009). If clinicians are forced to rely on symptoms to diagnose treatment failure, the patients they shift to a second-line regimen are already sick, and therefore less likely to survive (Athan, O'Brien *et al.* 2010; Fox, Sanne *et al.* 2010; Loubiere, Meiners *et al.* 2010; Phillips, Pillay *et al.* 2008). CD4 tests are relatively affordable and can sometimes detect a worsening immune system before there is a crisis, but CD4 tests have been shown to be unreliable for this purpose. Measuring viral load is used clinically in wealthy settings and allows rapid detection of failure, timely switching of regimens, and thus stalls the evolution of resistance (Keiser, Chi *et al.* 2011; Kimmel, Weinstein *et al.* 2010; Keiser, Tweya *et al.* 2009). Unfortunately, this expensive and complex diagnostic test is rarely available in resource-poor settings, which reduces both the cost of treatment but also its success rate. Some costs are driven by the drugs themselves in first-line regimens (Holmes, Coggin *et al.* 2010). Better quality drugs are recommended by newer guidelines, for example tenofovir rather than stavudine is now recommended as a first-line drug (World Health Organization 2010), but it is more expensive (Jouquet, Bygrave *et al.* 2011). Similarly, efavirenz is a safer drug in pregnant women than nevirapine, but is also

---

[1] Inferring the prevention benefit of scaling up treatment from this study is difficult because, for the sake of study design, the study was confined to stable serodiscordant couples. For example, people who declare themselves to be in stable partnerships and are willing to start treatment with high CD4 counts are likely to be more adherent to their medication and have fewer risky partnerships than would average patients with the same high CD4 counts.

more expensive. Other costs depend on the organization and management of facilities, local human resource costs, and decisions about who is qualified to deliver antiviral treatments (Long, Brennan *et al.* 2011; Sanne, Orrell *et al.* 2010; Babigumira, Castelnuovo *et al.* 2009; Shumbusho, van Griensven *et al.* 2009). Yet further issues are supply chain costs and management overheads, which may or may not improve the quality of the services (Babigumira, Castelnuovo *et al.* 2011; Babigumira, Sethi *et al.* 2009). In understanding the benefit to cost ratio of HIV treatment, the costs are obviously fundamentally important.

Clinical and public health decisions based upon who gains the most benefit from treatment are challenged in programs by our limited ability to identify those infected, link them into care, and maintain their treatment (Zachariah, Tayler-Smith *et al.* 2011; Braitstein, Brinkhof *et al.* 2006; Amuron, Namara *et al.* 2009; Zachariah, Harries *et al.* 2009). Inevitably there is unfairness in who receives treatment, since it will first be available where services can be organized and delivered (Cleary 2010; Cleary, Silal *et al.* 2010). Thereafter treatment decisions are driven by the clinician faced with the patient, not by how best to use scarce resources. This leads to less than optimal programs and also a failure to treat those newly in need if those already enrolled in treatment programs saturate available services (Cleary, McIntyre *et al.* 2008). This can be illustrated in our model where, without increased resources, many will continue to die. Further, we can illustrate the reduced incidence[2] of infections with improved coverage of treatment. Unfortunately, the model parameters available do not indicate at what point treatment for prevention will be adequate for HIV control and whether other investments are needed.

Methods

A model is used to calculate the discounted future costs of HIV treatment and the discounted future benefits of that treatment. These benefits include both the survival of the treated individuals and the reduction in spread of infection that is achieved through their treatment. In each sub-Saharan African country we calculate costs based on the relationship we derived between costs and GNI per capita and scale (i.e. the number being treated in a country). These country-level calculations are informed by the current incidence of HIV and how it relates to prevalence. The results presented for sub-Saharan Africa as a whole are the aggregation of the country-specific results.

Modeling the dynamics of treatment: uptake and coverage

Two of the most important policy decisions which affect the cost and the benefit of AIDS treatment are the threshold CD4 count at which a country declares its HIV-infected population to be medically eligible for publicly supported AIDS treatment, and the rate of treatment initiation it chooses or can achieve to apply to this medically eligible group. An HIV-infected individual is "in need" of anti-retroviral treatment once their immune system has been sufficiently damaged – as measured by their CD4 cell count. What constitutes "sufficient damage" depends upon the prevailing guidelines and standards of care adopted in a country. Individual countries can, and typically do, select a threshold level of CD4 somewhere between 200 and 350 cells per cubic micro-liter.

As HIV treatment is still scaling up, there is a reservoir of people in need who, according to the medical criteria in effect in any given country, should be treated immediately. This reservoir of people who need but do not receive treatment shrinks when some of them are recruited into treatment programs, and grows when previously HIV-infected people cross the threshold into needing treatment. The total number of people receiving treatment grows as new people are recruited, and shrinks when people fail treatment.

---

[2] In this paper we adopt the epidemiologist's definition for the term "incidence" as the flow of new infections during a period of time, typically a year. In contrast, the term "prevalence" denotes the stock of people infected at a point in time. In this paper we do not address issues related to the distribution of the costs and benefits of AIDS by individual or household characteristics, and therefore we have no call to use the term "incidence" in the sense it is typically used in the economics literature.

The coverage rate of AIDS treatment is conventionally defined as the percentage of all those alive and medically eligible for treatment at a particular time (UNAIDS 2009). As normative guidelines change, the criteria for when treatment is beneficial include more HIV infected people, and coverage therefore declines. Unfortunately, coverage of the medically eligible is a poor indicator of a country's policy success, because it excludes from the denominator all those who have died for lack of treatment. Once an initial cohort has been treated a country can maintain a high coverage rate by continuing this cohort on treatment, despite allowing large numbers to die without treatment. An indicator of treatment expansion that more closely characterizes a country's current national policy is the "uptake rate," defined as the proportion of those needing treatment and not receiving it who are added to treatment rolls in a given year. A high uptake rate necessarily generates a high coverage rate, but a high coverage rate can be achieved with relatively low uptake rates once there has been an initial high recruitment. In our model "coverage" is the dynamic consequence of the uptake rate and the relative survival of those on treatment and is an output of the model rather than an input. The costs of treatment and the benefits derived depend upon the number of people who are receiving treatment, although survival is worse in the first few months of treatment. Whether this poorer prognosis is associated with increased costs from the management required for more complex cases is unclear, because the attention these complex cases receive may vary greatly from one facility to the next.

In this paper we characterize alternative national policies by the two parameters: the median CD4 count at which patients are recruited to AIDS treatment, and the uptake rate among all patients who are eligible but not yet on treatment. We make the simplifying assumption that a country can manipulate these two parameters independently of one another: the first by promulgating guidelines regarding the threshold level of CD4, and the second by allocating treatment "slots" to treatment facilities and supplying those facilities with the corresponding quantities of anti-retroviral medications and complementary resources.[3] Increasing either the median CD4

count at recruitment or the uptake rate will engender both costs and benefits. Our purpose is to show how the choice among these alternatives affects the benefit to cost ratio of treatment.

For the purposes of our modeling exercise we are interested in two different measures of coverage. The first is coverage as normally defined, which is the proportion of those defined as needing treatment or eligible for treatment who are receiving treatment at a point in time. This definition corresponds to the way the term "coverage" is used by governments and implementing agencies. The second is the proportion under treatment of all those infected. We use this second definition of coverage to calculate the influence of treatment in reducing transmissibility.[4]

To model these processes of treatment uptake and patterns of survival, we represent the HIV infected population in a few categories: those infected and not yet in need of treatment; those in need of treatment; those treated using first-line regimens and those treated using second-line regimens. The flow of individuals between these categories is illustrated in Figure 3.1 and defined with the following equations.

---

[3] For a single health care facility with a low uptake rate in its catchment area and a low median CD4 count of recruitment to raise its median CD4 of recruitment without first raising its uptake rate among sicker patients would require it to prioritize some less sick patients (with higher CD4 counts) over sicker patients (with lower ones). Few clinicians or policymakers would agree to such a prioritization regardless of WHO or national guidelines calling for initiation at higher CD4 counts. However, given the heterogeneity of HIV epidemics within countries, a country could have some facilities with historically high uptake and coverage rates, while others have low uptake and coverage. If those facilities with high uptake rates begin to recruit at higher CD4 levels, the country as a whole would be observed to increase its median CD4 recruitment level while its national uptake rate remains low.

[4] The AIDSCost model used for these simulations allows the user to project the consequences for future infections and ART costs of the assumption that ART expansion changes the population's sexual behavior. The model characterizes this relationship as proportional to the proportion of all HIV-infected people receiving treatment. However, in this paper we suppress the function of this parameter, assuming that ART expansion has no direct effect on risk behavior, either positive or negative.

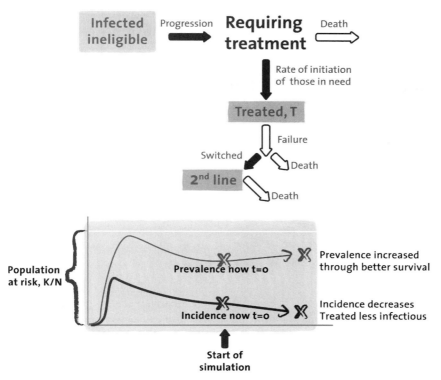

Figure 3.1 *Schematic diagram of model for projecting the cost of anti-retroviral therapy, accounting for its prevention benefits*

The difference equation for the stock of HIV infected who are not yet eligible for treatment is given in equation (1):

$$h_t = h_{t-1} + i_{t-1} - (erate * h_{t-1}) \qquad (1)$$

where *erate* is the rate at which the stock of infected become treatment eligible, which depends on a parameter of the model, *CD4*, the median CD4 rate at which patients are eligible for recruitment.[5] The stock of those eligible but not yet recruited into a treatment program evolves according to equation (2):

$$un_t = un_{t-1} + (erate * h_{t-1}) - \sigma * un_{t-1}$$
$$- ndrate * (1 - \sigma) * un_{t-1} \qquad (2)$$

where σ is the "uptake rate" at which eligible patients are recruited into the first year of ART and therefore leave the stock of those not yet recruited.

The parameter *ndrate* is the mortality rate among those not recruited and is also a function of the parameter *CD4*.[6]

The stock of those in their first year of first-line ART evolves according to:

$$a1_t = a1_{t-1} + \sigma * un_{t-1} - (1 - adrate1)$$
$$* a1_{t-1} - adrate1 * a1_{t-1} \qquad (3)$$

where *adrate1* is the rate at which patients fail treatment in their first year. Since the time-step in this

[5] At the default value of *CD4*, of 130, we assume the time to treatment eligibility would be approximately nine years, so that the value of *erate* is 0.111. We calibrate *erate* to other CD4 levels based on Collins (2009), which is available here: http://i-base.info/htb/5955.

[6] For the relationship between the parameter *ndrate* and the median CD4 of recruited patients, we rely on eART-linc (2008).

model is one year, the first term on the right-hand side of equation (3) cancels with the last two terms to ensure that all patients in their first year are new each year. The stock of those in their second and subsequent years of first-line ART increases by the number who do not fail treatment in their first year, but decrements due to a lower failure rate, *adrate2*:

$$a2_t = a2_{t-1} + (1 - adrate1)$$
$$* \, a1_{t-1} - adrate2 * a2_{t-1} \qquad (4)$$

The stock of those on second-line therapy augments by a proportion of those failing first line which is determined by the policy-selectable second-line coverage rate, *cvrg2*, and decrements according to a second-line failure rate, *bdrate*:

$$b_t = b_{t-1} + adrate2 * cvrg2 * a2_{t-1}$$
$$- bdrate * b_{t-1} \qquad (5)$$

Annual deaths are the aggregation of the deaths from each of these groups as follows:

$$d_t = ndrate * (1 - \sigma) * un_{t-1} + adrate1$$
$$* \, a1_{t-1} + adrate2 * (1 - cvrg2) * a2_{t-1}$$
$$+ bdrate * b_{t-1} \qquad (6)$$

Accumulated discounted years of death over the entire projection period are defined by the following double-summation:

$$YD = \sum_{t=2011}^{2050} \sum_{s=2011}^{t} \frac{d_s}{(1 + \tau)^s} \qquad (7)$$

where d is the discount rate and τ is the number of AIDS deaths in year s. Denoting the alternative scenarios by superscripts 0 (for the baseline or counterfactual) and 1 for a simulated investment program, an investment in AIDS treatment should reduce the number of years of death in the population. That is, it should be true that:

$$YD^1 < YD^0 \qquad (8)$$

so that the discounted benefits of the program can be measured by the discounted number of years of death averted. Since a year of death averted is a year of life saved, we define the present-discounted value of years of life saved as:

$$YLS = YD^0 - YD^1 \qquad (9)$$

We assume the coverage rate of second-line treatment in Africa will never exceed 10 percent during the projection period, and we do not model either the costs or the benefits of continued care and salvage regimens for those failing the second-line drug regimens.

The number of people infected with HIV is obviously a function of accumulated incidence, which depends on transmission from those already infected. To represent the recruitment of newly infected individuals and how this might change as a function of treatment coverage we use a very simple model based on the observed epidemiology of HIV in a baseline year.

Modeling the impact of treatment on new infections

Predicting the scale of an HIV epidemic is a hard problem, in part because patterns of risk behavior are intrinsically difficult to measure and bias-prone and in part because the pattern of spread is sensitive to small differences in risk behavior. Spread of HIV is driven by those with a high risk of acquiring and transmitting infection. Different patterns of risk behavior – numbers of sexual partners, numbers of people sharing injecting equipment, overlap between sexual partners, sexual practices, e.g., oral, anal, and vaginal sex – all vary across populations, meaning that not everyone is at risk of acquiring HIV and even fewer have the potential to spread infection. If there is a smaller higher-risk pool in one population, HIV will initially spread more rapidly, but in the longer run level off at a lower equilibrium infection rate. If risk is more evenly distributed, the epidemic will spread more slowly at first but then reach a dynamic equilibrium at a higher infection rate. Thus, there is great uncertainty predicting HIV epidemics from the start, but given that thirty years have passed and the HIV epidemic appears to have stabilized in many places, it is possible to assume a stable incidence and prevalence, and infer how much changes in pattern of risk might alter the incidence and prevalence of infection. Here we are assuming that countries with nascent and concentrated epidemics will not go on to suffer generalized HIV spread, and that generalized epidemics have reached their steady level. This could be changed exogenously by changes in risk behavior, but there is no reason for us to assume such changes.

The rate of new infections per susceptible individual, known as the incidence, depends upon a few fundamental parameters. These include the patterns of contacts among infected and susceptible persons, and on the infectivity of those infectious individuals. The duration of infection determines how long individuals stay in the infectious pool, and whether the infectious individual is treated determines how infectious they are. Heuristically we can build a model of HIV incidence that depends upon current prevalence;[7] we can then calculate how incidence would change if current risks of infectiousness changed across those infectious individuals. The fundamental problem is how to allow for heterogeneity in risk behavior across populations. Here we define a fraction of the population that has any risk of acquiring HIV. If this is a large fraction then a low incidence to prevalence ratio will generate the observed incidence, whereas if the fraction is limited a higher incidence to prevalence ratio at baseline can be assumed. This has important implications. We have an over-specified model where a parameter that we have no information on determines just how hard it is to control the spread of HIV. This allows us to do illustrative calculations, but does not allow us to say what is sufficient to bring HIV epidemics to a halt.

Our model of HIV transmission can be written down explicitly and related to standard epidemiological models. A standard simple model of a viral infection is given by the following two equations describing the rate of change of the numbers of susceptible and infectious in the defined at-risk population (Anderson, Medley et al. 1986; Anderson and Garnett 2000). Here S is susceptible, I infectious, and γ is the rate of entry "per person" into the at-risk population which is multiplied by the population size, N, where $N = S + I$. The parameter μ is the background mortality rate, α the death rate due to infection, and β a transmission coefficient. In the computer algorithm the patterns of entry and exit are determined by a more detailed model as described above. However, here we are most interested in the incidence term which

decrements the number of susceptibles in equation (10) and augments the number of infected in equation (11):

$$\frac{dS}{dt} = \gamma N - \beta S \frac{1}{N} - \mu S \qquad (10)$$

$$\frac{dI}{dt} = \beta S \frac{I}{N} - (\mu + \alpha)I \qquad (11)$$

There is a disease-free equilibrium where $I = 0$, which is unstable when $\beta/(\mu + \alpha)$, the basic reproductive number (which is denoted R_0), passes a threshold value of 1. The equilibrium steady state numbers of susceptible and infectious are given by: $S^* = N(\mu + \alpha)/\beta$ and $I^* = N^*((\gamma/(\mu + \alpha)) - (\mu/\beta))$. The endemic prevalence of infection can readily be calculated from the basic reproductive as $1 - (1/R_0)$ for this homogeneous population.

It is important to note that in a homogeneous population, where everyone has equal risk, infection spreads extremely widely with a modest basic reproductive number (Garnett 2002). This is obviously an invalid model for HIV where there is a great deal of heterogeneity in risk. In many models the detailed patterns of contact are represented. However, in developing a model to apply across Africa, where detailed behavioral data are often missing, we have chosen the parsimonious approach, employed in the UNAIDS Epidemic Projection Package, of dividing the population into those at risk and those not at risk (Brown, Grassly et al. 2006). If we assume that a fraction k of the population was at risk and we remove those already infected from this susceptible fraction, we have a revised simple set of equations:

$$\frac{dS}{dt} = k\gamma N - \beta S \frac{I}{N} - \mu S \qquad (12)$$

$$\frac{dI}{dt} = \beta S \frac{I}{N} - (\mu + \alpha)I \qquad (13)$$

$$\frac{dZ}{dt} = (1 - k)\gamma N - \mu Z \qquad (14)$$

In this case the susceptible numbers are given by the equation $S = Nk - I$ and infection saturates in this subset of the population.

[7] The term "prevalence" refers to the stock of infected people at a point in time. See n. 4 above.

In generating a parsimonious model of transmission we use the information currently available about transmission across most sub-Saharan African countries, the number infected, and the number newly infected in the most recent UNAIDS estimates to determine the epidemic potential of HIV in each country. We then assume that the relationship between incidence and prevalence will remain constant into the future unless there are changes in policy and the coverage of interventions. Thus, we adjust the simple models above to develop a new model which calculates the incidence in future years according to changes from a base year ($t = 0$).

The absolute number of infections during our base year, which is observed (or estimated) within a country as A_0, is also a function of the number susceptible and their risk:

$$A_0 = \beta(kN_0 - I_0)\frac{I_0}{N_0} = E_0(kN_0 - I_0) \quad (15)$$

We can set either k and derive E_0 or we can set E_0 and derive k:

$$E_0 = \frac{A_0}{kN_0 - I_0} \quad (16)$$

$$k = \frac{A_0 + E_0 I_0}{E_0 N_0} \quad (17)$$

We can then progressively calculate the absolute incidence rate at time t as a function of the number susceptible in the previous year, the prevalence of infection in that year, and how much the level of infectiousness has changed:

$$A_t = (kN - I_{t-1})\beta_t \frac{I_{t-1}}{N_{t-1}} \quad (18)$$

where β_t is a function of β_0 and $\beta_0 = E_0/(I_0/N_0)$, with the relationship also dependent on the coverage of treatment, circumcision, and other prevention interventions. In equation (18) we include the current numbers infected, I_{t-1}, which increases as improved survival is gained through treatment. This is then divided by the proportion infected at baseline, which is included in the expression for β_0. If the number infected rises, all else being equal, incidence will also rise. However, if treatment reduces transmissibility, we need to take this into account.

We also achieve this in our equations by comparing the ratio of transmissibility left at time $t - 1$ with that at time zero.

$$\beta_t = \beta_0 \left(\frac{\tau_{t-1}}{\tau_0}[1 - C][1 - e][1 + \delta\,\theta_{t-1}] \right) \quad (19)$$

The residual transmission in the presence of treatment τ_{t-1} is defined at baseline time $= 0$ and as for the previous year, $t - 1$ as a function of the fraction treated.

Where θ_{t-1} is the fraction with all those infected in the denominator and those on treatment in the numerator on treatment at time $t - 1$ (our second coverage definition above), g is the effectiveness of treatment in reducing the transmission probability of HIV and f is the fraction of infectiousness that can possibly be reduced by treatment as it occurs after the initial peak viremia. The parameter f should reduce as individuals have been on treatment for longer as they are remote from their primary viremia, so it represents a crude measure of the difficulty of eliminating infection through universal treatment at all CD4 counts where it is hard to identify all patients immediately. As treatment coverage increases, a smaller fraction of those infected are infectious. The ratio τ_{t-1}/τ_0 is a way of controlling for the numbers treated in the baseline year. The parameter f reflects the role of early infections which disproportionally transmit infection before people could reasonably be put on treatment (Powers, Ghani et al. 2011). The parameter g represents the effectiveness of treatment in reducing transmissibility.

The way this treatment effect works might best be illustrated with a numerical example: if $f = 0.7$ and $g = 0.7$, the number infected is 10,000 in year zero and for simplicity year $t - 1$, and that 1,000 are treated in year zero and 5,000 treated in year $t - 1$. This would set $\theta_0 = 0.1$ and $\theta_{t-1} = 0.5$; with $\tau_0 = 0.951$ and $\tau_{t-1} = 0.755$ and with $\tau_{t-1}/\tau_0 = 0.794$, this increase of treatment "coverage" from 10 percent to 50 percent would reduce incidence by 20.6 percent.

In considering the reduced transmissibility of those on treatment g it is worth noting that whilst in the HPTN-052 trial efficacy was over 90 percent, this only applied to couples where treatment successfully reduced the viral load (Cohen, Chen

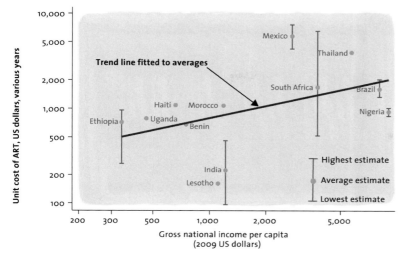

Figure 3.2 *Meta-analysis of studies of the cost per year of anti-retroviral therapy reveals heterogeneity within and between countries*

et al. 2011). Effectiveness will likely be much less than efficacy due to treatment failure, loss to care, the evolution of drug resistance, and viral blips due to poor adherence. We have made few assumptions about the relative efficacy of treatment in reducing transmissibility at different CD4 levels and about different treatment regimens. The parameter g is assumed identical for first- and second-line treatment. If second-line treatment is successful it should be equally efficacious through reductions in viral load; if it is unsuccessful then the patient will likely die.

In the broader transmission term, equation (19), C represents the product of the fraction of the population at risk that are men, the fraction circumcised, and the effectiveness of circumcision in reducing risk; e represents reductions in risk due to behavioral communication or condom social marketing, and represents the change in risk either increasing or decreasing resulting from coverage of treatment. There is debate over whether risk behavior will increase or decrease in response to the knowledge that anti-retroviral therapy is accessible and effective: in studies in Africa of self-reported risk, a decrease in risk behaviors has been observed (Gregson and Garnett 2010; Venkatesh, de Bruyn *et al.* 2010), but studies in Europe have argued, based on

trends in HIV infection rates, that there has been increased risk behavior (Bezemer, de Wolf *et al.* 2008).

Characterizing the unit cost of treatment

In determining what can be achieved for a given increment in spending on anti-retroviral therapy, we need to estimate the cost per person-year on treatment. This can be derived in three ways: 1) using commodity costs and prices for services to estimate what the cost should be; 2) using survey data measuring the actual costs of delivering ARVs in facilities; and 3) dividing current aggregate treatment expenditures by the number of people receiving treatment (Galarraga, Wirtz *et al.* 2011; Holmes, Coggin *et al.* 2010; Cleary, McIntyre *et al.* 2006, 2008). These methods generate somewhat different results. Figure 3.2 displays the estimates surveyed by Galarraga and co-authors, demonstrating a rough correlation with gross national income per capita. Figure 3.3 shows that PEPFAR budgeted expenditures display economies of scale (Institute of Medicine 2010). Both sources suggest that the average cost per patient-year in Africa varies between $200 and $1,000.

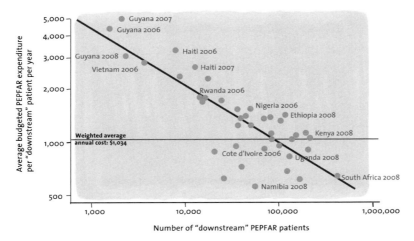

Figure 3.3 *Average unit treatment budgets reported by PEPFAR for 2006–2008 show mild economies of scale*
Source: *Institute of Medicine 2010.*

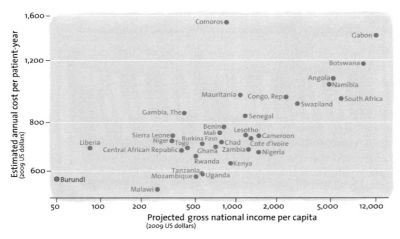

Figure 3.4 *Country-specific cost per person-year of treatment assumed in the projection model in 2012*

For the present exercise, we estimate unit costs by assembling several cost components. We assume that the average fixed cost per patient for a country with only 1,000 patients on treatment is $750, but that this amount declines by 14.2 percent for every doubling of the number of patients. Since several of our projection scenarios display remarkable growth in the number of patients, this assumption results in reducing the fixed cost per patient-year. We assume the variable cost per patient-year is indexed to a country's gross national income per

capita, and thus is higher for wealthier countries and grows as national economies grow. (We project economic growth in accordance with predictions of the World Bank.) To these average fixed and variable costs we add the annual drug costs per patient, which we derive from the most recent UNAIDS report on the epidemic. These costs too are positively correlated with a country's per capita income, as appears to be broadly true in reality. The result of these projections is displayed in Figure 3.4 for specific African countries in 2012 and in Table 3.1 for

Table 3.1 Cost per person-year in sub-Saharan Africa is modeled as varying by gross national income per capita, by drug regimen, and by scale of the national treatment effort

	Year	Component	Cost of treatment per person per year in sub-Saharan Africa (2009 US dollars)			
			Mean	Median	Minimum	Maximum
Cost of 1st-line treatment	2012	Drug	195.5	197.2	96.5	248.8
		Non-drug	517.1	441.1	355.1	1,133.4
		Total	712.5	631.1	482.6	1,345.0
	2050	Drug	235.5	244.9	150.4	260.1
		Non-drug	749.7	722.5	383.3	3,926.6
		Total	985.3	967.4	533.7	4,186.7
Cost of 2nd-line treatment	2012	Drug	1,569.4	828.6	2,426.8	1,373.8
		Non-drug	521.6	450.2	355.1	1,096.2
		Total	2,091.0	1,872.4	1,251.4	3,523.0
	2050	Drug	2,160.2	1,019.3	2,626.7	2,343.8
		Non-drug	750.5	722.5	383.3	3,926.6
		Total	2,910.7	3,067.1	1,402.6	6,553.3

Note: Means are weighted by number of people receiving either first- or second-line treatment in each country by year.

Source: Authors' estimates.

the average African patient in both 2012 and 2050. These procedures lead us to predict that, by the year 2050, the average cost of treatment in Africa will rise from its current level of $712 to $985. It can be debated whether costs should be adjusted for purchasing power parity. However, as we are concerned with the global resources available for treatment and the benefits they can generate, we choose not to so adjust.

Unlike early in the use of ARVs when the costs of the drugs themselves represented the majority of the annual treatment costs, current ARV treatment costs break down with approximately a third to drugs, a third to procurement and service delivery, and a third to laboratory tests. Thus, future cost savings may lie elsewhere than in the price of drugs. Costs are likely to vary according to how the ARVs are delivered and who delivers them. Currently the costs of second-line treatments are about two- or three-fold higher than first-line treatments. We use these modeled costs in our cost-benefit analysis of treatment.

Characterizing the simulated scenarios

Beyond contrasting two scenarios, with and without increased resources, choices can be made about who is treated and with what, which will influence the life years saved from given resources. We can contrast early versus late treatment; treatment with only first-line regimens, or treatment using second-line regimens; and treatment with different first-line drugs, i.e., regimens including tenofovir, or those that do not.

In analysis we can explore the impact of different levels of treatment uptake which leads to a cost due to the number of person years on treatment and a benefit, in terms of life years saved. This can be projected into the future in scenarios with and without given levels of treatment. To determine the benefits to be derived from $2 billion per year, we have to adopt a counterfactual for what future expenditure would be without this addition and what treatment uptake coverage would be without it. Two main choices appear possible. First, we could adopt the pessimistic assumption that donors will respect their existing commitments, but cease enrolling new patients. We call this the "zero uptake" counterfactual. Alternatively, we could more optimistically assume that the relatively high rates of patient recruitment seen in recent years will continue into the future. We call this second baseline possibility the "historical" counterfactual. The exercise of spending an additional $10 billion over five years begins with these two scenarios.

Figure 3.5 reports the results of applying our simulation model multiple times in order to

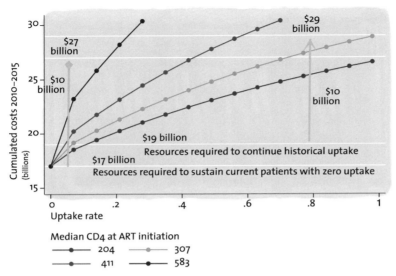

Figure 3.5 *The five-year cost of various combinations of uptake rate and median CD4 at initiation*

discover what $10 billion will buy. Our model estimates that the five-year cost of the zero uptake scenario in sub-Saharan Africa is about $17 billion, while the five-year cost of the continuation of historical trends would cost $19 billion over five years.[8] These alternative baseline spending levels are indicated by the horizontal lines in Figure 3.5. The figure also contains a line constructed to lie exactly $10 billion higher in relation to each of these starting points. There is such a line at $27 billion and one at $29 billion. The upward sloping curved lines in the figure display the relationship between spending and uptake rate that can be achieved when holding the median CD4 count constant. The lowest of the four lines shows that if the median CD4 rises only slightly to 204, expenditure will increase modestly with uptake, rising to touch the $27 billion mark when uptake approaches 1.0. Thus, from a starting point of zero uptake costing $17 billion, this line shows that an additional $10 billion allows virtually 100 percent uptake of those with a median CD4 of 200. Alternatively, if we look at the curve drawn for a median CD4 of 411 (the second curve from the top), we see that the $10 billion incremental expenditure up to the $27 billion ceiling for total cost will only get us to about 40 percent uptake, which is still a substan-

tial improvement over today's median CD4. These three scenarios are listed in the first three rows of Table 3.2.

Similarly, Figure 3.5 can be used to find what CD4 count and uptake rate combinations could be achieved if the $10 billion is added to the $19 billion projected to be flowing if uptake remains at its historical rate of growth. The answers are given in rows four through six of Table 3.2. At an uptake of 98 percent, a CD4 median of 307 will exhaust the $10 billion, whereas at an uptake rate of 25 percent, recruitment can be targeted at the quite high CD4 level of 583. These combinations can again be read from Figure 3.5.

In addition to these six scenarios, it is interesting for argument's sake to ask how the benefit to cost ratio would differ if both uptake and the recruitment threshold were pushed as ambitiously as possible. We call this the "universal access" scenario and compare it to the other scenarios under study. We are interested to see whether the universal access scenario can be argued to be superior on benefit-cost grounds even though it would increase

[8] Continuation at historical trends means that each country in Africa continues to add patients at an uptake rate equal to its achievements from 2008 to 2010.

Table 3.2 Alternative scenarios for computing the benefit to cost ratio of additional AIDS treatment expenditure

	Baseline expenditure 2011–2015	Uptake rate (sigma)	Median CD4 at treatment initiation (CD4)
Counterfactual			
Zero uptake	$17bn	0%	NA
Alternative ways to spend $10bn			
High uptake, low CD4	$27bn	98%	204
Lower uptake, high CD4	$27bn	40%	411
Counterfactual			
Historical uptake	$19bn	27%	130
Alternative ways to spend $10bn			
High uptake, low CD4	$29bn	98%	307
Lower uptake, high CD4	$29bn	25%	583
Universal access scenario			
High uptake, high CD4	$49bn	98%	800

five-year expenditure by about $30 billion over either of our two baseline counterfactuals.

Results

Suppose we ignore the prevention benefits of AIDS treatment and assume that every patient would die without treatment and survive if they receive it. In this simple but unrealistic world, the cost per additional year of life for AIDS treatment would simply be equal to the costs displayed in Table 3.1. Rather than use one of the available methods for estimating the dollar value of a life-year in sub-Saharan Africa, which would generate different values of life for each African country in our model, we conform to the rules of *RethinkHIV* by adopting the two alternative assumptions regarding the value of a year of life in sub-Saharan Africa that other authors are using: $1,000 and $5,000. If the value of a life is $1,000 per year, this naïve approach to the calculation of the benefits per dollar of additional AIDS

treatment cost yields a ratio of 1.4:1.0 for first-line treatment (= 1000/712.5) in 2012, and a ratio of 0.5:1 for second-line treatment (= 1000/2091). If a life is valued at $5,000 per life-year, these ratios become 7:1 and 2.4:1 respectively.

These naïve estimates are inadequate for several reasons. First, they ignore the potential for treatment optimization through the manipulation of several policy parameters, especially including the uptake rate and the CD4 at which patients initiate treatment. Second, they ignore the prevention benefits of treatment described above. Third, they ignore the spillover costs and benefits of AIDS treatment expansion on the rest of the health system. Our model incorporates the first two of these considerations, but the spillover costs and benefits on the health system are beyond the scope of this paper.

First, consider the role played by the country's choice of the CD4 count at which it initiates treatment. Figure 3.6 displays, in the top curve, the relationship recently estimated between a patient's life-expectancy at the time they initiate treatment and the CD4 count at which they initiate (Mills, Bakanda *et al.* 2011). Note that initiation at low CD4 counts near the right of the figure is associated with a much lower life-expectancy than initiation with a CD4 count above 150. One might expect that life-expectancy would continue to climb with initiation at even higher CD4 counts, but the study found to the contrary a statistically significant decline in life-expectancy at initiation CD4 counts above 250. This finding may be a statistical anomaly due to sampling error or to selection bias, due to sicker patients having initiated earlier. Or it may signal real difficulties with early initiation, such as poor adherence, or drug toxicity.

The bottom curve in Figure 3.6 displays the relationship between life-expectancy and CD4 count for people who do not initiate treatment (eART-Linc 2008). While the marked decline in life-expectancy as CD4 count declines is well known, the results of this study allow us to estimate how long a patient would have lived had he or she not initiated treatment at any given CD4 count.

A patient initiating treatment at a given CD4 count can expect an increase in life-expectancy equal to the difference between the top and bottom

Life-expectancy by CD4 count

by whether or not a person initiates treatment at that CD4 count
For age of infection 25–29

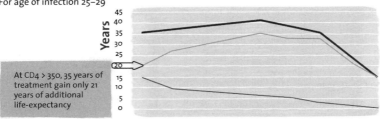

At CD4 > 350, 35 years of treatment gain only 21 years of additional life-expectancy

	350 and above*	275 to 349*	250 and above*	200 to 274*	150 to 249*	Less than 200*	100 to 149*	50 to 99*	Less than 50**
Life expectancy without ART*	14.6	9.8	8.6	7.4	6.3	5.2	2.85	1.675	0.5
Life expectancy with ART*	35.4	36.8	38.2	39.6	41	38.2	35.4	24.1	14.6
Years gained (using estimates which exclude Thailand)	20.8	27.0	29.6	32.2	34.7	33.0	32.6	22.4	14.1

The sources of the two sets of life-expectancy estimates reported in the top and bottom curves are denoted by the number of asterisks, with one asterisk indicating the eART-Linc study and two the Mills study. The authors have constructed the intermediate line as the difference between the two lines fro the cited studies.

Figure 3.6 *Years gained by an individual patient from anti-retroviral therapy by CD4 at treatment initiation defined as the difference between life-expectancy at that CD4 count with and without treatment. Curves are interpolated between CD4 ranges*
Sources: *Mills* et al. *(2011) and eART-Linc (2008).*

curves in Figure 3.6. This difference is graphed as the middle curve in the figure. Note that this curve lies well below the top curve for patients who initiate early, with a high CD4 count, and converges to the top curve as the CD4 count declines towards the right side of the figure.

The benefit-cost implications of this relationship are apparent. The top curve gives the expected years of AIDS treatment expenditure required to "purchase" an addition to life-expectancy represented by the middle curve. Thus, despite the greater life-expectancy of patients who initiate earlier which has been heralded in the literature, such patients consume more years of AIDS treatment for each year of life gained than do patients who initiate late in their disease progression. It's true that the cost of initiating a patient is potentially higher at lower CD4 counts, but this difference is thought to apply only to the first year of treatment

and is unlikely to outweigh the fact that early initiating patients consume thirty-five years of treatment expenditure for every twenty-one years of life gained. The effect is to multiply the above benefit to cost ratios by approximately 21/35 for early initiation, reducing the benefit to cost ratio for AIDS treatment, which suggests that, ignoring other considerations, countries achieve more benefits per dollar of treatment expenditure when they expand treatment first to those with the lowest CD4 counts. Only when a country has achieved nearly universal coverage of those with low CD4 counts should it consider allocating resources to recruit patients with higher CD4 counts.

Because a patient who strictly adheres to anti-retroviral therapy is less infectious than a patient who is not on therapy, and recent trial results described above confirm that this effect holds even at high CD4 counts, the future course of the HIV

AIDS treatment: Patients, mortality, and costs
Total for SSA

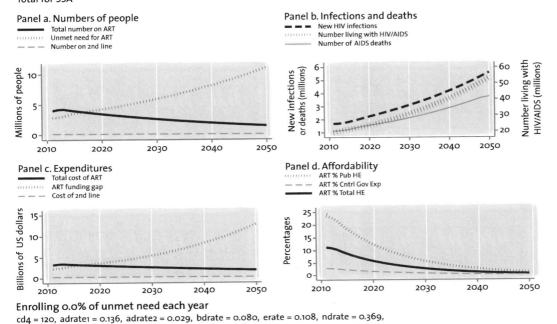

Panel a. Numbers of people
— Total number on ART
ⁱⁱⁱⁱⁱⁱⁱ Unmet need for ART
– – – Number on 2nd line

Panel b. Infections and deaths
▪ ▪ ▪ New HIV infections
ⁱⁱⁱⁱⁱⁱⁱ Number living with HIV/AIDS
‒‒‒‒‒ Number of AIDS deaths

Panel c. Expenditures
— Total cost of ART
ⁱⁱⁱⁱⁱⁱⁱ ART funding gap
– – – Cost of 2nd line

Panel d. Affordability
ⁱⁱⁱⁱⁱⁱⁱ ART % Pub HE
– – – ART % Cntrl Gov Exp
— ART % Total HE

Enrolling 0.0% of unmet need each year
cd4 = 120, adrate1 = 0.136, adrate2 = 0.029, bdrate = 0.080, erate = 0.108, ndrate = 0.369,
endogenous incidence maxep = 0, maxcp = 0, csp = 0.60, maxvp = 0, ve = 0, gp = 0.70,
maxdt = 0, maxdu = 0, iro = 0.20

Figure 3.7 *Zero uptake is a pessimistic counterfactual which avoids spending on AIDS treatment at the cost of millions of African lives.*
Source: *Authors' estimates using the AIDSCost model.*

epidemic is influenced by the uptake of antiviral treatment. However, because HIV is a slow disease, the benefits of resources spent to prevent HIV infection do not accrue within the five-year time horizon of the present exercise. Therefore, while we impose the $10 billion budget constraint over the years 2011 through 2015, we compute the present-values of the benefits and costs over the period 2011 to 2050. The benefit to cost ratio is the ratio of these two discounted numbers.

Before presenting the results of these calculations, we first present the full simulation results for four of the scenarios we are comparing. Figure 3.7 presents the simulation results for the most pessimistic scenario, the zero uptake counterfactual. Because no additional patients are being recruited, this scenario shows a declining number of persons on ART in panel a, while unmet need climbs to 10 million people by the year 2050. Panel b shows increasing AIDS deaths through the end of the

forty-year period, reaching almost 4 million per year from the current level of about 1 million. Panel c shows the spending of more than $3 billion per year, which accumulates to $17 billion by 2015, but falls to under $2 billion per year by the end of the period, as patients slowly fail treatment and no new patients are added. And panel d shows that total ART spending as a proportion of domestic resources falls from its high current level of 23 percent of public health expenditure and more than 10 percent of total health expenditure to lower and lower percentages, soon becoming affordable by national governments without donor support. This zero uptake scenario is parsimonious, but it causes almost a quadrupling of AIDS deaths, fails to stem the growth of infections, and amounts to a surrender to the AIDS epidemic.

Figure 3.8 presents the results of the historical uptake projection continued to the year 2050. In contrast to the zero uptake scenario, historical

AIDS treatment: Patients, mortality, and costs
Total for SSA

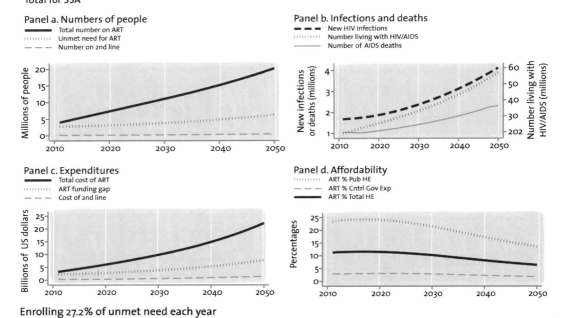

Enrolling 27.2% of unmet need each year
cd4 = 120, adrate1 = 0.136, adrate2 = 0.029, bdrate = 0.080, erate = 0.108, ndrate = 0.369, endogenous incidence maxep = 0, maxcp = 0, csp = 0.60, maxvp = 0, ve = 0, gp = 0.70, maxdt = 0, maxdu = 0, iro = 0.20

Figure 3.8 *Historical uptake expands treatment rolls and prolongs lives at the cost of an additional $15 billion per year by 2050, but total deaths rise almost as high as with zero uptake*
Source: *Authors' estimates using the AIDSCost model.*

uptake substantially grows the number of people on treatment, thereby reducing the unmet need for care, plotted by the dotted line in panel a. However, in this scenario, treatment does not expand fast enough to reduce the annual number of deaths from its current level. Because of increasing expenditure, which rises to $25 billion per year by the year 2050, panel c shows that ART spending would remain large in comparison to the average country's own budget for this forty-year period.

Figure 3.9 presents an analysis of the incremental $10 billion investment option, when it is assumed to be additional to the historical uptake counterfactual as portrayed in Figure 3.8. With a total of $29 billion to spend on AIDS treatment between now and 2015, the number of people on ART grows to 40 million by 2050, instead of 20 million in the historical uptake scenario of Figure 3.8. This

is good news for the public health of the country, since without the incremental money all of these people would have died. Panel b shows that this incremental spending pushes AIDS deaths sharply down to less than half their current level before they rebound due to the continually spreading epidemic. At the end of the period AIDS mortality remains at about 1 million deaths per year, less than a quarter of what they would be in the zero uptake scenario of Figure 3.7 and less than half of their value in the historical uptake scenario of Figure 3.8. Note that ART expenditures rise to above 50 percent of the African continent's public health spending by 2020 and then gradually return to their current proportion of public health spending by 2050.

Figure 3.10, the universal access option, is not a part of the present exercise, and is presented for comparison only. Note that in this scenario the

AIDS treatment: Patients mortality, and costs
Total for SSA

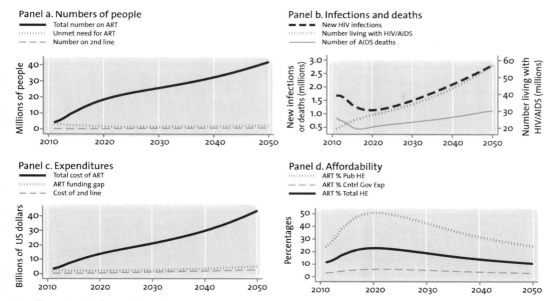

Panel a. Numbers of people
— Total number on ART
⋯⋯ Unmet need for ART
– – – Number on 2nd line

Panel b. Infections and deaths
– – – New HIV infections
⋯⋯ Number living with HIV/AIDS
— Number of AIDS deaths

Panel c. Expenditures
— Total cost of ART
⋯⋯ ART funding gap
– – – Cost of 2nd line

Panel d. Affordability
⋯⋯ ART % Pub HE
– – – ART % Cntrl Gov Exp
— ART % Total HE

Enrolling 98.0% of unmet need each year

cd4 = 307, adrate1 = 0.084, adrate2 = 0.027, bdrate = 0.080, erate = 0.198, ndrate = 0.111,
endogenous incidence maxep = 0, maxcp = 0, csp = 0.60, maxvp = 0, ve = 0, gp = 0.70,
maxdt = 0, maxdu = 0, iro = 0.20

Figure 3.9 *The high uptake scenario which costs $10 billion more than historical uptake greatly reduces unmet need and reduces the number of annual deaths in 2050 by about one million, but leads to an annual expenditure of almost $80 billion by the year 2050*
Source: *Authors' estimates using the AIDSCost model.*

number of people on treatment and the total ART expenditure both rise rapidly through 2015. By that year, ART expenditure attains peaks at 80 percent of African public health spending. But due to the prevention effect of putting 98 percent of HIV-infected patients on treatment, by the year 2050 there are cost savings. In this universal access scenario the costs in the year 2050 are about 25 percent less than in Figure 3.9, about $60 billion per year rather than $80 billion. Also in 2050 AIDS deaths per year are lower than they are in any of the other scenarios so far explored. In this situation, where heavy expenditure in the near term saves lives in the future, benefit-cost analysis is necessary to sort out the choice among alternatives.

Figures 3.11 and 3.12 present the cost-effectiveness and benefit-cost results for the scenarios described in Table 3.2. Each group of three bars is specific to a single counterfactual and a single discount rate. The first two bars in each group of three are for the two $10 billion scenarios we analyze, one with high uptake and low CD4, and the other the reverse. The third bar in each group presents the benefit to cost ratio of the three-times more expensive universal access policy. Figure 3.11 shows that, in comparison to the zero uptake counterfactual, the cost per life-year saved is lower at all discount rates for the $10 billion high-uptake, low-CD4 scenario than for the equal-cost low-uptake, high-CD4 scenario, as would be predicted from our analysis of the benefits of giving priority to those with low CD4 counts as explained by Figure 3.6. However, in comparison to the historical uptake scenario, the cost-effectiveness ranking of these two equal-cost

AIDS treatment: Patients mortality, and costs
Total for SSA

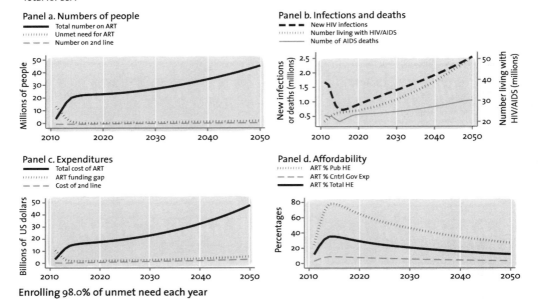

Enrolling 98.0% of unmet need each year

cd4 = 800, adrate1 = 0.004, adrate2 = 0.027, bdrate = 0.080, erate = 0.994, ndrate = 0.005, endogenous incidence maxep = 0, maxcp = 0, csp = 0.60, maxvp = 0, ve = 0, gp = 0.70, maxdt = 0, maxdu = 0, iro = 0.20

Figure 3.10 *The universal access scenario increases the number on ART in early years and requires increasing investment by $30 billion over the next five years, but achieves a 25 percent reduction in people living with AIDS by the year 2050*
Source: *Authors' estimates using the AIDSCost model.*

options is reversed, perhaps because the historical uptake has already achieved some of the most cost-effective health gains at low CD4 levels. Under our central assumption that anti-retroviral treatment reduces transmission of the average patient by 70 percent, the much greater expense of universal access does not achieve commensurate health improvements in comparison to either counterfactual at any discount rate. (Of each triple of bars in Figure 3.11, the third is always the highest.)

Figure 3.12 is the mirror image of Figure 3.11, with the height of each bar representing the benefit to cost ratio under the assumption that a life-year is valued at $5,000.[9] The figure shows that any of these investments has a somewhat higher benefit to cost ratio in comparison with a zero uptake than with the historical uptake. This pattern can be attributed to the phenomenon of dimin-

ishing returns. Spending $10 billion to add patients when none would otherwise be added reaps a higher return per dollar than adding $10 billion additional spending over and above the historical trend in each country. In infectious disease epidemiology, we can hope to achieve increasing returns to expanding investments when we push the reproductive rate of a disease down towards and below 1.0. Clearly none of these scenarios achieves that objective.

How much impact did the assumed HIV prevention benefits of ART have on these results? Figure 3.13 provides evidence on this question, by repeating the Figure 3.12 analysis four times,

---

[9] Since in this model the costs of treatment grow somewhat with increasing per capita income, it would be reasonable to allow the value of a life-year to grow as well. To do so would improve these benefit to cost ratios.

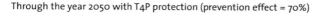

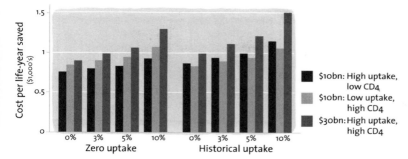

Figure 3.11 *Cost per life-year saved at a range of discount rates*
Source: *Authors' estimates using the AIDSCost model.*

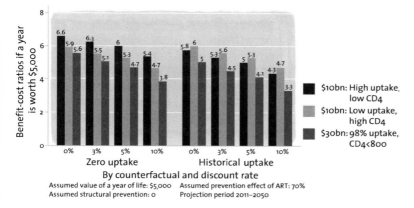

Figure 3.12 *Benefit to cost ratios for two $10 billion scenarios and one $30 billion scenario for two counterfactuals and two discount rates, assuming that a year of life is worth $5,000 and the prevention effect of ART is 70 percent.*
Source: *Authors' estimates using the AIDSCost model.*

with values of the prevention effect of ART ranging from 0.3 in the upper left to 0.9 in the lower right. Figure 3.12 is repeated in the lower left of Figure 3.13, for easy comparison with the others. Comparison of the four panels shows immediately that the benefit to cost ratios are greater when ART is assumed to have a stronger prevention effect. All of the benefit-cost numbers increase monotonically, from upper left to lower right, with the prevention effect of ART. Furthermore, the scenarios which are helped the most by assuming a strong prevention effect are the ones that expand treatment most vigorously. Universal access performs best relatively to the other scenarios when (a) the prevention effect

is strongest and (b) the discount rate is lower than 3 percent. However, even for the highest value of the prevention effect of 0.9, we do not see an order of magnitude improvement in the benefit to cost ratio of treatment, only a marginal improvement.

Finally, Figure 3.14 presents the results that are analogous to those in Figure 3.11, except with each year of life valued at $1,000 instead of $5,000. The pattern of the bars is identical to that in Figure 3.12, but the heights of the bars representing the benefit-cost calculations are one-fifth the size of the same bars in Figure 3.11.

If additional resources are used to treat those with higher CD4 counts while leaving those with

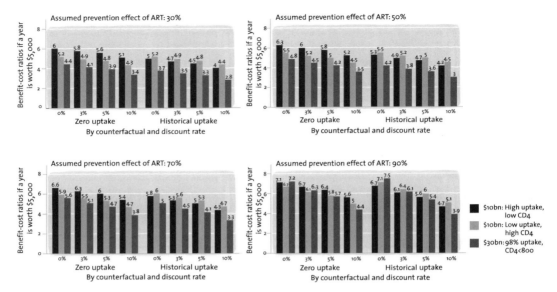

Figure 3.13 *Sensitivity of benefit to cost ratios to the prevention effect of ART, by counterfactual, discount rate, and scenario, assuming the value of a life-year is $5,000*
Source: *Authors' estimates using the AIDSCost model.*

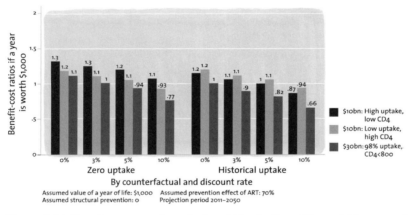

Figure 3.14 *Benefit to cost ratios calculated identically to Figure 3.11, except that each year of life gained is valued at $1,000*
Source: *Authors' estimates using the AIDSCost model.*

low CD4 counts untreated, then less than universal coverage will be achieved. Such a strategy fails to prevent a number of near-term deaths among the untreated with lower CD4 counts. In addition it does not achieve a great deal more in terms of HIV prevention, as those with lower CD4 counts are likely to be more infectious, apart from the period

of high viremia when it is unlikely patients will be identified to receive treatment.

Clearly, the costs of treatment will increase if more expensive drugs are used including both second-line and improved regimens. Currently second-line drugs are rarely used, which means they have little impact. However, if concerted efforts were made to employ second-line treatments and treatment failure grew over time, then they could constitute a major fraction of costs. This would leave fewer resources for first-line treatments and would decrease the overall benefit of programs in terms of life years saved.

Discussion

The costs of anti-retroviral treatment have dropped dramatically over the last fifteen years, allowing many more people infected with HIV to benefit from treatment (Mwagomba, Zachariah *et al.* 2010; Keiser, Anastos *et al.* 2008; Miiro, Todd *et al.* 2009). Concomitantly resources have been made available from both development aid for health and from national spending to increase numbers on treatment. Our results illustrate the dramatic difference that an extra $10 billion dollars over five years could make to treatment coverage. Such resources, if there were the capacity and the motivation to use them, could eventually achieve close to the universal coverage promised by world leaders. Unfortunately, although the benefit to cost ratios for these policies are greater than unity, the absolute projections show the number of AIDS cases and total AIDS expenditure on an accelerating trend, fast enough to more than keep pace with economic growth in many of these countries. These projections suggest that African countries hoping to reduce costs over the long run must necessarily invest in concomitant HIV prevention efforts in order to reduce the future growth in treatment need.

The costs per life year saved work out at close to $1,000 per year; thus if we value a life year at $1,000, then the benefit to cost ratio is about unity. If we value a life year at around $5,000, the benefit to cost ratio is about 5 relative to the historical counterfactual. This is favorable, but not the best buy in terms of investments in health. To argue for spending an additional $10 billion on AIDS treatment despite these relatively low estimated benefit to cost ratios would require marshaling a strong case that AIDS treatment has extremely large spillover benefits for the rest of society. In this paper we have included the spillover benefit on prevention, but found it to be insufficient to greatly increase the

benefit to cost ratio of treatment. Some of the other spillover benefits that have been adduced to AIDS treatment include: (a) a strengthened health system, newly competent at managing chronic progressive disease, (b) reduction in the years of orphanhood experienced by the children of deceased AIDS patients, (c) crowding out of poor quality informal AIDS treatment which would be likely to facilitate the appearance and spread of resistant strains of HIV, (d) improved social cohesion as the threat of early mortality is held at bay, (e) a more productive labor force, and (f) reduced gender violence.

Unfortunately, after thirty years of the AIDS epidemic, the evidence to support these beneficial spillovers is weak, and confined to specific settings. For example, the argument that AIDS treatment reduces the congestion in hospitals by shifting patients to outpatient clinics has some merit, but has rarely been quantified and is undercut by the observation that in the absence of anti-retroviral therapy, few African AIDS patients seek formal medical care. Some argue that AIDS treatment expansion has come at the expense of other more cost-effective and more equitably distributed health expenditures, such as immunization (Bongaarts and Over 2010). And others have suggested that African governments will increasingly resent the dependency of a large part of their adult population on foreign donors for their life-preserving daily medication (Lyman and Wittels 2010; Over 2009, 2011).

For the AIDS treatment community to compete successfully with other investment opportunities in today's fiscal climate will require new and more compelling demonstrations of the spillover benefits of AIDS treatment. Randomized controlled trials designed to test the existence and measure the extent of any of the hypothesized spillover benefits mentioned above could provide the information to enhance the benefit to cost ratios we estimate here and strengthen the argument for sustaining AIDS treatment funding. New research on so-called "combination prevention" may reveal synergies between AIDS treatment and other HIV prevention interventions that are sufficiently powerful to raise the benefit to cost ratio of the combined package to a far higher score. Over the longer run, Figures 3.8 and 3.9 both show AIDS treatment becoming increasingly affordable as African countries grow faster than their AIDS treatment expenditure burden. Thus, depending on the scenario, donors can be reassured that after the year 2020, AIDS treatment spending will begin to decline as a portion of African health budgets, and it will be possible for one African country after another to follow the lead of South Africa and Botswana in assuming responsibility for funding their own citizens' AIDS care.

There are important trade-offs in decisions about how best to deploy ARVs, which depend upon the perspective taken: do we wish to maximize utility or equity? Do we wish to privilege the patient in the care of a clinician or fairly share the benefits of health across populations? Choices along such dimensions often evolve without guidance from policy-makers. Our analysis of trade-offs between early versus late treatment illustrates that better care for some reduces the care available to others. In view of the prevention benefits of treatment, there are economic and public health arguments for allocating treatment resources to those patients who would otherwise be most likely to transmit the infection. And doing so would enhance the spillover benefits of treatment beyond those we have included in this model, but attaining these benefits would require us to reach those most at risk of transmitting with treatment programs. Other potential trade-offs to explore would likely have a short-term rather than longer-term impact, and include first-line drugs only, versus a more comprehensive and expensive pharmacopeia of first- and second-line drugs or even salvage regimens, and also the option of selectively substituting cheaper for better quality drugs.

In order to generate results applicable across the African continent and characterizing major decisions about treatment regimens, we have deliberately generated a parsimonious description of HIV progression, treatment, and transmission. The detailed assumptions about risks of morbidity, mortality, and transmission could be questioned. Thus, our results should be treated as crude estimates. More detailed analysis would require information on how the incidence of HIV is likely to change over time in different epidemiological settings. A major assumption here is that the current incidence to prevalence ratio for HIV infection is stable, and

that changes in the treatment of those infected influence this ratio in a predictable way. It has been argued that the availability of treatment allows people better knowledge of their infection and reduces risk behavior (Venkatesh, de Bruyn *et al.* 2010), but the opposite pattern of reduced fear of AIDS due to increased treatment has been observed elsewhere, with reductions in transmissibility being offset by increases in risk behavior (Bezemer, de Wolf *et al.* 2008). This behavioral response to reduced risk has been called "disinhibition" or "risk compensation" in the epidemiological and public health literature, and "moral hazard" in the economics and insurance literature. As anti-retroviral treatment is sustained and expanded in the coming decades, policy-makers will need information about the extent of such adverse behavioral responses and answers to other open questions in order to maximize the benefits to accrue from every dollar of AIDS treatment expenditure.

In summary, our results show that increased anti-retroviral treatment can yield benefits in excess of its costs, but also that we need HIV prevention that is able to control and substantially reduce the spread of HIV to make treatment affordable in the long term. Some have argued that the observed efficacy of treatment in reducing HIV transmissibility means that treatment "is prevention" and that scaled-up treatment should suffice. However, our analysis suggests that, with the parameters we use, this is not sufficient. If our parameterization were correct, treatment needs to be combined with other interventions and behavior changes such as adult male circumcision and greater condom use or reduced partner numbers, probably in combination, to dramatically reduce HIV incidence. We are also skeptical that prevention, in the absence of substantial treatment access, can succeed in reducing HIV incidence. Framing the resource allocation problem for AIDS in Africa as a stark choice between treatment and prevention ignores the proven and potential complementarities between the two. It has been cogently argued that treatment, via reduced stigma and greater knowledge of HIV, could act to help reduce risk behaviors. However, this result from treatment programs would have to be appropriately implemented and we lack good evidence on whether and how best this can be achieved. If it can,

Table 3.3 Parameters used in the AIDSCost projection program

Patient recruitment		Default value
Uptake of first-line treatment modeled as constant proportion, sigma, of unmet need, where sigma is constant across all countries and equal to:	$sigma$	User defined
The median CD4 count at ART initiation is:	$cd4$	130
Proportion of HIV-positive newly eligible for ART	$erate$	0.111
Incidence is modeled as endogenous to ART and affected by prevention scale-up		
Incidence rate in core group, Year 0	$ir0$	.2
Maximum HIV prevention effort	$maxep$	.6
Treatment effects		
Fraction transmission after primary infection	f	.7
Protection of treatment: $g = 1$ perfect	g	.7
Projection period		
First year of projections (projection take-off)	$takeoff$	2011
Last year of projections (projection horizon)	$horizon$	2050
Second-line treatment		
Second-line anti-retroviral therapy (ART) to start in year	$strtyr$	2009
Second-line ART to reach target in year	$trgtyr$	2020
Starting coverage rate for second-line ART[a]	$strtcov2$	Region specific
Target coverage rate for second-line ART	$trgtcov2$	0.10
Mortality		
Death rate of patients during their first year on first-line ART	$adrate1$	0.133
Death rate during subsequent years on first-line ART	$adrate2$	0.04
Death rate of patients on second-line ART	$bdrate$	0.04
Death rate of patients who are eligible for ART but are not enrolled in ART	$ndrate$	0.325
Cost computations based on following parameters		
Lower bound for first-line drug costs[b]	$rxc1lb$	$88
Upper bound for first-line drug costs	$rxc1ub$	$261
Lower bound for second-line drug costs	$rxc2lb$	$819
Upper bound for second-line drug costs	$rxc2ub$	$2,634
Number of bed-days per year per patient	$hsbedn$	1.56
Number of outpatient visits per patient	$hsvstn$	9.5
Average fixed non-drug cost at ART = 1,000	$nonrxcaf$	$750
Elasticity of average fixed cost of ART with respect to the number of ART patients	$scale$	−0.142

Notes: The parameter definitions and their default values in this table apply to AIDSCost Version 4.x. The table omits parameters set to zero in all the runs reported in this paper, such as those that apply to male circumcision or a hypothetical HIV vaccine.
[a] We assume those who fail first-line ART have only a 10 percent chance of access to second-line treatment. Increasing this proportion would decrease the benefit-cost ratio of any of the scenarios.
[b] Drug costs are assumed to vary across countries with the 2007 GDP per capita of the country according to the patterns observed by the World Health Organization in 2006 and then remain constant in any given country over time.

then the benefit to cost ratios shown in our analysis could be greatly improved, making anti-retroviral treatment a much better buy.

References

Amuron, B., Namara, G. *et al.* (2009). Mortality and loss-to-follow-up during the pre-treatment period in an antiretroviral therapy programme under normal health service conditions in Uganda. *BMC Public Health* **9**: 290.

Anderson, R. M. and Garnett, G. P. (2000). Mathematical models of the transmission and control of sexually transmitted diseases. *Sex Transm Dis* **27**(10): 636–43.

Anderson, R. M., Medley, G. F. *et al.* (1986). A preliminary study of the transmission dynamics of the human immunodeficiency virus (HIV), the causative agent of AIDS. *IMA J Math Appl Med Biol* **3**(4): 229–63.

Athan, E., O'Brien, D. P. *et al.* (2010). Cost-effectiveness of routine and low-cost CD4 T-cell count compared with WHO clinical staging of HIV to guide initiation of antiretroviral therapy in resource-limited settings. *AIDS* **24**(12): 1887–95.

Babigumira, J. B., Castelnuovo, B. *et al.* (2009). Potential impact of task-shifting on costs of antiretroviral therapy and physician supply in Uganda. *BMC Health Serv Res* **9**: 192.

Babigumira, J. B., Castelnuovo, B. *et al.* (2011). Cost effectiveness of a pharmacy-only refill program in a large urban HIV/AIDS clinic in Uganda. *PLoS One* **6**(3): e18193.

Babigumira, J. B., Sethi, A. K. *et al.* (2009). Cost effectiveness of facility-based care, home-based care and mobile clinics for provision of antiretroviral therapy in Uganda. *Pharmacoeconomics* **27**(11): 963–73.

Bendavid, E., Grant, P. *et al.* (2011). Cost-effectiveness of antiretroviral regimens in the World Health Organization's treatment guidelines: a South African analysis. *AIDS* **25**(2): 211–20.

Bertozzi, S. M., Martz, T. E. *et al.* (2009). The evolving HIV/AIDS response and the urgent tasks ahead. *Health Aff (Millwood)* **28**(6): 1578–90.

Bezemer, D., de Wolf, F. *et al.* (2008). A resurgent HIV-1 epidemic among men who have sex with men in the era of potent antiretroviral therapy. *AIDS* **22**(9): 1071–7.

Bongaarts, J. and Over, M. (2010). Public health. Global HIV/AIDS policy in transition. *Science* **328**(5984): 1359–60.

Braitstein, P., Brinkhof, M. W. *et al.* (2006). Mortality of HIV-1-infected patients in the first year of antiretroviral therapy: comparison between low-income and high-income countries. *Lancet* **367**(9513): 817–24.

Brown, T., Grassly, N. C. *et al.* (2006). Improving projections at the country level: the UNAIDS Estimation and Projection Package 2005. *Sex Transm Infect* **82** Suppl 3: iii34–40.

Cleary, S. (2010). Equity and efficiency in scaling up access to HIV-related interventions in resource-limited settings. *Curr Opin HIV AIDS* **5**(3): 210–14.

Cleary, S. M., McIntyre, D. *et al.* (2006). The cost-effectiveness of antiretroviral treatment in Khayelitsha, South Africa–a primary data analysis. *Cost Eff Resour Alloc* **4**: 20.

Cleary, S. M., McIntyre, D. *et al.* (2008). Assessing efficiency and costs of scaling up HIV treatment. *AIDS* **22** Suppl 1: S35–42.

Cleary, S., Silal, S. *et al.* (2010). Equity in the use of anti-retroviral treatment in the public health care system in urban South Africa. *Health Policy* **99**(3): 261–6.

Cohen, M. S., Chen, Y. Q. *et al.* (2011). Prevention of HIV-1 infection with early anti-retroviral therapy. *N Engl J Med* **365**(6): 493–505.

Dodd, P. J., Garnett, G. P. *et al.* (2010). Examining the promise of HIV elimination by test and treat in hyperendemic settings. *AIDS* **24**(5): 729–35.

Donnell, D., Baeten, J. M. *et al.* (2010). Heterosexual HIV-1 transmission after initiation of antiretroviral therapy: a prospective cohort analysis. *Lancet* **375**(9731): 2092–8.

eART-linc. (2008). Duration from seroconversion to eligibility for antiretroviral therapy and from ART eligibility to death in adult HIV-infected patients from low and middle-income countries: collaborative analysis of prospective studies. *Sexually Transmitted Infections* **84**(Supplement 1): 31–6.

Fox, M. P., Sanne, I. M. *et al.* (2010). Initiating patients on antiretroviral therapy at CD4 cell counts above 200 cells/microl is associated with improved treatment outcomes in South Africa. *AIDS* **24**(13): 2041–50.

Galarraga, O., Wirtz, V. J. *et al.* (2011). Unit costs for delivery of antiretroviral treatment and prevention of mother-to-child transmission of HIV: a systematic review for low- and middle-income countries. *Pharmacoeconomics* **29**(7): 579–99.

Garnett, G. P. (2002). An introduction to mathematical models in sexually transmitted disease epidemiology. *Sex Transm Infect* **78**(1): 7–12.

Granich, R. M., Gilks, C. F. *et al.* (2009). Universal voluntary HIV testing with immediate antiretroviral therapy as a strategy for elimination of HIV transmission: a mathematical model. *Lancet* **373**(9657): 48–57.

Gregson, S. and Garnett, G. P. (2010). Antiretroviral treatment is a behavioral intervention: but why? *AIDS* **24**(17): 2739–40.

Hendriks, J. C., Medley, G. F. *et al.* (1993). The treatment-free incubation period of AIDS in a cohort of homosexual men. *AIDS* **7**(2): 231–9.

Holmes, C. B., Coggin, W. *et al.* Use of generic antiretroviral agents and cost savings in PEPFAR treatment programs. *JAMA* **304**(3): 313–20.

Institute of Medicine. (2010). *Preparing for the Future of HIV/AIDS in Africa: A Shared Responsibility*. Washington, DC: Institute of Medicine.

Jouquet, G., Bygrave, H. *et al.* (2011). Cost and cost-effectiveness of switching from d4T or AZT to a TDF-based first-line regimen in a resource limited setting in rural Lesotho. *J Acquir Immune Defic Syndr*.

Keiser, O., Anastos, K. *et al.* (2008). Anti-retroviral therapy in resource-limited settings 1996 to 2006: patient characteristics, treatment regimens and monitoring in sub-Saharan Africa, Asia and Latin America. *Trop Med Int Health* **13**(7): 870–9.

Keiser, O., Chi, B. H. *et al.* (2011). Outcomes of antiretroviral treatment in programmes with and without routine viral load monitoring in southern Africa. *AIDS* **25**(14): 1761–9.

Keiser, O., Tweya, H. *et al.* (2009). Switching to second-line antiretroviral therapy in resource-limited settings: comparison of programmes with and without viral load monitoring. *AIDS* **23**(14): 1867–74.

Kimmel, A. D., Weinstein, M. C. *et al.* (2010). Laboratory monitoring to guide switching antiretroviral therapy in resource-limited settings: clinical benefits and cost-effectiveness. *J Acquir Immune Defic Syndr* **54**(3): 258–68.

Long, L., Brennan, A. *et al.* (2011). Treatment outcomes and cost-effectiveness of shifting management of stable ART patients to nurses in South Africa: an observational cohort. *PLoS Med* **8**(7): e1001055.

Loubiere, S., Meiners, C. *et al.* (2010). Economic evaluation of ART in resource-limited countries. *Curr Opin HIV AIDS* **5**(3): 225–31.

Lyman, P. N. and Wittels, S. B. (2010). No good deed goes unpunished. *Foreign Affairs* **89**(4): 74–84.

May, M., Boulle, A. *et al.* (2010). Prognosis of patients with HIV-1 infection starting antiretroviral therapy in sub-Saharan Africa: a collaborative analysis of scale-up programmes. *Lancet* **376**(9739): 449–57.

Miiro, G., Todd, J. *et al.* (2009). Reduced morbidity and mortality in the first year after initiating highly active anti-retroviral therapy (HAART) among Ugandan adults. *Trop Med Int Health* **14**(5): 556–63.

Mills, E. J., Bakanda, C., Birungi, J., Chan, K., Ford, N., Cooper, K. L., Nachega, J. B., Dybul, M. and Hogg, R. S. (2011). Life expectancy of persons receiving combination antiretroviral therapy in low-income countries: a cohort analysis from Uganda. *Annals of Internal Medicine* E-358. doi:10.1059/0003-4819-155-4-201108160-00358.

Mwagomba, B., Zachariah, R. *et al.* (2010). Mortality reduction associated with HIV/AIDS care and antiretroviral treatment in rural Malawi: evidence from registers, coffin sales and funerals. *PLoS One* **5**(5): e10452.

Over, M. (2009). Prevention failure: the ballooning entitlement burden of US global AIDS treatment spending and what to do about it. *Revue d'Economie du Developpement* **2009**(1–2): 107–44.

Over, M. (2011). *Achieving an AIDS Transition: Preventing Infections to Sustain Treatment*. Washington, DC: Brookings Institution Press.

Palella, F. J., Jr., Delaney, K. M. *et al.* (1998). Declining morbidity and mortality among patients with advanced human immunodeficiency virus infection. HIV Outpatient Study Investigators. *N Engl J Med* **338**(13): 853–60.

Phillips, A. N., Pillay, D. *et al.* (2008). Outcomes from monitoring of patients on antiretroviral therapy in resource-limited settings with viral load, CD4 cell count, or clinical observation alone: a computer simulation model. *Lancet* **371**(9622): 1443–51.

Powers, K. A., Ghani, A. C. *et al.* (2011). The role of acute and early HIV infection in the spread of HIV and implications for transmission prevention strategies in Lilongwe, Malawi: a modelling study. *Lancet* **378**(9787): 256–68.

Quinn, T. C., Wawer, M. J. *et al.* (2000). Viral load and heterosexual transmission of human immunodeficiency virus type 1. Rakai Project Study Group. *N Engl J Med* **342**(13): 921–9.

Sabin, C. A. and Phillips, A. N. (2009). Should HIV therapy be started at a CD4 cell count above 350 cells/microl in asymptomatic HIV-1-infected patients? *Curr Opin Infect Dis* **22**(2): 191–7.

Sanne, I., Orrell, C. *et al.* (2010). Nurse versus doctor management of HIV-infected patients receiving antiretroviral therapy (CIPRA-SA): a randomised non-inferiority trial. *Lancet* **376**(9734): 33–40.

Shumbusho, F., van Griensven, J. *et al.* (2009). Task shifting for scale-up of HIV care: evaluation of nurse-centered antiretroviral treatment at rural health centers in Rwanda. *PLoS Med* **6**(10): e1000163.

UNAIDS. (2009). *Report on the Global AIDS Epidemic.* Geneva: UNAIDS.

UNAIDS. (2010). *Outlook Report.* Geneva: UNAIDS.

Venkatesh, K. K., de Bruyn, G. *et al.* (2010). Decreased sexual risk behavior in the era of HAART among HIV-infected urban and rural South Africans attending primary care clinics. *AIDS* **24**(17): 2687–96.

Walensky, R. P. and Kuritzkes, D. R. (2010). The impact of the President's Emergency Plan for AIDS Relief (PEPfAR) beyond HIV and why it remains essential. *Clin Infect Dis* **50**(2): 272–5.

Walensky, R. P., Wood, R. *et al.* (2010). Scaling up the 2010 World Health Organization HIV Treatment Guidelines in resource-limited settings: a model-based analysis. *PLoS Med* **7**(12): e1000382.

Waning, B., Kaplan, W. *et al.* (2009). Global strategies to reduce the price of antiretroviral medicines: evidence from transactional databases. *Bull World Health Organ* **87**(7): 520–8.

Waning, B., Kyle, M. *et al.* (2010). Intervening in global markets to improve access to HIV/AIDS treatment: an analysis of international policies and the dynamics of global antiretroviral medicines markets. *Global Health* **6**: 9.

Wirtz, V. J., Forsythe, S. *et al.* (2009). Factors influencing global antiretroviral procurement prices. *BMC Public Health* **9** Suppl 1: S6.

World Health Organization. (2010). *Towards Universal Access: Scaling up priority HIV/AIDS interventions in the health sector Progress Report 2010.* Geneva: World Health Organization.

Zachariah, R., Harries, K. *et al.* (2009). Very early mortality in patients starting antiretroviral treatment at primary health centres in rural Malawi. *Trop Med Int Health* **14**(7): 713–21.

Zachariah, R., Tayler-Smith, K. *et al.* (2011). Retention and attrition during the preparation phase and after start of antiretroviral treatment in Thyolo, Malawi, and Kibera, Kenya: implications for programmes? *Trans R Soc Trop Med Hyg* **105**(8): 421–30.

3.1 Treatment

Perspective paper

ROBERT J. BRENT

This is one of the perspective papers dealing with the assessment paper on Treatment by Mead Over and Geoffrey Garnett – hereafter O&G – as part of *RethinkHIV* seeking how best to spend an extra $10 billion to combat HIV/AIDS in sub-Saharan Africa. The purpose of the perspective paper is to provide a counterbalance to the assessment paper by indicating areas of agreement, disagreement, and discussion.

The main focus of the assessment paper is on ARV treatment as prevention. O&G analyze this issue by recognizing that the drugs reduce the viral load and thereby reduce the transmission of the HIV infection to others, saving lives in the process. The transmission process they model specifies an effect on yearly infections that depends on the coverage of treatment in each period of time. The greater the coverage, the lower the transmission rate, the fewer the number of infections, and the greater the number of lives saved which, valued at a pre-assigned amount per life year saved, provides the benefits in *RethinkHIV*. It is the ability of the extra funds to increase coverage that enables the benefits to be obtained. How far coverage can increase the benefits due to the extra funds depends on the yearly costs of the treatment, which consist of the price of the drugs and the testing and delivery costs.

O&G find that treatment as prevention can produce benefit-cost ratios (BCRs) in the range 3 to 3.5 in one scenario ("zero uptake") and they are in the range 2.3 to 2.5 in the alternative scenario ("historical uptake"). In the sensitivity analysis, the B/C ratios never exceed 4. Our main contribution in this paper is to reconstruct their analysis using these ratios as benchmarks so that we can identify the types of assumption that can validate the O&G results. From there we add some new assumptions in the context of a particular type of treatment

intervention not covered explicitly in the assessment paper.

Because the main contribution of the O&G paper is to formulate and estimate a transmission rate for HIV infection that depends on time, it constitutes an important first step towards constructing a dynamic evaluation of HIV treatment. Given this, it seems useful to place their contribution within a more complete dynamic framework to help understand what the particular transmission mechanism specified contributes to the evaluation and to see also what is missing. The dynamic framework is presented below.

We provide a discrete time representation of the dynamic model used. This puts the evaluation of treatment into the context of an intervention for a single person receiving treatment, which performs the same function as the representative agent model in macroeconomics. We use the discrete time representation to highlight the importance of particular data assumptions and, in particular, the impact of using different discount rates. In this framework we interpret the enhanced ability of treatment to reduce infections in the O&G analysis to be an externality that magnifies the benefits that an individual receives. The existence of externalities is clearest in the case of the prevention of mother to child transmission (MTCT) and this is the intervention that will be evaluated. As we shall see, there will be two types of externality when women are treated, and this is not the case when men are treated. We thus introduce an important gender consideration that is missing from the assessment paper.[1] Below, we compare our results with others making similar calculations in *RethinkHIV*. The paper concludes

---

[1] Pregnant women are mentioned early in the assessment paper, but there is no further consideration anywhere else.

with a discussion section followed by the summary and conclusions.

Dynamic models of the effect of HIV treatment on infections

The model used in the assessment paper is basically an S-I (susceptible-infection) transmission system that is a staple in the epidemiological literature that has been developed by Gersovitz and Hammer (2004) for health economists. The dynamic framework below is a simplified version of the Gersovitz and Hammer model which is adapted to apply to HIV treatment. We call this the standard dynamic model of infections. We will not go very far with the analysis, just far enough to be able to reflect on the model presented in the assessment paper, which is the O&G model. Our analysis begins with the part of the standard model that explains how the flow of infections will change over time. We then present the same type of analysis as it appears in the O&G model. We then compare the two versions in terms of the number of infections that each will predict. After this we explain how the standard model analyzes interventions that will influence the flow of infections. We will show that the O&G model omits important mechanisms by which treatment affects infections.

The standard dynamic model of infections

The starting point is a number of population identities. The population, N, in any country affected by HIV is the sum of those susceptive to infection, S, and the number of persons infected, I:

$$N = I + S \tag{1}$$

The state variables are the infection rate (i.e., prevalence rate) and the susceptible rate defined as:

$$i = I/N \text{ and } s = S/N \tag{2}$$

The variables change over time as follows (using dots above variables to signify time derivatives). Population increases due to the birth rate ε and

decreases by the natural (not due to infection) death rate μ:

$$\dot{N} = (\varepsilon - \mu)N \tag{3}$$

Under random matching, the probability per contact of a susceptible meeting an infected person is i. Then Si is the total number of susceptibles having contact with an infected person. The transmission rate per contact is β. The rate of increase of transmissions from this rate applied to the number having contact with an infected person is βSi. Thus the number of infecteds increases over time by the number of new infections less the number of people who die anyway (μ) or because of AIDS (α):

$$\dot{I} = \beta Si - (\mu + \alpha)N \tag{4}$$

Lastly, the number of susceptibles increases naturally from population growth and decrease as some of them get infected or die naturally:

$$\dot{S} = (\varepsilon - \mu)N - \beta Si \tag{5}$$

The O&G model of infections compared

The assessment paper has equations similar to (4) and (5). Since the two equations are strongly interrelated, to make our points we need only focus on one of them, which will be the susceptibles equation. O&G's version of equation (5) is their equation (3), which we reproduce here as:

$$\dot{S} = k\gamma N - \beta Si - \mu S \tag{6}$$

where γ is the rate of entry per person into the "at risk" population and k is the fraction of the population at risk. For ease of comparison term by term we rewrite our equation (5) as:

$$\dot{S} = \varepsilon N - \beta Si - \mu N \tag{7}$$

There is no difference in the second terms of equations (6) and (7), but there are important differences in the first and third terms. These differences imply that the O&G model will underestimate the number of S and I and hence also underestimate the number of infections that a reduction in the transmission rate β will generate.

A comparison of the first terms reveals that O&G for some reason want to restrict entry into the numbers of people who are going to be judged as newly "at risk" in the population. They have applied the parameters $k\gamma$ to the population N instead of the birth rate ε as in the standard model. There are two restrictions imposed here and both of them are questionable in the context of the treatment intervention. The standard model assumes that everyone born is susceptible to infection sometime in their lifetime and this includes those newly born. In the O&G model only the fraction k is at risk. Given that the number of children infected with HIV is so high in SSA, not to have $k = 1$ is very strange. Even if $k = 1$ is adopted, the second difference is that O&G want to use the rate of entry into the risk population γ rather than the birth rate ε. It is difficult to know whether γ is going to be higher than ε because a definition of an "at risk" group is not given in the assessment paper.

In fact an estimate of k is not presented anywhere in the paper either. All we get is their equation (8), which tells us how one can *deduce* k from a knowledge of other parameters. This after-the-event approach shares the same basic weakness as the World Bank's and many other groups' strategy with HIV which seeks to target the high-risk groups first. As pointed out in Brent (2010a), in the context of a generalized epidemic as in an SSA country, one often does not know which group is to be considered "high-risk" *a priori*. For example, Pisani (2008) informs us that a schoolgirl in South Africa is ten times more likely to be infected with HIV than a prostitute in Beijing. In this particular case, schoolgirls are to be targeted as the "high-risk" group, and not prostitutes. Who would have thought that this would have been the case in advance of looking at the facts?

A comparison between the third terms of equations (6) and (7) again shows how the O&G model will underestimate the number of infections. The death rate μ is applied to S in O&G's equation (6), while it is applied to N in the standard model equation (7). Since N is greater than S by the number of I – see equation (1) – the O&G model reduces the number of S due to the death rate less than the stan-

dard model. So using equation (4) the lower value for S will generate a lower number of infections that can be reduced by treatment.

The standard and O&G dynamic models with interventions

We now introduce into the analysis control variables, variables under the control of the government via the expenditures that are incurred on them. In the context of *RethinkHIV*, the controls are the HIV interventions. These may be for prevention, treatment, or mitigation. Control variables affect the parameters in the system, i.e., ε, μ, β, and α. Typically prevention is targeted at the susceptibles and treatment to the infecteds. However, in the assessment paper the focus is on treatment as prevention, so in principle every parameter in the system can be affected by treatment T. We will assume:

$$\varepsilon = \varepsilon(T), \acute{\varepsilon} > 0 \tag{8a}$$

$$\alpha = \alpha(T), \acute{\alpha} < 0 \tag{8b}$$

$$\mu = \mu(T), \mu' = 0 \tag{8c}$$

$$\beta = \beta(T), \beta' < 0 \tag{8d}$$

In (8a) we recognize that HIV lowers the fertility rate. Therefore providing treatment will raise the fertility rate and with it the birth rate. A rise in the population will increase the number of infecteds directly, via I, and indirectly via the number of susceptibles S in (4). Equation (8b) focuses on the effect of treatment on the death rate of those living with HIV/AIDS.[2] The consequences can also be explained in terms of equation (4). The lower is α, the more people living with infections will go up in terms of N. Moreover, the more infecteds there are, the higher is i and the more new infections will take place via βS. This is of course the reason why HIV prevalence in the US is rising, even though the rate of new infections (incidence) has been staying relatively constant. People with HIV who do not die add to the number living with HIV and, because they are still around, they can give the virus to others. Equation (8c) acknowledges the

---

[2] Although overall effect of treatment is to increase life expectancy, for a few individuals ARV is fatal because of its toxicity.

possibility that there could be an impact on the death rate for those not infected with HIV who take treatment, for example as a pre-exposure prophylaxis; but at this point in time there is no firm general evidence that its impact is not zero. Lastly in the list of parameters affected by treatment we come to equation (8d). Treatment reduces the transmission mechanism β and will therefore reduce the number of new infections – see equation (4) – and so increase the number of lives saved.

Of the four possible effects of treatment listed in equations (8a) to (8d), only (8d) appears in the O&G model. The omission of equations (8a) and (8b) in particular reinforces our previous conclusion that the O&G model is underestimating the number of lives saved from treatment. In the previous paragraph we have explained how the number of lives saved increase due to treatment using models explaining the flow of infections. Here we just need to reinforce this conclusion by pointing out that equations (6a) and (6b) recognize the fertility effects of treatment. That is, increasing births and reducing deaths must increase the number of lives saved. Since the main contribution of the assessment paper is to model how treatment will change the transmission mechanism $\beta(T)$, we will now examine in detail O&G's formulation of equation (8d).

The O&G model's specification of the transmission mechanism

The O&G model's specification of the transmission mechanism and how it changes due to treatment is given in equation (19) in the assessment paper, which becomes our equation (9):

$$\beta_t = \beta_0(T_t/T_0)[1-C][1-e][1+\delta h_t] \qquad (9)$$

where β_t is the transmission rate in any year t, β_0 is the transmission rate in the base year prior to the expansion of treatment, τ_t is the treatment rate in any year t, τ_t is the treatment rate in the base year, C is the proportion by which circumcision reduces the transmission rate, e is the proportion by which educational programs reduce the transmission rate, and δ is the perverse incentive effect (the "moral hazard" effect), whereby increasing coverage h_t

in year t increases risky behavior leading to more infections.

The easiest way to interpret the role of equation (10) is to focus on the second terms of equations (6) and (7), which are identically the same, being βSi. If we ignore the first and third terms which we have already analyzed, we can replace both (6) and (7) by:

$$\dot{S} = -\beta Si \qquad (10)$$

Equation (10) just says that increasing infections lowers the number of susceptibles. In O&G's equation (19) they recognize that the effects in the square brackets lower the number of susceptibles and hence the transmission rate of HIV. Effectively they are defining an adjusted S which we will call S' and using this to replace equation (10) in the form:

$$\dot{S} = -\beta_t S'i \qquad (11)$$

where

$$S' = [1-C][1-e][1+\delta h_t]S \qquad (12)$$

and

$$\beta_t = \beta_0(T_t/T_0) \qquad (13)$$

We can therefore regard O&G's equation (19) as making a contribution by decomposing equation (11) into the two parts (12) and (13). Equation (12) reminds us that the transmission rate is reduced by treatment only after the effects of other behavioral interventions have first taken place. This is of course correct. But, O&G do not in fact make any of the adjustments implied by S' in (12), as they report that they have set all the variables in (12) (except for S) equal to zero in their simulations. This leaves only equation (13) left to understand and assess.

In equation (13), β_t starts off equal to β_0 and then changes according to τ_t/τ_0, which is the percentage change in the fraction getting treatment in any year relative to the base year. To determine the treatment fraction in any year, O&G use:

$$T_t = 1 - fgh_t \qquad (14)$$

As treatment coverage h_t changes over time, the extent of treatment is affected by f, the fraction of the transmission that takes place in the early stage of the infection when treatment is thought not to be effective, and g, the overall effectiveness of the treatments when they are given after the non-responsive stage. In their simulations, O&G assume that $f = 0.7$ and $g = 0.7$. Equation (14) then reduces to: $\tau_t = 1 - 0.49\, h_t$. To illustrate their methods, O&G consider the situation where the original coverage is $h_0 = 0.1$ and treatment is being scaled up so that coverage becomes $h_t = 0.5$. This means $\tau_0 = 1 - 0.49\,(0.1) = 0.951$ and $\tau_t = 1 - 0.49\,(0.5) = 0.0755$, which makes $\tau_t/\tau_0 = 0.794$. The result therefore of increasing coverage by 40 percentage points is to decrease infections by $1 - 0.794$, i.e., 20.6 percent. It is clear then from this calculation that the precise definition of τ_t is the fraction of people treated who are no longer infecting others. It represents the number of lives saved as a percentage of those infected.

In the context of this worked example, i.e., the 40 percentage points scaling up of coverage, O&G are estimating that for every two persons treated there will be one fewer person infected. We think this is an underestimate, not because of the estimate of g, but rather because of the assumed value for f. O&G are right that a value for g in the upper 90 percent range as claimed by Cohen, Chen et al. (2010) is not likely to be generalizable to the total population. While it is true that in the population as a whole there are going to be people who are so newly infected that they will either: (a) not know their HIV status and thus not know they need treatment or (b) are so infectious that treatment will not be minimally effective in reducing transmissions; but this does not mean that it is reasonable to assume that $f = 0.7$ for the purposes of the *RethinkHIV* policy experiment. An extra $10 billion is not going to be able to treat everyone who could possibly need treatment. At a cost of $1,374.7 per person (my estimate), $10 billion would cover 7.3 million people and there are over 22 million with HIV in SSA at this present time. So the 30 percent of people assumed untreatable for the f parameter is not likely to apply to the treatment scale-up for *RethinkHIV* policy. With $f = 1$, we have $\tau_t/\tau_0 = 0.698$ and not 0.794. Infections would be reduced by 30.2 percent and not just 20.6 percent.

To summarize our assessment of the O&G dynamic model of infections: we think that the model that predicts one fewer infections for two persons treated is an underestimate of the lives saved by treatment scale-up with the $10 billion budget as envisaged by *RethinkHIV* Policy. Benefit cost ratios of around 3 that follow from the O&G estimates of lives saved are therefore likely to be too low. We reach this conclusion for four main reasons:

- The O&G model restricts the population who can be infected to those who are high-risk. This ignores babies, for example, at a time when child infections are so large in SSA – there are 2.3 million currently infected.
- The number of S and I are underestimated relative to the standard model of infection flows. So a reduction in β would have a larger impact than assumed.
- The O&G model concentrates only on β_t and ignores all the other ways that treatment can impact the flow of infections, for example by increasing fertility.
- Finally, the O&G model regards 30 percent to be untreatable when the treatment scale envisaged will not attempt to reach this group. We think that $f = 1$ can be used instead of $f = 0.7$ and so more people can be treated effectively than is assumed.

A discrete time representation of the dynamic CBA framework

The continuous time, infinite horizon, dynamic framework provides some basic insights into evaluating HIV treatment, but it is also useful to look at the O&G assessment paper through the eyes of a discrete, finite time horizon formulation. To set the stage we first work through a present value CBA calculation where the prevention benefits of treatment are excluded, which is the reference point that the assessment paper used when first considering its benefit-cost calculations. This calculation is a fuller version of what O&G call "naïve estimates" of BCRs for treatment when introducing their results section. This first calculation serves to illustrate the main method that will be used in the rest of this perspective paper. In the process we can highlight the role and importance of discounting. Then we extend the calculations to fit in with the O&G analysis proper which involves including the prevention benefits of treatment for others which we interpret to be the positive externalities of treatment. Throughout our focus will be on what are the assumptions necessary to obtain B/C ratios equal to 3 and when should we expect higher ratios. In this section we will stick to the O&G context where treatment is to be applied to the general population. In the next section we will analyze results that apply just for the subset of treatment that targets prevention of MTCT.

Calculating benefits and costs when treatment does not prevent infection to others

In this exercise, as in O&G's results using the naive estimates, the time horizon is thirty-five years, the drugs add twenty-one years of life, but these added years only appear after fourteen years have elapsed. These years correspond to an initiation of ARVs when the CD4 count is greater than 350 as shown in Figure 3.5. The average cost per person year is the $735.5 first-line treatment amount given in Table 3.1. The yearly benefits use the upper bound $5,000 value. The calculations are shown in our Table 3.1.1. The present value sums are shown in the last row, with and without discounting.

In Table 3.1.1, the undiscounted B/C ratio is 4.09 ($105,000/$25,672.5), the B/C ratio with a 3 percent discount rate is 3.23 ($52,484/$16,234) and the B/C ratio with a 5 percent discount rate is 2.70 ($33,997/$12,611). The higher the discount rate, the lower is the B/C ratio. This result is because, for ARV treatment, where the costs are immediate and the benefits appear in the future only when the extended life expectancy is gained, the discounting affects costs and benefits asymmetrically.

To see this clearly, look at years 1 and 15. In year 1 there are costs of $734 but no benefits. By year 15 when the benefits start they are no longer worth $5,000. With a 3 percent discount rate they are worth $3,306 and with a 5 percent rate they are worth only half of $5,000 (i.e., $2,525). The role of the discount factor is crucial here as it serves to

lower the current values of benefits and costs. The discount factor attached to the second year of costs that occur in year 2 is 0.971 with the 3 percent rate and 0.952 with the 5 percent rate. So costs are not reduced by much. By contrast the present values of the second year of benefits are almost halved. The discount factor attached to the second year of benefits, which occur in year 16, is 0.661 with the 3 percent rate and 0.505 with the 5 percent rate.

The results of discounting on the B/C ratios presented in Table 3.1.1 appear again in the first row of numbers in Table 3.1.2. We see that these relate just to the case where treatment is initiated with a CD4 count greater than 350, giving thirty-five years of costs and twenty-one years of benefits, and where the costs are the lowest in O&G's Table 3.1, corresponding to 2010 first-line treatment values. In rows 2–4 of Table 3.1.2, with benefits throughout fixed at the upper bound $5,000 amount, we show the effects of discounting with the higher cost values presented by O&G. B/C ratios remain always above 1 (which is the cut-off value for an expenditure to be socially worthwhile) only for first-line treatment. For second-line treatment, B/C ratios exceed 1 only when the lower cost figure is used and the discount rate is not above 3 percent. The rest of Table 3.1.2 shows the results when treatment is initiated at CD4 counts other than at greater than 350. Table 3.1.2 confirms the soundness of the O&G strategy to start the scaling up of treatments with the group of people living with HIV/AIDS who have the lowest CD4 counts. B/C ratios are always higher the lower the CD4 count when treatment is initiated.

In the analysis that is to follow we are going to be using a special case of O&G's treatment fraction equation (14): $\tau_t = 1 - f g h_t$. Neither the transmission rate nor the coverage rate will vary by year. The fraction f, for the reasons explained previously, will be equal to 1. As we are considering a representative individual, the coverage rate is effectively going to be $h = 1$. As a result we are simply working with: $\tau = 1 - g$. So if a treatment is 30 percent effective, i.e., $g = 0.3$, then 70 percent of infections will still take place and benefits would be only 30 percent of the value that would exist if there were 100 percent effectiveness.

Table 3.1.1 Benefits and costs for first-line treatment with 2012 costs and no externalities

Year	Costs ($)	Benefits ($)	Discount factor at 3%	Discounted costs ($) 3%	Discounted benefits ($) 3%	Discount factor at 5%	Discounted costs ($) 5%	Discounted benefits ($) 5%
1	734	0	1.000	734	0	1.000	734	0
2	734	0	0.971	712	0	0.952	699	0
3	734	0	0.943	691	0	0.907	665	0
4	734	0	0.915	671	0	0.864	634	0
5	734	0	0.888	652	0	0.823	603	0
6	734	0	0.863	633	0	0.784	575	0
7	734	0	0.837	614	0	0.746	547	0
8	734	0	0.813	596	0	0.711	521	0
9	734	0	0.789	579	0	0.677	496	0
10	734	0	0.766	562	0	0.645	473	0
11	734	0	0.744	546	0	0.614	450	0
12	734	0	0.722	530	0	0.585	429	0
13	734	0	0.701	514	0	0.557	408	0
14	734	0	0.681	499	0	0.530	389	0
15	734	5,000	0.661	485	3,306	0.505	370	2,525
16	734	5,000	0.642	471	3,209	0.481	353	2,404
17	734	5,000	0.623	457	3,116	0.458	336	2,291
18	734	5,000	0.605	444	3,025	0.436	320	2,181
19	734	5,000	0.587	431	2,937	0.416	305	2,078
20	734	5,000	0.570	418	2,851	0.396	290	1,979
21	734	5,000	0.554	406	2,768	0.377	276	1,884
22	734	5,000	0.538	394	2,688	0.359	263	1,795
23	734	5,000	0.522	383	2,609	0.342	251	1,709
24	734	5,000	0.507	372	2,533	0.326	239	1,628
25	734	5,000	0.492	361	2,460	0.310	227	1,550
26	734	5,000	0.478	350	2,388	0.295	217	1,477
27	734	5,000	0.464	340	2,318	0.281	206	1,406
28	734	5,000	0.450	330	2,251	0.268	196	1,339
29	734	5,000	0.437	321	2,185	0.255	187	1,275
30	734	5,000	0.424	311	2,122	0.243	178	1,215
31	734	5,000	0.412	302	2,060	0.231	170	1,157
32	734	5,000	0.400	293	2,000	0.220	162	1,102
33	734	5,000	0.388	285	1,942	0.210	154	1,049
34	734	5,000	0.377	277	1,885	0.200	147	999
35	734	5,000	0.366	268	1,830	0.190	140	952
Sum	25,633	105,000		16,234	52,484		12,611	33,997

Note: The present value (PV) for a benefit or cost in any year is the product of the current value times the discount factor where $DF = (1 + \rho)^{-t}$.

Source: Constructed by the author using the CD4 >350 initiation timeline for benefits and costs given in Figure 3.5 of O&G.

Table 3.1.2 B/C ratios by CD4 count initiation and line of treatment with no externalities

Intervention	Years of benefits	Years of costs	Annual cost	Annual benefit	B/C ratio $\rho = 0\%$	B/C ratio $\rho = 3\%$	B/C ratio $\rho = 5\%$
			Initiation of treatment: CD4 > 350				
1st-line treatment							
2012 costs	21	35	$733.5	$5,000	4.09	3.23	2.70
2050 costs	21	35	$1,004.6	$5,000	2.99	2.36	1.97
2nd-line treatment							
2012 costs	21	35	$2,117.1	$5,000	1.42	1.12	0.93
2050 costs	21	35	$2,939.7	$5,000	1.02	0.81	0.67
			Initiation of treatment: CD4 < 350 & CD4 > 275				
1st-line treatment							
2012 costs	27	37	$733.5	$5,000	4.97	4.19	3.67
2050 costs	27	37	$1,004.6	$5,000	3.63	3.06	2.68
2nd-line treatment							
2012 costs	27	37	$2,117.1	$5,000	1.72	1.45	1.27
2050 costs	27	37	$2,939.7	$5,000	1.24	1.05	0.91
			Initiation of treatment: CD4 < 200				
1st-line treatment							
2012 costs	37	41	$733.5	$5,000	6.15	5.73	5.42
2050 costs	37	41	$1,004.6	$5,000	4.49	4.18	3.96
2nd-line treatment							
2012 costs	37	41	$2,117.1	$5,000	2.13	1.98	1.88
2050 costs	37	41	$2,939.7	$5,000	1.53	1.43	1.35
			Initiation of treatment: CD4 < 100 & CD4 > 50				
1st-line treatment							
2012 costs	22	24	$733.5	$5,000	6.25	6.05	5.90
2050 costs	22	24	$1,004.6	$5,000	4.56	4.41	4.31
2nd-line treatment							
2012 costs	22	24	$2,117.1	$5,000	2.16	2.09	2.04
2050 costs	22	24	$2,939.7	$5,000	1.56	1.51	1.47
			Initiation of treatment: CD4 < 50				
1st-line treatment							
2012 costs	14	15	$733.5	$5,000	6.36	6.26	6.19
2050 costs	14	15	$1,004.6	$5,000	4.65	4.57	4.52
2nd-line treatment							
2012 costs	14	15	$2,117.1	$5,000	2.20	2.17	2.15
2050 costs	14	15	$2,939.7	$5,000	1.59	1.56	1.54

Calculating benefits and costs when treatment does prevent infection to others

The calculations appearing in Tables 3.1.1 and 3.1.2 can be viewed as the CBA results for evaluating treatment that is solely for the benefit of the person who receives the drugs. In this case the medicine is targeting *primary* infection prevention. Another reason for administering ARVs is for *secondary* infection prevention, or preventing others getting infected. The O&G paper is mainly concerned with trying to capture the benefits of treatment that prevent secondary infections. This is the usual interpretation of what it means to employ the strategy of using "treatment as prevention." To move easily from our previous analysis of primary infection to incorporate also secondary prevention we will regard the prevention of infections of others as an externality of individual treatment. The prevention of others will be expressed in terms of the number of partners saved from HIV by the originally HIV-infected individual getting treatment. Every partner saved provides $5,000 worth of benefits. So we just apply multiples of $5,000 to the number of partners saved, to get the new benefit figures with the externality included.

The benefit figure of $5,000 that appears in both Tables 3.1.1 and 3.1.2 corresponds to the case where there are zero partners saved. For every partner saved, there is an extra $5,000 worth of benefits. This means that for one partner saved the benefits are $10,000, and for two partners saved the benefits are $15,000. Costs are not affected by the addition of the secondary benefits to the calculations. To see what impact adding the prevention of secondary infections makes to our previous analysis we will start with Table 3.1.1, which is summarized by the first line of Table 3.1.2. Note that the objective is to end up with B/C ratios that replicate O&G's results, i.e., are close to 3.

To replicate any particular set of results using our framework, we need a set of benefits and costs and a timeline that applies to these benefits and costs. The timeline will be as in Table 3.1.1, i.e., twenty-one years of benefits and thirty-five years of costs, as this already fitted in with O&G's naive estimates. For costs we will use O&G's Table 3.1. This has costs for first-line and second-line treatment for 2012 and 2050. We can use averages of the two periods to represent what is typical over the period. Mean first-line costs are $869.10 and they are $2,528.40 for the second-line drugs. Currently, only 3 percent of the treatments in SSA use second-line drugs. However, we can expect the share to rise over time. The Global Fund uses 5 percent. But if we are supposed to be working towards universal coverage we should expect the ratio to be higher than this. Medecins Sans Frontiers, in their longest running project in Khayelitsha in South Africa, found that 22 percent had to switch from first-line to second-line drugs.[3] Since the experience of South Africa is often going to be the upper bound for what is feasible with HIV/AIDS interventions in SSA, we will take the 20 percent figure as being what we can expect in the future for full scale-up. Taking the average for the cost of first-line treatment and adding this on to 20 percent of the second-line treatment average, we get $1,374.70 as the cost per treatment that we will be using to replicate the O&G results. Note that by working with the 20 percent figure we are deviating from the 10 percent second-line treatment assumption used in the assessment paper.

With the timeline and the costs fixed, we now turn to the benefits. As we explained earlier, the benefit values we will be using are going to be a function of the number of partners saved. $5,000 is the value of the life of the person him/herself and we then add $5,000 for every partner that is going to avoid transmission because of the original person being treated. In Table 3.1.3, we give results for one and for two partners saved. According to Oster (2009) who analyzed DHS surveys in fourteen SSA countries, only about 3 percent of women and 12 percent of men have multiple partners. Most people who have multiple partners report just two partners. It is reasonable to assume therefore that one or two partners saved would be typical in SSA. With two partners, B/C ratios would be in the range 3 to 10 with discount rates in the 3 percent to 5 percent range.

---

[3] The three percentages for second-line treatment coverage just cited come from the All Party Parliamentary Group on AIDS (2009), p. 12.

Table 3.1.3 B/C ratios by CD4 count initiation and line of treatment with externalities

No. partners saved	Years of benefits	Years of costs	Annual cost	Annual benefit	B/C ratio $\rho = 0\%$	B/C ratio $\rho = 3\%$	B/C ratio $\rho = 5\%$
Initiation of treatment: CD4 > 350							
2	21	35	$1,374.7	$15,000	6.55	5.18	3.14
1	21	35	$1,374.7	$10,000	4.36	3.45	2.10
Initiation of treatment: CD4 < 350 & CD4 > 275							
2	27	37	$1,374.7	$15,000	7.96	6.71	4.64
1	27	37	$1,374.7	$10,000	5.31	4.48	3.09
Initiation of treatment: CD4 < 200							
2	37	41	$1,374.7	$15,000	9.85	9.18	7.85
1	37	41	$1,374.7	$10,000	6.56	6.12	5.24
Initiation of treatment: CD4 < 100 & CD4 > 50							
2	22	24	$1,374.7	$15,000	10.00	9.68	9.04
1	22	24	$1,374.7	$10,000	6.69	6.45	6.03
Initiation of treatment: CD4 < 50							
2	14	15	$1,374.7	$15,000	10.18	10.02	9.72
1	14	15	$1,374.7	$10,000	6.79	6.68	6.48

We can immediately see in our replication of the O&G results in Table 3.1.3 a cause for disagreement with the O&G findings. To obtain B/C ratios of 3 we must restrict the initiation period only to those who initiate ARVs when the CD4 count is above 350. Even with just one partner saved, B/C ratios would in most cases exceed 3. This supports our conjecture earlier that the O&G model is likely to underestimate the B/C ratios of treatment. In the next section we focus just on a particular category of treatment where B/C ratios will be much higher than would be the case for treatment aimed at the population as a whole.

Mother to child transmission (MTCT)

The most obvious intervention that fits into the category of treatment as prevention, and not covered explicitly in the assessment paper, is that involved with giving ARV medications to pregnant women to prevent the transfer of HIV to their babies. According to Avert (2011a), without treatment, HIV is transferred during pregnancy, labor, and delivery to 15–30 percent of babies and during breastfeeding to a further 5–20 percent of babies. In 2009 around 400,000 children became infected with HIV, mainly through MTCT, about 90 percent in SSA.

In terms of the time horizon analysis we have just been using, the importance of considering treatment to reduce MTCT is that it is the intervention that has the longest period of benefits (the baby's expected lifetime gained by treatment) relative to the period of costs (the cost period is very short as many times a single dose is given to the mother and to the baby after delivery). So it has the potential to have the highest B/C ratio of any form of HIV/AIDS treatment.

In 2007, there were 1.3 million pregnant women who were HIV-positive needing ARVs for preventing MTCT in SSA. At the time there were 446,000 pregnant women who did receive ARVs for this purpose.[4] We will use the 1.3 million figure as the number of additional persons whose treatment can be funded as part of the $10 billion that we are considering to spend as part of *RethinkHIV*. There will be three alternative PMTCT programs that we will be evaluating in our CBA. Their range varies from the simplest, a single dose, to a full package of

---

[4] See Table 5.4 in UNAIDS (2009).

services lasting eighteen months. All the programs will involve other costs than the drugs themselves. For each program we will assume that the following non-drug costs are required to receive the full benefits that we will be assuming:[5]

- A screening test to learn each woman's HIV status (at a cost of $3.90 per woman).
- For each HIV-positive woman, testing and counseling (at a cost of $13 per woman).
- Family planning services for prevention of unintended pregnancies (at a cost of $20 per woman per year).
- For each HIV-positive woman, a CD4 screening, to determine eligibility for ARVs (at a cost of $20).
- Early infant diagnosis of HIV exposure (at a cost of $32.50).
- Cotrimoxazole prophylaxis for the postpartum treatment of infected infants (at a cost of $5).

The total of these non-drug costs is $94.40 per woman. However, the screening test to detect the HIV virus has to be carried out for all pregnant women, and not just those who eventually will be found to be HIV-positive. So the screening is a cost that applies to all pregnant women in SSA, which we will assume to be around 20 million per year. Since our CBA of MTCT is working on an average per infected pregnant woman basis, we have to calculate how many women need to be tested per HIV-positive pregnant woman. We have previously established (adding the 446,000 number of HIV-positive pregnant women who are on ARV medications to the 1.3 million needing treatment) that there are about 1.75 million pregnant women per year who are infected with HIV. Dividing 20 million by 1.75 produces approximately an 11 to 1 ratio. Thus for every person found infected with HIV, ten other pregnant women are required to have the screening test. At $3.90 per test, the total screening cost for other women is $39. Adding $39 to the $94.40 amount for a HIV-positive woman results in a total non-drug cost of $133.40 per woman treated.

We define "full benefits" to be the life expectancy that can be expected if PMTCT is 100 percent effective in reducing infection, i.e., one baby's life is saved for every mother treated. In all cases the full benefits from treatment will generate 0.3 of the value of a life year saved (which will continue to be $5,000) as this is the proportion of babies that would likely become infected in the absence of the intervention. So $1,500 will be the annual full benefits for 100 percent effectiveness. The number of years of expected life expectancy to be gained from PMTCT treatment depends on the life expectancy at birth with and without AIDS. Table 3.1.4, based on Velkoff and Kowal's (2007) Table 2, presents estimates of the life years gained by gender if there were no AIDS in the twenty-six countries in SSA where HIV has had the most impact on life expectancy. The average of the males gained is 11.64 years and the average for the females was 14.8, which makes the overall average around thirteen years. If a baby would have died after two years with AIDS, then the thirteen years of life gained would begin at year 3 and end at year 15.

The thirteen years of life years gained, and the $1,500 per year gained for the full benefits, will apply in the same way to all three PMTCT programs we will be evaluating. What differs by program will be the actual transmission rate that will be applied to the 100 percent effectiveness base and the drug costs of each program.[6] Note that the actual transmission rate for PMTCT does not, like the general case modeled by O&G, depend a lot on human behavioral responses to the HIV epidemic in terms of condom use, circumcision, etc. We will therefore model the change in babies infected as depending solely on the g effectiveness parameter in the O&G model which varies by PMTCT program.

The first program that we will be evaluating we will call the Nevirapine (NVP) program. This single dose drug reduces the chance of transmission by about half to 16 percent. With $g = 0.16$ instead of 0.30, the benefits per year would be reduced from the full benefit figure of $1,500 to approximately $750. Although the cost of NVP is miniscule at around five cents per dose, we have to add on the non-drug costs of $133.40 (as explained above) to produce a cost estimate of $133.45 per treatment.

[5] All of these cost figures come from Schwartländer et al. (2011).

[6] The estimates of the actual treatment effectiveness and the costs for the first two PMTCT programs examined below are taken from the All Party Parliamentary Group on AIDS (2009), p. 11.

Table 3.1.4 Differences in life expectancy at birth without and with AIDS for selected sub-Saharan countries in 2006

Country	Difference (in years) if there were no AIDS (male)	Difference (in years) if there were no AIDS (female)
Botswana	22.3	28.4
Burkina Faso	4.4	5.6
Burundi	7.0	9.0
Cameroon	5.5	7.2
Central African Republic	13.5	17.6
Congo	6.0	7.8
Cote d'Ivoire	6.2	9.3
Eritrea	3.9	5.3
Ethiopia	4.2	5.5
Gabon	9.4	12.0
Guinea Bissau	3.8	5.2
Kenya	8.5	10.7
Lesotho	22.7	29.5
Liberia	3.7	5.3
Malawi	13.5	17.6
Mozambique	12.5	15.0
Namibia	24.0	30.6
Nigeria	5.2	7.2
Rwanda	4.2	5.6
South Africa	20.6	28.7
Swaziland	38.9	43.1
Tanzania	7.0	9.0
Togo	5.8	7.6
Uganda	7.5	9.6
Zambia	13.3	16.6
Zimbabwe	29.1	35.7
Average number of years gained	11.6	14.8

Source: Based on US Census Bureau, International Programs. Table 2 of Velkoff and Kowal (2007).

The B/C ratios for the Nevirapine are presented in Table 3.1.5. At the 3 percent discount rate, the B/C ratio is 54.31 (and 67.44 without discounting and 47.44 at the 5 percent discount rate).

The second program we will call the Zidovudine (ZDV or AZT) program. This program used to be the WHO recommended regimen and involves the following combination: Zidovudine from six months' gestation, a single dose of Nevirapine at birth, and a week of Zidovudine and Lamivudine after delivery. This combination is obviously more difficult to administer and costlier than the single dose of Nevirapine. The drug costs are $24, and with the $133.4 of non-drug costs, the total is $157.4 as opposed to the $133.45 with Nevirapine. But it is also more effective than NVP. The number of babies who get infected after the ZDV combination is 10 percent, which means that it is 90 percent effective and $g = 0.03$. Multiplying the full benefit value of $1,500 by 0.9 gives a $1,350 figure for the benefits per year for this program. Table 3.1.5 shows that even though the costs are higher than for the Nevirapine program, the benefits are higher still, so the B/C ratio is greater at 82.89 with the 3 percent discount rate (and 102.92 without discounting and 72.40 at the 5 percent discount rate).

Lastly we will evaluate what we will call the WHO program as this is the regimen that fits in with the latest 2010 WHO guidelines. These guidelines are targeted at the 60 percent of women who are not yet recommended for treatment for themselves as their CD4 count exceeds 350. For the 40 percent of women who take ARVs for themselves, we will assume that they will follow the Zidovudine program with its costs.[7]

For the 60 percent of the women who are not yet on ARVs, there are two options, A and B. Option A involves a dual prophylaxis and option B has a triple prophylaxis. Of the 60 percent, the split is 36 percent on option A and 24 percent on option B. Option B costs more than option A. Schwartländer *et al.* (2011) have estimated the weighted average of the two options (using the percentage splits as the weights) to be $705 per woman. This cost includes drugs and non-drugs. The drug regimen lasts eighteen months as it includes twelve months of breastfeeding as recommended by the WHO. For simplicity, we will assume half of the costs take place in the

[7] When we assumed that Nevirapine was the program for the 40% of women who were already on treatment instead of the Zidovudine program, which we assumed in the text, there was only a difference of $10 in the costs, so the B/C ratios did not change greatly.

Table 3.1.5 B/C ratios for three prevention of MTCT programs

Intervention	Years of benefits	Years of costs	Annual cost	Annual benefit	B/C ratio $\rho = 0\%$	B/C ratio $\rho = 3\%$	B/C ratio $\rho = 5\%$
Nevirapine program	13	1	$133.45	$750	67.44	54.31	47.44
Zidovudine program	13	1	$157.40	$1,350	102.92	82.89	72.40
WHO program	13	2	$243.00	$1,500	37.04	30.27	26.69

first year and one-half in the second year. Putting all of the costs together involves a weighted average calculation. We take 0.4 of the $157.45 (which is the cost of the Zidovudine program) and add this to 0.6 of the $705 WHO program costs involving options A and B to obtain $486. Of this, $243 occurs in the first year and $243 in the second year. Given that the Zidovudine program already has 90 percent effectiveness and the WHO program is investing in a comprehensive set of additional drugs and services to enhance effectiveness, it is reasonable to assume 100 percent effectiveness and set $g = 0$, which means that the full benefits per year of $1,500 would apply. Because the costs are so much higher than for the Zidovudine program, and the benefits are only slightly larger, Table 3.1.5 shows that the B/C ratios are lower than for the Zidovudine program. The B/C ratio is 30.27 with the 3 percent discount rate (and 37.04 without discounting and 26.69 at the 5 percent discount rate).

To summarize our CBA of MTCT programs. The Zidovudine program had the largest B/C ratios and at 82.89 with the 3 percent discount rate is likely to have the highest ratio of all *RethinkHIV* interventions that are under evaluation for *RethinkHIV*.[8] Certainly, as far as the treatment inventions as a whole are concerned, as reflected by the B/C ratios coming from the O&G study, PMTCT should be given the highest priority. Our B/C ratios are for individual treatments. If the Zidovudine program can be scaled up to all of the 1.3 million pregnant mothers in 2007 keeping the ratios intact, PMTCT would cost $205 million and save around 390,000 lives.[9]

This cost of $205 million to save 390,000 babies' lives by treating 1.3 million pregnant women is per year. We also need to consider scaling up such that every pregnant woman with HIV now and in the future is going to be treated. If we assume that

there are going to be no new infections, as envisaged in the UNAIDS Treatment 2.0 initiative, then we are planning to regard all women currently living with HIV as future pregnant mothers.[10] In sub-Saharan Africa in 2009 there were 12.1 million such women. If the cost per woman treated is the same for all the 12.1 million as the figure we have just considered, i.e., $157.40 per woman, then the total cost would be $1.9 billion, nearly 20 percent of *RethinkHIV*'s $10 billion targeted budget, to save 3.63 million lives.

Realistically, though, there will be some additional women who will become newly infected, so elimination of MTCT using just treatment will cost more than $1.9 billion. Moreover, as pointed out by Lori Bollinger in her assessment paper covering MTCT, the necessary scale-up is only feasible if two impediments are removed, i.e., achieving improved access to antenatal care and the reduction of stigma associated with an HIV diagnosis. Extra resources are therefore also necessary to remove these two impediments in order to ensure that the high overall B/C ratios for MTCT will remain intact.

Treatment versus family planning to prevent MTCT

So far we have carried out the CBA as if the only ways to reduce or eliminate MTCT are to give

---

[8] Strictly, if PMTCT is to be evaluated as a separate program and not part of a $10 billion package, then the size of the net-benefits would be the appropriate CBA criterion. However, the rankings by net-benefits mirror that of the B/C ratios for the PMTCT programs.

[9] $205 million is 1.3 million times $1,557.40 and 1.3 million pregnant mothers times 0.3 (the mother to child transmission rate) equals 390,000.

[10] These numbers come from Avert (2011b).

pregnant mothers ARVs or to stop women getting infected in the first place (primary prevention). The ratio of women living with HIV/AIDS to the number of babies with HIV/AIDS, which was 7 to 1 in 2009, need not be a constant. An alternative strategy is to prevent the number of unwanted pregnancies that women living with HIV/AIDS have by investing and intervening through family planning (FP).

A central concept in the literature on the prevention of MTCT via FP is that of *unmet need* for contraception. Mahy *et al.* (2010) describe this as a common measure of access to FP, and define it as: "the proportion of sexually active, fecund women in a union who wish to stop or postpone childbearing and are not currently using contraception. The measure can be interpreted as the increase in contraceptive prevalence rates if all women were able to fulfil their preferences." The extent of unmet need in twenty-four of the countries with the largest numbers of HIV-positive pregnant women in 2009 is shown in Table 3.1.6. The table also shows the percentage of women using contraception and the percentage that would be using contraception in 2015 if the unmet need were satisfied.

We see in Table 3.1.6 that 25 percent of pregnancies would not have occurred if women had the contraception that they wanted. This means that 25 percent of MTCT in 2009 would have been averted with FP. Since the reduction in MTCT from ARVs was estimated by Mahy *et al.* (2010) to be 24 percent between 2000 and 2009 from these same countries, it would seem that FP would be more effective than ARVs in reducing MTCT.

To see how these effectiveness outcomes convert to cost-effectiveness outcomes, we need to factor in the costs. For ARVs we will use the cost figure for the WHO option A strategy described in our MTCT CBA given earlier, which was identified separately to be $237 by Schwartländer *et al.* (2011). This same study also put the cost of FP at $20 per woman. So with slightly greater effectiveness and much lower costs than ARVs, FP would be the more cost-effective intervention. This was the conclusion by almost every study in the literature of the comparison between these two interventions – see, for example, Sweat *et al.* (2004), Reynolds *et al.* (2006), and Hladik *et al.* (2009).

However, even though FP is judged to be more cost-effective than ARVs, this is not at all the same thing as saying that FP is more socially beneficial from a CBA perspective of MTCT. Note that the outcome variable that is used to compare FP with ARVs in the context of MTCT in the cost-effectiveness literature is the number of infant infections averted. When ARVs are involved, the reduction in number of infant infections is lives saved, and so fits exactly with the *RethinkHIV* policy guidelines. A life year saved can be valued at $5,000 (or $1,500 per 0.3 of a life year saved) to form the benefits, and with a comparison with the costs the B/C ratio can be formed. This is not the case with FP. The reductions in the number of infections that take the form of babies that are not born cannot be regarded as a "life year saved," even though they are life years saved from HIV. The easiest way to see this is to look back at Table 3.1.5 which summarized our B/C results for three PMTCT programs based on ARVs. The treatments provided thirteen years of added life expectancy on top of the two years that the infected baby otherwise would have had. On the other hand, with an infection averted by a baby not being born due to FP, there is no positive number of life years to consider. So there can be no benefits. There can only be costs with FP MTCT evaluations.

One could argue that mothers are better off by not having an unwanted pregnancy and not having an unwanted child. To quote Mahy *et al.* (2010): "by eliminating unmet need for family planning, women living with HIV would have the children they want when they want them." This then would be a benefit to be quantified by a CBA. For this purpose, the willingness-to-pay (WTP) for contraception could be used as a proxy measure of the benefits. But, the point is that WTP is not the CBA framework for benefit estimation in the *RethinkHIV* policy guidelines. This simply relies on life years saved, valued at $5,000 per year. Averting unwanted babies by FP does not supply added baby life years.

Treatment for all HIV-positive women versus treating just pregnant women

An alternative way of preventing MTCT using ARVs is to give them to infected women prior to

Table 3.1.6 Unmet need for family planning (FP) in the top 24 countries in SSA in 2009

Country	No. HIV+ women delivering in 2009	% women using contraception in 2009	% women reporting unmet need for FP in 2009	% women meeting unmet need in 2015
Nigeria	210,000	20	20	41
South Africa	210,000	62	14	76
Mozambique	97,000	26	18	44
Uganda	88,000	27	41	67
Tanzania	84,000	34	22	56
Kenya	81,000	41	25	65
Zambia	68,000	35	27	61
Malawi	59,000	37	28	65
Zimbabwe	50,000	61	13	74
DR Congo	36,000	27	24	52
Cameroon	34,000	35	20	55
Ethiopia	30,000	22	34	56
Cote d'Ivoire	20,000	31	28	58
Chad	16,000	11	21	32
Burundi	14,000	19	29	49
Lesotho	14,000	45	31	76
Ghana	13,000	31	35	67
Sudan	14,000	44	26	70
Botswana	13,000	63	27	90
Rwanda	11,000	23	38	61
Swaziland	9,300	54	24	78
Namibia	7,700	57	7	63
Burkina Faso	6,500	19	29	48
Average	51,543	36	25	61

Source: Based on Mahy *et al.* (2010), Table 1.

their becoming pregnant. If HIV-positive women are already on ARVs they will not have to be given treatment later when they become pregnant. This alternative fits in closely with the rest of this chapter, as we have already evaluated treatment in the context of no externalities (Tables 3.1.1 and 3.1.2) and then again when there are externalities (Table 3.1.3). We have also evaluated ARVs just in the context of MTCT (Table 3.1.5). The case we are dealing with combines the different types of analysis in a particular way. From the point of view of giving the mother ARVs on an ongoing

basis, rather than just prior to birth, the prevention of MTCT is an externality that will raise B/C ratios like any other positive externality. Because the ARVs will prevent MTCT for every baby that is born, the externalities will be greater the more children the woman has.

We will start with the calculations that were presented in Table 3.1.1. This was assumed to apply to anyone on HIV treatment and looked at the effect simply on the person themselves. Now we apply them to a woman who is affected. As there was nothing gender-specific in Table 3.1.1, we can still apply these results to any woman who is infected. The only difference to our calculations in terms of Table 3.1.1 is that we are not going to consider a series of different prices of treatment. We will just go with the first-line and 20 percent second-line treatment average costs that we used in Table 3.1.3 (i.e., $1,374.7). Now we introduce the possibility of childbirth. As in Table 3.1.1, and in the top parts of Tables 3.1.2 and 3.1.3, we are going to use the time horizon that corresponds with the initiation of ARVs when the CD4 count is greater than 350. This generates twenty-one years of benefits and thirty-five years of costs. The costs will not vary by year.

The benefits on the other hand will vary a lot by year. In Table 3.1.1 the benefits are zero for the first fourteen years, and from year 15 and thereafter equal to $5,000. This will be changed as we will add the benefits that exist because of avoiding having an HIV-infected baby. Following the time horizon used in Table 3.1.5, for each baby there will be two years of no additional benefits (the baby was expected to live two years anyway) and then thirteen years of benefits. We assume full effectiveness, in which case the $1,500 per child per year figure applies. We will assume that women have babies at two-year intervals starting from year 1. So there will be a series of additional two-year zero and thirteen-year $1,500 benefit cycles. We will make a set of calculations when there are zero, one, two, three, and four children to see what difference the number of children makes to the B/C ratios. For reference we present Table 3.1.7 which shows the four-baby upper bound case, so that one can readily see all the assumptions that are now being made different from Table 3.1.1. The first baby is assumed to be born in year 1, the second baby in year 3, the third baby in year 5, and the fourth baby in year 7. The benefits peak in year 15 at $11,000 because this is the first year that the mother's personal benefits of $5,000 appear, and there is $6,000 of benefits from the four babies. Once the effects of childbirth are over, in year 21, benefits revert to the levels in Table 3.1.1.

The total benefits of $109,302 and the total costs of $30,425 (or $3,123 annual average benefits and $1,374.4 annual average costs) at the 3 percent discount rate form a B/C ratio of 3.59, or 3.41 at the 5 percent rate, and these results appear in the first row of Table 3.1.8. As the number of

children a woman has decreases, so do the B/C ratios. The case of zero children is important, as this provides the benchmark for the evaluation. It is the B/C ratio that would apply if a man were taking the ARVs rather than a woman. The rest of Table 3.1.8 includes adding the number of partners saved by treatment, one or two, as in the calculations in Table 3.1.3. The full external benefits then of giving HIV-positive pregnant women treatment is that their children and their partners will not be infected. For males, the external benefits are restricted just to their sex partners. We see in Table 3.1.8 that for the case that we consider to be the maximum, where there are two partners and four children, the B/C ratio at the 3 percent rate is 6.93 and it is 6.18 at the 5 percent rate. Overall, the B/C ratios for women are double that for men if there are zero partners saved; the ratios are 50 percent higher if there is going to be one partner saved; and the ratios are a third higher when there are two partners saved.

Comparison of our results with other studies in *RethinkHIV*

By design there is a strong overlap between this paper and the two others by O&G and John Stover that are all devoted to treatment as prevention. In addition, because we have in our analysis extended O&G's work to include MTCT, we will also compare out results with the assessment paper on the Prevention of Non-sexual Transmission of HIV.

Comparison with the treatment as prevention papers

Stover summarizes O&G's results as giving B/C ratios in the range of 1.4–4.00 (when the additional year of life is valued at $5,000) and he states that his estimates are about five to six times higher. Our estimates are in between the two other sets, being in the range 5–8. Since there are these differences in the results, it is important to understand why these differences have occurred.

Stover attributes the main difference between his results and those of O&G to his assumptions about future costs per patient. O&G use a

Table 3.1.7 Benefits and costs when pregnant women are themselves treated and also prevent MTCT to four children

Year	Costs ($)	Benefits ($)	Discount factor at 3%	Discounted costs ($) 3%	Discounted benefits ($) 3%	Discount factor at 5%	Discounted costs ($) 5%	Discounted benefits ($) 5%
1	1,374.7	0	1.000	1,375	0	1.000	1,335	0
2	1,374.7	0	0.971	1,335	0	0.952	1,309	0
3	1,374.7	1,500	0.943	1,296	1,414	0.907	1,247	1,361
4	1,374.7	1,500	0.915	1,258	1,373	0.864	1,188	1,296
5	1,374.7	3,000	0.888	1,221	2,665	0.823	1,131	2,468
6	1,374.7	3,000	0.863	1,186	2,588	0.784	1,077	2,351
7	1,374.7	4,500	0.837	1,151	3,769	0.746	1,026	3,358
8	1,374.7	4,500	0.813	1,118	3,659	0.711	977	3,198
9	1,374.7	6,000	0.789	1,085	4,736	0.677	930	4,061
10	1,374.7	6,000	0.766	1,054	4,599	0.645	886	3,868
11	1,374.7	6,000	0.744	1,023	4,465	0.614	844	3,683
12	1,374.7	6,000	0.722	993	4,335	0.585	804	3,508
13	1,374.7	6,000	0.701	964	4,208	0.557	765	3,341
14	1,374.7	6,000	0.681	936	4,086	0.530	729	3,182
15	1,374.7	11,000	0.661	909	7,272	0.505	694	5,556
16	1,374.7	9,500	0.642	882	6,098	0.481	661	4,570
17	1,374.7	9,500	0.623	857	5,920	0.458	630	4,352
18	1,374.7	8,000	0.605	832	4,840	0.436	600	3,490
19	1,374.7	8,000	0.587	807	4,699	0.416	571	3,324
20	1,374.7	6,500	0.570	784	3,707	0.396	544	2,572
21	1,374.7	6,500	0.554	761	3,599	0.377	518	2,450
22	1,374.7	5,000	0.538	739	2,688	0.359	493	1,795
23	1,374.7	5,000	0.522	717	2,609	0.342	470	1,709
24	1,374.7	5,000	0.507	697	2,533	0.326	448	1,628
25	1,374.7	5,000	0.492	676	2,460	0.310	426	1,550
26	1,374.7	5,000	0.478	657	2,388	0.295	406	1,477
27	1,374.7	5,000	0.464	637	2,318	0.281	387	1,406
28	1,374.7	5,000	0.450	619	2,251	0.268	368	1,339
29	1,374.7	5,000	0.437	601	2,185	0.255	351	1,275
30	1,374.7	5,000	0.424	583	2,122	0.243	334	1,215
31	1,374.7	5,000	0.412	566	2,060	0.231	318	1,157
32	1,374.7	5,000	0.400	550	2,000	0.220	303	1,102
33	1,374.7	5,000	0.388	534	1,942	0.210	289	1,049
34	1,374.7	5,000	0.377	518	1,885	0.200	275	999
35	1,374.7	5,000	0.366	503	1,830	0.190	262	952
Sum	48,115	183,000		30,425	109,302		23,635	33,997

Source: Constructed by the author using the CD4 > 350 initiation timeline for benefits and costs when there are zero babies.

Table 3.1.8 B/C ratios for treating the pregnant mothers themselves with varying numbers of children

Number of children	Number of partners	Years of benefits	Years of costs	Annual cost	Annual benefit	B/C ratio $\rho = 3\%$	B/C ratio $\rho = 5\%$
4	0	33	35	$1,374.4	$3,123	3.59	3.41
3	0	33	35	$1,374.4	$2,752	3.17	2.99
2	0	33	35	$1,374.4	$2,359	2.71	2.52
1	0	33	35	$1,374.4	$1,942	2.23	2.01
0	0	33	35	$1,374.4	$1,405	1.73	1.44
4	1	33	35	$1,374.4	$4,528	5.21	4.74
3	1	33	35	$1,374.4	$4,157	4.78	4.32
2	1	33	35	$1,374.4	$3,764	4.33	3.85
1	1	33	35	$1,374.4	$3,347	3.85	3.34
0	1	33	35	$1,374.4	$2,810	3.45	2.88
4	2	33	35	$1,374.4	$6,028	6.93	6.18
3	2	33	35	$1,374.4	$5,657	6.51	5.76
2	2	33	35	$1,374.4	$5,169	5.95	5.18
1	2	33	35	$1,374.4	$4,847	5.57	4.78
0	2	33	35	$1,374.4	$4,499	5.18	4.32

Note: The annual benefits vary by year, so the figures in this column are the average benefits undiscounted over the 35 years.

Source: Constructed by the author.

40 percent increase in costs, while Stover assumes a 75 percent reduction. Stover makes the logical point that *if* there is to be a significant increase in coverage of ARVs in the future, then efficiencies have to be found that decrease the cost per patient. And *if* treatment becomes simpler, e.g., there is a single pill that has minimal side-effects and does not require much medical supervision, then the necessary efficiencies would occur. However, such a simple regime does not yet exist. If pharmaceutical companies come up with a simpler regime, there is no guarantee that the medications would not be priced considerably higher. It is true that ARV prices have fallen sharply in the past due to the existence of generic drugs. But there are patent agreements that have been signed (Trade Related Intellectual Property Rights agreements, or TRIPS) which, although in the past were circumvented, in the future will become more binding. Moreover, there already exist agreements (TRIPS plus) that have been made whereby developing countries will be given trade concessions only if they agree *not* to try to avoid complying with TRIPS by, for example, applying for patent "flexibilities" (exclusions). We

therefore cannot endorse the view that costs will decrease in the future as envisaged by Stover. This difference in the cost estimates explains why our B/C ratios are so much lower than Stover's.

Our estimates differ from those of O&G on both the costs and benefits (effects) sides. Although our costs are higher than O&G's, which would otherwise lower B/C ratios, our results are much (50 percent) higher than theirs because we believe that they have greatly underestimated the number of lives saved. On the costs side we use the $1,374.70 per annum figure rather than O&G's $1,000. This is because we anticipate the need for greater use of the much more expensive second-line drugs and we expect that expanded coverage would entail extending treatment to rural areas where delivery costs and patient transport costs would be much higher than for the urban areas currently dispensing the ARVs. On the benefits side we examined the O&G transmission model. We found (among a number of problems), by their focusing only on the high-risk groups, that they would be excluding a large number of people who otherwise could get infected, especially newly born infants.

Comparison with the prevention of non-sexual transmission papers

Lori Bollinger, in the assessment paper on Prevention of Non-sexual Transmission of HIV, evaluated the prevention of MTCT as one of four possible prevention interventions. We will just examine her MTCT intervention results. For comparison purposes we are going to focus only on her results that relate to 3 percent discounting and a $5,000 benefit per life year saved as we consider these to be the most relevant assumptions for *RethinkHIV*. Our 270,000 estimate of the number of infections averted by the prevention of MTCT was remarkably close to the 265,000 figure found by Bollinger. Also very close was our 1.3 million number of beneficiaries, just 0.09 million greater than her estimate. So any differences that may arise can be due only to the per person costs and effects that we are assuming.

In Bollinger's Table 2.7, she used 13.9 years of life gained for an infant in one set of results, and 7.0 years in another set. Based on our Table 3.1.4, we used an additional thirteen years above the two years that an infant would normally expect to live with AIDS, to obtain a fifteen-year evaluation time horizon. This time horizon sits nicely in the middle of the two estimates used by Bollinger, so this is not really a source of disagreement. A difference can be seen in her $237 cost per treatment figure (option A) relative to our $157.4 estimate. Our average cost is two-thirds of hers. If Bollinger had used our cost estimate, total costs would have been $82.35 million (i.e., 0.66 times $124 million) and her B/C ratio would have been 158 instead of her original estimate of 146 – a figure that is already extremely high, so making it even higher does not make much of a difference in terms of setting priorities for HIV interventions. On the other hand, if we had used Bollinger's cost amount, our B/C ratio would have been 55 instead of 83. This is not an insignificant reduction, but again, in terms of setting priorities for HIV interventions, 55 is very high and indicates a top-priority intervention.

What is a source of disagreement is the methodology used in Bollinger's assessment paper. For some reason she has interpreted the *RethinkHIV*

guidelines as saying that one has to add to the value of a life saved an amount equal to the ART cost savings arising from the prevention of each HIV infection. This must be a misinterpretation because this approach to benefit estimation involves double counting. In a cost-minimization setting one uses the cost savings to measure the benefits and compares this to the costs of the intervention. In a CBA, one estimates the benefits directly and values the lives that are saved using a shadow price of an infection averted, in this case $5,000. This $5,000 is the comprehensive value of the quantity and quality of a life saved. There is no need to add anything, certainly not the treatment cost savings, which is the alternative benefit measure approach if one were *not* going to value the lives saved directly. Adding the two alternative measures of benefits is therefore double counting.

Fortunately, because the prevention of MTCT is such a worthwhile intervention, factoring out the double counting does not make a lot of difference to Bollinger's results. For scenario III in her Table 2.7, she has $24,929 million as her total benefit figure and nearly the same amount, i.e., $24,125 million, as the value of years gained without the cost savings. Thus eliminating the double counting would make an inconsequential difference to the B/C ratio.

To summarize this section comparing our results with others in *RethinkHIV* who are evaluating similar interventions: we think B/C ratios in the range 5 to 8 are more reasonable than the alternatives given in the treatment assessment paper and the other treatment perspectives paper. Our range is in between the other two sets of estimates. For the prevention of MTCT, we agree with the Prevention of Non-sexual Transmission assessment paper that B/C ratios well in excess of 50 are what the evidence suggests. As 50 is even higher than the B/C ratio for male circumcision, the prevention of MTCT should be given the highest priority of all those considered by the expert panel. Note that male circumcision is highly effective in preventing male transmission of HIV from infected females; female transmission from an infected male is not nearly as effective. There is therefore a male bias with male circumcision. On the other hand, preventing the vertical transmission from the mother to the baby is fairer, as it is gender neutral. The baby prevented from infection is as likely to be a male as a female.

Discussion

We give some thought here to whether the benefits should be $1,000 or $5,000 per life saved, and to the role of discounting and how it can affect outcomes for treatment programs. It is important to have a clear understanding of what benefit figure is going to be used *and why* in order to ensure that double counting is not taking place in this CC policy exercise. Lastly, we deal with the need to give priorities to treatments that target females.

Choosing $1,000 or $5,000 as the value of a life year

We can use some CBA studies of interventions in Tanzania to provide some perspective on helping us decide the appropriate value to place on the outcome of a treatment intervention. The *RethinkHIV* guidelines refer to $1,000 being appropriate for a poorer SSA country and $5,000 for a richer country. Using income as the benchmark is consistent with the human capital (HC) approach for valuing benefits in CBA, which values a life according to the present value of a person's lifetime earnings.

Although this approach is very often used for CBAs in the health care field, it is not best practice in CBA viewed as applied welfare economics. Some people earn little (women in SSA) and some nothing at all (the unemployed, the elderly, and the infirm). In general we can regard the HC as providing a lower value for valuing benefits. When this benefit methodology was used to value female education as a way of preventing HIV transmission in Tanzania,[11] it valued a female's life to be worth $8,907, when it would have been worth in the millions in the US. However, this low valuation did not mean that the CBA was predestined to find that investing in female education in Tanzania would not be worthwhile. The B/C ratio was in fact in the range 1.3 to 2.9, so the investment was highly beneficial. This result came about because, even though the benefits of using the human capital approach

in a poor country were low, the costs were also very low in such a country. Seven years of primary education cost only $213.

The point that is being made here is that if the benefits are being measured in the context of low incomes and the costs are also being measured in the context of low incomes, then the CBA outcome need not be distorted by the use of the HC approach. But, as with treatment that we considering in this perspective paper, which is measuring benefits in local terms and measuring drug costs in the context of rich developed countries, then using the HC approach to value benefits is not going to be appropriate.

Best practice in CBA is to use the willingness to pay (WTP) approach. This is consistent with the welfare economics base behind most normative economic policy in the West.[12] This benefit methodology can be applied to intervention commodities, such as the provision of condoms in Tanzania, where a CBA found B/C ratios in the range 1.3 to 1.7 at the existing subsidized price,[13] or it can be applied directly to the value of a life saved from voluntary counseling and testing using the value of a statistical life (VSL) approach,[14] which obtained B/C ratios above 3 for both individual and dual testing scaled up to the population as a whole.

Note that the value of a life saved using the VSL approach in Tanzania was $38,900, over four times the value used for a life saved using the human capital approach. For CBAs in developed countries, there is a rule of thumb that the WTP approach gives estimates that are three times that of the HC approach.[15] This relationship is probably higher for developing counties, in which case if $1,000 is the HC valuation, then $5,000 would probably be a reasonable estimate using the VSL approach. For this reason we have used only the $5,000 benefit figure and not the $1,000 amount in all our calculations.

It is useful to compare this $5,000 figure with the value that was obtained using the revealed preference (RP) approach to carry out the value of a life

---

[11] See Brent (2009a).
[12] For an exposition of CBA that utilizes this welfare economic base, see Brent (2006).
[13] See Brent (2009b).
[14] See Schelling (1968).
[15] See Brent (2003), ch. 11.

year (strictly, a disability adjusted life year DALY as envisaged by the *RethinkHIV* guidelines).[16] The RP approach assumes that behavior reveals preferences. In this case the assumption is that the more that a decision-maker values something, the more that the person will spend money in obtaining it. Brent (2010b) did a statistical analysis of the spending decisions by the Global Fund when giving grants to African countries for HIV interventions and they implicitly valued a DALY at $10,000 when AIDS or malaria or TB was contributing to the DALY, and at $6,000 when any other disease was contributing to the DALY. The standard DALY value of $6,000 is close to the $5,000 figure that we are recommending. Since the AIDS DALY is worth more than this according to the Global Fund's preferences, we can be sure that our $5,000 valuation for benefits is not too high.

Interpreting the $5,000 benefit amount to be the value of a statistical life, i.e., what a poor country with $1,000 per capita income would be valuing the avoidance of the risk of losing someone from AIDS, is important because it provides clearcut guidelines related to when double counting of benefits can be said to be taking place. The VSL is a comprehensive measure of benefits; it does not need augmenting. Hence in the previous section of this paper when we compared our results on MTCT with those in the assessment paper by Bollinger, we suggested that adding treatment cost savings to the $5,000 figure was double counting. Similarly, both the Bollinger assessment paper and the one by Behrman and Kohler raised the question as to whether the production losses from a person affected by HIV/AIDS needs to be added to the $5,000 benefit amount. Again the answer is "no"; production effects are already included as part of the VSL. Note that when the CC guidelines for valuing benefits are fully adhered to, and the evaluator is applying the $5,000 figure not to the number of lives saved, but to the number of DALYs, the DALY measure itself already includes the lost production effects *implicitly*. DALYs weight a person's years of life expectancy differently, according to the age of the person losing the life years. Years at the beginning and at the end of the life cycle are given lower weights than in the middle years (an inverted U-shaped, age-weighting func-

tion). Because the middle years lost are the ones where a person is most productive, this is consistent with allowing for production effects.[17]

As a final postscript to this discussion, it is necessary to point out that ignoring WTP and using a fixed value to apply to numbers of lives saved to estimate the benefits, as suggested by the *RethinkHIV* guidelines, will not always work. As we realized in this paper, when we carried out a comparison of the evaluation of treatment versus family planning in the context of MTCT, not every intervention explicitly can be reduced to saving lives. It may be that lives are not saved, but lives (albeit with HIV infection) are simply not being created. In this case, one has to directly find out what a woman is willing to pay for FP and use this to measure the benefits.

Evaluating treatment as prevention and the role of discounting

Having a dynamic perspective of CBA enables one to have a deeper understanding of the essential similarities and differences between treatment and prevention in terms of carrying out a CBA of health care interventions. In any intervention numbers are important. Prevention usually involves a large number of people taking a precautionary action that involves costs in exchange for a fewer number of persons receiving the benefits in terms of avoiding the adverse effects of an illness or disease. In the case of HIV/AIDS prevention, the costs involve potentially everyone getting tested or taking condoms in order that some of them do not get infected

---

[16] We will refer again to the role of DALYs for evaluating treatment in the Summary and Conclusions section.

[17] Note that Murray and Acharya (1997), who were the ones who first developed the DALY concept, gave higher weights to middle age years because people at this stage of their lives have more social responsibilities (others depend on them for care and direction) and not because they are more productive. But, nonetheless, this is still consistent with giving higher weights to more productive years even though Murray and Acharya explicitly wanted to avoid this interpretation. They are, as we are, against using the HC approach. But, in any interpretation of age weighting, there is no scope to add forgone production to the $5,000 DALY value. It is ruled out and, if it were not ruled out, it has already been included implicitly (which is our argument).

with the virus. Numbers are also important for HIV treatment, but it is in terms of numbers of years and not numbers of persons. For any one person on treatment, a larger number of years have to be devoted to incurring the costs of medications than the years of extra life expectancy that is generated by the drugs. This was the central feature that drove the calculations presented in this discussion paper.

Linked to the number of years that are involved with the costs is whether the intervention is a one-time or continuous activity. In many CBAs outside the health care field (for example building a bridge or school), there is a large upfront cost incurred in the first period and the evaluation task is to convert a future stream of benefits to be comparable to the current costs (i.e., the present value of the benefits must be calculated). In our evaluation of MTCT we considered both cases, one where treatment was just during the birth of the baby, and again when treatment was given to mothers even prior to the pregnancy when they were being treated in their own right.

It is the context of differing numbers of years of benefits and costs, and whether costs are a one-time or continuous expense, that the impact of discounting for the evaluation of treatment can be understood. As we saw in Table 3.1.1 and repeated in the first row of Table 3.1.2, the fact that benefits come in year 15 and are therefore heavily discounted while the costs are experienced in all years, means that discounting is going to have a large impact when initiation is with a CD4 count of greater than 35. In the first segment in Table 3.1.2, we see that the B/C ratio is greater than 1 only if there is no discounting – see the last row which corresponds to second-line treatment and 2050 costs. This was true when there were twenty-one years of benefits and thirty-five years of costs. In the middle segment, where benefits are for thirty-seven years and follow more closely the forty-one years of costs, the impact of discounting is very small. With 2050 costs, the B/C ratio is 1.56 with no discounting and very close to the 1.43 and 1.35 with 3 percent and 5 percent discounting respectively. When we reach the fifth and final segment of Table 3.1.2, discounting has almost no impact in affecting B/C ratios. When it comes to considering the evaluation of treatment that is initiated with a CD4 count <50,

the *RethinkHIV* experts panel need not agonize over what is the appropriate discount rate, whether 3 percent, which is current practice for health care evaluations, or whether 5 percent, which used to be the rate most often used. These generalizations hold also for Table 3.1.3 where externalities are also included.

In the evaluation of PMTCT programs, there is (are) only one (or two) years of costs and these are incurred in the beginning year(s). Discounting will not impact costs. But, the benefits flowing over thirteen years are greatly affected by the choice of discount rate. Fortunately the best MTCT program has enormously high value B/C ratios even at the 5 percent rate, i.e., it is 72.40, so again the *RethinkHIV* experts panel do not need to agonize over whether to give the highest priority to MTCT programs on the basis of which discount rate to use.

Women and HIV in SSA

A glaring omission from the assessment paper is any allowance for equity considerations, whether they be related to individual, regional or gender inequalities. We will just focus on gender inequality.

Worldwide, 52 percent of adults living with HIV in low- and middle-income countries are women, while 58 percent of those receiving treatment are women. So outside of SSA, the ratio of women to men receiving treatment is in line with gender HIV prevalence.[18] But in SSA 60 percent of the HIV infections involve females. It is likely that in SSA the women's share is not in line with prevalence; especially as some treatment programs require co-payments for costs of diagnosis, treatment or care, or need to know the insurance status of patients. Women have fewer resources and are less likely to have insurance than men, and would therefore be at a disadvantage. In addition, sometimes requirements are made for those initiating treatment that they disclose their status to at least one person. Such criteria may limit access to care and treatment for women because of fear of violence from partners.[19]

---

[18] See WHO (2009).
[19] Again, see WHO (2009).

However, even if 60 percent of ARVs do go to women in SSA, an argument could be made that the share should be even higher. MTCT is very high in most countries and in many countries MTCT government programs allegedly give priority to the prevention of MTCT, yet there were an estimated 370,000 children who contracted HIV during the perinatal and breastfeeding period, most of them in SSA. In addition, there were 90,000 AIDS-related deaths among children in SSA in 2009.[20] The clearest sign that prevention of MTCT must have been inadequate is the CBA results we found in this perspective paper. If B/C ratios of 70 to 100 can be obtained for the prevention of MTCT, then this is direct evidence that resources must have been used for lower priority interventions in the past.

In this perspective paper we have come up with an externalities argument as to why females should always be given priority over males in the allocation of ARV treatments: women have children; men do not. While it costs the same to give treatment to women as men, there will always be more persons who do not get infected and hence higher benefits from treating women, if the number of sex partners is the same. While there is evidence that males do have more partners than females in SSA, the difference is very small. Earlier we referred to the study by Oster (2009) which reported that men only have 9 percentage points more partners than females, which would not make up for the advantage of a female having just one child whose life would be saved.

Summary and conclusions

The assessment paper on Treatment finds that if an extra $10 billion is spent on expanding ARV provision, then the B/C ratio generated by this intervention would be in the range 2 to 3 (see Figure 3.11). This would mean that additional benefits would be $20 to $30 billion, which makes HIV treatment a highly socially worthwhile investment. The strategy that achieved this outcome would be to expand treatment first to those with CD4 counts less than 50 and work up the CD4 initiation list until the budget was exhausted.

The dynamic model of infections that was used by Over and Garnett to produce the estimated number of lives saved by treatment was similar in structure to the standard epidemiological model, but it did have some important differences that suggest that the assessment paper underestimated the true benefits of treatment. For example, the assessment paper model did not allow for fertility effects of treatment. If there would have been more people infected than was predicted, then there would be more lives that could have been saved when increased treatment coverage takes place.

In our simplified version of the dynamic model, which focused on a representative individual on treatment and allowed for different treatment effectiveness by considering varying amounts of partners whose lives would be saved from treatment, we were able to replicate the assessment paper's findings only under very restrictive circumstances – see Table 3.1.3. First of all there would have to be only one sex partner. If someone had any other partner than their spouse or regular partner, then B/C ratios less than 3 could not be obtained. Second, the discount rate would have to be 5 percent and not 3 percent. And finally, the CD4 count at initiation would have to be less than 350.

A useful way of summarizing Table 3.1.3 is to recognize that scaling up treatment would involve starting with the CD4 <50 group and then moving up the list of five groups until one reached the CD4 >350 group. Since all five groups' results would be a part of this process and should be included, one can take the average of the five group B/C ratios to obtain the overall result. With one partner, the average B/C ratio is 5.44 at the 3 percent discount rate and 4.59 at the 5 percent discount rate, and with two partners the average B/C ratio is 8.15 at the 3 percent discount rate and 6.88 at the 5 percent discount rate.

If the number of lives saved is underestimated in the assessment paper, the benefits are going to be underestimated. The numerator part of the B/C ratio will be low. To know whether the ratio as a whole will be too low, we also need to consider whether the costs in the denominator of the ratio have been appropriately estimated. O&G come up

[20] See UNAIDS (2010).

with a figure of $1,034 as the average treatment cost per year – see Figure 3.3. They obtain this figure on the assumption that there will be economies of scale with treatment, i.e., a 10 percent increase in scale will lead to a 3 percent reduction in average cost. They refer to cross-section data in Figure 3.3 to support their claim that economies of scale exist. But, there are two main reasons for doubting that there will be falling average costs with treatment scale-up. The cross-section analysis is not relevant and treatment side-effects are not recognized, as we now explain.

First, health care facilities in SSA are mainly in the urban areas, where population densities are high. Rural areas are underserved. To expand treatment in SSA will involve going into the rural areas, where transport costs will inhibit uptake. These transport costs, including the opportunity cost of time, need to be factored into the average cost estimates. Assume that half of a typical SSA country lives in rural areas. The cross-section data analyzed in Figure 3.3 have countries expanding treatment so that costs approximate the experience of South Africa, where there were 971,556 persons on ARVs, out of a population of 2,600,000 that needed to be treated, according to WHO 2010 guidelines. We are assuming therefore that the costs that South Africa is experiencing are mainly urban treatment costs. Now take the case of Swaziland which has 47,241 on ARVs and 80,000 are needed. The thought experiment in the assessment paper is that Swaziland scaling up towards 80,000 will be like moving towards South Africa's near million on ARVs. But the reality is that all of Swaziland's expansion will involve going into the rural areas, where average costs are much higher than in the urban areas.[21]

The second problem with the assessment paper's costs assumption is that it ignores the fact that ARV treatment has enormous adverse side-effects that reduces people's tolerance and hence adherence to treatment. The assessment paper points out that thirty-eight out of fifty countries surveyed by the WHO had started replacing Stavudine, d4T, a staple of first-line treatments, with a less toxic option. The point simply is that as scaling-up takes place, more people will need to be treated with second-line (and third-line) drugs that are much more expen-

sive (double the cost, according to the assessment paper). This means that it is very unrealistic for the assessment paper to assume that only 10 percent of the people on treatment will be on second-line drugs when there is going to be such a large scale-up. In our CBA calculations we attempted to partially correct for the underestimation of costs in the assessment paper by replacing their $1,034 figure with our $1,375 estimate, which is a third higher. We obtained this amount by assuming 20 percent of treatment will use second-line drugs. As we pointed out earlier, when we were explaining the justification for the numbers determining the B/C ratios in Table 3.1.3, some programs in South Africa already treat 20 percent of the infections with second-line drugs.

To summarize so far: we suggest that the estimates in our Table 3.1.3 are more reliable on both the benefits and costs sides, and so the B/C ratios we found in the range 3 to 10 are better predictors of outcomes than the 2 to 3 range in the assessment paper.

Up to this point we have been assuming that *all* of the $10 billion is to be spent on treatment. We will now consider the results we found when only a part of the funds was going to be spent on treatment. In the presence of a budget constraint, and with the assumption that all projects are independent and divisible, the correct CBA procedure is to calculate the B/C ratios for all types of intervention, i.e., prevention, treatment, and mitigation, and to rank them from highest to lowest. Then one starts funding with the interventions with the highest B/C ratio and then works down the list until the total budget is exhausted.[22] We have argued in this perspective paper that MTCT is likely to have the highest B/C ratios of any treatment program because it will give the largest number of years of benefits (additional life expectancy) for the least number of years of costs (in most cases just one year of costs). In fact, it is highly likely that the B/C ratios for MTCT will be the largest for any type of intervention that the *RethinkHIV* initiative will be considering. B/C

---

[21] The ARV figures in this paragraph are from UNAIDS (2009).

[22] For a proof that this is the correct CBA procedure when there is a budget constraint, see Brent (1998), ch. 2.

ratios for three alternative prevention of MTCT programs listed in Table 3.1.5 are in the range 27 to 103. For the best alternative MTCT via a Zidovudine program, the B/C ratios are in the range 72 to 103. A strong case can be made that if $2 billion of the $10 billion is devoted to treating 12.1 women currently pregnant and likely to be in the future, then this will save 1.25 million babies' lives and around $200 billion of benefits.

Prevention of MTCT is concerned with saving the lives of the children of the pregnant mothers. If one is also concerned with treating the mothers themselves, then the evaluation framework changes considerably to be a mix of the analyses in Tables 3.1.3 and 3.1.5. The results are shown in Table 3.1.8. Costs need to be incurred in every year for the person treated. In Table 3.1.7 we see that (undiscounted) costs over the woman's lifetime amount to $25,633. So treating 11.6 million women would far exceed the $10 million budget. In fact, it would not be feasible to fund the 1.6 million women who are currently pregnant and are infected with HIV. Instead there could be only 390,122 people treated with the funds available.

So the question is: who should be the 390,122 people that receive treatment for the $10 billion? The answer is clear according to Table 3.1.8. The benefits of treatment depend on the size of the externalities, which is determined by the number of partners and children who are not infected because the drugs prevent the transmission of the virus to them. Men, like women, can have sex partners, but cannot have children. So the externalities are larger for women for a given number of partners. The male treatment B/C ratios correspond to the three rows in Table 3.1.8 where there are no children. We see that for no partners, the B/C ratio for women with four children are double that for males when the discount rate is 3 percent.[23] For one partner, which is the norm in SSA, the B/C ratio is 26 percent higher if a female has two children and has treatment, and is 51 percent higher if a female has four children and has treatment. The answer then is that treatment should first be given to females.

The fact that there is no analysis of treatment by gender in the assessment paper is a major omission. The transmission rate from males to females is three times that from females to males,[24] yet the trans-

mission coefficient β_t has no gender component in equation (9). It would have been a simple matter to have disaggregated the S and the I in equations (6) and (7) and used a β three times larger when attached to the female term $S_f i_f$.

The other major omission from the assessment paper that affects all their results is that they did not follow the *RethinkHIV* guidelines and convert their outcome measure of lives saved to disability adjusted life years (DALYs). This omission probably affects the results for treatment much more than it would any of the other interventions that the *RethinkHIV* experts are considering. Anti-retroviral drugs have highly adverse side-effects, due to their toxicity. For example, they lead to lipodystrophy and impotence in males. Whether one is using DALYs, or their inverse, quality adjusted life years (QALYs), these side-effects greatly reduce the quality of a life year saved *even if* we assume that people do not stop taking their medications because of their existence (which we know does take place). In a CBA of ARVs for older adults in New York City, Brent (2011) and Brent *et al.* (2011) found that the medications reduced the quality of life by 27 percent for those who were not depressed. Multiplying all benefits in O&G's paper by 73 percent would reduce all their B/C ratios by approximately a quarter.

This would also be the case with our Tables 3.1.3 and 3.1.8. Females and males alike would have their quality of life greatly reduced by treatment. However, this would *not* be the case with our evaluation of the prevention of MTCT and our results given in Table 3.1.5. Prevention for a pregnant woman is a one-off intervention in this context. When successful, neither the mother nor the baby has to take ARV medications in the future, so neither of them will have their quality of life reduced. This reinforces our main recommendation in this perspective paper that the first $2 billion of the additional funding should be devoted to the prevention of MTCT

[23] Obviously, for women to have children, they must have had sex partners in the past. So the table with 0 partners is to be understood as the number of partners a woman will have in the future.

[24] See Stillwaggon (2006).

as this treatment intervention is likely to have the highest B/C ratio of any intervention.

References

Avert. (2011a). Preventing mother-to-child transmission of HIV (PMTCT). Downloaded from www.avert.org/motherchild. htm (accessed September 9, 2011).

Avert. (2011b). Sub-Saharan Africa HIV & AIDS statistics. Downloaded from www.avert. org/africa-hiv-aids-statistics.htm (accessed September 9, 2011).

Brent, R. J. (1998). *Cost-Benefit Analysis for Developing Countries*. Cheltenham: Edward Elgar.

Brent, R. J. (2003). *Cost-Benefit Analysis and Health Care Evaluations*. Cheltenham: Edward Elgar.

Brent, R. J. (2006). *Applied Cost-Benefit Analysis*. 2nd edn. Cheltenham: Edward Elgar.

Brent, R. J. (2009a). A cost-benefit analysis of female primary education as a means of reducing HIV-AIDS in Tanzania. *Applied Economics* 41(14): 1731–43.

Brent, R. J. (2009b). A cost-benefit analysis of a condom social marketing program in Tanzania. *Applied Economics* 41: 497–509.

Brent, R. J. (2010a). *Setting Priorities for HIV/AIDS: A Cost-Benefit Approach*. Cheltenham: Edward Elgar.

Brent, R. J. (2010b). An implicit price of a DALY for use in a cost-benefit analysis of ARVs. *Applied Economics* 43: 1413–21.

Brent, R. J. (2010c). A social cost-benefit criterion for evaluating voluntary counselling and testing with an application to Tanzania. *Health Economics* 19: 154–72.

Brent, R. J. (2011). The effects of HIV medications on the quality of life of older adults in New York City. *Health Economics* (forthcoming).

Brent, R. J., Brennan, M. and Karpiak, S. E. (2011). Using a happiness index to measure the benefits for a cost-benefit analysis of anti-retrovirals for older adults with HIV in New York City. Fordham University, New York.

Cohen, M. S., Chen, Y. Q. *et al.* (2010). Prevention of HIV-1 infection with early antiretroviral therapy. *N Engl J Med* 365(6): 493–505.

Gersovitz, M. and Hammer, J. H. (2004). The economic control of infectious diseases. *The Economic Journal* 114: 1–27.

Hladik, W., Stover, J., Esiru, G. *et al.* (2009). The contribution of family planning towards the prevention of vertical HIV transmission in Uganda. *PLoS One* 4, Issue 11, e7691.

Mahy, M., Stover, J., Kiragu, K. *et al.* (2010). What will it take to achieve virtual elimination of mother-to-child transmission of HIV? An assessment of current progress. *Sexually Transmitted Infections* 86 (Suppl 2): ii48–ii55.

Murray, C. J. L. and Acharya, A. K. (1997). Understanding DALYs. *Journal of Health Economics* 16: 703–30.

Oster, E. (2009). *HIV and Sexual Behavior Change: Why not Africa?* University of Chicago and NBER.

Pisani, E. (2008). *The Wisdom of Whores: Bureaucrats, Brothels and the Business of AIDS*. New York: W.W. Norton & Company.

Reynolds, H. W., Janowitz, B., Homan, R. *et al.* (2006). The value of contraception to prevent perinatal HIV transmission. *Sexually Transmitted Diseases* 33: 350–6.

Schelling, T. C. (1968). The life you save may be your own. In Chase, S. B., Jr. (ed.) *Problems in Public Expenditure Analysis*. Washington DC: Brookings Institution, 127–61.

Schwartländer, B., Stover, J., Hallet, T. *et al.* (2011). Towards an improved investment approach for an effective response to HIV/AIDS. *The Lancet*, doi:10.1016/S0140-6736(11)60702-2. There is online supplemental material (26/05/2011) for this article that is referred to in our paper.

Stillwaggon, E. (2006). *AIDS and the Ecology of Poverty*. New York: Oxford University Press.

Sweat, M. D., O'Reily, K. R., Schmid, G. P. *et al.* (2004). Cost-effectiveness of Nevirapine to prevent mother-to-child transmission in eight African countries. *AIDS* 18: 1661–71.

The All Party Parliamentary Group on AIDS. (2009). *The Treatment Timebomb. Report of the Inquiry of The All Parliamentary Group on AIDS into Long-term Access to HIV Medicines in the Developing World*, July.

UNAIDS. (2009). *Towards Universal Access: Scaling Up Priority HIV/AIDS Interventions in the Health Sector. Progress Report 2009*.

UNAIDS. (2010). *Report on the Global AIDS Epidemic 2010*.

Velkoff, V. A. and Kowal, P. R. (2007). *Population Aging in Sub-Saharan Africa: Demographic Dimensions 2006*, U.S. Census Bureau, Current

Population Reports, P95/07-1, U.S. Government Printing Office, Washington, DC.

WHO. (2009). *Integrating Gender into HIV/AIDS Programmes in the Health Sector: Tool to Improve Responsiveness to Women's Needs.* Geneva.

WHO. (2010). *Antiretroviral Drugs for Treating Pregnant Women and Preventing HIV Infection in Infants: Towards Universal Access.* Geneva.

Treatment

Perspective paper

JOHN STOVER

In their paper for *RethinkHIV*, "Treatment," Over and Garnett estimate benefit to cost ratios for anti-retroviral treatment (ART) in sub-Saharan Africa (SSA). They use an epidemiological simulation model to determine the number of HIV infections over time and the effects of various ART scale-up scenarios on new infections, AIDS deaths, and life years gained. They apply the model to a number of countries in SSA and aggregate the results to the entire region. Their specific purpose is to estimate the benefits and benefit to cost ratios of applying an additional $2 billion per year to ART programs from 2011 to 2015. They compare the benefits of scaling up ART to two counterfactual scenarios: one where those currently on treatment receive continued support but no new patients are added, and one where the historical trend in scale-up is maintained.

A unique feature of Over and Garnett's work is their approach to estimating future ART costs per person. Their approach recognizes that drug and service delivery costs may decline with scale and increase with gross national income (GNI) per capita. They estimate that average costs for first-line treatment in SSA may rise from about $712.50 in 2012 to almost $1,000 by 2050.

For both counterfactual scenarios, Over and Garnett calculate results for two ways of spending $10 billion: one focuses on providing treatment for those with the lowest CD4 counts and achieves full coverage for those newly needing treatment, and a second scenario that makes treatment available to those with higher CD4 counts but achieves lower coverage of those newly needing treatment. A third scenario removes the funding constraint and allows early initiation of treatment such that the median CD4 count at treatment initiation increases to 800 compared to 200–300 and 410–580 under

the two scenarios that are limited to an additional $10 billion.

The authors estimate a benefit to cost ratio for ART of 5–6.3 when discount rates are 3–5 percent and an additional life year is valued at $5,000, and 1–1.3 when an additional year of life is valued at $1,000. They conclude that spending an additional $10 billion on ART provides significant benefits but is not necessarily the best health investment. They point out that such a program would provide additional benefits not captured in their analysis in terms of strengthening the health system.

Key issues in assessing future costs and benefits

Over and Garnett have applied an appropriate epidemiological model to estimate the impact of ART in a number of countries in SSA, have based their parameter values on the latest research findings, and they have developed an innovative approach to projecting cost per patient into the future. Their sensitivity analysis captures the main uncertainties regarding who would benefit from the additional funding. However, there are at least two aspects of the analysis that might be done differently and could affect the findings: (1) examining whether treatment costs per patient will inevitably rise in the future, and (2) whether the approach to simulating national epidemics is the best way to determine the impact of an additional $10 billion over five years. This paper will focus on these two issues.

Future costs of ART per patient

The annual cost per ART patient has declined dramatically since ART was first introduced in the

1990s. Costs per patient were initially as high as $20,000 in the most developed countries, but have declined to well below $1,000 in low-income countries today. This decline was driven by the availability of generic drugs, and negotiations with manufacturers that resulted in lower prices in low-income countries. The decline in ARV prices has continued over the past few years, although at a slower pace. The annual cost of the most common first-line regimens in low-income countries has declined by 54 percent, from 2006 to 2009 (WHO 2010). As a result, in many countries the costs of laboratory monitoring and service delivery are higher than ARV costs. The US-funded President's Emergency Response to AIDS Relief (PEPFAR) has found that its costs per patient have dropped considerably as programs have scaled up. In Uganda, for example, financial costs per patient dropped by 54 percent over 18–24 months (Macro International 2009). The program documented declines in both investment and recurrent costs per patient, as volumes expanded.

Since resources available for HIV have been stagnant the last few years, many are concerned that we will not be able to keep expanding access to all who need treatment unless the cost per patient drops significantly. In response, the World Health Organization (WHO), UNAIDS, and other organizations have launched an initiative called Treatment 2.0 (UNAIDS 2009). This initiative envisions a simplified approach to treatment that includes: a combination first-line pill that is easy to take, has low toxicity, and is effective against resistance; reductions in the cost of monitoring through less expensive tests (such as point-of-care dipsticks for CD4 and viral load monitoring) and reduced need for frequent tests; and rationalized service delivery that requires fewer monitoring visits and uses physicians only for essential tasks. These changes could lead to a significant reduction in costs per patient. An initial analysis done for UNAIDS' new investment framework envisions cost per patient dropping from about $570 in 2010 to $150 by 2020 (Schwartländer *et al.* 2011). Drug costs are reduced through volume production of a standard regimen. A very effective first-line regimen would significantly reduce the need for routine CD4 counts or viral load test. Service delivery costs could fall to

Table 3.2.1 Potential reductions in treatment cost per patient

Component	2009	2020
First-line ARVs	$155	$57
Second-line ARVs	$1,680	$295
Laboratory tests	$180	$24
Service delivery	$180	$30
Procurement as percentage of drug costs	20%	5%

one-third of current values with a more effective and tolerable first-line regimen. Changes in specific components are shown in Table 3.2.1.

If the goals of the Treatment 2.0 initiative can be achieved, it would lead to costs per ART patient that would be only $150 by 2020, significantly below the $1,000 per patient for first-line therapy envisioned by Over and Garnett for 2050.

Life years gained by treatment

This analysis is supposed to determine the benefits of an extra $2 billion each year for five years, from 2011 to 2015. It is more difficult to address this question for treatment than it is for almost any other area of HIV programs. To precisely answer this question we should calculate the benefits of providing ART to additional patients for five years only, after which support is stopped. In that case the years of life gained would be small because not all those receiving treatment during the five-year period would have died without treatment. In addition any prevention benefits of treatment would not be captured, since infections averted during 2011–2015 would only result in life years gained after 2015. More importantly one can never imagine such a scenario, since starting someone on treatment implies a moral obligation to continue that treatment for as long as the patient needs it. Over and Garnett project their simulation model to 2050 in order to capture all the benefits of increased expenditure, but even then they may not capture all the benefits unless the increase in patients happens very early in the period.

An alternative approach is to examine the benefits and costs of a single patient starting on treatment

Adult CD4 Model

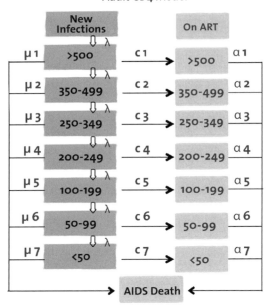

Figure 3.2.1 *A model for tracking the effects of ART initiation at different CD4 counts*

Table 3.2.2 Years of survival on ART for a person starting treatment at age 35 by CD4 count at initiation

CD4 count at treatment initiation	First-year survival rate	Subsequent annual survival rate	Median number of years on ART	Median years of survival without ART
<50	0.154	0.083	7	1.5
50–99	0.087	0.048	12	1.7
100–199	0.051	0.029	18	2.2
200–249	0.044	0.025	21	3.0
250–349	0.038	0.022	22	4.4
350–500	0.032	0.019	24	6.5
>500	0.026	0.016	26	11.5

today. That implies a commitment to continue treatment well beyond 2015, but we can assume that the additional funds available in 2011–2015 represent an allocation that can be invested today and spent in the future as needed. We can calculate the present day benefits and costs of starting one person on treatment and continuing treatment until the patient dies. The discounted costs represent the amount that needs to be obligated today to ensure future treatment needs are met. These calculations can be performed by tracking a newly infected person by CD4 count and describing the annual probability of death, progress to the next lowest CD4 category, or starting on ART. An outline of the model is shown in Figure 3.2.1.

The survival of a person starting on ART ($\alpha 1$ to $\alpha 7$, in Figure 3.2.1) is determined by their CD4 count at treatment initiation. Mortality rates in the first year and subsequent years on treatment have been estimated for East Africa by the IeDEA Consortium using data from treatment cohorts (Yiannoutsos 2008). These rates apply to all patients on treatment, including both first- and second-line, so this model does not distinguish between the two. Patients are also subject to non-AIDS mortality ($\mu 1$ to $\mu 7$, in Figure 3.2.1). These calculations use typical non-AIDS mortality rates for a person starting treatment at age thirty-five. Non-AIDS mortality is a relatively minor factor during the first five years of treatment (0.75 percent per year), but becomes more important as survival on ART lengthens and the patient ages (0.85 percent at 40–44, 1.0 percent at 45–49, 1.2 percent at 50–54, and 1.5 percent at 55–59). The resulting years of survival on ART are shown in Table 3.2.2.[1]

The survival of an HIV-positive person who does not receive ART is determined by the rates of progression from one CD4 category to the next and by mortality rates at each CD4 count. These rates have been estimated to match the survival pattern for untreated people with HIV from the ALPHA network (Todd *et al.* 2007) (a consortium of cohort studies) and the distribution of CD4 counts for the HIV-infected population not on ART from the Kenya AIDS Indicator Survey of 2007 (Ministry of Health, Kenya, 2008), as described elsewhere (Stover *et al.* 2011).

The difference between survival with and without ART for people in each CD4 count category is the additional years of life gained by ART. These are discounted at 3 percent annually to produce the

[1] These calculations are implemented in an interactive internet-based model that can be accessed at www.FuturesInstitute.org by selecting Policy Tools and ART Cost Model.

Table 3.2.3 Discounted years of life gained, costs, and discounted cost per year of life gained by CD4 count at ART initiation

CD4 count at treatment initiation	Discounted years of life gained	Present value of treatment costs	Cost per life year gained
<50	8.3	$3,260	$395
50–99	14.1	$4,360	$310
100–199	20.3	$5,300	$260
200–249	22.5	$5,580	$250
250–349	21.2	$5,850	$280
350–500	22.2	$6,100	$275
>500	22.5	$6,300	$280

final estimates of years of life gained by ART due to reduced mortality.

There will also be gains due to the effect of ART on reducing infectiousness and thus averting transmission to uninfected individuals. This effect is more difficult to capture in a model that follows a single infected individual. A simple approach is to recognize that according to UNAIDS in 2009, there were 20.5 million adults living with HIV in SSA, and 1.5 million new infections. So, on average, each HIV-infected person accounts for 0.074 new infections per year. If ART reduces infectiousness by about 70 percent (as estimated by Over and Garnett), then the annual number of infections averted by ART per HIV-infected person becomes 0.052. If an infection averted gains about eleven years of life (the median survival of an untreated person), or 9.5 years when discounted at 3 percent, then each year of ART produces about 0.5 additional years of life. This benefit can be added to the years of life gained by the infected individual to determine the total life years gained by ART for initiation at each CD4 count.

Results

The present values of the costs of treatment are determined by the number of years of treatment and the cost per patient for each year from Table 3.2.1. The results are shown in Table 3.2.3.

The average benefit of scaling up ART will depend on the mixture of CD4 counts for new patients. An ideal distribution would first provide treatment for all those in need at CD4 counts <50, then for those with CD4 counts <100, etc., but this ideal will not be achieved, because not everyone who is HIV-positive has been identified or has access to treatment. Two other allocation approaches are possible: (1) the likelihood of getting on ART is proportional to the unmet need (everyone who is eligible for treatment has an equal chance of starting on treatment regardless of CD4 count) and (2) the likelihood of getting on ART is proportional to expected mortality without ART (those with lower CD4 counts and higher expected mortality have a better chance of starting on treatment). When compared to actual data on CD4 counts at treatment initiation the first approach tends to over-estimate the chance of getting started at high CD4 counts and the second approach tends to over-estimate the chance of getting started at low CD4 counts, but the average of the two approaches closely approximates the actual distributions observed in South Africa. When eligibility is defined as CD4 counts under 350 and the CD4 distribution of HIV-positive patients not on ART is similar to the distribution found in the Kenya AIDS Indicator Survey, the resulting distribution of new ART patients is 27 percent at <50, 20 percent at 50–99, 24 percent at 100–99, 10 percent at 200–49, and 19 percent at 250–349. The resulting weighted discounted cost per life year gained is $310.

The final benefit to cost ratios for treatment are 3.3 when a year of life is valued at $1,000, and 16 when a year of life is valued at $5,000.

Discussion

Over and Garnett estimate the benefit to cost ratio for ART at 1–1.3 when discount rates are 3–5 percent and an additional year of life is valued at $1,000, and 5–6.3 when an additional life year is valued at $5,000. This alternative analysis finds benefit to cost ratios that are about three times higher. The difference is mainly due to assumptions about the future costs of treatment per patient.

Over and Garnett assume that costs per patient will decline with higher volumes but that these scale effects will be overwhelmed by the effects of increasing GNI per capita such that per patient costs will increase by about 40 percent from 2010 to 2050. This paper uses the assumptions of the Treatment 2.0 initiative to project that improvements and drugs and service delivery will result in a decrease in per patient costs of 75 percent.

The future may lie somewhere in between. It is difficult to imagine that we can achieve significantly higher coverage of ART in the future without finding efficiencies that reduce the cost per patient. Whatever changes do take place are unlikely to be uniform across all countries. Some countries will continue to be dependent on funds from PEPFAR and the Global Fund while others, such as Botswana and South Africa, will increasingly take over treatment of financing. The tremendous variation across countries in the cost per patient treated that currently exists will probably narrow, as approaches are standardized and more countries obtain the best possible prices for ARVs.

In almost any analysis, ART will clearly be a cost-effective way to reduce deaths due to AIDS, but will generally be more expensive than purely preventive interventions with high effectiveness. Nevertheless, the current distribution of expenditures between prevention and treatment indicates that cost-effectiveness is not the only criteria used today to allocate HIV funds. We will need to find the right balance between preventing new infections and providing life-saving treatment for those already infected.

References

Macro International. (2009). *The Cost of Comprehensive HIV Treatment in Uganda. Report of a Cost Study of PEPFAR-Supported HIV Treatment Programs in Uganda.* Macro International. September.

National AIDS and STI Control Programme, Ministry of Health, Kenya. (2008). *AIDS Indicator Survey 2007: Preliminary Report, National AIDS and STI Control Programme*, Ministry of Health, Nairobi, Kenya.

Over, M. and Garnett, G. (2011). A cost-benefit analysis of AIDS treatment in sub-Saharan Africa, draft report, prepared September.

Schwartländer, B., Stover, J., Hallett, T. *et al.* (2011). Towards an improved investment approach for an effective response to HIV/AIDS. *Lancet.* Published online June 3. doi:10.1016/S0140-6736(11)60702-2.

Stover, J., Bollinger, L. and Avila, C. (2010). Estimating the impact and cost of the WHO recommendations for antiretroviral therapy. *AIDS Research and Treatment* 2011, Article ID 738271, 7 pages. doi:10.1155/2011/738271.

Todd, J., Glynn, J. R., Marston, M. *et al.* (2007). Time from HIV seroconversion to death: a collaborative analysis of eight studies in six low and middle-income countries before highly active antiretroviral therapy. *AIDS* **21**, supplement 6, pp. P–S63.

UNAIDS. (2009). Treatment 2.0.

WHO. (2010). *Towards Universal Access: Scaling Up Priority HIV/AIDS Interventions in the Health Sector. Progress Report 2010.* Geneva: World Health Organization.

Yiannoutsos. (2008). PLoS ONE.

Strengthening health systems

Assessment paper

WILLIAM P. MCGREEVEY, WITH CARLOS AVILA
AND MARY PUNCHAK

Executive summary

RethinkHIV seeks answers to the question: "How can additional spending, $2 billion per annum over five years, a total of $10 billion, best be spent across a range of treatment, prevention, research, etc., measures in sub-Saharan Africa (SSA) to respond to HIV/AIDS?" Among the prospective options is an effective bridging between actions focused specifically on HIV/AIDS, and actions that aim to strengthen health systems. The strengthening health systems component considers below these possible solutions:

- Universal testing, informing, and counseling can be achieved with a voucher of $5 paid to each of the 400 million adults who accept to learn their HIV status. The cost is substantial at $2 billion, but benefits of knowledge could cut new infections by a quarter million annually, and the B/C ratio would range between a low of 2.5 and a high of 15.
- Deployment of community health workers to the rural population at a cost of $2.64 billion could cut maternal deaths by 0.3 million annually and child deaths by millions more, with B/C ratios ranging from about 1.1 to 9.5.
- Reducing the opportunistic infection of crypto-coccal meningitis (CM) at a cost of $1.5 billion can yield a ratio of benefits to costs between 2.7 and 20.
- An Abuja Goals Fund (AGF) can offer a cash on delivery (COD) incentive for meeting-agreed goals of spending 15 percent or more of public revenues on public health, yielding a ratio of benefits to cost between 1.1 and 8.

The analysis of these solutions applies cost-benefit analysis (CBA) to provide guidance for resource allocation at the margin between these and other potential solutions to health deficiencies in SSA. Each of the solutions reviewed offers positive returns of benefits compared to the incremental costs that would be incurred to implement them (see Table 4.1). The analysis considers scenarios in which the value of a year of life is set at $1,000 or $5,000 to include the range of income levels in SSA. The net present value (NPV) of future years of life is assessed using both a 3 percent and a 5 percent discount rate. Once these values for a life-year are adjusted to yield net present values of all the years of life that can be saved by a solution, we calculate the ratio of these two measures of benefits to the costs identified.

Summary of findings

As expected, the benefit to cost ratios varied substantially between the four solutions. The highest ratio of benefits to cost appears to derive from optimal treatment of the opportunistic infection, crypto-coccal meningitis, which without treatment puts as many as 32 million persons at risk in SSA. A lower but still positive ratio of benefits to costs emerges from using a cash on delivery bonus to countries that move toward the Abuja goal of more spending on public health. Other solutions lie between these high and somewhat lower results.

All four solutions show promise of implementation at a cost per disability adjusted life year (DALY) below the limits suggested for the $1,000 and $5,000 values of a life-year used in this exercise. Solutions that focus on young adults were deemed in the analysis to yield the best results in terms of life-years gained with the application of each solution. Solutions that combine HIV/AIDS prevention, family planning, and reproductive health appear to be particularly strong choices.

In aggregate, the costs for these proposed solutions would require a significant share of the proposed $10 billion to be made available. They are not equally advantageous. One solution would supply the rural poor with upgraded and more numerous community health workers to assure them of basic maternal and child care and expanded knowledge of HIV status. The poor can reasonably hope that their governments will be encouraged to reallocate public resources toward public health needs once an Abuja Goal Fund offers added incentives to governments to encourage matching rhetoric and reality.

Introduction

HIV/AIDS is a health challenge of global significance, but its greatest impact has been, and will continue to be, on the health of sub-Saharan Africa. After several decades of success in raising life expectancy since many countries in the region achieved independence, AIDS has driven down life expectancy at birth from greater than sixty years to less than fifty years in countries of eastern and southern Africa.

The combination of personal behavior change, government action, and donor support now show signs of meeting the challenge of the epidemic. Incidence is on the decline. Treatment now becomes prevention, and male circumcision shows promise as a new mode of prevention of sexual transmission. More AIDS-positive persons are living longer lives thanks to anti-retroviral therapy (ART). Since the United Nations General Assembly Special Session on AIDS (UNGASS) in June 2001, substantial financial resources have contributed to a reduction in deaths associated with AIDS.

In this paper, we examine selected cases of policy actions, interventions, and solutions that bridge the objective of health systems strengthening (HSS) with that of continuing the fight against HIV/AIDS in sub-Saharan Africa. We find that incentives that encourage demand for selected HIV/AIDS interventions also contribute to health system objectives. Incentives can be blended as well to promote more effective and complementary supply improvements. Providing subsidized care by reduc-

ing or even eliminating user fees is in effect a price-reduction incentive. This paper identifies four specific interventions that repay costs with substantial benefits in terms of better overall health indicators and reduction of HIV.

Conditional cash transfers (CCTs), a demand-side intervention, can be adapted to serve the joint objectives. Other demand-side interventions can complement conditional cash transfers, e.g., by promoting a new focus on "cash-on-delivery" (COD) forms of donor assistance. Donor agencies, especially the World Bank, are also testing methods of results-based financing (RBF). This new approach is in the process of emerging and being subjected to monitoring and evaluation. The signs are positive that benefits of new guidelines for assistance will yield attractive ratios of benefits to costs.

Refocusing preventive care on service provision that blends concern with family planning and reproductive and sexual health can also help end the anomalous situation in which a large share of HIV-positive persons in the region do not know their status and hence may become ill and infect others unknowingly with HIV. The search for and identification of that small minority of patients infected with *Cryptococcosis neoformans*, an opportunistic infection associated with AIDS patients with very low CD4 cell counts, can be a cost-effective intervention that will depend on effective build-up and deployment of health personnel able to apply a simple test and provide AmB/5FC to those few beneficiaries whose lives can be saved.

A revamped public health system built on a cadre of community health workers is now seen by UNAIDS and cooperating agencies as a sound means to upgrade preventive services at modest cost and promote voluntary testing and counseling that can reduce the spread of HIV.

Cost-benefit analysis can demonstrate the soundness of health system strengthening as a complementary intervention along with other more HIV/AIDS-focused interventions.

Previous health systems analysis

An earlier work, *Global Crises, Global Solutions* (Lomborg 2004), included a chapter on communicable diseases that focused on three "solutions" or opportunities: malaria control, HIV/AIDS control, and strengthening basic health services. After reviewing these and fourteen other proposed solutions, an expert panel rated control of HIV/AIDS highest priority and control of malaria fourth highest of seventeen challenges and opportunities. Scaled-up basic health services ranked twelfth. It is thus fitting that this work focusing on HIV/AIDS and HSS in sub-Saharan Africa builds on these earlier analyses.

A subsequent review of the proposed solutions by UN health sector representatives in October 2006 approved the general approach taken in *Global Crises, Global Solutions*. They ranked strengthening health systems at the top of their priority list. As representatives of national governments on the receiving end of assistance, they expressed the need for comprehensive, system-wide support. Over the next several years, a British-led effort, International Health Partnership (IHP+), also pressed for procedures and plans that would support sector-wide improvements; that leadership was in turn backed by major donors including some, such as PEPFAR, the Global Fund, and GAVI, that in principle operate more like "vertical" than horizontal or sector-wide programs (see Avila 2009).

In support of these complementary objectives a High Level Taskforce on International Innovative Financing for Health Systems (HLT) reviewed modes of finance, new sources of funding, and best means to implement programs aimed at improving health in low-income countries. The Taskforce sponsored the efforts of specialists to recommend how best to spend additional resources once available. That was the task of Working Group 1, Constraints to scaling-up and cost.

As co-director of that working group, Professor Anne Mills, London School of Hygiene and Tropical Medicine (and co-author of an earlier *Global Crises, Global Solutions* chapter), prepared an overview of issues facing the effort to strengthen health systems. Data include selected scenarios of aggregate health system strengthening costs. The analysis estimates parameters for annual spending requirements for sub-Saharan Africa. For seven years, 2009 to 2015, total requirements appear to range from just under $100 billion at the low end to $170 billion at the high end. Spending on a per person basis ranges from a low of only $3 for the World Bank's marginal budgeting for bottlenecks

(MBB) minimum scenario in 2009 to a high of $54 under the MBB maximum scenario by the year 2015. A simplifying assumption may be that annual spending of $20 billion added to current outlays, for a total of about $52 billion annually, should yield the prospective benefits identified in the high level review exercise.

The need to add financing to strengthen health systems is so apparent that one easily understands the demand from public health advocates that more of the substantial increment available for HIV/AIDS since 2001 must support this broader health sector objective. Commitments to aid made in 2005 at the Gleneagles G8 meetings may be falling well short of intentions, perhaps by as much as $19 billion in the current fiscal year. Thus the issue of how and what to fund is as great as ever: what actions in favor of both strengthening health systems and fighting HIV/AIDS can offer benefits adequate to repay the costs incurred?

Bongaarts and Over (2010) argue that the cost of universal access to treatment is unsustainable. The AIDS share of health assistance was already "too high" in 2007, they argue, claiming 23 percent of funds then available, at a time when deaths attributable to AIDS were less than 5 percent of all deaths in developing countries. "In a few African countries, foreign HIV/AIDS assistance exceeds the entire budget of the Ministry of Health."

In 2009 the leaders of UNAIDS, the Global Fund, GAVI, and PEPFAR (Piot and others 2009) argued that a third of their assistance is supporting health system strengthening as well as the specific objectives of AIDS support:

> Although AIDS has exposed weaknesses in health systems, funds for this disease are making a major contribution to the strengthening of health systems.

> The Global Fund and PEPFAR are now among the biggest investors in health systems, joining other funds such as the GAVI Alliance. Although drugs and other commodities account for nearly half of Global Fund spending, 35 percent of the Fund's financing for AIDS, tuberculosis, and malaria contributes directly to supporting human resources, infrastructure and equipment, and monitoring and evaluation: all key components of health systems. Overall, the Fund has committed more than $4 billion in these three areas. From 2004 to 2009, on

Table 4.1 Overview of solutions with potential impact on supply, demand, and price, and cost-benefit prospects

Solution	Impact on...	Persons affected (millions)	Cost, $ millions	B/C ratio range	Comments
1. CCTs for VCT	Demand	400+	2,000	2.5–15	Eliminate 0.25 million infections
2. CHWs, all	Supply	100+	2,640	1.1–9.5	Front-line workers
3. CRAG to prevent CM	Supply OIs	32+	1,500	2.7–20	CRAG, test & treat
4. Abuja Goals Fund	Supply	500+	1,000	1.1–7.7	Upgrade HIV, basic health services

Source: Authors' estimates as described in Appendix tables.

the basis of conservative estimates, PEPFAR will commit more than $4 billion to health systems, including more than $1 billion in 2009 alone.

The authors go on to present details on health infrastructure, workforce, and freeing up of health facilities, thanks to the efforts to strengthen health systems by using HIV/AIDS-specific funding provisions. A recent aids2031 summary paper identified substantial sums allocated by the principal donors to strengthening health systems (Avila *et al.* 2009):

- PEPFAR – $638 million of the money it obligated in 2007 was devoted in full or in part to capacity-building activities.
- The Global Fund expected (in mid-2008) to spend $363 million on actions that will strengthen health systems in recipient countries.
- The GAVI Alliance pledged on May 23, 2008 to "increase its funding for health system strengthening to $800 million" (Avila *et al.* 2009).

Broadly speaking these commitments have continued despite the global recession. *The Economist* on June 4, 2011, p. 90, went so far as to identify these agencies, substantially supported by US government-funded allocations, among the heroes in the history of AIDS. Continued dedication of the UK-led International Health Partnership (IHP+) further complements these efforts.

HIV/AIDS spending contributes to HSS

WHO defines health systems as "all organizations, people and actions whose primary intent is to promote, restore or maintain health." Health system strengthening includes cross-cutting activities that reinforce the whole system, including governance,

human resources, and information systems. Potential beneficial solutions could include governance-planning, health infrastructure build-up, expanded workforce, better information systems, and improved procurement and supply of medicines.

UNAIDS has compiled evidence to support the argument that HIV/AIDS program spending does contribute to the general objectives of health systems strengthening. Among nearly forty interventions that promote prevention, care, and treatment of HIV/AIDS, the following also contribute to HSS objectives:

- Universal precautions.
- Safe medical injections.
- Blood safety.
- Patient transport and emergency rescue.
- Operations research.
- Drug supply systems.
- Information technology.
- Upgrading laboratory infrastructure and new equipment.
- Upgrading and construction of infrastructure and new health centers.
- Human resources training.
- Research.

Analysts then reviewed actual outlays for all programs included in the National AIDS Spending Assessment (NASA) for major world regions (see Figure 4.1). In only two of the nine regions, Latin America and Oceania, did the share of HSS-assisting expenditures fall below a third. It is over half in East Asia, Middle East and North Africa, and South and Southeast Asia.

Nearly 40 percent of AIDS spending in SSA supports HSS objectives. Priority areas include upgrading lab infrastructure, staff training, drug

Table 4.2 Health spending ratios, major world regions, 2000, 2008

Ratio indicators	WHO Africa region		LICs		Lower MICs		Upper MICs		High-income countries	
	2000	2008	2000	2008	2000	2008	2000	2008	2000	2008
Health as % GDP	5.5	6.0	4.6	5.4	4.4	4.3	5.9	6.3	10.0	11.1
Govt share, all health	43.7	49.8	37.1	40.5	37.1	45.4	54.0	57.2	59.3	62.2
Govt health as % all govt	8.2	9.6	7.7	8.9	7.1	7.8	9.0	9.9	15.3	16.7
External as % all health	6.6	9.5	11.0	16.4	1.1	1.0	0.6	0.2	0.0	0.0

Source: WHO Health Statistics, 2011, p. 136.
Acronyms: LICs = low-income countries; MICs = middle-income countries, lower and upper. WHO Africa region includes Maghreb countries north of the Sahara.

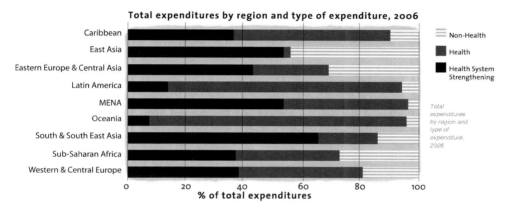

Figure 4.1 *NASA-identified total AIDS spending by type of expenditure, health systems strengthening, health sector, and non-health, nine low- and middle-income regions, 2006, percentage distribution. Number of countries: sub-Saharan Africa (17), Latin America (12), Eastern Europe and Central Asia (10), South and South East Asia (5), Caribbean (4), East Asia (2), MENA (3), Oceania (1), Western and Central Europe (1).*
Source: *UNAIDS, based on results from National AIDS Spending Assessment data; included in Avila et al. (2009).*

supply systems, construction of new health centers, operations research, and blood safety. This "vertical" program offers important "horizontal" and "diagonal" support to health improvements more generally.

However, many specialists express doubt about the extent to which HIV/AIDS spending supports broader objectives. The number of approved Global Fund grants for HSS was fewer in the most recent year (2010) than in previous years, according to a brief note in *Global Fund Observer*:

Health systems strengthening
The number of cross-cutting health systems strengthening requests recommended for funding dropped to 11 in Round 10, from 17 in Round 9 and

25 in Round 8. The two-year cost of the approved proposals in Round 10 dropped to $128 million, from $363 million in Round 9 and $283 million in Round 8. The Global Fund says that these drops are likely due to a range of factors, including availability of funding from other sources, previously approved requests, and proposals not being of the best quality. (*Global Fund Observer*, May 24, 2011)

These changes suggest that HIV/AIDS supporters face a continuing challenge as they seek to combine "vertical" assistance with the "horizontal" task of strengthening health systems. This combination of efforts can then yield a satisfactory "diagonal" blend of donor support.

Increased health spending, 2000–2008

Spending on health in sub-Saharan Africa, and for most regions and countries, has risen substantially in this new century (see Table 4.2). For the WHO Africa region, which includes North Africa as well as sub-Saharan Africa, several health spending indicators have increased, including the health share in total GDP, government's share of total health spending, the health share in all government spending, and external assistance as a share of all health spending. The direction of change has been the same for all low-income countries, most of them being in sub-Saharan Africa.

The picture of overall health financing has grown more positive and data on health status improvements since the 1990s are positive, too (United Nations 2011). SSA is supplying more funds to support health system strengthening now than it did in past years. Donors are contributing a larger share of aggregate health spending than they were at the start of this century. The funding base is increasing. A substantial part of the reason for that increase is the supply of donor assistance for HIV/AIDS programs.

A principal challenge now has two parts. First, donors and governments in Africa need to continue to raise their commitment to financing health care and strengthening the system as a whole. Second, greater efficiencies remain to be developed, particularly the effective extension of basic services to rural areas. In the longer term of half a century or more, part of the "efficiency solution" will lie in the continued process of rural-to-urban migration. Costs of reaching and providing services to those in need will decline as the friction of distance falls with concentration of more people in cities. For those advantages to unfold as they have in what are now high-income and middle-income countries, spending on urban health will require safe water and sanitation and safe means of transport to reduce the still-high levels of infectious and communicable diseases (ICDs) and injury in the low-income countries of sub-Saharan Africa. These changes are costly but practical and will yield benefits that can amply repay costs incurred. These supply-side improvements then need to be supported by continuing expansion of incentives to spur demand for

Table 4.3 Return on investment in the proposed UNAIDS framework

Benefit identified	2011–2015	2011–2020
Total infections averted	4.2 million	12.2 million at a cost of $2,450 each
Infant and child infections averted	680,000	1.9 million at a cost of $2,180 each
Life years gained	3.7 million	29.4 million at a cost of $1,060 each
Deaths averted	1.96 million	7.4 million at a cost of $4,090 each

Source: Schwartländer *et al.* 2011, Annex Table 2.

better health systems as well as for an effective use of HIV/AIDS services. It is to that topic we now turn.

UNAIDS – a new approach and its expected returns

In April 2011, UNAIDS released an analysis demonstrating that a basic spending program, combined with "critical enablers" and support from "synergies with development sectors," would cost about $17 billion in 2011, $22 billion in 2015, at its peak, and $19 billion in 2020. What are the expected returns on these investments? Reduced infections, gains in years of life lived, and deaths averted appear in the estimates of benefits (see Table 4.3).

These results can be turned into an aggregate cost-benefit analysis by comparing the costs estimates in Table 4.3 for deaths averted to two ranges of benefits, namely when the value of a year of life is given as $1,000, appropriate for low-income countries in sub-Saharan Africa, and $5,000, more fitting for Botswana, Namibia, and South Africa, the somewhat better-off countries of the region.

Deaths averted in the 2011–2020 period are 7.4 million. (For purposes of this analysis there is no discounting of future-year lives saved over the framework period of a decade.) The cost of averting these deaths is set at $4,090 per death averted, for a total expenditure of $30.3 billion. The benefits derive from the estimated value of averting each of these deaths. For purposes of analysis, $1,000 and

$5,000 are presented as lower- and upper-bound estimates of the value of a year of life saved. When discounted at 3 percent, and assuming that all lives saved occur at age twenty-two, then the aggregate benefits of the interventions, at their lower- and upper-bound levels, are $185 billion and $925 billion, respectively.

The estimated ratios of benefits to costs derived from these data are B/C = 6.1 at the lower bound, and B/C = 30.5 at the upper bound. These findings will be compared later in this paper against other estimates that focus more explicitly on health system strengthening as a complement to HIV/AIDS programs. We do not propose to assess this comprehensive plan as one of the solutions offered here. It may be useful, however, as a basis for comparison with the B/C ratios estimated for specific solutions discussed below.

A final word on these aggregate estimates. Global resource needs estimates first appeared at the time of the UNGASS meetings held in mid-2001 (Schwartländer et al. 2001). These quantitative targets and scenarios supported scientists' arguments in favor of allocating more resources for the fight against AIDS. Establishment of the Global Fund to Fight AIDS, Tuberculosis and Malaria followed soon after UNGASS. The USA PEPFAR program came soon after that. The establishment of explicit costing estimates proved to be a key reason for the success of the global effort to address the HIV/AIDS epidemic. Emphasis on resource needs and sound estimation of the potential effectiveness of spending have been major sources of support for programs and their financing. Without the estimates of the kind discussed here, there may never have been a concerted effort to address this global health challenge.

Priority setting, other approaches

Dean Jamison (Lomborg 2010, pp. 325–6, Table 17.6) lists seven intervention areas as key investment priorities for disease control:

- Tuberculosis: appropriate case finding and treatment.
- Heart attacks (AMI): acute management with low-cost drugs.

- Malaria: prevention and ACT treatment package.
- Childhood diseases: expanded immunization coverage.
- Cancer, heart disease, other: tobacco taxation.
- HIV: prevention package.
- Injury, difficult childbirth, other: surgical capacity at the district hospital.

B/C ratios range from a high of 30:1 to a low of 10:1. HIV prevention is one of the seven investment priorities; several of the others would serve as complementary health strengthening interventions that also support HIV prevention, e.g., tuberculosis treatment, in light of the co-infection frequencies in Africa; childhood immunization practices that can include testing services that could support VCT for HIV; and malaria prevention and treatment, as this disease may also have co-infection implications. The summary tables in this report draw substantially on the analysis provided by Jamison in that report.

Valuing benefits of lives saved

Analysts building on the work of Viscusi (1986, 1993), Nordhaus (2003, 2008), Cutler (2004, 2008), and others have placed the value of a statistical life in the USA at more than $7 million. Viscusi and Aldy (2003) show further that revealed preference in other countries indicate lower values of a statistical life but in amounts that reflect other countries' lower levels of income and wealth. Shillcutt et al. discuss twice per capita GNI as a "threshold" level for an acceptable price for value of a statistical life (Shillcutt et al. 2009, pp. 3–4).

Using the proposed value of a DALY as $1,000 and $5,000 for low and high estimates, we can then prepare a simple table showing how undiscounted and discounted values of a life saved compare under these circumstances (see Tables 4.9 and 4.10, which are based on the more detailed Table 4.8).[1]

---

[1] For sub-Saharan Africa as a whole, the 2009 GNI per capita, Atlas method was $1,125, and by purchasing power parity (PPP) method was $2,051 (World Bank WDI 2011, p. 12). GNI per capita for South Africa was $5,760 by Atlas, and $10,050 by PPP. One of the lowest GNI per capita amounts was for Burundi, at $150.

Table 4.4A Estimated benefits of saving lives, assuming adult DALYs valued at $1,000, and infant DALYs valued at $500, with discount rates of 0, 3 percent, 5 percent, and 10 percent, $000

Discount rate	Infant	Age 22	Age 50
0	33	43	15
3%	15	25	13
5%	10	18	11
10%	5	10	8

Table 4.4B DALYs valued at $5,000 and infant DALYs valued at $2,500

Discount rate	Infant	Age 22	Age 50
0	163	215	75
3%	72	123	64
5%	48	90	56
10%	25	50	41

Source: Details in Table 4.8. All estimates assume life continues from age at which life is saved by the intervention to age 65. The value of an infant life-year is 0.5 value of an adult life-year.

The "most-valued" persons in the age distribution are young adults. At the same time they are also the persons most at risk of HIV/AIDS infection and death. Infants are "more valuable" than older adults only at very low discount rates of 0 and 3 percent. They are less valuable than all adults at high discount rates (5 percent and 10 percent). This is broadly compatible with the observed underspending in African countries on low-cost health interventions that could save many more children's lives than is now current practice.

So-called "hyperbolic discounting," as the example of a discount rate of 10 percent per annum shown in the tables can indicate, reflects a tendency to over-value the present at cost to future concerns. Such very high discounting of the future may be common among the poor. Many Africans face a high degree of uncertainty about the future in part because of their poverty and dependence on factors like weather and risks of drought and must thus focus on the present at the cost of preparing for an uncertain future. Without discounting, the life of a person aged 50 is worth less than half the life of an infant even when each life-year of an infant

is counted as only half that of the adult. But with discounting, the older person's life is worth 60 percent more than that of the infant under conditions of 10 percent discounting, a rough equivalent of "hyperbolic discounting." This behavioral feature may help explain health care spending decisions that lead to what better-off persons in developed countries would deem as inadequate attention to the health needs of the young.

Deeply discounting the future, a common enough practice whenever there is substantial uncertainty, has an inordinate and unwelcome influence on many private and public choices. Saving, investing, protecting one's health, and getting an education may all be under-supported when doubts about the very possibility of survival are at stake. Reducing uncertainty is broadly recognized as a means to increase subjective well-being (Graham 2009). Investing in health and reducing health risks can confront discounting practices that support underinvestment, producing a virtuous circle of better health and more effective spending on health improvements that matter most.

Advances in estimating health benefits

The five pages of references to the Mills and Shillcutt paper in *Global Crises, Global Solutions* does not include key papers that have advanced our understanding of the benefits derived in financial terms from the additions of lives saved and life-years gained from selected interventions. Their work focuses, as do many of the leading works in the area of cost-effectiveness of health interventions, on disability-adjusted life years (DALYs) gained. There is of course controversy about valuing life and life years that can be gained from a host of interventions.

DCP2 and health sector priority setting

By 2005, there was already broad though not universal agreement among health economists that lives and life-years saved are sound measures of benefits to be derived from health investments (cf. Behrman 1998, ch. 1; Jamison *et al.* 2006a, 2006b).

Despite the advantages offered by CBA, its use has been on a long-term decline in the World Bank:

> The percentage of Bank projects that are justified by cost-benefit analysis has been declining for several decades, owing to a decline in adherence to standards and to difficulty in applying cost-benefit analysis...
>
> [T]he percentage of projects with such analysis dropped from 70 percent to 25 percent between the early 1970s and the early 2000s... A little more than half of this decline was due to an increase in projects in sectors at the Bank that tend not to apply a cost-benefit analysis to their projects... [M]ost of the improvement in project performance ratings that has occurred at the Bank in the past 20 years has been in the five sectors that tend to apply cost-benefit analysis. (Warner 2010, p. ix)

In lending operations for education, health, nutrition, population, and public sector governance, a mere 1 percent of projects approved over the nearly forty years of Bank lending reported economic rates of return (ERR). Such rates, when present, are an indication that a BCA has been performed (Warner 2010, Table 2.1, p. 7 and related text). In most cases, this result suggests, the Bank did not conduct such analysis for these so-called "soft sector" projects. Given that such analysis was shown in the Warner analysis to greatly improve project performance, the absence of it in these sectors is a source of regret.

Details by solution

Solution 1: Conditional cash transfers (CCTs)

> Conditional cash transfers (CCTs) that induce all adults to seek testing and hence reduce the current high prevalence of HIV-positive persons ignorant of their status.

Four decades ago, in the 1970s, the Indian government provided in-kind grants to men who accepted a vasectomy. The government's purpose? Reduce what many viewed as too-high fertility. But whatever the effects on the birth rate in India (it was small), there arose a storm of opposition, claiming that the grants were coercive. Very poor people sacrificed their capacity to have more children in exchange for current payments. The Chinese government used a different approach in the 1970s. It offered no incentive for couples to conform to its new one-child policy. It imposed controls and enforced them with some vigor. World opinion was even more outraged against this form of coercion than it was against Indian government vasectomy incentives.

Not so many years later, in the mid-1990s, Mexico's government upped the ante on incentives. Families got cash payments in exchange for ensuring their children attend school at least 85 percent of required days. Separate payments went to women who sought and received antenatal and neonatal care. There, few if any complaints of coercion arose. The conditional payments have now spread to many countries (they were even tried, though soon abandoned, in New York City).

How well did they work? As with all topics in health policy, views differ. One of the originators has written of its success (Levy 2006). Karlan and Appel warmly agree in their book, *More than Good Intentions* (2011, pp. 201–5, 231–5). Banerjee and Duflo, leaders of the MIT Poverty Lab, are not so sure: payments may be less important than alerting families to their own actions that can promote or impede their children's health and education (see their *Poor Economics, a Radical Rethinking of the Way to Fight Global Poverty*, 2011).

As these and other authors are wont to remind us, details matter. Applying CCTs to strengthen health systems and address the HIV/AIDS epidemic will require careful thought. Payments must not be allowed to be, or even appear to be, coercive. They must not endanger human rights by focusing on any "key" groups or most-at-risk populations. Any system of payments, incentives, and actions must be designed to avoid the opposition that surrounded the earlier attempts in China and India to reduce fertility.

The solution proposed here: offer a voucher worth $5 to every adult aged eighteen to forty-nine in exchange for agreeing to be tested, counseled, and as necessary treated for HIV/AIDS. The one-time cost of this voucher if all eligible persons accept would be about $2 billion. As the discussion below argues, the benefits could exceed these costs by a factor of 2:1, just in considering the reduction in new infections. There will also be contingent benefits in reduced numbers that eventually require ART and in the ramping up of basic health services needed to provide testing and related support services to the dispersed, largely rural population of Africa. Perhaps most importantly, this testing-for-all strategy avoids the stigma and human-rights violations that confound any proposal to focus on most-at-risk populations.

The proposal by Granich *et al.* (2008) for universal voluntary testing goes much farther than the cash transfer proposed here. Granich recommends moving immediately to ART for all persons found to be HIV-positive. Garnett and Baggaley (2009) in commenting on this plan urge caution; voluntary testing might lead to coercive therapy. The payment recommended here should be provided for testing and counseling but leave treatment and other behavior change as personal, informed choices.

CCTs as a path to knowing

Far too many Africans who are HIV-positive do not know it. Reports in demographic and health surveys (DHS) show that three-quarters or more of all HIV-positive persons in countries surveyed are not aware of their status. This lack of knowing varies widely among nine countries surveyed in sub-Saharan Africa, "with more than 20 percent of people living with HIV being aware of their HIV status in four countries (up to 31.4 percent in Rwanda) and less than 20 percent in five countries. The median percentage in the nine African countries is 16.5 percent."[2] Health systems remain far from achieving a "test and treat" objective for addressing efforts to prevent the further spread of HIV. This "not knowing" must be a key factor that permits the numbers of new infections to continue to exceed each year's additions to the number of persons treated with ART in the region.

How CCTs might work

Many poor rural Africans live on less than a dollar a day, spend more than three-quarters of their resources on food and basic shelter, and live many hours' walk from the nearest modern health facility. The combination of poverty and isolated rural

location causes them to procrastinate and not seek health care beyond what can be provided by a nearby traditional healer. It is thus no surprise that with an infection like HIV, that can remain undetected for years, many who are infected do not know it. Only the presence of a visible threat such as a sexually transmitted disease like syphilis or gonorrhea will cause the ill person to seek diagnosis, care, and treatment. If that health-seeking behavior also includes a test for HIV, then potential sexual partners of that person may in future benefit from NOT being at risk of transmission, assuming that behavior change results from a positive diagnosis.

Where CCTs have worked in Africa

In rural Malawi, Rebecca Thornton studied a demand-side performance-based incentive (PBI) by randomizing the distribution of vouchers to clients, worth up to a day's wage, redeemable upon submission to an HIV test and receipt of their results at a nearby voluntary counseling and testing (VCT) clinic. She found that while there was substantial demand for HIV testing even in the absence of cash incentive, any positive amount nearly doubled uptake of HIV testing. She also found that HIV-positive respondents who learned their test results were significantly more likely to purchase condoms in follow-up interviews. She concludes that even small cash incentives might be useful in overcoming inertia or stigma-related costs in learning HIV status, and may even be marginally useful in condom uptake, thereby averting further infections (Thornton, 2005).[3] Provision of basic and accessible clinic services for HIV testing can equally strengthen the health system. Such an incentive can yield benefits that more than repay its costs.

Also in Malawi, Baird, Chirwa, McIntosh, and Ozler (2009) randomized a conditional cash transfer that sought to estimate the effect of receiving a small cash payment conditional on girls' school attendance. Some girls received the cash

---

[2] WHO 2008, *Toward Universal Access*, p. 54 and Table 3.3.
[3] We are indebted to Mead Over for calling these examples to our attention in his papers and presentations through the Center for Global Development (Over 2008, 2010). Several of his works are included in the list of references to this paper.

regardless of whether they went to school, others only if they went to school, and others received nothing. The authors found that one year after the intervention, cash transfers led not only to increases in self-reported school attendance but also to declines in early marriage, pregnancy, sexual activity, risky sexual behavior, and coital frequency for the sexually active.

As for using conditional cash transfers for HIV prevention, Medlin and de Walque (2008), after surveying the literature, suggest that the best proxy on which to condition transfers might be new sexually transmitted infections (STIs), as they are transmitted by similar risk behavior as HIV. They are in some cases easier to observe and, unlike HIV, some are curable. By conditioning the transfer on a reversible event (STI infection), instead of an irreversible one (HIV infection), a conditional transfer program can continue to provide rewards for safe behavior to people who have previously failed the condition, a group of particular interest for curbing the epidemic.

The results of this randomized trial are encouraging in another respect: they refute the assertion that is sometimes made that poor African women have little or no physical control over their own sexual risk. In another randomized study that demonstrates how much control women can have even in the absence of an income transfer, Dupas has shown that the information that older men are more likely to be HIV infected has led young poor African women to reduce the frequency with which they have sex with older men (Dupas 2010). Focusing on persons who must seek treatment for STIs can be just as stigmatizing as focusing on those who agree to be tested for HIV. Even though this approach "works," it is basically fraught with the implication that the beneficiaries of the cash transfer are "different" from the population as a whole.

A promising, preliminary study appeared at the recent XVIII International AIDS Conference. The Schooling, Income, and HIV Risk (SIHR) study in Malawi assigned 3,796 young women aged 13–22 randomly to two groups, with half the women receiving cash payments of varying amounts. Interviewed 18 months after the project start-up, girls in the cash group who were in school at the start of the study had a 60 percent lower HIV prevalence compared with schoolgirls who received no payments. This result was probably due to a reduction in transactional sex with older men. These results held even for girls who received cash with no school attendance requirements (unconditional cash). The effect increased with payment size; extreme poverty may thus have influenced girls' sexual choices.

The RESPECT study in Tanzania examined the effect of CCTs as an incentive for young people to stay free of STIs. Investigators randomly assigned young men and women aged 18–30 years to a control group or CCT group. Participants in the cash group were eligible to receive a payment of $20 every four months if they had negative laboratory tests for curable STIs: prevalence of STIs declined in the cash group compared with the control group. In contrast, a study in Malawi found that a one-time cash reward for maintaining HIV-negative status for one year had no measurable effect.

The examples above show that CCTs can work. But they can also be stigmatizing unless carefully designed. It may now be time to take a more universal approach to offering a voucher for performance. Proposals from WHO scientists have been urging expanded testing for some time (Granich *et al.* 2008), and UNAIDS offers continuing support so long as rights are respected (Schwartländer *et al.* 2011).

Why universal adult testing for HIV?

Consider the less-stigmatizing procedure of universal adult testing: provide a voucher worth five US dollars equivalent in local currency to any and all who agree to be tested and then to hear test results and participate in appropriate counseling. Payment need not be conditioned one way or the other on the test outcome or further behavior; the only purpose is to increase knowledge.

In light of the millions of persons who will have to be tested, there are obvious implications for increased near-term demands on the health sector and its personnel. There are about 400 million adults in the region that could take the tests and receive the vouchers. Would the benefits repay such high costs? Could health systems handle the very heavy service load such testing would imply?

Linkage to social enablers

Note that the improved investment approach promoted by UNAIDS and others already proposes annual resources required above $16 billion annually (Schwartländer *et al.* 2011, Table 2) and a substantial part of that goes to provider-initiated counseling and testing. "Program enablers include incentives for program participation, methods to improve retention of patients on anti-retroviral therapy, capacity building for development of community-based organizations, strategic planning, communications infrastructure, information dissemination, and efforts to improve service integration and linkages from testing to care" (Schwartländer *et al.* 2011, pp. 4–5).

Spending in these areas would amount to over a third of total requirements. The cost-benefit analysis must then move to address the question of whether a cash transfer might complement the proposed social or program enablers. Since this approach of providing a cash incentive for such testing has been tried and proven to work, the authors must acknowledge that a certain amount of guesswork underlies the estimate suggested below. What can be confirmed without qualification is that current approaches of a purely voluntary nature are not working; something else has to be tried, and an incentive for testing that does not stigmatize any specific group may just be the right way to begin.

For all low- and middle-income countries, this new UNAIDS program seeks to cut new infections from about 2.5 million annually in 2011 to one million by 2015. Suppose that the proposed voucher could be credited with cutting a quarter of a million infections annually. That reduction in new infections is here conceived as the incremental benefit of the conditional cash transfer. That benefit would constitute one-sixth of the projected reduction in new infections annually. This crude estimate is at best a guess at how much of a contribution to reduced incidence this modest payment can make. Current efforts to induce people in SSA to undertake voluntary counseling and testing are having at best very modest success, as indicated by the high numbers of persons ignorant of their HIV status. Thus, this solution is offered on grounds that some additional direct incentives for testing and counseling are worth investigating.

Equally, we can have no prior certainty about how many infections averted can be attributed as an incremental benefit to be associated with the incremental cost derived from the payments made to adults to undertake the testing and receipt of information about their status with respect to HIV. Further, the incremental reduction in new infections will have the important secondary effect of reducing the number of persons who, years later, will need treatment for opportunistic infections and anti-retroviral therapy (ART). The cost savings derived from this reduced incidence of HIV add to the incremental benefits deriving from this conditional payment to these millions of adults. The specific amounts attributable to the cash transfer are again a matter of guesswork. With these caveats in mind, we proceed to examine this scenario.

For each of the presumed quarter million infections avoided, this solution saves varying amounts determined in a two-way relationship between the presumed value of a life year and the assumed discount rates used to evaluate future years of benefits, both life-years saved and OIs and ART costs avoided (see Table 4.9). In these scenarios, the four resultant B/C ratios range from a low of 2.5 to a high of 15. All four combinations yield benefits that more than compensate for costs.

This solution holds an appeal by reason of its potentially striking impact on new infections, on the demands it makes to strengthen the health sectors as a whole for participating countries, and its inclusion of the whole population of sub-Saharan Africa into participation in the fight against AIDS.

If a quarter million deaths are averted at a cost of $2 billion, the cost per death averted is then $8,000 ($2 billion/0.25 million lives saved = $8,000). Assume the person saved by this intervention is age twenty-two so that the present discounted value of that saved life is twenty-five years at a 3 percent discount rate and eighteen years at a 5 percent discount rate. Thus the cost/DALY ranges from $320 with a 3 percent discount rate for future years of life to $444 with a 5 percent discount rate (see Table 4.9). This cost would appear reasonable when compared to the range of values of a year of life that appear in Table 4.8.

Does it make sense to test 400 million adults, or can a far more limited but effectively targeted number of persons be offered the CCT voucher? Targeting can quickly devolve into a human rights issue inasmuch as the most-at-risk populations may be further stigmatized by the very existence of such a payment. Thus the starting point, to avoid the possible stigma generated by a program "targeted" on high-risk groups, must be the whole population.

It is not essential that all testing begin in all countries. The nine countries in eastern and southern Africa with HIV prevalence rates above 10 percent among adults aged fifteen to forty-nine might be an appropriate place to start.[4] There need be no stigma or discrimination attached to a national program in those countries. In those countries the number of now unaware HIV-positive persons would be significantly higher than in countries with lower prevalence rates in, for example, West Africa. Thus the benefits of increased knowledge would be greatest in these nine countries.

In the event, smaller numbers may fit the requirements in selected countries or even regions within countries where presumed prevalence is so low as to vitiate the testing procedure. But as a starting point, the program should be universal. It may in any case prove useful to begin this cash transfer plan in eastern and southern African countries with high rates of prevalence, hence gaining useful knowledge more quickly there than in lower-prevalence West African states.

Some readers may suggest that the benefits of mass testing would not be adequate to repay such a high cost. Of these 400 million adults only 17–18 million of them, less than 5 percent of the total, will be discovering that they are HIV-positive.[5] If all these persons then abstain from sexual contact, the next year's incidence of new infections should fall precipitously from an otherwise anticipated nearly two million.[6]

These considerations only serve to emphasize further how important it may be to increase the share of all Africans aware of their status and hence able to benefit from care and to take measures to protect their partners. Without effective health system strengthening, those changes will be difficult to implement. Thus even treatment for opportunistic infections that burden those persons who have moved to full-blown AIDS can work more completely and effectively in a strengthened health care

system. Such treatments may fail badly where the overall system fails.

Recall that South Africa's President, Mr. Jacob Zuma, has himself submitted to HIV testing and has urged his fellow countrymen to join him in such testing. Thus there is already senior leadership in support of the proposed solution offered here.

Solution 2: Upgrade health worker skills and services

> Enhance numbers, training, and skill development for community health workers to strengthen basic health services and test and treat for HIV/AIDS.

The success of Solution 12 will depend on health system strengthening (HSS) and having adequate health human resources. This staffing requirement has gained particular attention in the work of several international health agencies:

- The Commission on Macroeconomics and Health (CMH) led the way more than a decade ago in defining the health care needs summarized in the Millennium Development Goals (MDGs).
- International Health Partnerships (IHP+) focus on requirements across the board to achieve HSS objectives.
- The Platform for Health System Strengthening moves a step closer to developing country government control over the way forward and some means to remove user fees.
- The High Level Taskforce (HLT) urges "Promoting the retention and motivation of health workers particularly in underserved areas" (Mills 2009).
- The Earth Institute Technical Task Force Report, *One Million Community Health Workers* (CHW

---

[4] These countries include Swaziland, Botswana, Lesotho, South Africa, Zimbabwe, Zambia, Namibia, Mozambique, and Malawi, as listed in Table 1.1 of Chapter 1.

[5] The UNAIDS 2008 report placed the number of HIV-positive persons in sub-Saharan Africa at 22 million, of which about four to five million were aware of their status, so that the numbers to be discovered were just under 20 million.

[6] Professor Alan Whiteside has suggested a one-month sexual abstinence period as a method to break the cycle of infection.

2011), provides detailed estimates of costs for all SSA of expanded rural health services.

The bridge between HSS and HIV/AIDS can best be crossed with enough personnel to be able to conduct tests and report diagnoses for very large numbers of persons, including the rural poor. Because of poor nutrition, long distances from the sites of health care services, and levels of uncertainty that may lead to simply putting off the search for care, the rural poor are those most at risk to a range of infectious and communicable diseases.

The World Bank *Voices of the Poor* project interviewed thousands of poor people in sixty countries. Their report is a clarion call for more effective attention to the health needs of the poor, including better access to health workers and health services:

> Distance to health-care facilities, problems and costs of reaching them, and lack of medicines often make obtaining treatment difficult.
>
> In Africa and elsewhere, people report a sheer lack of health posts, clinics and hospitals – and discouraging distances to the ones that exist. Rural areas suffer the most marked lack of services. In discussing problems in obtaining medical care, participants in parts of Ethiopia, Ghana, Malawi, Somaliland and Zambia mention the long distances that have to be traversed more often than problems of cost or quality . . . In Malawi an increase in disease, especially HIV/AIDS, has made the lack of accessible facilities a more pressing problem. (Narayan *et al.* 2000, p. 101)

The shortage of health workers is particularly critical in countries experiencing severe HIV/AIDS epidemics. WHO identifies five countries – CAR, Lesotho, Malawi, Mozambique, and Zambia – in which adult HIV prevalence rates exceed 10 percent and the shortage of health workers is acute (Herbst 2008, p. 329). The Food and Agricultural Organization (FAO) estimates that more than two-thirds of the population of the twenty-five African countries most affected by HIV live in rural areas (FAO 2008). In contrast, medical doctors (MDs) live in the cities. For example, patient load in Maputo City is 342/MD, but on average in the Mozambique countryside that ratio is 6,496/MD (Hagopian *et al.* 2008). "Such patient loads exceed any reasonable standards" (Herbst 2009, p. 329).

Moreover, there is a serious "performance problem": in the five countries identified by WHO above, an average 35 percent absentee rate among health workers is the norm. Researchers in many low-income countries have found similar slacking of effort in many low-income settings. The World Bank's *World Development Report 2004, Making Services Work for Poor People*, gave ample attention to the problem. Since then, the *randomistas*, proponents of randomized controlled trials, have studied the staffing problem in detail (Banerjee and Duflo 2011; Karlan and Appel 2011). Too often, skill requirements do not match salaries. Workloads set by managers exceed the skills and capacities of community health workers. Too often, the details of actual practice in Africa's health sectors do not fit service-provision norms.

There remains the persistent problem of retaining newly trained health staff, whose skills are rewarded at far higher wages outside the public health sector. This applies especially in high-income countries. A study of final-year medical students in Ethiopia finds that more than 40 percent of students choose jobs outside the health sector upon graduation (Herbst *et al.* 2008, based on Serneels *et al.* 2005).

To what level of skill do these front-line health workers need to be trained? With two-thirds of Africans resident outside urban areas, it is to rural areas that most newly trained community health workers will have to be assigned. They will have to be workers committed to working among their neighbors, most of whom will be part of the large majority of the rural poor. This new group of community health workers will have to be recruited in full recognition of their work being more closely tied to the needs of their own communities.

Strengthening health services in rural areas

UNAIDS recently drew on an Earth Institute study of what costs would be incurred to put in place an adequate human resource base (CHW Technical Task Force 2011). A community health worker (CHW) can take care of over 500 rural households per year, at a per-person cost of about $5 per annum. The cost to serve sub-Saharan Africa's 530 million rural persons is about $2.64 billion per annum. This amount is then a small share, about 4 percent, of the needed annual health spending for the region of around $52 billion identified by the Task 1 report of the HLT (Mills 2009). The Earth Institute study goes on to estimate that extending HIV testing once a year to all HIV-negative persons above the age of fourteen would add about $2.50 per person serviced by the CHW program (CHW Technical Task Force 2011, p. 60). The cost of providing community health workers need not be a barrier. What must be assured is that there are adequate benefits to repay such costs.

The Malawi case was developed to assess specific contributions that the new staffing plan could make to strengthening family planning services and reducing the risks of maternal to child transmission of HIV. It did not include the additional costs and benefits of universal testing and treatment, services discussed here as part of Solution 1 in the preceding section.

The protocol referred to as Option B+ provides that all HIV-positive pregnant women, regardless of their CD4 cell count, will continue to receive ART for life (Fasawe *et al.* 2011). The study estimates that Option B+ can save more than 100,000 life years above the natural progression expected if the mothers only receive PMTCT prophylaxis. The generalized cost-effectiveness ratio for Option B+ was $697 per maternal life year saved. Moreover, if the cost and outcomes from mothers and children are added using Option B+, then 331,000 life years would be saved and the cost-effectiveness ratio would improve to $261 per life year. This amount is well below the $1,000 as the value of a life year used throughout this paper and for this *RethinkHIV* exercise in general. A reasonable conclusion is that the integration of family planning and ART services shows considerable benefits. Option B+ would require further financial resources, but it will also save societal resources in the long term.[7]

Reducing maternal mortality

Malawi has seen a reduction in maternal mortality in the last decade, as it fell by half between 1998 and 2008. Coverage of ART among pregnant women has also increased from 10 percent in 1999 to 58 percent by the end of 2009. These coverage improvements demonstrate successful national

efforts in reducing disparities in safe motherhood within the country.

Preventing unintended pregnancies among women living with HIV

Adding family planning to the menu of sexual and reproductive health services can provide substantial clinical, health, and human development benefits:

> The majority of people living with HIV in Africa – 61 percent – are women. Women age 15–25 are three times more likely to be HIV+ than men their age . . . Furthermore, women with HIV have a 20–45 percent chance of passing the virus on to their children. The feminization of the epidemic in Africa may be the single most important reason for linking HIV/AIDS and SRH programs. (Lule 2009, p. 372)

An effective family planning strategy requires community mobilization to increase the uptake of family planning services. If 90 percent of the unmet need for family planning were to be met among women living with HIV, the cost per DALY averted would fall below $70, well within the acceptable cost-effectiveness range (see Joshi 2011). Reducing the unmet need for family planning is a more cost-effective strategy than delivering just ART to HIV-positive women. Even at lower levels of family planning service provision, the relative cost-effectiveness demonstrated in the Fasawe (2011) study remains high.

Assessing benefits and costs of staff expansions

The solution under discussion here is massive expansion of the number of community health workers who would provide basic health services in rural areas, especially focused on family planning and reproductive health. The Malawi exercise provides a template for a scenario of expansion of

---

[7] Estimates derived from this modeling are comparable to previously published estimates that range from $60 to $274 per DALY. Sweat and colleagues (2004) derived an estimate range of $58 to $310 per DALY averted across seven countries in sub-Saharan Africa; another study done in Tanzania by Robberstad *et al.* (2010) reported a cost-effectiveness ratio of $162 per DALY averted.

the CHW build-up to continental scale. At an estimated cost of $5 per person served, the 530 million rural persons in sub-Saharan Africa could be provided with CHWs at a total cost of $2.64 billion. The full benefits of their efforts can be summarized as follows:

- reducing maternal deaths by 0.3 million with a net present value of $25,000 (low estimate) and $123,000 (high estimate) each;
- reducing infant infections with HIV by PMTCT programs could save up to 0.1 million infant lives with a net present value of $15,000 (low estimate) and $72,000 (high estimate) each;
- meeting the currently unmet need for family planning can reduce total births by ten million; and
- CHWs can contribute to reducing other infectious and communicable diseases via health promotion activities.

We focus here on the reduction of infant and maternal deaths associated with the reduction of unmet need for family planning. Note that the specific benefits cited above refer to reduced numbers of infant infections with HIV in response to fuller availability of PMTCT. The substantial benefits of PMTCT are the subject of another paper in this collection (2.0 Bollinger).

The sum of the full value of benefits 1 and 2 cannot all be attributed to increased provision of services by CHWs. We estimate that half of the value of benefits 1 and 2 can be attributed to the incremental services provided by CHWs (see Table 4.10). The resultant B/C ratio estimates range from a low of 1.1 when net present value is estimated with a $1,000 value of a year of life discounted at a 5 percent discount rate, to 9.5 with a lower 3 percent discount rate and the higher $5,000 for the value of a year of life.

These ratios of benefits to costs are substantial, and they will be larger, the larger are the collateral benefits implicit in items 3 and 4, not to mention the merits of family planning now reaching women who express need for it.

The cost per death averted is about $16,000 ($2.64 billion/(0.3m women + 0.05m infants) * 1/2 = $15,857). Net present value of costs per DALY range from about $587 to $825, depending

on the lower 3 percent or higher 5 percent discount rate used for future years of life gained.

Whether presumed incremental benefits will in fact be forthcoming depends fundamentally on the "truth" of the assumed value of the upgrade of basic service availability. Will these additional community health workers really add value? Is such a system subject to extension into fairly remote rural areas where supervision is difficult?

The most recent update on progress toward MDG 2015 objectives underlines the large remaining gap between goal and progress through 2008 in SSA. Maternal deaths per 100,000 births fell from 870 in 1990 to 640 in 2008, a 26 percent decline (United Nations 2011, p. 28). However, the 2015 goal is much lower. Fewer than half of SSA births are attended by skilled personnel, and the region continues to have the highest level of unmet need for family planning and reproductive health services (United Nations 2011, pp. 30, 33).

A recent review sponsored by the World Bank demonstrates that family planning programs are very cost-effective while generating both direct and indirect benefits. The author summarized other studies in these words:

> By offering FP services at voluntary counselling and testing sites in the 14 countries with high HIV prevalence, child HIV infections could be averted at a cost of $489, and child deaths could be averted at a cost of $278 per event – well below the cost of averting these events using traditional PMTCT services. In addition, these family programs would avert orphans at a cost of $278, and maternal deaths at a cost of $1,284 per event. In terms of DALYs the benefits of such programs are even more startling: while HIV services cost approximately $27 per DALY, the reduction of mother–child transmission costs about $5 per DALY. (Joshi 2011)

Even though these programs offer positive returns, family planning has declined in donor emphasis as HIV/AIDS assistance has risen:

> Unfortunately, funding for family planning programs has faltered for more than a decade. Between 1995 and 2008, while funds committed by donors and developing countries to HIV and AIDS programming increased by nearly 300 percent, funds devoted to family planning declined by some 30 percent. As a result, many countries are less able

to provide family planning services today than they were a decade ago, and much of the earlier commitment has waned. There are indications that fertility declines are levelling off or even being reversed in some countries. (Bongaarts and Sinding 2009, p. 43)

Few programs in public health have the potential to complement each other as well as family planning and HIV/AIDS prevention services. With continued high fertility and unmet need for family planning, both programs need strengthened health care systems if they are to flourish in SSA, the region with highest fertility and highest HIV/AIDS prevalence. Combined programs need to reach beyond the easiest households to reach in major cities to the under-served countryside. It is hard to imagine an upgrade to health services and an improvement in health outcomes without effectively reaching rural Africa.

Solution 3: Test for cryptococcal antigen (CRAG)

Test for cryptococcal antigen (CRAG) to support focused treatment of an opportunistic infection.

An opportunistic infection associated with HIV, cryptococcal meningitis (CM), is a major threat to health in sub-Saharan Africa. It killed over six thousand persons in South Africa in a recent year and threatens the lives of an estimated 720,000 in the region as a whole. "When comparing the estimate of deaths in sub-Saharan Africa with other diseases excluding HIV, deaths associated with cryptococcal meningitis are higher than tuberculosis (350,000) and approach the number related to childhood-cluster diseases (pertussis, poliomyelitis, diphtheria, measles, and tetanus, 530,000 death combined), diarrheal diseases (708,000), and malaria (1.1 million)" (Park *et al.* 2009, p. 527). Lives can be saved with a newly developed optimum treatment strategy. It identifies the presence of cryptococcal antigen (CRAG) among those who are HIV-positive with very low CD4+ cell counts. The small percentage found with CRAG is then treated with amphotericin B and 5-flucytosine (AmB/5FT). Most survive for an average of eleven years. Full testing of 32 million persons in SSA, followed by focused

treatment on the small minority with CRAG, about 0.7 million persons, can yield very positive benefit to cost ratios (Punchak 2011).

The effectiveness of this solution will depend in substantial measure on early identification of the small group likely to fall victim to CM. Thus, an expansion of the tested population, an expansion that will require strengthening the health system to permit it to manage such testing, depends on better staff and inclusion of a larger share of the population among those tested. This solution thus relies on both effective HIV/AIDS programs and expansion and improvement of the testing capacity of the health system as a whole. The best approach to identifying candidates for CRAG will be to focus on those most obviously ill yet uncertain of the cause of their illness. A share of such persons, perhaps a significant share, will be persons with low CD4 cell counts below 100 and hence persons at great risk of death from an opportunistic infection associated with HIV and AIDS. Testing for CD4 cell count can be made a part of the overall testing expansion provided under Solution 1 above, and it will be strengthened with the enhanced provision of community health workers suggested as a key part of Solution 2.

Evidence presented here depends largely on data and analysis generated in the Republic of South Africa (see Table 4.5). There is reason to believe findings about this solution in this one country will apply in varying degrees to other SSA countries. Poorer countries may well have more of their people in extreme distress due to opportunistic infections yet may remain undiagnosed and untreated except for minimal palliative care. This possibility adds yet more support for an expanded effort to test and treat a larger share of adults in sub-Saharan Africa who may be ill yet not know the cause of their illness. Expansion of basic test-and-treat capacity to rural Africa is an essential part of the next phase of addressing the HIV/AIDS pandemic.

Cryptococcosis neoformans is an opportunistic fungus that affects immuno-compromised individuals, causing the human cryptococcosis infection, common in SE Asia and Africa; as many as 700,000 deaths annually may be attributed to this opportunistic infection. It is a major cause of

Table 4.5 Disease statistics for HIV/AIDS infected population of South Africa, all sub-Saharan Africa

Indicators	South Africa	All SSA	Source/comments
Population, millions	49.3	800	World Development Indicators
CM cases, most recent year	6,309	720,000	DOH, Rep of S. Africa; Park *et al.* 2009
Mortality rate, CM cases, %	64	73.6	DOH, Rep of S. Africa; Park *et al.* 2009
HIV infected, %	11.3	2.8	UNAIDS 2008
% CD4+<100 cells/ul of treated	41		Lawn *et al.*
Need screening with CRAG, millions	0.85	32	Author estimates
Need to treat with AmB+5FC	6,309	720,000	Same as CM cases identified
Need to treat with fluconazole, millions	0.85	32	Author estimates

Source: Punchak 2011, based on Dept of Health, Republic of South Africa; World Bank World Development Indicators, UNAIDS, Lawn *et al.*, author estimates.

AIDS-related death even in developed countries, and is linked to intracranial pressure as a result of cryptococcal meningitis (Bicanic *et al.* 2005).

Untreated CM is uniformly fatal; infection is usually diagnosed at a late stage, but if the cryptococcal antigen is detected early, treatment can reduce mortality and gain life-years for the infected person (Perfect *et al.* 2010).

Researchers in SSA are at work to determine if screening the group at risk for developing cryptococcosis for the cryptococcal antigen, and then providing *only those who test positive* with the optimal drugs, would be cost-effective (Meya *et al.* 2010). Screening the group at risk for the cryptococcal antigen, and treating only those relatively few persons identified as positive with the optimal treatment, yields the best ratio of benefits to costs.

Costs and benefits of CRAG

Even at the point of initial testing, when the CD4+ cell count is below 100, patients will survive for two years on average with only palliative care. Screening the 32 million persons in the at-risk group will cost $6 per test, totaling about $200 million. Identifying that small minority testing positive for CRAG, and treating only that group, can increase average life span of the estimated 0.72 million at-risk persons to 11.6 years (Meya *et al.* 2010). That process along with treatment will cost $1,810 per person for this smaller group, a total of $1.3 billion. This cost includes one CRAG screening test for 32 million persons, a two-week supply of AmB/5FC for the many fewer, approximately 0.7 million,

in need of this targeted treatment, and an eight-week supply of fluconazole. Once this treatment is completed, it does not need to be repeated.

The benefit is $1,000 or $5,000 per year for the 9.6 additional years of life gained by the 0.7 million who will benefit from treatment (see Table 4.11). With this discounting the benefits for SSA as a whole range from $6 billion (with a value of a year of life of $1,000 and a discount rate of 5 percent) to $30 billion (with a value of a year of life of $5,000 and a discount rate of 3 percent), yielding B/C ratios ranging from a low of 2.7 to a high of 20. The cost per death averted is $2,083.[8] The cost/DALY discounted at 3 percent and 5 percent ranges from $260 to $347.

The success of this intervention depends on reasonably complete access to and knowledge of how likely patients are to proceed from *C. neoformans* to CM and hence near-term risk of death. Persons with CD4+ cell counts at levels below 100 may show such significant symptoms of illness that they seek health care. Thus the share of these most ill persons that are ignorant of their HIV status is probably low. Recall, nonetheless, that over two-thirds of Africa's population lives in rural and isolated areas at some distance from any health care service points.

---

[8] Cost per death averted is lower than for other solutions discussed here, in large part because the solution adds fewer additional years of life, only about ten more years, than do the other solutions that cause a young adult to survive to age sixty-five.

These considerations only serve to emphasize further how important it is to increase the share of all Africans aware of their status and hence able to benefit from care and to take measures to protect their partners. The problem of CM would appear to be far greater in sub-Saharan Africa beyond South Africa's borders than in that country alone, which has made the most progress in developing this treatment protocol. Without effective health system strengthening, those changes will be difficult to implement. Thus even treatment protocols against opportunistic infections that burden those persons who have moved to full-blown AIDS can work more completely and effectively in a strengthened health care system. They may fail badly where the overall system fails.

There are still ways to improve treatment. In South Africa, only 37 percent of HIV-positive persons receive ART therapy; only that percentage of patients have their CD4+ cell levels tracked. Thus currently, many potential beneficiaries are at risk, unidentified, and untreated. Identification and treatment can cut mortality rates in South Africa substantially; achieving that objective will require far better coverage via test-and-treat protocols that need to reach all persons at risk of being HIV-positive. Expanding the numbers and skills of community-directed health workers would enhance the performance of a more comprehensive test-and-treat strategy.

Upgrading the quality and quantity of diagnosis and treatment for opportunistic infections will require strengthening health systems overall. In that respect, HSS is an essential component of better HIV/AIDS programs as well.

Solution 4: "Cash on delivery" (COD) through an Abuja Goal Fund (AGF)

> Offer "cash on delivery" (COD) through an Abuja Goal Fund (AGF) as an incentive to induce countries to raise public health spending and strengthen health partnerships in ways that also strengthen health and HIV/AIDS programs.

Solution 1 would provide individual vouchers that promote demand for testing to identify millions of adults who are HIV-positive but do not know it. Solution 2 promotes an increase in the supply of basic health service personnel. Solution 3 targets specific testing services for OIs that harm those with diseases linked to HIV/AIDS but require an upgrading of health services generally. Solution 4 suggested here would promote upgrades in the financing of public health by governments. This solution would make payments to governments in exchange for progress toward the agreed goal of allocating at least 15 percent of public spending to health services. Payment would flow through a to-be-established Abuja Goal Fund (AGF) endowed initially with a billion dollars. Disbursements would be made against actual, agreed progress in allocating more public funds for public health in countries that agree to pursue this goal.

Subsidiary agreements about the nature and content of spending objectives could be negotiated between AGF managers and governments seeking funds. The incentive provided to governments with AGF funds need not imply a specific commitment of these payments to the provision of health services. The purpose of the COD payment is to induce an SSA government to devote its own financial resources to the health sector, not to pay for any specific health program, except the overall increase in public funding for the sector. Thus, in the BCA analysis of this solution, there is the (untested) assumption that the incentive of untied AGF resources will induce greater spending on health in line with objectives set out in the MDG framework, the IHP+ approach, and the Platform for Health Strengthening now being rolled out in selected countries.

Background on Abuja

In April 2001 representatives of all African governments pledged to achieve what has come to be called the Abuja goal for health spending. Few countries have actually achieved that goal (see Figure 4.2). More could do so. This solution would create a fund that would disburse against confirmed progress in raising the spending share from its current level (the health share in 2009, for example) to an agreed higher share in 2012 and years beyond through 2015. The way such a fund might work in one country, Uganda, appears in the appendix to this chapter.[9]

The majority of sub-Saharan African countries still remain well short of an agreed goal, the Abuja target, established a decade ago to raise public health spending to 15 percent of all government spending. As of the year 2008, for which reasonably complete data are now available, seven countries had reached and exceeded that target level: Rwanda, Tanzania, DRCongo, Liberia, Burkina Faso, Zambia, and Djibouti. Five of these seven countries may have met the Abuja goal thanks to considerable donor assistance, which provided over a third to nearly two-thirds of health financing among five of the larger countries.[10] More than thirty other countries still fell below that target level in their public spending on health. The median and unweighted mean for all countries is 10 percent of total government spending. Most countries are still well below the target public spending level for the health sector.

How can countries be induced to make progress toward the Abuja commitment? Can movement toward that commitment strengthen the health system and support the MDG of turning back the HIV/AIDS epidemic? We argue in favor of this approach, fully recognizing doubts among those who reject such incentives as inadequate to cause ministries of finance to act positively.

Once such a fund is created other interested donors could add to it. Disbursements could begin in 2013 (against progress in the 2012 budget appropriation) and continue into the future. The target shares would be a subject for agreement between national governments and fund management. Disbursements would follow the principle of cash on delivery, i.e., presentation and agreement by both parties that verify progress (Barder and Birdsall 2006).

Current World Bank results-based funding (RBF) programs follow related procedures (Savedoff 2010). A platform approach inspired by the International Health Partnerships (IHP+) and the High Level Taskforce cited earlier is already functioning in Ethiopia and Nepal (Glassman and Savedoff 2011).

In some respects at least, these new modes of financing parallel other donor practices. The Global

Table 4.6 Selected health benefits of health system strengthening

Additional deaths averted in 2015	Calculated, millions	WHO	MBB
Under-5 deaths averted (including newborn, infant, and neonatal) adjusted downward by 0.5	4	3.9m	4.3m
Maternal deaths averted	0.3	322,000	259,000
HIV deaths averted	0.1	193,000	74,000
Tuberculosis deaths averted	0.25	265,000	235,000
Total deaths averted (sum of first four rows above)	4.65		
Decrease in number of births due to increased use of family planning	10	11m	9m

Source: HLT Group 1 (Mills) report, Table 9, p. 57. The column, Calculated, millions, adjusts original estimates in the WHO and MBB columns via the reduced valuation of infant and child deaths and an approximation of the mean between the WHO and MBB estimates.

Fund seeks proposals covering five years but disburses only for the first two years. GF then reviews progress with recipient country coordinating mechanisms and agrees to further disbursement depending on progress made. GF principles require it to "leverage additional resources" beyond its own grants (Post and McGreevey 2005). In fact, it is a continuing challenge for donors to avoid having their external funds "crowd out" support by governments. One estimate is that it would require $1.4 in donor funds just to cover the $1 of reduced health spending by SSA governments, as finance ministries divert money away from health to other purposes (Lu *et al.* 2010). This problem has been the subject of review at the World Bank for more than two decades (for a recent review see Tandon 2009).

[9] Dugger (2011), citing the work of Lu *et al.* (2010), describes a serious incident in Uganda demonstrating lack of emergency obstetric care and suggests that donor assistance may have led to a reduction in public support for the health sector from the government's own resources.

[10] The donor share is only 18.8 percent and 29.2 percent in DR Congo and Burkina Faso, respectively, according to the source. One may perhaps suspect that either donor shares or public-sector commitment to health spending might be incorrectly stated in these cases.

The World Bank has for years operated structural adjustment lending approaches that make disbursement conditional on agreed goals and progress toward those goals. The highly indebted poor countries initiative (HIPC) exchanges debt forgiveness against country pledges to increase public social spending. These examples suggest ample opportunity to provide attractive incentives to SSA governments that will induce them to shift priorities in favor of basic health. Similarly, AGF would not directly finance any health care services. Instead, it offers an incentive to a government to augment its own funding for health. The successful countries can avert many deaths that might otherwise occur as they strengthen health systems and build up the necessary staff support. To begin estimating benefits from the incentive effect of AGF, consider what potential benefits of the Taskforce total could be scored as deriving from the AGF incentive.

Incremental costs in 2015

Data developed by HLT Group 1 follow the decade-earlier Commission on Macroeconomics and Health (CMH) in proposing to more than double spending on health in the SSA region. They refer to an additional $29 per capita beyond current spending on health of about $25 per capita. Total health spending in the region would rise from its current level of about $24 billion to a total of $52 billion to be spent on all SSA health care in 2015 (HLT Group 1 report 2009).[11]

What incremental benefits can arise from this additional spending? The answer provided by HLT Group 1 can be summarized as additional deaths averted in the single year 2015 (see Table 4.6). Both WHO and the World Bank marginal budgeting for bottlenecks analysis (MBB) have provided best estimates of under-five, maternal, HIV, and TB deaths that can be averted.

A total of about 4.65 million deaths will be averted, and hence 4.65 million lives saved in the year 2015. Most of the lives saved, 86 percent of the total, are for children under age five. The value of lives saved might thus range from a low of $20,000 per life saved to a high of $100,000 per life saved, amounts when future years are discounted at 3 percent that lie mid-way between the values for infants and young adults in Table 4.8.

For this exercise, we adjusted the number of under-five deaths to be consistent with the approach described earlier in the preceding text. The sum is then estimated as 2.65 million deaths averted in that single future year. This number of deaths averted then helps specify the incremental benefits deriving from the increased spending to strengthen health systems. Such strengthening also clearly contributed to reducing deaths from HIV/AIDS.[12] Thus the calculated lower- and upper-bound estimates of benefits are $93 billion and $465 billion, respectively (see Table 4.12).

These amounts for benefits, when divided by the incremental costs drawn from the HLT Group 1, yield B/C ratios in the range of 1.1 to 7.7. Cost per DALY ranges between $600 and $1,000. Those amounts are broadly comparable to, if somewhat below, levels identified for other solutions and interventions under discussion here. Cost per death averted would be about $11,000 ($29 billion/2.65 million deaths averted = $10,943).

The HLT Group 1 report goes on to assess the plausibility of the cost and impact estimates and compares the cost per death averted derived from the cost and impact estimates done for the essential package in the World Bank, *World Development Report 1993, Investing in Health*. Updated to 2005 prices, the cost-per-death averted of the WDR package is $9,000. The estimates here look plausible for a broad set of interventions that address the main causes of the burden of disease. They require broad systems development, including buildings, staff, and management, to deliver the whole set

---

[11] Assume, along with UN and World Bank projections, a 2015 population of just under one billion for SSA and hence total health expenditure, when per capita spending is $54, of $52 billion, half of which is incremental, additional spending recommended by the HLT Group 1 report.

[12] There are in addition substantial reductions in morbidity and improved individual well-being and quality of life benefitting millions of people. In the WHO approach an extra 56m women would have access to safe birth attendance and antenatal care, and their babies would receive quality care at birth and during the neonatal period. In the MBB approach an additional 17 million women would receive antenatal care in 2015, and 16 million would benefit from safe birth attendance. Moreover, the strengthened national health systems would enable sustained health improvements into the future.

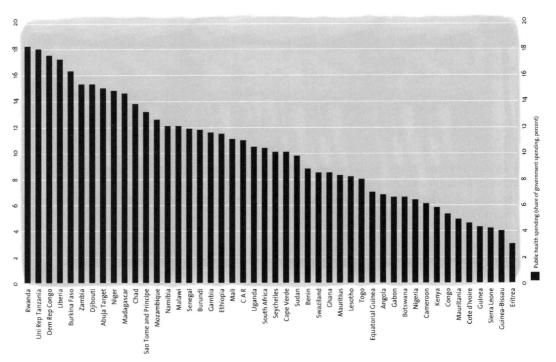

Figure 4.2 *Reaching the Abuja goal: by 2008, seven countries had, 38 had not*
Source: WHO Health Statistics, 2011, *pp. 128–34. No data for Somalia and Zimbabwe.*

at the same time. Averted deaths are only one element of the broad health gains that could be created by scaling up interventions and the health system platform.

Are the estimates reasonable? Do they complement other solutions focused more directly on HIV/AIDS? The HLT taskforce authors raise questions of their own:

> The hoped-for health benefits may also appear high. The deaths averted represent a roughly two thirds average reduction in child and maternal mortality from the 2005–2008 baseline over a six-year period. Rapid reductions are possible. For example, Eritrea managed to reduce the under-five mortality rate from 147 deaths per 1000 live births in 1990 to 70 in 2007 . . . The infant mortality rate also declined significantly over this time period . . . Tanzania managed to reduce its rate of under-five mortality from 157 to 116 deaths per 1000 live births over the same period. (HLT Group 1 report, p. 59)

The earlier Commission on Macroeconomics and Health (CMH) estimated annual economic benefits of $360 billion for a similar upgrade of future health spending. That earlier estimate lies above the range of the benefit estimates in Table 4.12. The highest estimate there is a net present value of life-years saved of $223 million for the combination of a life-year valued at $5,000 and a discount rate of 3 percent for future life-years.[13]

An issue for this solution is whether and how the AGF incentive can be said to help achieve these benefits along with the direct costs for service delivery. Since the AGF does not yet exist, there is no way to "prove" that it will contribute, much less to show with certainty "how much" its existence can

---

[13] If, as an alternative evaluation, the analysis did not discount the future years of life of infants by half, then the much larger total of $368 million would emerge from the analysis. This comparison underlines the significant role played by the decision to reduce the estimated value of future life-years of the very young when compared to those of adults.

contribute to the prospective benefits of HSS. At best one can say, "Incentives matter, and governments respond positively to them." That much we know from responses to HIPC, structural adjustment lending, and IHP+.

Central to this analysis is the presumption that the additional investments in service delivery really will work as planned. There are many skeptics and even some evidence from trials that suggest that success if achieved will be far from universal (Banerjee and Duflo 2011; Karlan and Appel 2011; and earlier analyses by Filmer and Pritchett 1999). Even at the higher prospective estimate of the value of life used here, and with the modest discount rate of 3 percent, the B/C ratio is not notably high when compared to some "vertical" programs or HIV prevention measures.

The advantage that AGF can bring to the table is that the nearly forty governments in sub-Saharan Africa that have not reached Abuja goals can set their own plans and priorities before the Fund and its staff, and work out plans consistent with national goals. This "hands-off approach" is consistent with cash on delivery and results-based financing approaches, according to one recent overview of the new Platform meant to replace excessive donor involvement in what must be national governments' policies and actions (Glassman and Savedoff 2011).

Conclusions and recommendations

In the preceding pages we examined four possible solutions to strengthen health systems and support the ongoing effort to turn back the pandemic of HIV/AIDS in sub-Saharan Africa. In general, these solutions offer positive returns of benefits compared to the costs that would be incurred to implement them (see Table 4.7). Their costs per DALY, shown separately, are reasonable as well.

The recently issued UNAIDS scenario, when applied to SSA, calls for spending $22 billion annually (first rising then falling in the years 2012 to 2020). It will reduce the incidence of new infections and extend the lives of persons who are already HIV-positive.[14] Estimates of lives saved and costs incurred yield cost per death averted of $4,090 (see Table 4.2 above). This cost is well below the lower

value of a life saved at age twenty-two and extended to age sixty-five (discounting future years at 3 percent or even at 5 percent as in Tables 4.9 and 4.10). The new strategy from UNAIDS suggests a B/C ratio of 6 to 30. These are very positive results.

How well do the four solutions that combine the strengthening of health systems and HIV/AIDS efforts compare to the UNAIDS scenario? The B/C ratios for these four approaches range from a low value of 1.1:1 to a high value of about 20:1. Cost per DALY ranges from about $250 to $1,000. Costs per death averted, with future years of life assumed to begin at age twenty-two in most cases, and discounted at 3 percent and 5 percent, range between $2,000 and $16,000. Details appear in the main text and annex tables.

Various studies used to support DALY estimates for strengthening health systems, improving family planning and reproductive health, reducing maternal deaths, improving treatment for OIs, and generally upgrading health systems range from well under $100 per DALY to over $1,200. The UNAIDS new approach offers a B/C ratio ranging from 6 to 30, a cost per DALY of $1,060, and a cost per death averted of $4,090. A comparison of this new approach to the proposed solutions may show that some solutions that provide *both* health system strengthening and HIV/AIDS prevention, care, and treatment offer somewhat better B/C ratios and costs per DALY and per death averted. Donor policies that blend vertical and horizontal approaches into a diagonal approach may be most advantageous. Much will depend on the efficacy of implementation.

Some of these cost estimates lie below the UNAIDS cost of saving a year of life, others above. In virtually all cases, there are possible ancillary, uncalculated benefits of these solutions. There may also be unintended consequences of some interventions. The incentives made explicit in conditional cash transfers and cash on delivery may cause unanticipated behavioral changes by persons and governments. Once such payments occur they may

---

[14] Over the 2011 to 2020 period the new strategy can save 29.4 million life-years at an average cost of $1,060, roughly equivalent to the lower-bound value of a life-year used in this paper.

Table 4.7 Solutions with potential impact on supply, demand, b/c, cost per DALY, and cost per death averted

Solution	Impact on...	Persons affected (millions)	Costs ($bn)	B/C	C/DALY ($)	C/DA ($)
UNAIDS new scenario	Incidence, prevalence		22/yr	6 to 30.5	1,060	4,090
Proposed solutions						
1. CCTs for VCT	Demand for prevention	400	2	2.5–15	320–444	8,000
2. Upgrade health workers & services	Supply of CHWs, esp. rural areas	100+	2.6	1.1–9.5	587–825	15,857
3. CRAG: prevent CM	Opportunistic infections	32+	1.5	4–25	260–347	2,083
4. COD for AGF	Supply of public health services	300+	1	1.1–7.7	627–915	10,943
All HSS + HIV/AIDS	Supply, demand, incentives	400+	5			

Source: Authors' estimates. For details on b/c ratios, see Appendix Tables. C/DALY = cost per disability life-year saved; C/DA = cost per death averted. Cost/DALY and cost per death averted from Schwartländer 2011, UNAIDS scenario, and Table 4.2 in text above; solution 1 assumes 1/6 of infections proposed to be averted by UNAIDS new approach attributable to CCT offered, with cost per deaths averted discounted at 3 percent; solution 2 from Joshi (2011), for child and maternal deaths averted, life-years saved; solution 3 from Punchak (2011) based in Rep of South Africa data in Excellent (2010), others; solution 4, from HLT Taskforce 1, Appendix 2 on deaths averted; solution 5, life-years averting poverty = life-years assumed saved. For additional sources, see text.

be demanded in the future when they cannot be further supported.

The best B/C ratios among these solutions arise from optimal treatment for the estimated 0.7 million persons in SSA with risk for cryptococcal meningitis. The other interventions also offer good value for money with ratios of benefits to costs exceeding 1.

The prospects for each of the four solutions presented in outline in Table 4.7 can be illuminated with the following summary descriptions:

- Universal testing, informing, and counseling can be achieved with a voucher of $5 paid to all those who accept to learn their status. The cost is substantial at $2 billion, but benefits of knowledge could cut new infections by a quarter million annually in the effort to turn back the epidemic, and the health system's capacity to test and treat a range of ICDs would grow as well.
- Deployment of community health workers to the vast rural population at a cost of $2.64 billion could cut maternal deaths by 0.3 million annually and child deaths by millions more, with B/C ratios ranging from 2 to 12, and we estimated that half the overall benefits from strengthening rural health service delivery could be attributable to this health outreach program. Reducing the opportunistic infection of cryptococcal meningitis at a cost of $1.5 billion will require fuller

health systems and can include enhanced attention to TB, XDR TB, and other illnesses, and still yield a ratio of benefits to costs between 2.7 and 20.

- Creating an Abuja Goals Fund (AGF) can call attention to the need to increase government health spending, giving incentives to enhance government spending with a $1 billion fund that would offer cash on delivery (COD) for meeting agreed goals of spending more public money on public health. The ratio of benefits to cost is positive though somewhat lower than the other solutions reviewed here.

The solutions vary widely in the number of persons they can be expected to affect. The cash transfer for testing and counseling might reach all adults, about 400 million persons. Treatment for those at risk of cryptococcal meningitis would lead to testing for about 30 million persons and an actual intervention for fewer than one million but could extend lives that would otherwise be lost for a decade. Specialized testing for CM might affect fewer at-risk persons than other solutions but it could be consistent with the cash transfers recommended in exchange for widespread counseling and testing.

Cash on delivery for Abuja goal progress might be easiest to negotiate with governments that would welcome a cash incentive in exchange for upgrading public health provision in line with

Table 4.8 Value of lives saved in infancy (where each year of an infant's life = 0.5 of an adult life-year), at age 22, and age 50, when value of current disability-adjusted life-year is $1,000 and $5,000, and discounted to present value at 3 percent, 5 percent, and 10 percent, $000

Value, lives saved, by age of person saved	VSL=$1, undiscounted	VSL=$5, undiscounted	VSL=$1, disc@3%	VSL=$5, disc@3%	VSL=$1, disc@5%	VSL=$5, disc@5%	VSL=$1, disc@10%	VSL=$5, disc@10%
Life saved as an infant*	65	325	29	144	19	96	10	50
Life-year of infant = 0.5 adult life-year	33	163	15	72	10	48	5	25
Life saved at age 22	43	215	25	123	18	90	10	50
Life saved at age 50	15	75	13	64	11	56	8	41

Source: Based on a table in Excel workbook, "CCC VSL Disc.xls."

commitments already made. An upgrade of public health spending by 50 percent – that is, from just 10 percent of total government spending where it lies on average now, to 15 percent of total government spending – could have a very wide impact.

Appendix: Uganda and AGF, a potential case study?

Uganda recently allocated 10.5 percent of its public spending to the health sector, 4.5 percentage points short of the 15 percent Abuja goal. Assume the government proposes to raise its share to 13 percent in 2012, 14 percent in 2013, and 15 percent in 2014, and maintain that share into the future. Spending on public health will have to rise from about $220 million now, to over $300 million by 2014.

Uganda proposes to increase its health spending to $250 million in 2012, $275 million in 2013, and $300 million in 2014. AGF agrees to disburse $3 million by June 30, 2013 if the Ugandan government reaches or exceeds the 2012 target. Additional disbursement of $4.5 million and $8 million occur at the midpoints of 2014 and 2015, respectively, if Uganda meets the next-year goals. Total AGF disbursements to Uganda, 2013 through 2015, would total $15.5 million if, and only if, all Abuja targets are met on time.

Similar outlays for thirty countries would total about half a billion dollars. Sums could be larger if additional donors agree to join AGF. Goals and timing would be adapted to each country's capacity to increase its health share.

Table 4.9 Incremental B/C ratio ranging from 2 to 15, cost per DALY ranging from $320 to $444 for spending $2 billion to test, inform, and counsel all SSA adults on their HIV status, cutting expected new infections by 0.25 million annually to yield benefits of $6.25 billion (low) or $32 billion (high)

	Benefits $ bn			B/C ratios		C/DALY $		
Value life-yr.	3% disc.	5% disc.	Costs $ bn	3% disc.	5% disc.	3% disc.	5% disc.	Cost/ death averted
$1,000	6	5	2	3.2	2.5	320	444	$8,000
$5,000	31	23	2	15	11	320	444	

Source: Authors' estimates allocating a share of all infections averted to the proposed cash transfer. See Table 4.8 for the $25,000 and $123,000 estimated value of life of a young adult discounted at 3 percent per annum.

Table 4.10 Benefits and costs to expand community health workers, $ billions, cost/DALY ($)

	Benefits $ b			B/C ratios		C/DALY $		
Value life-yr.	3% disc.	5% disc.	Costs	3% disc.	5% disc.	3% disc.	5% disc.	Cost/ death averted
$1,000	5	3	2.64	1.9	1.1	587	825	$15,857
$5,000	25	15	2.64	9.5	5.7	587	825	

Source: Authors' estimates based on data in HLT Taskforce 1 report (Mills 2009). Only benefits from averting deaths included, using the average of WHO and World Bank MBB estimates of deaths averted with adjusted value of child deaths.

Table 4.11 B/C ratio ranging from 4 to 25 for CRAG testing and treatment among 0.72 million in SSA, extending lives by 9 years at cost/DALY beyond age 22, B, C values in $ billions, C/DALY ($)

Value life-yr.	Benefits $ bn			B/C ratios		C/DALY $		Cost/ death averted
	3% disc.	5% disc.	Costs	3% disc.	5% disc.	3% disc.	5% disc.	
$1,000	6	4	15	4.0	2.7	260	347	$2,083
$5,000	30	20	1.5	20.0	13.3	260	347	

Source: Punchak 2011, Table 5; calculated from Meya (2010), Excellent (2010). Future years discounted at 3 percent for value of life-year $1,000 and 5 percent for value of life-year $5,000.

Table 4.12 Incremental B/C ratios for spending an additional $29 billion on basic health system strengthening in 2015

Value life-yr.	Benefits $ bn			B/C ratios		Cost/ DALY		Cost/ death averted
	3% disc.	5% disc.	Costs	3% disc.	5% disc.	3% disc.	5% disc.	
$1,000	46	31	29	1.6	1.1	627	915	$10,943
$5,000	223	155	29	7.7	5.3	627	915	

Source: Authors' estimates based on data in Task Force 1 of HLT group. Only benefits from averting deaths included, using the average of WHO and World Bank MBB estimates of the value of deaths averted adjusted downward for under-five deaths as in Table 4.8.

References

Aids 2031 Costs and Financing Working Group. (2009). *Synthesis Report*. Washington DC: Results for Development.

Ainsworth, M., World Bank and Operations Evaluation Dept. (2005). *Committing to Results: Improving the Effectiveness of HIV/AIDS Assistance. An OED Evaluation of the World Bank's Assistance for HIV/AIDS Control*. Washington DC: World Bank, www.worldbank.org/oed/aids/docs/report/hiv%5Fcomplete%5Freport.pdf.

Amico, Aran, C. and Avila, C. (2010). HIV spending as a share of total health expenditure: an analysis of regional variation in a multi-country study. *PLoS One* **5**(9): e12997.

Avila, C. *et al.* (2009). *HIV and AIDS Programs: How they Support Health System Strengthening.* Working Paper. Washington DC: Results for Development Institute.

Avila, C. *et al.* (2010). *Post-Crisis AIDS Financing: Smarter Choices, Integration and Efficiency.* Geneva: UNAIDS.

Baird, S., Chirwa, E., McIntosh, C. and Ozler, B. (2009). *The Short Term Impacts of a Schooling Conditional Cash Transfer Program on the Sexual Behavior of Young Women.* Washington DC: World Bank.

Banerjee, A. V. and Duflo, E. (2011). *Poor Economics, a Radical Rethinking of the Way to Fight Global Poverty.* New York: Public Affairs.

Barder, O. and Birdsall, N. (2006). Payments for Progress: A Hands-Off Approach to Foreign Aid. CGD Working Paper 102.

Belli, P., Anderson, J. R., Barnum, H. N., Dixon, J. A. and Tan, J. P. (eds.) (2001). *Economic Analysis of Investment Operations: Analytical Tools and Practical Applications.* Washington DC: World Bank, WBI Development Studies.

Bicanic, T. and Harrison, T. S. (2005). Cryptococcal meningitis. *Br Med Bull* **72**: 99–118.

Biesma, R., Harmer, B. R., Walsh, A., Spicer, N. and Walt, G. (2009). The effects of global health initiatives on country health systems: a review of the evidence from HIV/AIDS control. *Health Policy Plan* **24**(4): 239–52.

Birdsall, N. and Savedoff, W. (2010). *Cash on Delivery: A New Approach to Foreign Aid, with an Application to Primary Schooling.* Baltimore, MD: Brookings Institution Press.

Boehme, C. *et al.* (2011). Feasibility, diagnostic accuracy, and effectiveness of decentralized use of the Xpert MTG/RIF test for diagnosis of tuberculosis and multidrug resistance: a multicentre implementation study. *The Lancet* April 30; **377**: 1495.

Bollinger, L. (2011). *Prevention of Non-Sexual Transmission of HIV.* Assessment Paper.

Bongaarts, J. and Over, M. (2010). Global HIV/AIDS policy in transition. *Science* **328**, June 11: 1359–60.

Bongaarts, J. and Sinding, S. (2009). A response to critics of family planning programs. *International Perspectives on Sexual and Reproductive Health* **35**(1): 40–3.

Briscombe, B. and McGreevey, W. (2010). *Costs and Benefits Study of the NHIS/MDG Maternal and Child Health Project.* Washington DC: Futures Group.

Canning, D. (2006). The economics of HIV/AIDS in low-income countries: the case for prevention. *Journal of Economic Perspectives* **20**(3): 121–42.

CHW Technical Task Force. (2011). *One Million Community Health Workers: Technical Task Force Report*. New York: The Earth Institute, Columbia University.

Cutler, D. (2004). *Your Money or Your Life*. New York: Oxford University Press.

Cutler, D. M. (2008). Are we finally winning the war on cancer? *Journal of Economic Perspectives* **22**(4): 3–26.

Cutler, D. M., Deaton, A. and Lleras-Muney, A. (2006). The determinants of mortality. *Journal of Economic Perspectives* **20**(3): 97–120.

Cutler, D. M. and Miller, G. (2005). The role of public health improvements in health advances. *Demography* **42**(1): 1–22.

de Lalla, F., Pellizzer, G., Vaglia, A., Manfrin, V., Franzetti, M., Fabris, P. and Stecca, C. (1995). Amphotericin B as primary therapy for cryptococcosis in patients with AIDS: reliability of relatively high doses administered over a relatively short period. *Clin Infect Dis*. **20**(2): 263–6.

Department of Health, South Africa. www.doh. gov.za/.

de Savigny, D. and Adam, T. (eds.) (2009). *Systems Thinking for Health Systems Strengthening*. Geneva: WHO Press.

Dodd, P. J., Garnett, G. P. and Hallett, T. B. (2010). Examining the promise of HIV elimination by "test and treat" in hyperendemic settings. *AIDS* **24**(5): 729–35.

Dromer, F., Bernede-Bauduin, C., Guillemot, D., Lortholary, O.; French Cryptococcosis Study Group. (2008). Major role for amphotericin B-flucytosine combination in severe cryptococcosis. *PLoS One*. 6; **3**(8): e2870.

Dugger, C. W. (2010). Maternal deaths focus harsh light on Uganda. *The New York Times*, July 30, A1.

Dupas, P. (2010). Do teenagers respond to HIV risk information? Evidence from an HIV Field Experiment in Kenya. www.nber.org/papers/w14707.

Eichler, R. and Glassman, A. (2008). *Health Systems Strengthening Via Performance-Based Aid: Creating Incentives to Perform and to Measure Results*. Baltimore, MD: Brookings Institution.

Eichler, R. *et al*. (2009). *Performance Incentives for Global Health: Potential and Pitfalls*. Baltimore, MD: Brookings Institution Press.

England, R. (2007). Are we spending too much on HIV? *British Medical J*. **334**.

Epstein, H. (2007). *The Invisible Cure: Africa, The West, and the Fight Against AIDS*. New York: Farrar, Strauss and Giroux.

Fasawe, O. *et al*. (2011). Economic evaluation of policy options to prevent mother-to-child HIV transmission in Malawi: cost-effectiveness analysis of Option B+. Draft. Geneva: UNAIDS.

Fernald, L. C. *et al*. (2009). 10-year effect of Oportunidades, Mexico's conditional cash transfer programme, on child growth, cognition, language, and behaviour: a longitudinal follow-up study. *The Lancet* **374**: 1997–2004.

Filmer, D., Hammer, J. and Pritchett, L. (2000). Weak links in the chain: a diagnosis of health policy in poor countries. *The World Bank Research Observer* **15**(2): 199–224.

Filmer, D., Hammer, J. and Pritchett, L. (2002). Weak links in the chain II: a prescription for health policy in poor countries. *The World Bank Research Observer* **17**(1): 47–66.

Filmer, D. and Pritchett, L. (1999). The impact of public spending on health: does money matter? *Social Science and Medicine* **49**(10): 1309–23.

Fiszbein, A. *et al*. (2009). *Conditional Cash Transfers: Reducing Present and Future Poverty*. Washington DC: World Bank, policy research paper.

Fox-Rushby, J. A. and Hanson, K. (2001). Calculating and presenting disability adjusted life years (DALYs) in cost-effectiveness analysis. *Health Policy and Planning* **16**(3): 326–31.

Garnett, G. P. and Baggaley, R. F. (2009). Treating our way out of the HIV pandemic: could we, would we, should we? *Lancet* **373**: 9–11.

Glassman, A. and Savedoff, W. (2011). The health systems funding platform: resolving tensions between the aid and development effectiveness agendas. Draft. Washington DC: Center for Global Development.

Global Fund Observer. (2011). Brief note on decline in HSS components of approved grants.

Gottret, P., Waters, H. and Schieber, G. (eds.) (2008). *Good Practices in Health Financing: Lessons From Reforms in Low- and Middle-Income Countries*. Washington DC: World Bank.

Gottret, P. *et al.* (2009). *Protecting Pro-Poor Health Services During Financing Crises, Lessons From Experience*. Washington DC: World Bank.

Graham, C. (2009). *Happiness Around the world: The Paradox of Happy Peasants and Miserable Millionaires*. Oxford University Press.

Granich, R. M. *et al.* (2008). Universal voluntary HIV testing with immediate anti-retroviral therapy as a strategy for elimination of HIV transmission: a mathematical model. *The Lancet online*, Nov 28.

Guthrie, T. *et al.* (2010). *The Long Run Costs and Financing of HIV/AIDS in South Africa*. Washington DC: Results for Development Institute.

Hecht, R. (ed.) (2010). *Costs and Choices: Financing the Long-Term Fight against AIDS*. Washington DC: Results for Development Institute.

Hecht, R. *et al.* (2010). Critical choices in financing the response to the global HIV/AIDS pandemic. *Health Affairs* **28**(6): 1–15.

Herbst, C. H. *et al.* (2009). HIV/AIDS and human resources for health. In Lule, E. L., Seifman, R. M. and David, A. C. (eds.). *The Changing HIV/AIDS Landscape: Selected Papers for the World Bank's Agenda for Action in Africa, 2007–2011.*

IHP+ the International Health Partnership. (April 2008). *Update 7.*

IHP+ the International Health Partnership. (May 2008). *Progress Report to World Health Assembly.* (Accessed May 4, 2009.)

IHP+ the International Health Partnership. (January 2009). *Country Progress Reports: Kenya, Mozambique, Ethiopia, Zambia, Madagascar, Burundi, Cambodia, Mali & Zambia.* (Accessed August 3, 2009.)

IHP+ the International Health Partnership. (January 2009). *Update 1.* (Accessed August 3, 2009.)

IHP+ the International Health Partnership. (March 2009). *Update 15.* Available from www. internationalhealthpartnership.net/ ihp_plus_documents.html. (Accessed May 4, 2009.)

IHP+ the International Health Partnership. (2009). 4th progress report – ministerial review meeting February 4–5 (2009): 15.

IHP+ the International Health Partnership. IHP+. International Health Partnership objectives. Available from www. internationalhealthpartnership.net/

ihp_plus_about_objectives.html. (Accessed August 3, 2009.)

IHP+ Advisory Group. (2011). *IHP+ Results: Strengthening Accountability to Achieve the Health MDGs. Annual Performance Report 2010.* London: Responsible Action UK.

Jamison, D. T. (2010). Disease control. In Lomborg, B. (ed.). *Smart Solutions To Climate Change: Comparing Costs and Benefits.* Cambridge University Press.

Jamison, D. T. *et al.* (eds.) (2006a). *Disease Control Priorities in Developing Countries* (2nd edn). Washington DC: World Bank and Oxford University Press.

Jamison, D. T. *et al.* (eds.) (2006b). *Priorities in Health.* Washington DC: World Bank.

Jarvis, J. N., Lawn, S. D., Vogt, M., Bangani, N., Wood, R. and Harrison, T. S. (2009). Screening for cryptococcal antigenemia in patients accessing an anti-retroviral treatment program in South Africa. *Clin Infect Dis.* **48**(7): 856–62.

Joshi, S. (2011). How effective are family-planning programs at improving the lives of women? Some perspectives from a vast literature. Draft. Washington DC: Georgetown University.

Karlan, D. and Appel, J. (2011). *More than Good Intentions: How a New Economics is Helping to Solve Global Poverty.* New York: Dutton.

Kenny, C. (2011). *Getting Better: Why Global Development Is Succeeding – and How We Can Improve the World Even More.* New York: Basic Books.

Kranzer, K. (2011). Improving tuberculosis diagnostics and treatment. *The Lancet* April 30; **377**: 1467.

Levy, S. (2006). *Progress against Poverty: Sustaining Mexico's Progresa-Oportunidades Program.* Washington DC: Brookings Institution Press.

Lomborg, B. (ed.) (2004). *Global Crises, Global Solutions.* Cambridge University Press.

Lomborg, B. (ed.) (2006). *How to Spend $50 Billion to Make the World a Better Place.* Cambridge University Press.

Lomborg, B. (ed.) (2007). *Solutions for the World's Biggest Problems: Costs and Benefits.* Cambridge University Press.

Lu, C., Schneider, M., Gubbins, P., Leach-Kemon, K., Jamison, D. and Murray, C. J. L. (2010). Public financing of health in developing countries: a cross-national systematic analysis. *Lancet* **375**: 1375–87.

Lule, E. L., Seifman, R. M., and David, A. C. (2009). *The Changing HIV/AIDS Landscape: Selected Papers for the World Bank's Agenda for Action in Africa, 2007–2011*. Washington DC: World Bank.

Mathers, C. *et al.* [WHO]. (2009). *Global Health Risks: Mortality and Burden of Disease Attributable to Selected Major Risks*. Geneva: WHO.

McCoy, D. and Brikci, N. (2010). Taskforce on innovative international financing for health systems: what next? *Bulletin of the World Health Organization* **88**: 478–80.

McGreevey, W. (2009). Fiscal space and HIV and AIDS resource needs estimates, 2010–2030 – a report for UNAIDS Resource Tracking Unit. Mimeo. Washington DC: Georgetown University.

McGreevey, W. and MacKellar, L. (2007). Economic rate of return report: economic analysis of the Lesotho health project. Mimeo. March.

McNeil, D. G. (2010a). At front lines, AIDS war is falling apart. *The New York Times*, May 9.

McNeil, D. G. (2010b). U.N. reports decrease in new H.I.V. infections. *The New York Times*, November 24.

McNeil, D. G. (2011). Two studies show pills can prevent H.I.V. infection. *The New York Times*, July 14.

Medlin, C. and de Walque, D. (2008). *Potential Application of Conditional Cash Transfers for Prevention of Sexually Transmitted Infections and HIV in Sub-Saharan Africa*. Washington DC: World Bank Policy Research Working Paper No. 4673.

Meya, D. B., Manabe, Y. C., Castelnuovo, B., Cook, B. A., Elbireer, A. M., Kambugu, A., Kamya, M. R., Bohjanen, P. R. and Boulware, D. R. (2010). Cost-effectiveness of serum cryptococcal antigen screening to prevent deaths among HIV-infected persons with a CD4+ cell count < or = 100 cells/microL who start HIV therapy in resource-limited settings. *Clin Infect Dis.* 15; **51**(4): 448–55.

Micol, R., Tajahmady, A., Lortholary, O., Balkan, S., Quillet, C., Dousset, J. P., Chanroeun, H., Madec, Y., Fontanet, A. and Yazdanpanah, Y. (2010). Cost-effectiveness of primary prophylaxis of AIDS associated cryptococcosis in Cambodia. *PLoS One.* 9; **5**(11): e13856.

Milanovic, B. (2011). *The Haves and the Have-Nots, a Brief and Idiosyncratic History of Global Inequality*. New York: Basic Books.

Mills, A. (2009). *Constraints to Scaling Up and Costs. Working Group Report*. Taskforce on innovative international financing for health systems.

Mills, A. and Shillcutt, S. (2007). Communicable diseases. In Lomborg, B. (ed.). (2006). *How to Spend $50 Billion to Make the World a Better Place*. Cambridge University Press, pp. 19–37. Longer version appears in *Global Crises, Global Solutions*, pp. 62–114.

Narayan, D., Chambers, R., Kaul Shah, M. and Petesch, P. (2000). *Voices of the Poor, Crying Out for Change*. Washington DC: Oxford University Press for World Bank.

Nordhaus, W. D. (2003). The health of nations: the contribution of improved health to living standards. In Murphy, K. M. and Topel, R. H. (eds.). *Measuring the Gains from Medical Research: An Economic Approach*. University of Chicago Press.

Nordhaus, W. D. *et al.* (2008). The question of global warming: an exchange. *The New York Review of Books* **55**: 14.

Nossiter, A. (2011). In Sierra Leone, new hope for children and pregnant women. *The New York Times*, July 18.

Ooms, G. *et al.* (2008). The "diagonal" approach to Global Fund financing: a cure for the broader malaise of health systems? *Globalization and Health 4*: **6**, i7 p.

Over, M. (2008). *Prevention Failure: The Ballooning Entitlement Burden of U.S. Global AIDS Treatment Spending and What to Do about It*. Washington DC: Center for Global Development.

Over, M. (2010). *Using Incentives to Prevent HIV Infections*. Washington DC: Center for Global Development.

Park, B. J. *et al.* (2009). Estimation of the current global burden of cryptococcal meningitis among persons living with HIV/AIDS. *AIDS 2009*, **23**: 525–30.

Perfect, J. R., Dismukes, W. E., Dromer, F., Goldman, D. L., Graybill, J. R., Hamill, R. J., Harrison, T. S., Larsen, R. A., Lortholary, O., Nguyen, M. H., Pappas, P. G., Powderly, W. G., Singh, N., Sobel, J. D. and Sorrell, T. C. (2010). Clinical practice guidelines for the management of cryptococcal disease: 2010 update by the infectious diseases society of America. *Clin Infect Dis.* **50**(3): 291–322.

Piot, P., Kazatchkine, M., Dybul, M. and Lob-Levyt, J. (2009). AIDS: lessons learnt and myths dispelled. *TheLancet.com online*, March 20.

Post, S. and McGreevey, W. (2005). *Additionality: Dimensions, Issues and Indicators. Measuring the Systems Effect of the Global Fund with a Focus on Additionality, Partnerships, and Sustainability.* Geneva: The Global Fund.

Punchak, M. (2011). Cost-effectiveness of cryptococcal antigen screening of at-risk HIV/AIDS patients in South Africa in order to save lives associated with human cryptococcosis. Draft. London: LSHTM.

Raja, S. and Bates, J. (2009). Strengthening health systems: the role of supply chains in addressing the HIV epidemic. In Lule, E. L., Seifman, R. M. and David, A. C. (2009). *The Changing HIV/AIDS Landscape: Selected Papers for the World Bank's Agenda for Action in Africa, 2007–2011.* Washington DC: World Bank, pp. 411–26.

Robberstad, B. and Evjen-Olsen, B. (2010). Preventing mother to child transmission of HIV with highly active antiretroviral treatment in Tanzania – a prospective cost-effectiveness study. *Jaids – Journal of Acquired Immune Deficiency Syndromes* **55**(3): 397–403.

Roberts, M. J., Hsiao, W., Berman, P. and Reich, M. R. (2004). *Getting Health Reform Right: A Guide to Improving Performance and Equity.* New York: Oxford University Press.

Savedoff, W. (2010). Basic economics of result-based financing in health. Mimeo. Bath, Maine: Social Insight.

Scharfstein, J. A., Paltiel, A. D. and Freedberg, K. A. (1997). The cost-effectiveness of fluconazole prophylaxis against primary systemic fungal infections in AIDS patients. *Med Decis Making.* **17**(4): 373–81.

Schwartländer, B. *et al.* (2001). AIDS. Resource needs for HIV/AIDS. *Science* **292**(5526): 2434–6.

Schwartländer, B. *et al.* (2011). Towards an improved investment approach for an effective response to HIV. *The Lancet online*, June 3.

Serneels, P. *et al.* (2005). An honorable calling? Findings from the first wave of a cohort study with final year nursing and medical students in Ethiopia. Policy Research Working Paper No. 3686.

Shillcutt, S. D., Walker, D. G., Goodman and Mills, A. J. (2009). Cost-effectiveness in low- and middle-income countries: a review of the debates surrounding decision rules. *Pharmacoeconomics* **27**(11): 903–17.

Sloan, D. J., Dedicoat, M. J. and Lalloo, D. G. (2009). Treatment of cryptococcal meningitis in resource limited settings. *Curr Opin Infect Dis.* **22**(5): 455–63.

Tandon, A. (2009). Development assistance for health: some recent trends and implications. Mimeo. Washington DC: World Bank.

Task Force on Innovative International Financing for Health Systems. (2009). *More Money for Health, and More Health for the Money.* Geneva: WHO.

The Economist. (2011). AIDS: The 30 years war. June 4, pp. 11, 89–91.

The New York Times. (2011). The value of Medicaid, an editorial. *The New York Times*, July 18, A16.

Thornton, R. (2005). *The Demand for and Impact of Learning HIV Status: Evidence from a Field Experiment.* Southern African Regional Poverty Network.

United Nations. (2011). *The Millennium Development Goals Report.* New York: United Nations.

Viscusi, W. K. (1993). The value of risks to life and health. *Journal of Economic Literature* **31**(4): 1912–46.

Viscusi, W. K. and Aldy, J. E. (2003). The value of a statistical life: a critical review of market estimates throughout the world. *The Journal of Risk and Uncertainty* **27**(1): 5–76.

Warner, A. (2010). *Cost-Benefit Analysis in World Bank Projects.* Washington DC: Independent Evaluation Group, World Bank.

World Health Organization. (2007). *Everybody's Business: Strengthening Health Systems to Improve Health Outcomes. WHO's Framework for Action.* Geneva: World Health Organization.

Strengthening health systems

Perspectives for economic evaluation

Perspective paper

TILL BÄRNIGHAUSEN, DAVID E. BLOOM,
AND SALAL HUMAIR

Thirty years into the HIV epidemic, and in spite of significant progress against the disease in the last decade, HIV still causes enormous human suffering, extracts a huge financial cost, and imposes a daunting challenge for the future – 33 million people living with HIV (UN 2011b), 2.6 million new HIV infections, and 1.8 million HIV-related deaths in 2009 (UNAIDS 2010); annual global spending approximately $16 billion (UNAIDS 2011a); and resource needs projected at $22 billion/year by 2015 (for the UNAIDS strategic investment priorities (Schwartländer *et al.* 2011)), or as much as $35 billion/year by 2031 under a different investment trajectory (Hecht *et al.* 2009).

Extraordinary commitment, great gains

The past decade has seen the emergence of extraordinary global political commitment for fighting the HIV epidemic, unprecedented increases in donor funding for HIV, and exceptional progress in translating funding into programs and results. The global commitment was manifested in multiple UN General Assembly declarations recognizing HIV/AIDS as a "global crisis" (UN 2001), resolving to achieve universal access to anti-retroviral treatment (ART) by 2010 (UN 2006), and pledging to intensify efforts to eliminate HIV (UN 2011b). This global resolve translated to a nearly ten-fold increase in global spending on HIV from 2001 to 2010 (from $1.6 billion to $16 billion), fueled by bilateral donors (e.g., US President's Emergency Plan for AIDS Relief (PEPFAR)), multilateral institutions (e.g., the Global Fund to Fight AIDS,

Tuberculosis and Malaria (the Global Fund)), and private philanthropic organizations (e.g., the Bill and Melinda Gates Foundation (BMGF)). The result was a nearly 22-fold increase in the number of people receiving ART from 2001 to 2010 (about 6.6 million by the end of 2010) (UNAIDS 2011a) and an estimated 17 percent decline in the number of new infections from 2001 to 2008 (UNAIDS 2010).

New challenges

But the gains of the last decade are fragile, and barring new technological breakthroughs for fighting HIV, the coming decade could be very different for three reasons: (i) an expanding gap between available treatment resources and stated goals; (ii) flat-lining or declining donor support for global HIV programs; and (iii) the emergence of new demands on the global health community, such as the rise in non-communicable diseases in the developing world. The expanding gap between available and desired treatment resources comes from multiple sources: the new UN goal of achieving universal coverage by 2015 (UN 2011b); WHO's revised ART eligibility guidelines (from CD4 count$<200/\mu$l to CD4 count$<350/\mu$l) (WHO 2010) that have increased the number of people needing ART worldwide from 10 to 15 million (WHO *et al.* 2010); and the emergence of new evidence that treatment is a highly effective form of prevention (Cohen *et al.* 2011; Lancet Editorial 2011), which has led to a chorus of calls for expanding the use of ART for prevention much earlier in the progression of the disease (Economist 2011; Sidibé 2011; UNAIDS 2011a). Flat-lining or declining funding is a direct result of the global financial crisis that began in 2008; and although the UN General Assembly has just pledged to close the $6 billion gap between current funding ($16 billion in 2010) and the estimated need for 2015 (UN 2011), the fulfillment of this pledge remains uncertain as the world economy continues to be buffeted by new crises in Europe, the United States, and Japan. The emergence of new demands on the global health community was prominently highlighted by the UN General Assembly's High-Level Meeting in September 2011 on prevention and control of non-communicable diseases. The UN Secretary General's request seeking commitments for addressing non-communicable diseases at a priority level compatible with other diseases like HIV (UN 2011c), and the General Assembly's resolution reaffirming commitment to strengthening national health systems (rather than a particular disease like HIV) (UN 2010), could further contribute to shifting donor foci and funds away from HIV.

Increasing debates, shifting structures

In this environment, the HIV community is increasingly asking if past strategies for dealing with HIV through stand-alone interventions are still adequate, or if a more sustainable approach is to integrate HIV programs with other health care delivery. Of particular interest is the debate as to whether (i) HIV programs should be fully integrated with the primary health care system, (ii) it would be better to move toward "selective integration" of HIV services with other disease-specific programs within the overall health system, (iii) there should be "selective expansion" of current HIV programs to include synergistic HIV-related and -unrelated services for patients receiving ART (e.g., STI treatment, reproductive health services, treatment of cardiovascular diseases or mental health disorders), or (iv) HIV funding should be used to spur development in other sectors (e.g., in sex equality, education, and social protection) (Schwartländer *et al.* 2011).

For example, the Thematic Panel Discussion at the 2011 UN High-Level Meeting on AIDS recently examined how to integrate HIV with TB, sexual and reproductive health, and maternal and child health services (UN 2011a). And the recent UN declaration on HIV (UN 2011b) explicitly commits to redoubling efforts to strengthen health systems in developing countries through several initiatives (e.g., decentralizing HIV programs and/or integrating HIV programs with primary care programs).

In fact, the shift towards health systems strengthening (HSS) is already happening within initiatives previously dedicated only to HIV-specific interventions. For instance, PEPFAR, which has allocated more than $32 billion since 2004 for bilateral HIV programs (PEPFAR 2011), and the Global Fund,[1] which has committed approximately $22 billion since 2002 for HIV (The Global Fund 2011b), have recently started to invest more in HSS as part of their HIV portfolio investments. More specifically, PEPFAR has recognized the need to incorporate a health systems perspective into its programs, and has committed to training 140,000 health care workers, managers, administrators, and planning experts needed for critical functions of the health system (PEPFAR 2009a). One of its five goals for 2010 through 2014 is to integrate HIV programs with broader global health and development programs (PEPFAR 2009b). The US Global Health Initiative (GHI), the new umbrella organization for US global health engagements, includes strengthening health systems as a core objective (US Global Health Initiative 2011b). GHI activities encompass assistance for a broad range of areas, such as improving research and regulatory capacity, improving human resources, and supporting policy changes outside the health sector that can help improve health outcomes (US Global Health Initiative 2011a). The Global Fund is now seeking proposals for HSS interventions that cut across diseases, e.g., upgrading primary health care facilities, and reinforcing planning and policy-making

---

[1] PEPFAR has also contributed about $6 billion to The Global Fund since 2004, in addition to the $32 billion it allocated for bilateral programs.

capacities of ministries of health (The Global Fund 2011a).

Perspectives for evaluating health systems interventions

The growing focus on HSS simultaneously with HIV interventions has the potential to improve the effectiveness, efficiency, and sustainability of HIV programs. But two perspectives need to be kept in mind in setting expectations for (i) when positive impact on HIV programs can be achieved through HSS, and (ii) what interventions can be envisaged within the rubric of HSS, and what challenges they pose for the evaluation of costs and benefits.

Setting expectations: one structure does not fit all

The potential of HSS to improve HIV programs is unlikely to be realized through the undifferentiated integration of HIV programs into countries' general health care systems. A single structure (e.g., stand-alone HIV programs or HIV care delivered solely through the general primary health care systems) will not necessarily be well suited to all contexts. Donors and governments should carefully consider the characteristics of a particular setting to determine which mix of integration will work best there, assessing intervention feasibility and efficiency, as well as the flexibility in adjusting interventions and the ease of evaluating intervention impact (Bärnighausen *et al*. 2011).

Feasibility

A focus on one particular structure may not be feasible, for political or humanitarian reasons. For instance, in Nigeria and Pakistan, vertical polio campaigns almost ground to a halt in the face of religious and political opposition; and against similar opposition, stand-alone HIV programs could also become inaccessible or at best inefficient. On the other hand, in public health emergencies requiring rapid humanitarian responses, such as large unmet need for HIV treatment, stand-alone programs may be the only feasible option since they can be rapidly brought to scale, whereas HSS may take an unacceptably long time.

Technical efficiency

Stand-alone HIV interventions can be efficient for their specific focus, but inefficient at the health system level and at the societal level. *Increased* efficiency can result from health workers specializing and adapting their workflow to HIV treatment and prevention. *Decreased* efficiency can result at the level of the overall health care system from duplication of functions that are required in providing care for more than one disease, such as drug supply chains, laboratory facilities, and patient-record keeping. Inefficiency at the societal level can result because many HIV-infected patients suffer from diseases that are biologically or behaviorally related to HIV infection or treatment, e.g., opportunistic infections and cardiovascular diseases. HIV-infected patients who must travel between different facilities to receive complete care have to invest more time and money utilizing needed care than patients who can receive all their care in one place.

Flexibility

Stand-alone HIV programs may not be flexible enough for evolving health goals, even though they may be appropriate in the short term. The narrow scope of isolated delivery programs is likely to be especially problematic when a population's health care needs and demands are changing rapidly – for example, in countries undergoing rapid socioeconomic development with changing lifestyles, health risk-taking, and care-seeking behavior. In some situations, HIV programs may also draw resources such as health care workers away from general health systems, weakening the delivery of general health care. Furthermore, an excessive HIV focus may distract from long-term planning priorities, such as training an appropriate generalist health care workforce. But a positive effect from HIV programs is also possible if they can provide the motivation and resources to build specific types of capacity that can benefit the entire health system, as in the PEPFAR-supported USAID/DELIVER PROJECT for drug supply chains.

Evaluation

The emphasis on HSS instead of a narrower focus on HIV programs may also impede rigorous evaluation of program impact. Donor organizations increasingly require evaluation of interventions' impact on population health. Health systems interventions such as building infrastructure, training health care workers, or integrating HIV programs into general health care systems are often difficult to evaluate, because their effects are realized over the medium and long term – and because they affect multiple disease outcomes, they are insufficient on their own to guarantee that effective HIV treatment and care is delivered. The simultaneous trends toward HSS and better evaluation of impact thus run counter to one another, and both donors and governments need to carefully consider the increased difficulty of evaluating impact when shifting focus from HIV programs to HSS (Bärnighausen et al. 2012).

For these reasons, estimates of the impact of HIV interventions that seek to also strengthen health systems are difficult to obtain, making it difficult to do a comprehensive analysis of their costs and benefits. In the section *Evaluating costs and benefits*, we highlight the kind of issues that arise in doing a cost-benefit analysis for such interventions, by looking at some specific interventions identified by McGreevey et al. (2011) for the *RethinkHIV* project. We highlight both general issues raised when evaluating such interventions, and particular issues that are illustrated by the McGreevey et al. analyses.

Envisaging interventions: level and scope of intervention, and issues in evaluation

A framework is needed to guide the debate about HSS interventions, because a wide variety of HSS interventions that entail quite different costs, consequences, risks, and implementation challenges are being discussed in the literature (McGreevey et al. 2011; Schwartländer et al. 2011; UN 2011a). We discuss such a framework below, which can help clarify the goals of particular HSS interventions and thus help understand the issues involved in their evaluation.

Level and scope of interventions

HSS interventions may be envisaged as HIV-focused non-structural (HIVNS), HIV-focused structural (HIVS), or general structural (GS). HIVNS interventions aim towards expanding prevention, diagnosis, treatment, or care services for HIV *within* the structure of existing HIV programs, however these programs may be organized. Examples of such interventions include the conditional cash transfer intervention to incentivize people to get tested for HIV and the cryptococcal meningitis testing/treatment intervention proposed in McGreevey et al. (2011). HIVS interventions aim to expand HIV services through new structures, or to admit more services within HIV programs, or to integrate HIV programs into general health systems, thus affecting the structure of current HIV programs. Examples of such interventions include the training and deployment of community health workers to deliver HIV treatment as proposed by McGreevey et al. (2011), or addition of HIV-related or -unrelated services to HIV programs as by Schwartländer et al. (2011). GS interventions aim to broadly improve the functioning of the health system, with the hope that such strengthening can lead to improved HIV-related outcomes. GS interventions are essentially horizontal interventions, which aim to deliver care for several diseases simultaneously (Bärnighausen et al. 2011). Examples of GS interventions include the setting up of an independent fund to incentivize governments in sub-Saharan Africa to increase their allocations for health, as proposed in McGreevey et al. (2011).

Evaluating benefits

The focus of HSS interventions is progressively broadened when moving from HIVNS to HIVS to GS interventions, making the evaluation of their benefits increasingly difficult. HIVNS interventions focus on narrow sets of health outcomes (e.g., mortality and morbidity in HIV-infected individuals), while HIVNS and GS interventions are intended to affect a wider range of health outcomes. Full evaluation of GS interventions is more difficult than full evaluation of HIVNS interventions, because wider populations with a larger set of morbidities and causes of mortality have to be observed. A narrow evaluation of GS interventions that focuses only on HIV-infected persons or a select set of measures (e.g., maternal mortality, or under-five mortality) is not useful for many decision-making purposes because large components of the total effect might be neglected, e.g., a health worker intervention may save many life-years in diseases not considered.

Evaluating costs

A further complication arises when deciding which costs to include in the evaluation of different interventions. HIV-focused programs are commonly financed exclusively by one agency. Where multiple funders contribute to such programs, the contributions of the different agencies are often clearly visible to all funders. For instance, in South Africa, both PEPFAR and the South African government contribute to the funding of the public-sector ART program (Houlihan *et al.* 2011). This joint effort is coordinated and both parties can easily obtain information on financial outlays contributed by the other parties (Bärnighausen *et al.* 2011b). In contrast, in some types of horizontal programs, it may be much more difficult for the primary funder to obtain realistic estimates of the financial contributions of other agencies, because these programs will likely require more diverse sets of inputs and because these inputs will not be utilized exclusively by the horizontal programs. For instance, programs improving the supply chains of medicines to primary care clinics will likely require support by health workers in central pharmacies and by the health workers in the primary care clinics receiving the medicines. However, these health workers will only spend some portion of their time supporting the supply chain intervention. This portion is unlikely to be known without additional research effort, such as time-motion studies or health worker interviews. GS interventions are thus likely to imply substantially increased difficulty in determining an intervention's cost-benefit ratio.

Differing time-lags and levels of certainty

HIVNS interventions will commonly generate health impacts more quickly than horizontal ones. This occurs because interventions solely focused on benefitting HIV-infected populations generally need to be in place before an HIVNS intervention (e.g., ART delivery) can begin. By contrast, HSS interventions such as GS interventions require years of investment before the end results are visible, because, e.g., an investment into medical or nursing education will require many years before doctors and nurses become available to deliver ART. Similarly, the establishment of an electronic patient record system may require procurement of laptops, development of software, health worker training, and field testing before it can contribute to the quality or efficiency of ART delivery and improve health outcomes in patients. The longer the time lags between intervention and outcomes, the more complicated it will be to determine the costs and benefits of the intervention.

Even if GS can be rigorously evaluated, we may learn less from the evaluation results than in the case of the evaluation of HIVNS interventions, because GS interventions are commonly mediated through longer causal chains than HIVNS ones, and the number of factors that can modify intervention effects will likely increase. Take, for instance, a training program to increase the capacity of district health managers to plan the delivery of HIV programs. For this GS intervention to have an effect on population health, it will be necessary for district health managers to be trained and acquire new skills, and be willing to use their new skills. The impact on health outcomes will then further depend on the ability of the manager to effect changes in the actual delivery of ART. It is this actual delivery, on the other hand, which is usually the starting point for the evaluation of HIVNS programs such as ART programs. Thus, the mediating steps from the district health worker intervention to a health impact are many more than those from the ART program to health impact, and contextual factors influencing district health managers' capacity to use newly acquired skills will likely increase the heterogeneity of effects across settings (Bärnighausen *et al.* 2012).

Differences in mediating factors will lead to heterogeneity in estimated impacts across settings. The larger the number of mediating factors between the intervention and the outcome, the more resources will be required to either observe or control for all mediating factors. As the number of mediating factors will commonly increase as the intervention structure changes from HIVNS to GS, it is likely that impact evaluation that can shed light on the effects of programs across settings or populations will be more complex and require more resources for GS than for HIVNS interventions.

Evaluating costs and benefits

McGreevey *et al.* (2011) were commissioned by *RethinkHIV* to assess the costs and benefits of viable HIV interventions that also strengthen general health systems, under the assumption that an additional $2 billion per year can be spent on these interventions for the next five years in sub-Saharan Africa. The authors discuss four specific interventions and the magnitude of resources required for each:

- Conditional cash transfers (CCTs) to motivate adults to seek HIV testing, and thus reduce the number of HIV-infected people unaware of their status. The cost to test 400 million adults using a $5 voucher per person is estimated at $2 billion. The main benefit considered is a reduction in new infections by about 0.25 million annually.
- Deploy a large number of rural community health workers (CHWs) for HIV testing, diagnosis, and early stage treatment, as well as for delivering other basic health services, such as unmet need for family planning among rural women (particularly those tested to be HIV-infected). The cost is estimated at $640 million. The main benefit considered is a reduction in maternal deaths by about 0.3 million annually, and a reduction in infant mortality by 0.1 million lives annually (through reduction in infant HIV infections).
- Test HIV-infected people for cryptococcal meningitis (CM), an opportunistic infection associated with HIV, and treat those found to have CM. The cost is estimated at $1.3 billion. The benefits considered are an increase in life expectancy of people infected with CM by an average of 9.6 years.
- Provide cash on delivery (COD) to governments to increase the share of health spending in their overall public spending so they meet the Abuja

goals (15 percent of public spending on health), with the hope that strengthened health systems will also lead to better HIV treatment results. The benefits considered include under-five, maternal, HIV, and TB deaths averted, and a decrease in fertility rate.

For each intervention, the authors provide a qualitative discussion and calculate a cost-benefit ratio under at least one central assumption – e.g., assuming that CCTs can reduce annual infections by 250,000 annually, or assuming that 90 percent of the unmet need for family planning could be eliminated among women living with HIV. They then use available estimates about the number of lives saved, infections averted, etc., and the value of life and disability-adjusted life years (DALYs) suggested by *RethinkHIV*, to compute a benefit to cost ratio. The paper highlights considerable variation in the benefit to cost ratios of the interventions, but concludes by noting that the benefits collectively outweigh the costs.

General issues

As the authors note, these interventions involve unequal effort, target different population segments (e.g., all vs. women only), and affect different aspects of HIV (e.g., prevention vs. treatment), which makes it difficult to compare their cost-benefit ratio. In addition, the exact impact of such interventions, i.e., which specific aspects of the health system will be strengthened and by how much, is difficult to gauge. For instance, two of the interventions are explicitly focused on the demand side of HIV programs (CCTs and CM testing), and it is hard to be exact about how much they will strengthen general health systems. The two other interventions (training CHWs and COD) are focused on HSS, but operate at very different levels (CHW is focused only on HIV, and COD is focused on the entire health system). Therefore, it is hard to predict their impact because they are separated from the final health outcomes by many mediating steps.

Unintended consequences

Even if we could account for some consequences, the other difficulty in doing a cost-benefit analysis is that interventions for HSS could have a range of unintended consequences that may be difficult to identify and to quantify. Foreseeable consequences could include excessive resources required to manage the demand generated by the CCTs, or the negative social and political costs if enough resources are not made available to treat people who discover that they are HIV-infected, or an open-ended financial commitment to keep offering incentives for coming years. Unintended consequences may arise if CCTs lose their effectiveness over time, or if they "spoil the well," i.e., create an expectation that desirable behavior must be financially rewarded, thus reducing the likelihood of behavior change if a financial reward is not offered (de Walque *et al.* 2011). Our knowledge of the benefits and harms of individual-level financial incentives for changing behaviors that lead to improved HIV-related health outcomes is still evolving (Aidstar-One 2011), as is our understanding of government-level financial incentives (Over 2010).

Scale of intervention

The other challenge in cost-benefit analysis of the interventions proposed by McGreevey *et al.* is the different scales of implementation. The scale at which an intervention is implemented (e.g., offering CCT to everyone, or 80 percent of those in need of testing) affects its cost-benefit calculations, if either the effectiveness of an intervention is a non-linear function of the resources allocated to the intervention, or the costs are non-linearly increasing in the scale of the intervention. In such cases, the cost-benefit calculation will produce different values for the same intervention delivered at different scales. While the debate about how to account for issues of scale in cost-benefit and cost-effectiveness analyses for HIV interventions continues (Committee 2008; Kumaranayake 2008; Moatti *et al.* 2008), it is prudent to compare multiple cost-benefit values at differing scales of a given intervention to provide better guidance to policy-makers.

Implementation time

The proposed interventions also have very different times for implementation. These differing time-horizons can lead to two kinds of problems in cost-benefit calculations. First, the longer time period for health system interventions to take effect means

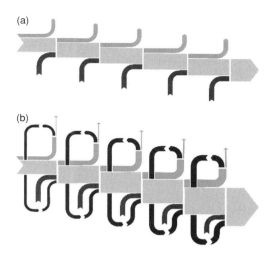

Figure 4.1.1 *(a) Model that does not incorporate feedback due to reduced mortality because of ART. (b) Model that does incorporate feedback due to reduced mortality because of ART*[2]

that discounted future benefits are likely to assess HSS interventions unfavorably against solely HIV-focused interventions. Second, accumulating benefits over time requires that we accommodate positive and negative feedback loops created by the interventions themselves.

Feedback

We know that provision of ART at a moderate to high coverage level produces a positive feedback loop that significantly increases future resources required for increasing coverage (Bärnighausen *et al.* 2007, 2009, 2010c). This feedback can be substantial, and models that do not account for it can significantly mis-estimate the costs and benefits of the interventions. Figures 4.1.1 and 4.1.2 show the magnitude of the effect feedback has on human resource requirements for ART, due to the mortality reduction effects of ART. Similar feedback loops may occur in other forms, e.g., the feedback

---

[2] Time is in years from left to right. The population needing ART is represented by the thickness of the main flow – if we consider the thickness of the starting flow from the left as 100 percent then about 30 percent more people are added to the pool requiring ART each year (These figures reflect approximately the 9 million needing ART globally, to which about 2.7 million new people needing ART are added each year (WHO 2009).

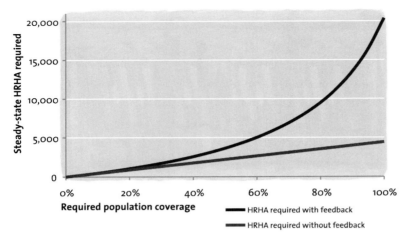

Figure 4.1.2 *Human resources required to provide universal ART coverage for SSA, expressed as a function of population ART coverage*

from ART to reduction in future HIV infections, or from changes in behavior due to prevention interventions to future infections (Bärnighausen *et al*. 2010a, 2010b).

Such difficulties raise the need for models more sophisticated than static cost-benefit calculations, for capturing time-varying intervention effects of HSS interventions. These models will have to be more powerful than the already existing tools at the HIV community's disposal. For instance, while a range of models specific to HIV are available for estimating time-varying effects of HIV interventions, they only consider a limited set of AIDS-related outputs (mortality, new infections, etc.) – e.g., epidemiological models, micro-simulations, and system dynamics models (Brown *et al*. 2010; Dangerfield *et al*. 2001; Stover *et al*. 2010a), and the freely available UNAIDS Spectrum modeling tools (Stover *et al*. 2010b; UNAIDS 2011b). Extending them to consider a broader range of outputs affected by HSS interventions offers an opportunity for productive original research.

Target populations and priority setting

When comparing the benefits and costs of different health interventions, it is crucial to consider to whom they accrue. In adding benefits and costs across different population groups, cost-benefit analysis always implies distributional value choices. For instance, weighting everybody equally

in the analysis, as McGreevey *et al.* do, implies an egalitarian position. However, health policy-makers and societies commonly consider targeting particular populations in priority setting for the health sector, e.g., "vulnerable populations" or populations suffering from particularly severe diseases (Jehu-Appiah *et al.* 2008). The four interventions considered by McGreevey *et al.* benefit very different populations: HIV-infected people suffering from cryptococcosis (CM testing), pregnant women and children (CHW), and the general population (COD and CCT). If policy-makers and societies indeed give priority to particular populations (such as pregnant women, children, or HIV-infected individuals) a comparison of the results of cost-benefit analyses of interventions affecting different populations would only be meaningful, if the results accounted for these preferences.

Specific issues

In spite of such difficulties, McGreevey *et al.* (2011) present a cost-benefit ratio for each intervention under particular assumptions. For example, for CCTs, they assume providing a $5 voucher to 400 million people to get tested will reduce infections by 0.25 million annually; for CHW training, they assume spending $640 million can eliminate 90 percent of the unmet need for family planning; for CODs, they calculate benefits assuming a $1 billion endowment fund can be used to

Table 4.1.1 A framework for thinking about HSS interventions and the challenges they raise for cost-benefit analyses

	HSS Interventions Framework			Impacts on evaluation and cost-benefit analysis		
Acronym	Type of intervention	Main aim	Examples	Benefits	Costs	Time lag and uncertainty
HIVNS	HIV non-structural interventions	Expand prevention, diagnosis, treatment, or care services for HIV within the structure of existing HIV programs	Conditional cash transfer intervention to incentivize people to get tested for HIV (McGreevey et al. 2011) and cryptococcal meningitis testing/treatment (McGreevey et al. 2011)	Limited in number, easier to evaluate (AIDS-related mortality etc.)	Limited number of sources of cost information and more control over cost information because of funding structure, costs incurred closer to program delivery	Causal chains from intervention to ultimate effects short
HIVS	HIV structural interventions	Expand HIV services through new structures, or to include more services within HIV programs, or to integrate HIV programs into general health systems, thus affecting the structure of current HIV programs	Training, deployment of community health workers to deliver HIV treatment (McGreevey et al. 2011), addition of HIV-related or -unrelated services to HIV programs (Schwartländer et al. 2011)	Some benefits easier to evaluate (AIDS-related mortality etc.), others difficult (counseling for STI, how much benefit displaced from other STI interventions)	Some costs easier to measure, others difficult	Causal chains from intervention to some effects short, other effects long
GS	General structural interventions	Broadly improve the functioning of the health system, with the hope that such strengthening can lead to improved HIV-related outcomes	Setting up an independent fund to incentivize governments in sub-Saharan Africa to increase their allocations for health (McGreevey et al. 2011), creating a health insurance system	Most benefits difficult to evaluate (prevention and treatment across many diseases, long-term behavioral change at both individual and population level)	Costs often difficult to identify conceptually, measure because of many different contributors, and attribute to different causes (training of doctors as a case)	Causal chains from intervention to ultimate effects long

incentivize governments in sub-Saharan Africa to spend up to $52 billion on health.

Some of these assumptions appear optimistic, such as being able to meet 90 percent of the family planning need in HIV-infected women through CHWs immediately, assuming that CHWs can also deliver ART, or that we can incentivize governments to spend $52 billion on health using an endowment fund of $1 billion. For comparison, Schwartländer *et al.* (2011) assume 80 percent ART coverage as a measure of widespread treatment, and assume that 86 percent ART coverage can be reached universally after ten years. Since ART coverage and family planning are linked in the CHW intervention, family planning coverage could follow a similar trajectory, and maintaining this coverage could require a long time horizon. Similarly, for the endowment fund, it might be useful to do a historical comparative study on how far external donor flows have increased country allocations to specific or general health priorities. In general, at this stage the evidence base for the impact of HSS interventions is not strong, and cost-benefit calculations must rely on strong assumptions without empirical support. One way to address this problem is to do a sensitivity analysis of costs and benefits around the assumptions. But such sensitivity analysis is typically most useful when there are non-linear, dynamic, or feedback effects (i.e., either the effects or the costs are non-linear as a function of the scale of implementation, or across time), otherwise both costs and effects are simply linear in the assumed effect sizes and sensitivity analysis does not generate new insights.

The proposed interventions also illustrate why one needs to consider carefully the pathways to intervention effects more broadly when reasoning about the impact on health systems. For instance, for CCTs, it is not clear how the reduction in infections by 0.25 million will occur. Presumably that will require some other form of prevention intervention or treatment with its attendant costs, since there is hardly any evidence that simply being aware of HIV status can reduce new infections significantly. Those extra costs will affect the cost-benefit calculations significantly. It is also not clear how the demand for testing generated by the vouchers will be met. Is the capacity to provide the additional

testing and counseling services already available, or will capacity need to be expanded, requiring further expenditures, to accommodate the 400 million people who are willing to be tested because of the intervention?

For long-lasting interventions, such as the creation of the Abuja Fund, focusing only on direct recurring costs of the interventions (as opposed to other administrative or capital costs) may be dictated by necessity at this stage, but other costs will need to be considered at least qualitatively to determine if a proposed intervention is realistic in a given country. For instance, a country with a very high degree of corruption would offer a difficult challenge in monitoring the use of resources disbursed under the Abuja Fund, and may require the setting up of costly independent monitoring and evaluation structures.

Finally, the cost-benefit ratio alone is not sufficient to distinguish between interventions, without considering other factors. For instance, CM testing will benefit a small minority of people who are HIV-infected, so its cost-benefit ratio alone is not a good indicator for comparison with other interventions thought to benefit many people.

Conclusions

The recent shift towards funding HSS as opposed to funding only stand-alone HIV interventions has the potential to increase the effectiveness, efficiency, and sustainability of HIV programs. But several issues arise when considering when and how to combine HSS interventions with HIV-focused programs, and how to evaluate their costs and benefits. First, the combination needs to be designed taking into account each country's circumstances. Second, HSS interventions can differ substantially in scope or scale, raising different challenges in the evaluation of costs and benefits. Finally, a full evaluation of an intervention needs to take into account issues such as feedback resulting from the intervention itself; and unintended consequences that can have major implications, particularly for the cost-benefit analyses of interventions such as those proposed by McGreevey *et al.* Dynamic models that incorporate both feedback and unintended consequences are essential for a proper cost-benefit accounting of HSS interventions.

References

Aidstar-One. (2011). *Debate Five: The Ethics of Material Incentives for HIV Prevention.* Emerging Issues in Today's HIV Response Debate Series (available at www.aidstar-one.com/events/emerging_issues_todays_hiv_response_debate_series/ethics_material_incentives_hiv_prevention). AIDSTAR-One, John Snow, Inc. for USAID.

Bärnighausen, T., Bloom, D. E. and Humair, S. (2007). Human resources for treating HIV/AIDS: needs, capacities, and gaps. *AIDS Patient Care and STDs* **21**: 799–812.

Bärnighausen, T., Bloom, D. and Humair, S. (2009). *A Mathematical Model for Estimating the Number of Health Workers for Universal Antiretroviral Treatment.* National Bureau of Economic Research (NBER) Working Paper #15517.

Bärnighausen, T., Bloom, D. and Humair, S. (2010a). Assessing the impact of the global financial crisis on ART programs: a behavioral feedback model. Oral presentation at the 11th International Congress of Behavioral Medicine (ICBM), August 4–7, 2010, Washington, DC.

Bärnighausen, T., Bloom, D. and Humair, S. (2010b). The sustainability of anti-retroviral treatment: the case of South Africa. Oral presentation at International AIDS and Economics Network, August 16–17, 2010, Vienna.

Bärnighausen, T., Bloom, D. and Humair, S. (2010c). Universal antiretroviral treatment: the challenge of human resources. *Bull World Health Organ* **88**: 951–2.

Bärnighausen, T., Bloom, D. and Humair, S. (2011). Going horizontal – shifts in funding of global health interventions. *New England Journal of Medicine* **364**: 2181–3.

Bärnighausen, T., Bloom, D. and Humair, S. (2012). Health systems and HIV treatment in sub-Saharan Africa: matching intervention and program evaluation strategies. *Sex Transm Infect* **88**(2): e2.

Brown, T., Bao, L., Raftery, A. E., Salomon, J. A., Baggaley, R. F., Stover, J. and Gerland, P. (2010). Modelling HIV epidemics in the antiretroviral era: the UNAIDS Estimation and Projection package 2009. *Sexually Transmitted Infections* **86**: ii3–ii10.

Cohen, M. S., Chen, Y. Q., Mccauley, M., Gamble, T., Hosseinipour, M. C., Kumarasamy, N., Hakim, J. G., Kumwenda, J., Grinsztejn, B., Pilotto, J. H. S., Godbole, S. V., Mehendale, S., Chariyalertsak, S., Santos, B. R., Mayer, K. H., Hoffman, I. F., Eshleman, S. H., Piwowar-Manning, E., Wang, L., Makhema, J., Mills, L. A., De Bruyn, G., Sanne, I., Eron, J., Gallant, J., Havlir, D., Swindells, S., Ribaudo, H., Elharrar, V., Burns, D., Taha, T. E., Nielsen-Saines, K., Celentano, D., Essex, M. and Fleming, T. R. (2011). Prevention of HIV-1 infection with early antiretroviral therapy. *New England Journal of Medicine*, 0.

Committee, E. S. (2008). Informing scale-up and resource allocation: the use of economic analysis. *AIDS* **22**: S5–S6, 10.1097/01.ids.0000327617.93737.82.

Dangerfield, B. C., Fang, Y. and Roberts, C. A. (2001). Model-based scenarios for the epidemiology of HIV/AIDS: the consequences of highly active anti-retroviral therapy. *System Dynamics Review* **17**: 119–50.

De Walque, D., Kazianga, H. and Over, M. (2011). *Antiretroviral Therapy Awareness and Risky Sexual Behaviors: Evidence from Mozambique.* Working Paper 239. Washington, DC: Center for Global Development.

Economist. (2011). AIDS: the 30 years war. *The Economist*, June 2.

Hecht, R., Bollinger, L., Stover, J., McGreevey, W., Muhib, F., Madavo, C. E. and De Ferranti, D. (2009). Critical choices in financing the response to the global HIV/AIDS pandemic. *Health Aff (Millwood)* **28**: 1591–605.

Houlihan, C. F., Bland, R. M., Mutevedzi, P. C., Lessells, R. J., Ndirangu, J., Thulare, H. and Newell, M.-L. (2011). Cohort Profile: Hlabisa HIV treatment and care programme. *International Journal of Epidemiology* **40**: 318–26.

Jehu-Appiah, C., Baltussen, R., Acquah, C., Aikins, M., D'Almeida, S., Bosu, W., Koolman, X., Lauer, J., Osei, D. and Adjei, S. (2008). Balancing equity and efficiency in health priorities in Ghana: the use of multicriteria decision analysis. *Value in Health* **11**: 1081–7.

Kumaranayake, L. 2008. The economics of scaling up: cost estimation for HIV/AIDS interventions.

AIDS **22**: S23–S33, 10.1097/01.aids. 0000327620.47103.1d.

Lancet Editorial. (2011). HIV treatment as prevention – it works. *The Lancet* **377**: 1719.

McGreevey, W., Avila, C. and Punchak, M. (2011). Strengthening health systems for HIV/AIDS in sub-Saharan Africa: Preliminary note for Copenhagen Consensus Center. Copenhagen Consensus Center.

Moatti, J. P., Marlink, R., Luchini, S. and Kazatchkine, M. (2008). Universal access to HIV treatment in developing countries: going beyond the misinterpretations of the "cost-effectiveness" algorythm. *AIDS* **22**: S59–S66, 10.1097/01.aids.0000327624. 69974.41.

Over, M. (2010). *Using Incentives to Prevent HIV Infections*. Working Paper. Washington, DC: Center for Global Development.

PEPFAR. (2009a). The U.S. President's Emergency Plan for AIDS Relief: Five-Year Strategy, Annex: PEPFAR's Contributions to the Global Health Initiative (December 2009). Washington, DC: The U.S. President's Emergency Plan for AIDS Relief.

PEPFAR. (2009b). The U.S. President's Emergency Plan for AIDS Relief: Five-Year Strategy, Executive Summary of PEPFAR's Strategy (December 2009). Washington, DC: The U.S. President's Emergency Plan for AIDS Relief.

PEPFAR. (2011). Making a Difference: Funding (updated February 2011). Available: www.pepfar.gov/press/80064.htm (accessed March 21, 2011).

Schwartländer, B., Stover, J., Hallett, T., Atun, R., Avila, C., Gouws, E., Bartos, M., Ghys, P. D., Opuni, M., Barr, D., Alsallaq, R., Bollinger, L., De Freitas, M., Garnett, G., Holmes, C., Legins, K., Pillay, Y., Stanciole, A. E., Mcclure, C., Hirnschall, G., Laga, M. and Padian, N. (2011). Towards an improved investment approach for an effective response to HIV/AIDS. *The Lancet* **377**: 2031–41.

Sidibé, M. (2011). The 4th decade of AIDS: what is needed to reshape the response. *UN Chronicle* **XLVII** No. 1 2011 (15.05.2011).

Stover, J., Johnson, P., Hallett, T., Marston, M., Becquet, R. and Timaeus, I. M. (2010a). The Spectrum projection package: improvements in estimating incidence by age and sex, mother-to-child transmission, HIV progression in children and double orphans. *Sexually Transmitted Infections* **86**: ii16–ii21.

Stover, J., McKinnon, R. and Winfrey, B. (2010b). Spectrum: a model platform for linking maternal and child survival interventions with AIDS, family planning and demographic projections. *International Journal of Epidemiology* **39**: i7–i10.

The Global Fund. (2011a). *The Global Fund's Approach to Health Systems Strengthening (HSS): Information Note*. Geneva: The Global Fund to Fight AIDS, Tuberculosis and Malaria.

The Global Fund. (2011b). *Making a Difference: Global Fund Results Report 2011*. Geneva: The Global Fund to Fight AIDS, Tuberculosis and Malaria.

UN. (2001). Declaration of Commitment on HIV/AIDS. New York: United Nations General Assembly Special Session on HIV/AIDS, June 25–27, 2001.

UN. (2006). Declaration of Political Commitment on HIV/AIDS. New York: United Nations General Assembly High Level Meeting on HIV/AIDS, May 31–June 2, 2006.

UN. (2010). Resolution 64/265: Prevention and Control of Non-Communicable Diseases. New York: United Nations General Assembly Sixty-Fourth Session, Agenda Item: 114, May 20, 2001.

UN. (2011a). Panel 5: Integrating the AIDS Response with Broader Health and Development Agendas, Moderated by Laurie Garrett. New York: United Nations 2011 High Level Meeting on AIDS, June 10, 2011.

UN. (2011b). Political Declaration on HIV/AIDS: Intensifying Our Efforts to Eliminate HIV/AIDS. New York: United Nations General Assembly High Level Meeting on HIV/AIDS, June 8–10, 2011.

UN. (2011c). Report of the Secretary General: Prevention and Control of Non-Communicable Diseases, May 19, 2011. New York: United Nations General Assembly Sixty-Sixth Session, Item 119 of the preliminary list, September 19–20, 2011.

UNAIDS. (2010). *Getting to Zero: 2011–2015 Strategy Joint United Nations Programme on HIV/AIDS (UNAIDS)*. Geneva: Joint United Nations Programme on HIV/AIDS (UNAIDS).

UNAIDS. (2011a). *AIDS at 30: Nations at the Crossroads*. Geneva: Joint United Nations Programme on HIV/AIDS (UNAIDS).

UNAIDS. (2011b). *Spectrum/EPP 2011* [Online]. Joint United Nations Programme on HIV/AIDS (UNAIDS). Available: www.unaids.org/en/dataanalysis/tools/spectrumepp2011/ (accessed September 15, 2011).

US Global Health Initiative. (2011a). GHI: Building On and Expanding Existing Platforms. Available: www.ghi.gov/what/platforms/index.htm (accessed August 23, 2011).

US Global Health Initiative. (2011b). The Plan. Available: www.ghi.gov/about/ghi/index.htm (accessed August 23, 2011).

WHO. (2010). *Antiretroviral Therapy for HIV Infection in Adults and Adolescents: Recommendations for a Public Health Approach*. Geneva: World Health Organization.

WHO, UNAIDS and UNICEF. (2010). *Towards Universal Access: Scaling Up Priority HIV/AIDS Interventions in the Health Sector. Progress Report 2010*. Geneva: World Health Organization.

Strengthening health systems

Perspective paper

NICOLI NATTRASS

This perspective paper reflects on the methodology employed by McGreevey *et al.*, comments critically on their proposed solutions, and offers an alternative suggestion: support the Global Fund in its efforts to involve communities in the AIDS response.

Methodological issues

This section considers two methodological concerns about the McGreevey *et al.* paper: their monetization of a human life year; and the way they extrapolate costs and benefits to the entire African continent without taking into account regional differences.

Why monetize the value of a life year?

McGreevey *et al.* employ cost-benefit analysis where the value of a disability-adjusted human life year lost (DALY) is assumed to lie between $1,000 and $5,000, i.e., lower and upper bounds conforming to average per capita incomes in low and rich countries respectively. In Table 4.8, they value adult DALYs at $1,000 and infant DALYs at $500 and then apply different discount rates to infants, adults aged twenty-two, and adults aged fifty. The result is a calculation which incorporates a set of judgements about the value of people at different ages – judgements which should be left up to policy-makers rather than buried in an obscure technical calculation.

Benefit-cost analysis should rather be presented in as simple and as clear a way as possible – and in a manner which facilitates discussion about the social choices involved in evaluating one intervention over another. The clearest metric is cost per life saved, or cost per life year saved, in the current

period. One could also present cost per DALY – but in doing so, policy-makers need to be made aware of the assumptions about the value of human life lived at different ages that are already built into the calculation. For benefit-cost calculations over time, future costs can be discounted by an interest rate – ideally linked to a measure of expected inflation. If policy-makers choose to apply the same discount rate to future years of life, this should be their choice. They may well choose to value current and future years of life on a different basis to cost estimates.

Extrapolating to the whole of Africa without taking into account country differences

The second methodological issue concerns the way in which Africa-wide estimates of the cost of programs or interventions are arrived at by multiplying per person costs (either based on pure assumption or on the basis of single country studies) by the relevant number of adults in Africa. For example, in estimating the costs of rolling out a new cohort of rural community health workers across Africa, data from Malawi are simply extrapolated to the entire continent by multiplying purported per person costs in that country by the number of African adults. Such an exercise is ultimately meaningless not only because the level of economic development (and health systems capacity) varies dramatically across Africa (see Table 4.2.1), but because the number of HIV-positive people is highly concentrated in East and Southern Africa. As shown in Figure 4.2.1, South Africa has more than a quarter of the total HIV-positive African population, and nine countries account for over three quarters of the total. Costs and benefits are thus likely to vary significantly across Africa. Single

Table 4.2.1 Development indicators for the nine countries highlighted in Figure 4.2.1

Country	GNI per capita (2010)	Literacy rate	Poverty head-count ratio	Life expectancy at birth	Births with skilled health staff	HIV prevalence (15–49)	% of young women (men) ever tested for HIV
Kenya	$780	87%	46%	55	44%	6%	18% (13%)
Malawi	$330	74%	52.4%	54	54%	11%	5% (4%)
Mozambique	$440	55%	54.7%	48	55%	12%	13% (6%)
Nigeria	$1,180	61%	54.7%	48	39%	4%	5% (5%)
South Africa	$6,100	89%	23%	52	91%	18%	n/a
Uganda	$490	73%	24.5%	53	42%	7%	n/a
Tanzania	$530	73%	33.4%	56	43%	6%	15% (11%)
Zambia	$1,070	71%	59.3%	46	47%	14%	13% (7%)
Zimbabwe	$460	92%	72%	45	60%	14%	n/a

Sources: World Bank Data (http://data.worldbank.org/), UNAIDS (www.unaids.org/en/dataanalysis/tools/aidsinfo/countryfactsheets/).

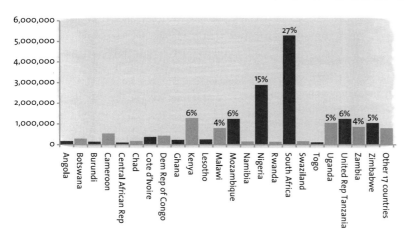

Figure 4.2.1 *Number of HIV-positive people in countries with 1 percent or more of the total sub-Saharan African HIV-positive population in 2009 (percent share indicated for the largest nine)*
Source: *UNAIDS (www.unaids.org/en/dataanalysis/epidemiology/).*

Africa-wide ball-park estimates make no sense in this context.

Addressing the HIV epidemic in Africa ought to take cognizance of where most of the HIV-positive people are – and the specific socio-economic challenges facing those countries as well as their level of development. Table 4.2.1 reports key development indicators for the nine countries highlighted in Figure 4.2.1. It shows that gross national income

(GNI) per capita ranges from $330 in Malawi to $6,100 in South Africa, and health system capacity ranges from a low of 39 percent of women giving birth in the presence of skilled health care workers in Nigeria, to 91 percent in South Africa. It also shows that the countries face different HIV disease burdens (with HIV prevalence ranging from 4 percent in Nigeria to 18 percent in South Africa). The fact that life expectancy at birth is lower in South

Africa than it is in Malawi reflects this high burden of HIV – both in absolute terms and as a share of the total population. The key take-home message is that not only is the distribution of HIV-positive people highly concentrated in Africa, but that the high-burden countries face different scales of the epidemic and have very different labor markets and economic and institutional capacity to respond. HIV-related and health systems support thus has to be calibrated to country-level requirements.

In short, extrapolating on the basis of the Malawian experience – where the levels of economic development (and wage costs) are relatively low, the burden of HIV relatively high (which means it has a relatively high social purchase) – to the whole of Africa is unhelpful, even for calculating ball-park estimates. At the very least, they should include specific country estimates for South Africa and Nigeria – and ideally also for Tanzania, Kenya, and Mozambique.

The proposed solutions

McGreevey *et al.* propose four solutions. Two entail improving health services and access to them (a test for the cryptococcal antigen and a new cohort of community health workers). The other two solutions are explicitly incentive-based: a $5 payment to Africans for HIV testing; and results-based donor funding to incentivize African governments to spend more on health. I comment briefly on the first two, and then spend more time exploring the appropriateness of their incentive-based proposals.

Strengthening health services and improving access to them

In "Solution 2" McGreevey *et al.* argue for the deployment of a new group of community health workers to the rural population of Africa. They draw on the case of Malawi to argue that this had benefits in terms of reducing births, maternal deaths, and infant HIV deaths – and that the program can be replicated across Africa. Promoting family planning, maternal health, and mother to child transmission prevention is a good idea – as is doing this through a new cohort of community health workers. But it is unrealistic to assume that the costs and the benefits can be extrapolated

across Africa in this way. Malawi is a relatively small, impoverished, low-wage country. Wage rates for community health workers in other countries – especially the high HIV prevalence countries of Southern Africa – are likely to be much higher, and where large distances are involved in servicing rural areas, logistical costs will probably also be substantially higher. Furthermore, the benefits will vary from country to country, depending on HIV prevalence and the existing level of fertility. There is no easy "one size fits all" approach to estimating costs and benefits of such interventions across Africa. The benefit-cost estimates are best disregarded.

In "Solution 3" McGreevey *et al.* propose that money be allocated for testing for the cryptococcal antigen (CRAG) in order to identify those at risk of developing cryptococcal meningitis, and to treat the disease in the early stages when outcomes are much more positive. The case seems compelling, but I am not in a position to comment on the medical costs involved, or on whether the costs and benefits are realistic on an Africa-wide basis. Clearly the benefit to cost ratios will be much higher in countries with high HIV prevalence rates (notably Southern Africa) – and it may well be the case that the costs are prohibitively high (relative to the benefits) in the low HIV prevalence countries in the West and North.

The use of incentives in driving change

The "big idea" in McGreevey *et al.* is the use of incentives to change the behavior of people and governments. They propose two solutions in this respect: a voucher worth $5 for every adult in Africa who comes in for an HIV test (Solution 1); and donor funding for health to governments conditional on progress towards the Abuja goal of 15 percent of domestic budgetary spending on health (Solution 4).

McGreevey *et al.* believe that the $5 voucher will incentivize and facilitate people to take the step of testing for HIV – and that in this regard, it could serve as one of the "critical enablers" indentified by Schwartländer *et al.* (2011) as being necessary for a successful AIDS response. More specifically, the authors propose that every adult aged eighteen to forty-nine be given a voucher[1] worth $5 in exchange for being tested, counseled, and if necessary treated. They argue that this avoids stigmatization because there is no explicit targeting. But this is not the case. In practice, a $5 voucher will result in a form of self-targeting which targets the poor (richer people will not be incentivized to spend their time in a queue just to obtain a $5 voucher). This will, of course, vary from country to country, where one would also expect more people (including the relatively better off) in countries like Malawi and Mozambique to be incentivized by a $5 voucher than would be the case in a middle-income country like South Africa (see Table 4.2.1). Where HIV is associated with poverty, then this probably does not matter. However, the empirical evidence suggests that HIV is not only, or even primarily, a disease of poverty in Africa, and that it is often the case that people at the higher end of the income distribution have higher HIV prevalence rates (e.g., Gillespie et al. 2007; Nattrass 2009).

McGreevey et al. go on to assume that not only will this intervention be successful at reaching all adults, but that this will cut new HIV infections by a quarter of a million (i.e., result in a 20 percent reduction in the number of expected annual infections in Africa). This impact is totally unrealistic given the lack of supporting evidence for this. Padian et al. (2010) have shown that the only systematic evidence on HIV prevention impacts comes from biomedical interventions such as male circumcision, mother to child transmission prevention, and anti-retroviral treatment. The absence of evidence in support of HIV testing as a prevention intervention is not, of course, evidence of the absence of any positive impact. The point is that the positive impact of HIV testing on behavior change has not yet been demonstrated – and thus the assumed benefits of this intervention are pure conjecture.

There is, however, a bigger problem with this proposal – namely that it will be logistically impossible to implement. How does one stop poor people doing many tests, in order to accumulate cash? If the program is to be offered to all adults (aged 18–49) on a single day, it is safe to assume that there will be insufficient health personnel to provide the necessary services (no matter what is assumed about other programs upgrading health services).

If it is to be run over a period of time, then how does one prevent corruption and multiple testing? Are ID documents to be marked? If so, what are the legal and social ramifications of that? Given these problems and complexities, the benefit to cost ratios presented by McGreevey et al. seem totally overblown – as is the claim that the initiative will bring "the whole population of sub-Saharan Africa into participation in the fight against AIDS."

Finally, there is also a very real danger that monetizing the incentive for HIV testing could undermine other efforts to encourage people to know their status as an act of civic duty as well as individual responsibility. For example, at six day-care centers in Haifa, a fine was imposed on parents who were late picking up their children at the end of the day. Parents responded to the fine by doubling the amount of time they arrived late. When after twelve weeks the fine was revoked, their enhanced tardiness persisted – the fine seemed to have undermined the sense of ethical obligation the parents felt to avoid inconveniencing the teachers and led them to think of lateness as a commodity that could be purchased. Bowles (2008) argues that this is an example of how preferences adapt to circumstances – and why we should be concerned about "incentivizing" individuals to act out of monetary considerations rather than social responsibility. Incentives can reframe the way that people understand appropriate behavior, and those who gain pleasure from acting in a socially responsible way may lose the incentive and the signal to do so when the action becomes rewarded. By contrast, game theoretic experiments which punish people for anti-social behavior generate feelings of shame, and subsequent changes in behavior (see summary in Bowles 2008). It may well be that a society-wide "know your status" campaign drawing in community leaders at all levels would not only be cheaper, but much more effective than the $5 voucher proposal.

Cash on delivery through an "Abuja Goal Fund"

The second incentive-based intervention proposed by McGreevey et al. is their "Solution 4" to promote

---

[1] Why a voucher and not cash? This is never explained or justified.

results-based donor funding through a new institutional vehicle they call the "Abuja Goal Fund." Their suggestion is that donor funding to African governments be conditional on progress towards the Abuja goal of allocating 15 percent of public spending on health, and that the Abuja Goal Fund be set up with an initial endowment of $1 billion. Drawing on work by the High Level Taskforce on Health Systems Strengthening, they suggest that encouraging African governments to move towards this goal could have substantial benefits in terms of preventing child and maternal deaths, tuberculosis deaths, and HIV deaths, and decreasing the number of births.

The key idea here is that the fund would be used to "induce" African governments to allocate more of their own resources to health, and that target shares (and its progress over time) would be the subject of negotiation between the Abuja Goal Fund and the country government concerned. They argue that such results-based funding practices are already evident in the Global Fund (which makes future tranche payments contingent on adequate progress) and that World Bank structural adjustment lending (in which loans were made conditional on policy changes) also serves as a relevant precedent. They note that it is difficult to know exactly how an Abuja Goal Fund would contribute to the process, but that "incentives matter and governments respond positively to them."

Precisely how the conditional grants will be monitored and managed is left unspecified. At no point do McGreevey *et al.* squarely face the tension between what country governments wish to do and what donors essentially impose on them through "incentivized" lending. They merely state, in a very unconvincing manner, that their proposal is a "hands off" approach. They are also silent on the political-economy of why most African country governments have not already allocated 15 percent of their budgets to health. In some (probably most) countries, it could be that governments are pursuing other objectives and that the citizenry would prefer more resources for health. But it may also be the case that some African country governments are reflecting a more wide-spread view among the citizenry that other spending priorities are more important. If the former, then an Abuja Goal Fund

would be a progressive intervention; but if the latter, then it could easily lose legitimacy, in the same way that the IMF and the World Bank have through their conditional lending programs. In countries where most people believe that the government is spending enough on AIDS or health relative to other concerns, then – irrespective of the country's prior commitment to the Abuja goal – there is very real political danger in using a mechanism such as the Abuja Goal Fund to coerce (albeit through incentives) changes in government policy. In such circumstances, we should either opt to allocate health resources to other countries, and/or to support civil society organizations to build popular support for, and understanding of, the need to prioritize health.

What do Africans think about health as a priority? The only systematic survey of African public opinion is that by the *Afrobarometer* project. In its 2005/6 round of surveys in eighteen countries, respondents were asked what they thought the country's most pressing problems were and whether they thought that more or less should be allocated to fighting AIDS.

More specifically, Question 66 asked:

Which of these statements is closest to your view?

- A: The government should devote many more resources to combating AIDS, even if this means that less money is spent on things like education.
- B: There are many other problems facing this country beside AIDS; even if people are dying in large numbers, the government needs to keep its focus on solving other problems.

The results, depicted in Figure 4.2.2, show that respondents in most countries typically favored option A (more resources to AIDS, even if it means fewer for other priorities like education), but that in Botswana, Ghana, Kenya, Madagascar, Malawi, Namibia, Zambia, and Zimbabwe, more than 50 percent of respondents agreed with option B (keep the government focus on other priorities). Note that these results cannot be interpreted as meaning that respondents wished to see fewer resources going to AIDS or health – it simply shows that in these countries there is a clear majority in support of continuing to focus on other priorities (i.e., not

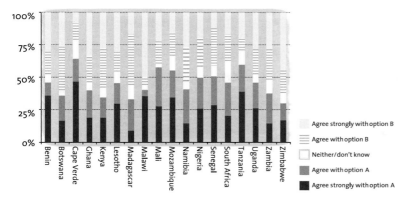

Figure 4.2.2 *Responses to the Afrobarometer Survey (2005/6) to Question 66*

restructuring the government budget towards more spending on health).

Afrobarometer provides some sense of what people considered to be the three most important problems facing their country in 2005/6. Table 4.2.2 shows that most people cited poverty and income-related issues, with health/sickness/AIDS typically coming in third (in the total sample, poverty/famine was mentioned 18 percent of the time, unemployment/income 17 percent, followed by health/sickness/AIDS 12 percent of the time). In the case of Malawi, which is poor, lacks safe water supplies, and is prone to famine, it is unsurprising that poverty and famine was the overwhelmingly largest concern (30 percent), followed by water supply (10 percent) and health/sickness/AIDS (8 percent). Dionne *et al.* report that Malawians are aware of the vast inflows of donor money for AIDS and suspect the government of creaming off some of this money. Given this context, it is hardly surprising that more respondents in Malawi (50 percent) than in any other African country sampled said they *strongly* supported option B.[2]

Table 4.2.2 also shows that, by 2008, Botswana and Zambia had already achieved the Abuja goal – hence the majority view in favor of keeping government focused on other priorities is unsurprising. And in South Africa, where progress towards the Abuja goal has been slow, and the burden of AIDS high, the relatively low support for keeping governments focused on other priorities is also unsurprising. Nudging countries like South Africa and Nigeria towards higher health spending is thus unlikely

to result in a groundswell of popular protest. But the results for Kenya and Malawi suggest that this may not be the case in these countries. Despite relatively low levels of government spending on health, a majority of respondents supported the government's current prioritization of other priorities over AIDS spending. "Inducing" these governments to change their spending patterns dramatically (in Kenya's case, almost tripling the share going to health) may well be seen as an unacceptable imposition of Western values over African priorities – and if this is used by politicians to drum up support, it could delegitimize existing health projects.

Note that the questions asked by the *Afrobarometer* are far from perfect, and the data is relatively dated. Even so, it points to the need to take popular opinion seriously. Just because governments in the past agreed to the Abuja target does not necessarily mean that there is popular support for it today.

Returning to the issue of political legitimacy for health care reform, McGreevey *et al.*'s casual acknowledgement of World Bank structural adjustment lending as a form of results-based funding seems innocent of the political baggage with which it was and remains accompanied in Africa. When

---

[2] Dionne *et al.* claim that we can "conclude with confidence that rural Malawians, like the critics of AIDS exceptionalism, would prefer fewer resources be allocated to AIDS and more to other critical day-to-day problems" (ibid.: 11). Note that the *Afrobarometer* data do not support this view. At most the data suggest that respondents would like to see more resources going to other priorities.

Table 4.2.2 Perceived most important problems facing governments (Afrobarometer 2005/6)

Country (2005 HIV prevalence rate)	Poverty/famine (% below poverty line)*	Unemployment/ income (unemployment rate)*	Health/sickness/AIDS	Water supply	Economic management	Infrastructure	Education	Agreed with option B Question 66 (do not shift more resources to AIDS)	% of health expenditure in total govt expenditure (2008)
Benin (1.8%)	8.0% (33%)	11.5% (n/a)	15.3%	10.0%	5.3%	10.4%	10.7%	49.1%	8.8%
Botswana (24.1%)	15.3% (47%)	27.1% (24%)	16.4%	7.8%	1.6%	3.0%	8.9%	61.5%	16.6%
Cape Verde (<1%)	13.9% (30%)	29.1% (21%)	9.9%	6.3%	1.4%	3.8%	6.6%	21.5%	10.1%
Ghana (2.3%)	7.9% (31%)	18.9% (20%)	10.6%	8.3%	5.6%	8.9%	15.3%	54.9%	8.5%
Kenya (6.1%)	14.5% (50%)	14.4% (40%)	11.4%	7.8%	5.9%	6.7%	8.7%	58.5%	5.8%
Lesotho (23.2%)	18.9% (49%)	23.9% (45%)	6.9%	9.8%	0.8%	8.4%	3.5%	47.0%	8.2%
Madagascar (0.5%)	18.3% (50%)	14.2% (n/a)	10.1%	4.0%	6.3%	10.7%	5.6%	56.6%	14.6%
Malawi (14.1%)	30.6% (55%)	5.1% (n/a)	7.5%	9.6%	3.2%	4.4%	6.2%	56.6%	12.1%
Mali (1.7%)	36.4% (30%)	6.4% (15%)	12.0%	9.8%	1.1%	4.8%	6.6%	40.0%	11.1%
Mozambique (16.1%)	14.5% (70%)	17.4% (21%)	17.2%	9.5%	2.1%	4.3%	10.6%	33.6%	12.6%
Namibia (19.6%)	8.2% (50%)	26.4% (35%)	11.9%	5.7%	2.5%	2.2%	11.6%	53.7%	12.1%
Nigeria (3.9%)	23.9% (60%)	18.7% (n/a)	4.9%	3.7%	6.2%	4.5%	7.3%	42.3%	6.4%
Senegal (0.9%)	17.1% (54%)	13.4% (48%)	18.0%	4.7%	3.8%	4.4%	7.9%	41.2%	11.9%
South Africa (18.8%)	10.5% (50%)	23.4% (26%)	13.0%	6.1%	1.9%	5.4%	4.3%	38.0%	10.4%
Tanzania (6.5%)	10.3% (36%)	6.1% (n/a)	16.7%	10.0%	2.8%	12.2%	9.5%	30.4%	18%
Uganda (6.7%)	19.9% (35%)	7.9% (n/a)	15.5%	10.3%	2.7%	5.8%	11.2%	48.5%	10.5%
Zambia* (17.0%)	22.3% (86%)	19.8% (50%)	9.7%	8.2%	2.4%	6.2%	12.8%	52.3%	15.3%
Zimbabwe (20.1%)	28.9% (70%)	15.2% (70%)	7.4%	2.5%	15.2%	0.6%	2.5%	63.4%	n/a

Sources: Afrobarometer (2005/6). Available at www.afrobarometer.org/data.html; WHO Health Statistics 2011: www.who.int/whosis/whostat/EN_WHS2011_Full.pdf.
* CIA Factbook (2005): www.umsl.edu/services/govdocs/wofact2005/. Note the figures for poverty and famine in Mali are for urban areas only.

African governments have been forced to adopt unpopular policy changes (for example, cutting food subsidies, increasing user fees for schooling and health) as part of their World Bank and IMF managed structural adjustment, this has often generated spontaneous popular protests and given African politicians a convenient scapegoat. The Abuja Goal Fund runs a similar danger. Precisely because it sets out to induce governments to change, and offers funding only with strings attached – and in a very public way – there is a serious danger that it could backfire – especially if more donor funding for health is channeled through such an ultimately coercive institution.

Another problem with the Abuja Goal Fund idea is that it does not confront the fact that extra spending on health may well be leveraged out of governments, but at the cost of welfare and other pro-poor programs. For instance, if there is a strong government coalition in favor of policies that benefit the elite (perhaps through industrial policies, highly subsidized tertiary education, urban housing, etc.) then an unintended and unanticipated consequence of incentivizing governments to spend more on health could be that they either spend less on pro-poor projects (such as emergency job creation programs) and/or spend more on hospitals and high-end medical equipment which cost a great deal (thereby helping achieve the Abuja target by virtue of the expense) but which continue to benefit the elite, at the cost of broad-based health care. Monitoring by, and negotiations with, officials in the Abuja Goal Fund could perhaps prevent such responses – but it will be difficult (government spending is fungible) and expensive in terms of the additional bureaucracy involved.

An alternative approach: support the Global Fund

RethinkHIV wants to know how an additional $10 billion can best be spent in sub-Saharan Africa to respond to HIV/AIDS. Building better and more integrated health systems on the back of the AIDS response is an obvious area to focus on. As McGreevey *et al.* correctly point out, we need stronger health systems, better diagnostic tools,

and greater community involvement – both on the supply side (community health workers) and the demand side (access to health services). They are also correct to highlight the issue of incentives, both on the side of people taking responsibility for their own health care, and on the part of government in shaping the public health policy. But they are, in my view, mistaken to suggest that we need new top-down innovative mechanisms, such as the $5 HIV testing vouchers and new institutions – notably the Abuja Goal Fund. Rather, we should be supporting domestic organizations to promote HIV awareness and responsibility, and we should be supporting *existing* innovative international institutions such as the Global Fund which already engages successfully with stakeholders at all levels, thereby mitigating some of the political-economic problems touched on above.

Incentives need to be taken seriously – and optimally in an explicitly political frame. As the World Development Report for 2004, *Making Services Work for Poor People*, found, adopting old-style public administration approaches to health planning without being alert to the "underlying patterns of accountability and incentives" which affect implementation is doomed to failure (World Bank 2004). And as a recent evaluation of World Bank health funding concludes, "the most pervasive lesson from the Bank's experience with health reform is that failure to assess fully the political economy of reform and to prepare a proactive plan to address this issue can considerably diminish prospects for success" (World Bank Independent Evaluation Group 2009). Improving health outcomes is as much a political challenge as it is a technical/planning challenge.

Civil society organizations and patient advocate groups are important in terms of mobilizing the citizenry to take responsibility for their own health care – and to demand better services from government. The AIDS response has been crucial in this respect. Patients on anti-retroviral treatment, precisely because the long-term management of HIV is handled as a chronic illness, have an ongoing incentive to fight for anti-retroviral treatment *and* more effective health systems. As Yu *et al.* noted in their assessment of the evidence on the relationship between AIDS spending and health systems:

AIDS activists increasingly advocate for the right of access to universal primary health care. They have also changed the dynamics between health care providers and clients, thus helping prepare health systems for the delivery of chronic care, which requires much more give-and-take between care providers and their clients than does the delivery of acute care. Indeed it is the activism for AIDS that has created solidarity about health as a concern for humanity, and as part of the evolving paradigm on globalization. (Yu *et al.* 2008)

International AIDS activists have also played a key role in driving down drug prices, challenging intellectual property, and forging international solidarity on AIDS (Smith and Siplon 2006). In sharp contrast to health interventions which either attempt to coerce governments by inducing them to change their spending priorities (such as the Abuja Goal Fund) or which simply rely on the good will and capacity of governments to deliver health care to a passive and poor citizenry, AIDS patient groups have built organizations and created political spaces for demanding health care from their governments.

This is most obvious in South Africa, where the Treatment Action Campaign (TAC) waged a successful social and political battle in support of evidence-based approaches to HIV prevention and treatment. In the early 2000s, President Mbeki and his Health Minister Manto Tshabalala-Msimang raised questions about the science of HIV and actively blocked the use of anti-retrovirals for HIV prevention and treatment in the public sector (see e.g. Nattrass 2007; Geffen 2010). It was only after sustained pressure from the TAC and its allies that Mbeki and Tshabalala-Msimang were forced to change policy. International pressure also helped, but ultimately the battle was won on the domestic political front as the TAC mobilized support from the trade union movement, health care professionals, people living with HIV, and sympathetic individuals in national and local government structures. Indeed, the political costs to Mbeki were such that they contributed substantially to his subsequent removal as president.

The TAC was effective on a range of levels, from high-profile legal action, to mass marches, and to the building of community-based branches

in strategic parts of the country. Donor funding was crucial in supporting these activities. The local level activities were vitally important too – and continue to be – as it is through direct action by affected patient groups that the health sector can be held to account.[3] Indeed, TAC branches have transformed the relationship between citizen and state in ways which make the building of better health systems more likely. As Jonny Steinberg observes with regard to the rollout of anti-retroviral treatment in Lusikisiki (rural Eastern Cape):

> The idea of demanding that a drug be put on a shelf, or that a doctor arrive at his appointed time, is without precedent. The social movement to which AIDS medicine has given birth is utterly novel in this part of the world, the relationship between its members and state institutions previously unheard of. (Steinberg 2008)

In short, supporting civil society organizations in high prevalence countries (such as the TAC in South Africa and the AIDS Support Organization (TASO) in Uganda) can be just as important as supporting governments to undertake health care reforms. Furthermore, by strengthening a cadre of domestic activists to hold governments to account, one can avoid the political costs of having international donor organizations being seen to be strong-arming governments to redirect funding away from domestic priorities.

Supporting domestic patient advocate groups can also help promote greater awareness of HIV and the need to adopt preventative measures. Helen Epstein argues compellingly that it was TASO and related grass-roots activism in Uganda which brought about behavior change (Epstein 2007). A similar case can be made for South Africa. For example, multivariate regression analysis of survey data from Cape Town shows that simply having

---

[3] Information can be found on the TAC website (www.tac.org.za) about the ongoing activities of TAC branches in urban and rural areas. TAC activists collect information about stock outages, organize protests in towns and outside clinics when services fail, and they provide "treatment literacy" education and support to people living with HIV. Local branches are also active in pushing for integrated TB and HIV health services, for national health insurance, and for better maternal and child care.

heard of the TAC significantly increased the likelihood of respondents practicing safe sex (Grebe and Nattrass 2011). Changing social attitudes from the ground up surely is a better idea than trying to pay people for once-off HIV testing (as in the $5 voucher proposal) – especially given the risk that people may then continue to demand to be paid for HIV testing, rather than take responsibility for doing it themselves on a regular basis. Supporting grass-roots initiatives which help reframe the way people see the AIDS epidemic – for example, buying into HIV science rather than Mbeki's AIDS denialism, or accepting that HIV testing is both a private and a public responsibility – should be of central importance in the ongoing AIDS response.

The international AIDS response has catalyzed new and innovative international institutions such as UNAIDS and the Global Fund – both of which involve NGOs, civil society, and patient stakeholder groups in decision-making at all levels – including in the country co-ordinating mechanisms through which Global Fund grants are channeled (Global Fund 2009; UNAIDS 2011). The Global Fund already allocates about a third of its funding for health systems strengthening and, as McGreevey *et al.* acknowledge, it already operates a system of results-based financing where grants are paid out in tranches depending on progress. According to an internal assessment, 94 percent of its African AIDS programs were successful and helped build better health systems (Global Fund 2009). This stands in sharp contrast with World Bank AIDS projects, 82 percent of which were assessed as having performed inadequately due to inappropriate design, too many actors, and inefficient monitoring (World Bank Independent Evaluation Group 2009, p. 38).[4]

There are various reasons why the Global Fund is successful, including performance-related disbursements – but it is support from UNAIDS and strong commitment to building capacity and ensuring genuine country ownership which is key. UNAIDS has brokered and funded the creation of technical support facilities in various regions to assist countries in their programs and applications to the Global Fund. Even during the Mbeki presidency, when relations between state and civil society were strained over HIV (putting corresponding

pressure on the country co-ordinating mechanism), Global Fund money was nevertheless successfully channeled to South Africa. Importantly, Global Fund grants funded the first pilot anti-retroviral treatment project in Khayelitsha, an innovative partnership involving local government, Medécins Sans Frontières (MSF), and the TAC.[5] Tshabalala-Msimang threw obstacles in the path of donor funding (for example, she blocked a Global Fund grant to KwaZulu Natal for over a year, by refusing to sign the necessary documents), but eventually folded in the face of domestic political pressure (Nattrass 2007). The key point here is that international pressure helps, but ultimately this has to be in partnership with strong domestic constituencies, if it is to have sustainable positive effects.

Supporting community organizations, of course, has its own major challenges. There is a persistent lack of capacity amongst African NGOs, as well as the ever-present problem of misappropriation of funds. However, it is important to acknowledge that institutions like the Global Fund have already developed networks and processes to address this. More recently (in 2009–10), the Global Fund started the development and implementation of the Community Systems Strengthening Framework to help civil society engage more

---

[4] It should, however, be noted that many of the underperforming projects were "emergency operations for HIV/AIDS in Sub-Saharan Africa at the height of the epidemic, with widespread civil instability in the region, food shortages, internal displacement and millions of refugees" – World Bank spokesman quoted in *The Guardian*, May 1, 2009: www.guardian.co.uk/business/2009/may/01/world-bank-health-aid-poverty.

[5] In 2001, Medécins Sans Frontières in collaboration with the Provincial Administration of the Western Cape launched a pilot anti-retroviral program in Khayelitsha, an African township on the outskirts of Cape Town. It was subsequently highlighted by the WHO in its *Perspectives and Practice in Anti-retroviral Treatment* – a series aiming to show that anti-retroviral treatment could be provided successfully to people with AIDS "even in the most resource-constrained settings" (MSF *et al.* 2003, p. 1). The Khayelitsha project demonstrated early on very good adherence to treatment regimens and excellent clinical outcomes (ibid.; Coetzee *et al.* 2004). It also showed how international NGOs, local government, and civil society could collaborate in innovative pilot projects even in the face of an unsupportive national political context.

actively with the Global Fund and obtain much needed funding (UNAIDS 2011, p. 7). Ultimately the Global Fund is successful primarily because of the innovative way that it and UNAIDS genuinely forge country ownership through supporting both states and civil society. UNAIDS reports that staff in their country offices spend up to 50 percent of their time supporting countries in the effective use of Global Fund grants, and that the technical support facilities helped unblock implementation challenges in twenty-seven countries in 2010 (UNAIDS 2011, p. 16). The Global Fund can thus draw on a range of established technical offices in ways which even the World Bank cannot.

We should be supporting this international global infrastructure to do what it is already doing – not setting up rival institutional mechanisms, such as the Abuja Goal Fund. The $10 billion should be given to the Global Fund specifically to help it build better health systems on the back of the AIDS response – and to ensure that funding for patient advocate groups continues – especially in Southern Africa, where most HIV-positive people reside.

References

Bowles, S. (2008). Policies designed for self-interested citizens may undermine the "moral sentiments": evidence from economic experiments. *Science* **320**(5883): 1605–9.

Coetzee, D., Hildebrand, K., Boulle, A., Maartens, G., Louis, F., Labatala, V., Reuter, H., Ntwana, N. and Goemare, E. (2004). Outcomes after two years of providing anti-retroviral treatment in Khayelitsha, South Africa. *AIDS* **18**: 887–95.

Dionne, K., Gerland, P. and Watkins, S. (2009). AIDS Exceptionalism: The View from Below. Paper presented at the Population Association of America Meeting, Detroit, Michigan, April 30–May 2. Available at: http://kimg.bol.ucla.edu/aids_exceptionalism.pdf.

Epstein, H. (2007). *The Invisible Cure: Africa, the West and the Fight against AIDS.* New York: Farrar, Straus and Giroux.

Geffen, N. (2010). *Debunking Delusions: The Inside Story of the Treatment Action Campaign.* Cape Town: Jacana Press.

Gillespie, S., Kadiyala, S. and Greener, R. (2007). Is poverty or wealth driving HIV transmission? *AIDS* **21**, Supplement 7: s5–s16.

Global Fund. (2009). Scaling Up for Impact: Results Report 2008, Global Fund. Available at: www.theglobalfund.org/documents/publications/progressreports/ProgressReport2008_en.pdf.

Grebe, E. and Nattrass, N. (2011). AIDS conspiracy beliefs and unsafe sex in Cape Town. *AIDS and Behavior*, published online: May 3. doi: 10.1007/s10461-011-9958-2.

McGreevey, W., Avila, C. and Punchak, M. (2011). Strengthening Health Systems. Draft paper for *RethinkHIV*, August.

MSF, UCT, PAWC. (2003). *Antiretroviral Therapy in Primary Health Care: Experience of the Khayelisha Program in South Africa (Case Study).* Geneva: WHO. Available at: www.who.int/hiv/pub/prev_care/en/South_Africa_E.pdf#search= 22khayelitsha%20best%20practice%20antiretroviral%22.

Nattrass, N. (2007). *AIDS Denialism and the Struggle for Anti-retrovirals in South Africa.* Pietermaritzburg: University of KwaZulu-Natal Press.

Nattrass, N. (2009). Poverty, sex and HIV. *AIDS and Behavior* **13**: 833–40. doi: 10.1007s10461-009-9563-9.

Padian, N., McCoy, S., Balkus, J. and Wasserheit, J. (2010). Weighing the gold in the gold standard: challenges in HIV prevention research. *AIDS* **24**: 621–35.

Schwartläander, B. *et al.* (2011). Towards an improved investment approach for an effective response to HIV/AIDS. *The Lancet*, published online June 3.

Smith, R. and Siplon, P. (2006). *Drugs into Bodies: Global AIDS Treatment Activism.* Westport, CT: Praeger.

Steinberg, J. (2008). *Three Letter Plague: A Young Man's Journey through a Great Epidemic.* Johannesburg: Jonathan Ball.

UNAIDS. (2011). *Maximising Returns on Investments: UNAIDS Support to Countries to Make Global Fund Money Work.* Geneva: UNAIDS.

World Bank. (2004). *Making Services Work for Poor People: World Development Report for 2004.* Washington DC: World Bank.

World Bank Independent Evaluation Group. (2009). *Improving Effectiveness and Outcomes for the*

Poor in Health, Nutrition and Population: An Evaluation of World Bank Group Support Since 1997. Washington DC: World Bank.

Yu, D., Souteyrand, Y., Banda, M. A., Kaufman, J. and Perriëns, J. H. (2008). Investment in HIV/AIDS programs: does it help strengthen health systems in developing countries? *Globalization and Health*; doi:10.1186/144-8603-4-8.

Social policy

Assessment paper

ANNA VASSALL, MICHELLE REMME, AND
CHARLOTTE WATTS

The HIV/AIDS epidemic is now in its thirtieth year. Over the past decade remarkable progress in addressing the consequences of HIV has been made, with nearly five million people on anti-retroviral treatment. However, prevention efforts have been less successful: globally there are approximately 7,000 infections daily, with the numbers of newly infected outnumbering those newly being put on treatment. Sub-Saharan Africa continues to bear the brunt of the HIV epidemic, with HIV prevalence rates of up to 26 percent in some countries (UNAIDS 2010a). Despite these challenges, there are also marked successes, with declines in rates of new HIV infections in many regions globally, including in sub-Saharan Africa. These declines are likely to be the result of large-scale HIV prevention efforts, as well as more fundamental changes in sexual behavior that have evolved as communities respond to the realities of the HIV epidemic and the toll that it is taking.

In sub-Saharan Africa, HIV transmission is largely heterosexual, although the role of transmission among men who have sex with men, and among injecting drug users, is also starting to be acknowledged. Established responses to addressing the heterosexual transmission of HIV include behavioral change communication programs, interventions focused on key at-risk populations (such as sex workers and their clients), male circumcision, HIV testing and counseling, condom promotion, and the treatment of sexually transmitted infections. Some of these interventions have been considered in other *RethinkHIV* papers, and are likely to remain central to a comprehensive HIV response. Although *RethinkHIV* focuses on sub-Saharan Africa in its entirety, the epidemic varies considerably by setting. In practice the optimal mix of interventions implemented in any setting will vary, and be influenced by the extent to which, at a population level, HIV infection is largely concentrated amongst vulnerable groups such as sex workers, men who have sex with men, or injecting drug users (a concentrated HIV epidemic), or more widely generalized in the population (a generalized HIV epidemic).

Over the past decade the HIV prevention landscape has continued to advance. Trial findings showing that male circumcision is protective against HIV infection has led to the widespread scale-up of male circumcision in generalized HIV epidemic settings. With recent scientific evidence showing that the early provision of anti-retroviral treatment significantly impacts on HIV transmission, the boundaries between HIV treatment and prevention have also become less distinct. Indeed, following the launch of new findings at the Rome International AIDS Society Conference in July 2011, there is now widespread discussion about the immense promise of anti-retroviral-based HIV prevention programming. This includes ART-based topical microbicides for women, the early provision of ART for those identified as being HIV infected, and the daily, oral prophylaxis use of ARVs for prevention. Trials to assess the potential impact of a slow release, ART vaginal ring are also underway.

However, when we review priorities for future HIV/AIDS investment in sub-Saharan Africa, it is important to be sanguine about the challenges. Economic and social factors continue to fuel HIV risk behaviors and undermine proven HIV interventions. Although condoms are highly effective at preventing HIV transmission, women still have very limited options to protect themselves from HIV. Stigma and the fear of the repercussions of finding out one's HIV status make many people reluctant to get tested, so although HIV testing is the cornerstone of all ART-based interventions, many fear the social consequences of being diagnosed HIV-positive. Weak health systems, cost and capacity constraints continue to make the large-scale ongoing delivery of HIV testing and anti-retroviral use for both prevention and treatment challenging to scale up and sustain.

Given these challenges above, this paper presents an analysis of the costs and benefits of interventions that seek to address some of the underlying social drivers of HIV vulnerability, and the social barriers to achieving a high coverage of proven HIV interventions. Specifically, we consider interventions to address the following four social drivers of HIV vulnerability:

1. Widespread problematic alcohol use that helps fuel men's and women's engagement in risky sexual behaviors, and undermines core HIV prevention messaging. A systematic review of twenty African studies found that alcohol drinkers had a 57 percent to 70 percent greater risk of HIV infection than non-drinkers (Fisher *et al.* 2007).
2. Transactional sex between young girls and older men, that provides one of the main bridges of HIV infection from older sexually active cohorts into uninfected newly sexually active adolescent cohorts. Current HIV prevalence data, for example, shows that eight fold more girls than boys are HIV-infected before age twenty-four in some sub-Saharan African settings (UNAIDS 2010).
3. Established social norms about gender roles and behaviors, including norms about masculinity that condone multiple sexual partnerships by men and permit some forms of domestic violence. These limit women's ability to negotiate or influence the circumstances of sex or address violence in their lives. For example, in South Africa, women in violent relationships are at 34 percent higher risk of incident HIV infection than other women (Jewkes *et al.* 2010).
4. Stigma and discrimination towards people infected with or affected by HIV, limiting their ability to access or benefit from HIV services, or ensure that HIV programs and policies are responsive to their needs (Nyblade 2004; Schwartländer *et al.* 2011). The active involve-

ment of those most vulnerable to HIV is central to an effective HIV response, with a study in Kenya finding four times higher levels of condom use in communities with strong community mobilization and involvement (Schwartländer *et al.* 2011).

Aims of analysis and description of policy interventions

Main aims

Our central hypothesis is that there are important social policy interventions that could have significant long-term impact on the HIV epidemic at a comparatively low cost, and that are likely to have both HIV and development-related benefits. The focus of these upstream interventions (structural interventions) in particular is on changing the circumstances in which risk behaviors occur. Governments, academia, and international development agencies have started to highlight several structural interventions that have the potential to mitigate some of the structural HIV risks through economic empowerment, social protection, financial incentives, and transformative processes (Blankenship *et al.* 2006; Gupta *et al.* 2008; Kim *et al.* 2008, 2011; Padian *et al.* 2011; Temin 2010; Cohen *et al.* 2004).

Drawing upon the growing literature on this issue, detailed analyses that have fed into a global investment plan for HIV (Schwartländer *et al.* 2011), and the results from several relatively recent intervention studies conducted in sub-Saharan Africa, this paper estimates the costs and benefits of the following four interventions:

- **Increasing alcohol taxes**, to reduce levels of problematic alcohol use, with the aim of reducing levels of risky sexual behavior, in addition to other health benefits and raising tax revenue.
- **Keeping girls in secondary school**, through the use of conditional cash transfers, with the aim of reducing levels of transactional sex between adolescent girls and older men, as well as generating broader educational-related development benefits.

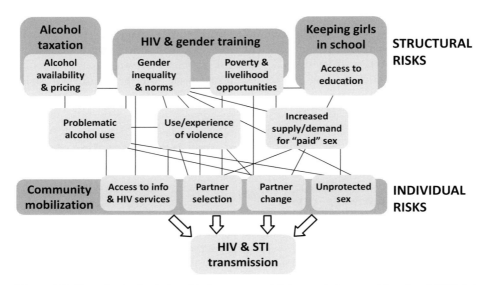

Figure 5.1 *Hypothesized relationship between social factors being considered and HIV risk*

- **Adding participatory gender and HIV training to existing microfinance and livelihood programs** with women and/or men, with the aim of ensuring that the potential synergies between poverty alleviation, gender equity, and HIV prevention programs are effectively realized and lead to reductions in levels of domestic violence against women.
- **Investing in community mobilization and stigma reduction**, involving those who are most vulnerable to or affected by HIV, to reduce community stigma and discrimination, and support communities to negotiate safer sexual behaviors and access services, including HIV testing and ART.

Figure 5.1 shows their hypothesized relationship to the more proximal, individual determinants of HIV risk.

Rationale for selection of interventions

The interventions were selected following a detailed review of the literature and consultations with HIV experts. As a first step, our review sought to identify the areas of social policy that had the most potential to impact the HIV epidemic. Subsequently, once we had identified the forms of social

policy intervention to focus on, we conducted a more detailed literature review of each focal intervention area, to identify the variables to use in our modeling analyses.

The initial round of reviews identified an emerging body of literature on the importance of structural drivers and social policy interventions, and helped us to map out key dimensions of HIV vulnerability and intervention options. This literature highlighted a consistent, albeit short, list of possible intervention options, with varying levels of evidence about their effectiveness in reducing high-risk sexual behaviors and impacting on the incidence of HIV.

The first area identified was a group of recent innovative experiments using financial incentives to motivate safe sexual behaviors for HIV prevention that have received considerable attention. For example, based on the hypothesis that economic instability and poverty drive risk behavior, conditional cash transfers (CCTs) are being provided to adolescent girls to stay in school, and to both men and women for remaining STI or HIV-negative, in Malawi and Tanzania (Baird *et al.* 2010; Kohler and Thornton 2010).

Legislative reform and community-focused interventions to reduce HIV-related stigma and discrimination and enhance social capital also emerged as being critical to ensuring that communities are able to access and benefit from HIV-related services (Schwartländer *et al.* 2011). We identified a body of literature describing programmatic experience on how to reduce HIV stigma and mobilize communities to generate positive social capital, reduce stigma and discrimination and transform norms around sexual behavior, and strong examples of situations where widespread shifts in the patterns of sexual behavior have occurred (Blankenship *et al.* 2006; Gupta *et al.* 2008).

We also identified several publications and policy literature describing the importance of social protection policies, to mitigate the impact of HIV on those affected by HIV and AIDS, including households with HIV-infected members, orphans and vulnerable children, and elderly caregivers. Although the importance of these policies for reducing future vulnerability to HIV infection was stressed, we found relatively limited data on the likely scale of these prevention impacts (Adato and Bassett 2009). However, in addition, we found an emerging body of evidence on the impact of different forms of participatory interventions that seek to promote gender-equitable relationships, and reduce levels of physical and sexual violence in relationships, built on the back of broader social protection efforts. In particular, we identified two rigorously conducted cluster randomized controlled intervention trials from South Africa that demonstrated significant impacts on levels of domestic violence and HIV-related risk (Jewkes *et al.* 2005; Pronyk *et al.* 2004).

Although less discussed in the field of structural HIV interventions, there was also a large body of literature focusing on the issue of problematic alcohol use, and potential intervention options. This included detailed reviews of the effectiveness and cost-effectiveness of interventions aimed at reducing the harm caused by alcohol, that considered action in the areas of education and information, the health sector, community action, drink-driving, availability, marketing, pricing, harm reduction, and illegally and informally produced alcohol. This literature, much of which came from outside the field of HIV, included both empirical evaluation studies as well as economic modeling analyses.

From this initial scoping exercise, cost and outcome data from a limited number of evaluation studies and reviews were repeatedly cited in the literature. These included the results from a randomized controlled trial to assess the impact of a conditional cash transfer intervention to keep girls in school in Malawi, that showed a significant impact on HIV prevalence; and the results from a cluster randomized controlled trial of an enhanced microfinance, HIV, and gender training intervention in rural South Africa, that had significant impacts on women's experience of domestic violence. We also drew upon reviews and secondary analyses of data that explored the effects of adding community mobilization intervention components to ongoing HIV programs in India, South Africa, and Tanzania; and meta-analyses that concluded that policies to make alcohol more expensive and less available are highly cost-effective strategies to reduce harmful alcohol use (Anderson *et al.* 2009), which led us to focus on the intervention of increased alcohol taxation.

As this is an emerging field of work, these studies strongly influenced our choice of social intervention options, as they provided sources of empirical data that could be used in this quantitative modeling analysis. Unfortunately, given the relatively limited body of empirical data that we were able to draw upon, we were not able to also explore the potential merits of different intervention approaches to each social driver – such as different approaches to keeping adolescent girls in school, or to reducing levels of domestic violence. However, when going through the process of selection, we tried to be strategic in our choices, aiming to identify important but relatively neglected opportunities that could be used to help rethink the HIV prevention landscape, to help ensure that future HIV responses more comprehensively respond to the social drivers of HIV infection. It should be noted, for example, that the opportunity and potential scope of benefits associated with each form of intervention considered differs widely:

- Alcohol taxation has the potential to have a widespread effect on levels of problematic alcohol use at very low cost.
- Investments to keep girls in secondary school have the potential to not only impact on HIV, but also have multiple important development gains.

- The addition of participatory HIV and gender training to livelihoods programs adds value to large-scale investments and initiatives to reduce poverty and achieve the Millennium Development Goals (MDGs) at potentially low incremental cost.
- Investment in community mobilization and stigma reduction will help ensure that communities and those most vulnerable to HIV infection are able to benefit from investments in core HIV programming and service provision, and ensure that these services are responsive to their needs.

It was therefore felt that, broadly, this selection of interventions would provide a good illustration of the range of potential interventions possible.

In summary, given the relative infancy of this field, the main purpose of our section and subsequent analysis is to explore the potential importance of different forms of social policy interventions to impact HIV, by examining a set of illustrative interventions, based on where the evidence currently exists. For this reason, our conclusions should be seen as exploratory, rather than providing definitive conclusions on the economically optimal mix of social interventions possible.

Evidence on effectiveness, cost-effectiveness, and cost-benefit analysis of each intervention

Reduced problematic alcohol use through increased taxation

There is consistent evidence that alcohol consumption, and in particular problematic alcohol use, is associated with higher HIV prevalence, unprotected sex, and poor medication adherence, as well as biological factors that may synergistically increase HIV acquisition and onward transmission (Hahn and Woolf-King 2011). This association is substantiated in sub-Saharan Africa, where a systematic review found that drinkers had 57–70 percent greater chance of being HIV-positive than non-drinkers in bivariate and multivariate analyses, controlling for confounders (Fisher *et al.* 2007).

However, as much of the data on association between alcohol and HIV comes from cross-

sectional data, it has proven more difficult to establish causality (Cook and Clark 2005; Kalichman *et al.* 2007; Fisher *et al.* 2007), with some suggesting that any association reported could be due to confounding factors. In particular, it has been argued that personality types could lead to an association between alcohol and HIV, with people who naturally have sensation/risk-seeking tendencies being more prone to both excessive alcohol consumption and risky sexual behavior (Rashad and Kaestner 2004; Kalichman *et al.* 2008; Shuper *et al.* 2010).

Stronger evidence of causality may be obtained from prospective longitudinal data that demonstrates that problematic alcohol consumption precedes HIV risk behaviors or infection, and from experimental studies that show that reductions (or increases) in alcohol use do in turn lead to reductions (or increases) in HIV risk (Leigh and Stall 1993; Halpern-Felsher *et al.* 1996; Weinhardt and Cary 2000; Woolf-King and Maisto 2011). Moreover, evidence of a plausible causal pathway, and of a dose-response relationship (so that those who drink more are at greater HIV risk than those who only drink a little), are also important criteria used to establish causality (Shuper *et al.* 2010). There is good evidence of a dose-response relationship, with heavy or symptomatic drinkers having higher odds of HIV infection than less heavy drinkers (Fisher *et al.* 2007). This is supported by a coherent theoretical pathway that has also been empirically established, with evidence of the direct pharmacological and psychological disinhibitory behavioral impact of alcohol consumption (Crowe and George 1989; Steele and Josephs 1990).

There is also some data suggesting that alcohol consumption (the cause) does indeed precede risky sex and HIV incidence (the effect). For example, Baliunas *et al.* (2010) reviewed African studies with incident HIV as an outcome, thereby making temporality a precondition for inclusion. This study found that those who drank before or during sexual intercourse were at an 87 percent increased risk for HIV infection. However, event-level methods that analyze diary entries and control for personality factors tend to show more equivocal results (Weinhardt and Carey 2000; Woolf-King and Maisto 2011).

Lastly, a causal relationship is supported by evidence suggesting that changes in the cause leads to changes in effects – in this case, that interventions that impact on alcohol use lead to reductions in HIV or other sexually transmitted infections (Shuper *et al.* 2010). In particular, Chesson *et al.* (2000) present evidence from the United States indicating that rates of sexually transmitted diseases (STDs) were responsive to alcohol regulation, with a beer tax increase of $0.20 per six-pack (accompanied by similar increases in wine and liquor taxes) being associated with an 8.9 percent reduction in gonorrhoea and a 32.7 percent reduction in syphilis.

Given these findings, a potentially important but untapped area of intervention for HIV are efforts to reduce problematic alcohol use. Despite the evidence from industrialized countries that shows that pricing and taxation policies can have a significant impact on problematic alcohol use, these forms of intervention have not been considered in SSA for HIV prevention. To date, evaluation studies of interventions that seek to directly influence the behaviors of drinkers or providers in sub-Saharan Africa do not appear promising, with trials of educational interventions targeted at drinkers through drinking establishments having no effect at all in Zimbabwe (Fritz *et al.* 2011) and weak and non-durable effects on the heaviest drinkers in South Africa (Kalichman *et al.* 2008).

In contrast, structural interventions, such as regulating the availability, price, and advertising of alcohol, seem to have potential. Indeed, a detailed analysis by the World Health Organization (WHO) concluded that regulating financial accessibility to alcohol through taxation can be a highly cost-effective policy intervention (Chisholm *et al.* 2004; WHO 2005). Later work also highlights the potential of taxation to have a strong impact on problematic drinking in the longer rather than shorter run, and to delay the start of drinking and finally to delay the progression of young people towards drinking larger amounts (Anderson *et al.* 2009). Overall, in Africa sub-region E,[1] Chisholm *et al.* find that the health effect of taxation was high, with 1,506 to 1,688 DALYs averted per one million people and thus cost-effectiveness was also high at $87 to $97 per DALY averted. A cost-effectiveness analysis of HIV prevention interventions in the United States concluded that alcohol taxation was one of the most cost-effective and under-utilized interventions, with an estimated cost-effectiveness ratio of $1,500 per infection averted (Cohen *et al.* 2004).

Global cost-effectiveness analysis found that such interventions led to a greater averted disease burden in the male population, as approximately two-thirds of the total population-level health gain was among men (Chisholm *et al.* 2004). Importantly for our analysis, only the direct effects of alcohol use on morbidity and mortality were taken into account. If HIV infections averted were considered, the cost per DALY averted may have been even lower, particularly in sub-region E, which also happens to include some of the countries with the highest HIV-related adult mortality rates.

In addition to cost-effectiveness evidence, negative externalities of hazardous alcohol use represent a market failure, which is a central justification for government intervention. Excise taxes are levied on so-called "sin" goods, such as alcohol, are therefore set to reflect the external costs associated with hazardous consumption. Moreover, the relative ease of taxing alcoholic drinks, and the inelastic demand for them in most developing countries, make excise taxes a popular source of tax revenue. A recent study found that, in Europe, alcohol excises are typically set too low, since the external costs far exceed the effective excise level (Cnossen 2007). A related analysis in South Africa compared alcohol-related excise and VAT revenues to public spending to deal with the consequences of alcohol abuse and conservatively estimated a shortfall of 1.1 billion ZAR (about $138 million) (Budlender 2009). Another study in South Africa estimated the economic costs of problem drinking to be in excess of $1.7 billion per year (2 percent of GNP), roughly three times the amount of revenue generated by excise taxes (Parry 2000). Thus, there appears to be scope for increasing these excises to better reflect actual external costs in SSA (Volkerink 2009).

[1] WHO's Global Burden of Disease Africa sub-region E includes the following countries: Côte d'Ivoire, Democratic Republic of Congo, Eritrea, Ethiopia, Kenya, Lesotho, Malawi, Mozambique, Namibia, Rwanda, South Africa, Swaziland, Uganda, United Republic of Tanzania, Zambia, Zimbabwe.

However, health, revenues, and economic impact are likely to be strongly influenced by current high levels of unrecorded consumption, and the ability to substitute taxed for untaxed alcohol consumption (which may also be toxic) in SSA. With a widespread availability of substitutes, in some countries there may be a heightened "Laffer curve" effect, where at high prices overall tax revenues may fall, as consumers switch to unregulated sources of alcohol. Moreover, the global analysis described above also found that, in Africa sub-region D,[2] taxation had a limited effect on hazardous alcohol consumption, with 64 to 99 DALYs averted per one million population, and that this was largely due to high current levels of unrecorded consumption. The concomitant cost-effectiveness ratios ranged from $1,719 to $2,662 per DALY averted, which can only be considered cost-effective in a limited number of African countries (Chisholm *et al.* 2004).

Studies from Tanzania and Kenya find a high degree of substitutability within the beverage industry (Okello 2001; Osoro *et al.* 2001). In Tanzania, a 1 percent increase in the price of commercial beer is accompanied by a 2.7 percent increase in the quantity of local brew demanded. Although this does indicate high cross-price elasticity of demand between beverages, a shift to the local brews may represent shifting to beverages with lower alcohol content. The health risks of substitution will occur in countries where there is a more significant supply of home-made spirits and adulterated industrial alcohol, although there is only anecdotal evidence of the severity of such cases, and little data available. Moreover, current trends in alcohol consumption suggest that in sub-Saharan Africa there is a distinct shift away from traditional home-brews to market beers, with the consumption of market beers being associated with a higher social status (Bird and Wallace 2010; Parry *et al.* 2005). This may mitigate this substitution effect.

A number of analysts have also explored where different African countries lie on this so-called Laffer curve for excise taxation, in order to determine whether there is still scope to increase excise rates, without reducing tax yields. Studies in Tanzania and Kenya find inelastic price elasticities of demand for most alcoholic beverages considered, particularly beer (with the exception of Guinness in Kenya). Higher excise rates on these goods would therefore be expected to optimize tax revenue. According to the study in Tanzania and simulations based on its findings in other SSA countries, the revenue-maximizing tax rate has not yet been reached (Bird and Wallace 2010). Data from Kenya, however, suggests that taxes on market beer were along the downward slope of the Laffer curve and would need to be reduced to 62.5 percent in order to optimize tax revenue (Karingi *et al.* 2001). The different situations in Kenya and Tanzania in part are likely to reflect (or may cause) differing levels of unrecorded consumption, at 60 percent and 30 percent respectively.

Work by Anderson *et al.* (2009) suggests several potential interventions for countries with high levels of unrecorded consumption, such as tax enforcement. These were found to be highly cost-effective, although the analysis only covers the Americas, Europe, and western Pacific regions. Others point to the possibilities of differential pricing of more alcohol beverages (Bird and Wallace 2010). However, while acknowledging the potential of these additional interventions, where unrecorded consumption and substitution may be issues, some economists remain skeptical about their feasibility of implementing them in some African contexts (Bird and Wallace 2010).

Finally, it is important to consider the distributive effects of any taxation. In general, evidence suggests that lower-income urban individuals are likely to bear a relatively larger share of the tax burden, making such taxes regressive (Bird and Wallace 2010). However, the more heavy drinkers within this group are disproportionately affected, and the apparent relationship between socioeconomic status and an increased risk of alcohol-related problems suggests that lower-income persons suffer more from alcohol problems and their consequences (Parry *et al.* 2005). By inference, although the poor will bear more of the costs,

[2] WHO's Global Burden of Disease Africa sub-region D includes the following countries: Angola, Benin, Burkina Faso, Cameroon, Cape Verde, Chad, Equatorial Guinea, Gabon, Gambia, Ghana, Guinea, Guinea-Bissau, Liberia, Madagascar, Mali, Mauritania, Mauritius, Niger, Nigeria, Senegal, Sierra Leone, Togo.

they are also likely to reap a larger share of the benefits of reduced problem drinking, that may neutralize the regressive nature of increased alcohol taxes. Nevertheless, the distributional aspect of alcohol taxation needs to be considered, and particular care needs to be taken to mitigate any higher levels of substitution in lower-income groups.

Keeping girls in school using conditional cash transfers

The primary constraint to female school attendance in sub-Saharan Africa is the high cost of schooling, including school fees, uniforms, and textbooks (Pettifor *et al.* 2008). Young women are also more often taken out of school to contribute financially to the household or care for siblings and sick family members. Successful interventions to address these economic barriers would need to reduce the financial cost of schooling, as well as the opportunity costs to households. Such interventions have been implemented, including waiving secondary school fees for girls, providing free uniforms and other supplies, or introducing unconditional cash transfers for the poorest households, resulting in increased enrollment, reduced drop-out rates, and even reduced marriage and pregnancy rates among girls in certain cases (Adato and Bassett 2009; Duflo *et al.* 2006; Hallfors *et al.* 2011).

Proven successful in Latin America, conditional cash transfers are also being experimented with in sub-Saharan Africa as a demand-side intervention to reduce the opportunity costs to parents of sending girls to school. By virtue of their conditionality, such transfers directly compensate households for these opportunity costs and increase the "price" of risky sex for schoolgirls, as pregnancy could lead to school expulsion and loss of the cash transfer. This partially serves to counter the effect of time discounting, by bringing the rewards of risk reduction closer to the present, rather than avoiding AIDS many years in the future. The income effect also appears to have a more direct impact on sexual behavior by reducing the girls' reliance on age-disparate relationships for economic support (Baird *et al.* 2010a).

A conditional cash transfer (CCT) intervention in Malawi paid girls to stay in school and resulted in girls in the cash group being 60 percent less likely to be HIV infected after 18 months, with the effect being attributed to reductions in transactional sex with older men. Importantly, there was no difference in effects between girls receiving conditional and non-conditional grants. However, there was a dose response effect with payment size, suggesting that poverty was an important motivation for transactional sex, and that the impact on HIV incidence was achieved through the reduction in poverty. Baird *et al.* (2012) calculate a cost per HIV infection averted through the conditional cash transfer scheme in Malawi of $5,000–$12,500.

In terms of the use of CCT to prevent HIV through other pathways (with less evidence), a randomized trial in Tanzania suggested that men and women receiving financial incentives had a 25 percent lower incidence of STIs than controls, while another scheme in Malawi that paid men and women to maintain their HIV-negative status for one year noted no effect (Kohler and Thornton 2010). Given that these are preliminary results, we focus on the more promising CCT to keep girls in school, which is also supported by evidence on gender income inequality being a structural driver. For example, a cost-benefit analysis of female secondary education in Tanzania concluded that the net benefit of investing in keeping girls in secondary school was between 1.3 and 2.9, based on HIV infections averted and increased earnings (Brent 2009). Similarly, a study in Uganda found that there were substantial additional returns to schooling through its effects on HIV prevention in particular. The labor market rate of return to education alone was estimated at 10.23 percent, while the additional rate of return from reduced HIV prevalence was found to be between 1.31 percent and 3.51 percent (De Walque 2002).

Finally, it should also be noted that in a 2008 Copenhagen Consensus Challenge paper, female education through conditional cash transfers was proposed as a key intervention for promoting women's empowerment and gender equality more broadly. It found a net benefit ranging from 3.0 to 26.1, which did not incorporate any HIV benefit (King *et al.* 2007).

Adding gender and HIV training onto livelihood programs

A range of interventions have been implemented to promote women's economic empowerment in sub-Saharan Africa and thereby potentially trigger a positive income effect on HIV (Blankenship *et al.* 2006; Kim *et al.* 2008). However, although microfinance, agricultural extension, and subsidized agricultural inputs have had positive effects on poverty and food security, we found no evidence that these interventions alone have influenced sexual behavior and HIV transmission (Davis *et al.* 2010; Denning *et al.* 2009; Pronyk, Hargreaves and Morduch 2007).

The best-documented intervention in SSA, which sought to combine an economic empowerment component with an HIV prevention component, is the Intervention with Microfinance for AIDS and Gender Equity (IMAGE) in South Africa. IMAGE added a ten-session participatory training curricular onto existing microfinance activities, with the sessions being conducted prior to the microfinance loan group meetings.

This combined approach significantly reduced levels of intimate partner violence and improved household well-being, social capital, and gender equity (Kim *et al.* 2009; Pronyk *et al.* 2006). Younger participants also reported reduced HIV risk behaviors, and an increased uptake of HIV testing. In contrast to the stand-alone HIV or gender training interventions, IMAGE was able to access and maintain a sustained contact with intervention participants for over a year, thanks to its concurrent concern for addressing the immediate economic priorities of participants. Moreover, detailed analyses of the findings suggest that the impacts achieved were primarily as a result of the combined benefits of the microfinance and training components of the intervention. This illustrates how such livelihood programs provide a critical opportunity to add further gender and HIV-related intervention activities, which are able to engage with participants over an extended period of time (Kim *et al.* 2009).

The benefits associated with engaging, in a participatory and ongoing manner, is also supported by the findings from a somewhat similar gender training program, Stepping Stones. Stepping Stones has been implemented in over forty countries since the mid-nineties, targeting both men and women, as a fifty-hour participatory HIV prevention stand-alone program that aims to improve sexual health through building more equitable gender relationships. A randomized controlled trial of this intervention showed significant impacts on herpes (HSV-2) over two years (Jewkes *et al.* 2008), as well as significant reductions in the reported levels of intimate partner violence perpetrated by men. In this case, where women had received the gender training, but there had been no economic component, the intervention did not impact significantly on their experience of partner violence.

Given the complex relationship between income and HIV incidence and the lack of evidence on the impact of economic empowerment and livelihood interventions alone on sexual behavior and HIV transmission, we build our analysis upon the IMAGE model in South Africa, drawing also from the impact findings for Stepping Stones with men. The microfinance component of the IMAGE intervention identified women above eighteen years and living in the poorest households as eligible loan recipients and control participants. Loan centers of about forty women met fortnightly to repay loans, apply for additional credit, and discuss business plans. These meetings served as avenues for introducing the Sister-for-Life participatory learning program to address HIV infection and intimate partner violence (Kim *et al.* 2007). In the first phase, ten one-hour training sessions were conducted, covering topics such as gender roles, communication, domestic violence, and HIV infection. In the second phase, women recognized as "natural leaders" by their peers undertook another week of training and then worked with their centers to address priority issues, through wider community mobilization engaging both youths and men in the intervention communities. The training curriculum was delivered alongside microfinance services over a twelve-month period (Kim *et al.* 2007).

We therefore model combining "piggy-backing" training focusing on HIV and gender relationships onto livelihood interventions that have an income effect, considering both the addition of the training for women (as in IMAGE) and with men (extrapolating from Stepping Stones about the benefits of working with men). For men, the underlying assumption is that the livelihoods activity provides a framework within which issues of gender and HIV can be explored, and that the combination of reduced household economic stress and gender training will impact on their perpetration of intimate partner violence. For women, our assumption with this approach is that a livelihood intervention that increases women's income can be expected to have a similar impact on intimate partner violence (IPV) as the IMAGE intervention, if administered with a gender and HIV training curriculum.

As with keeping girls in school, it should be noted that more broadly livelihood interventions have also shown to have multiple economic benefits. Although there is relatively limited data specific to Africa, impact assessments of microfinance schemes in Uganda and South Africa have found an enhanced household capacity to meet basic needs (including food) and to accumulate valuable assets (Barnes *et al.* 2001; Kim *et al.* 2009). Other successful income-generating models in SSA are largely agriculture-based, as more often than not agriculture represents the mainstay of the economy and rural livelihoods. Low yields and high food prices over the past few years have further exacerbated food insecurity and left 239 million people undernourished (FAO 2010). Limited access to improved agriculture technologies, inputs, credit, and extension are the key barriers to a Green Revolution in Africa (Denning *et al.* 2009), and women are particularly disadvantaged.

The Farmer Field School (FFS) is an innovative, participatory, and interactive agricultural extension model, initiated in Asia and subsequently replicated across the world (Braun *et al.* 2006). Based on hands-on farmer experimentation sessions and non-formal training (Anandajayasekeram *et al.* 2007), the approach has expanded its crops focus to include a wide range of topics such as livestock, community forestry, water conservation, food security, health, and HIV. An impact evaluation conducted in Kenya, Uganda, and Tanzania revealed a 61 percent increase in agricultural income and a more substantial impact among female-headed households (187 percent), compared to a non-participating control group.

Agricultural productivity in SSA is being further compromised by poor access by smallholder farmers to improved seed and fertilizer, in tandem with declining soil fertility. Based on this reality, there has been a return to government subsidies as an effective policy instrument for improving food security, as evidenced by Malawi's internationally acclaimed farm input subsidy program, which has transformed Malawi from a net importer of maize to a net exporter (Dorward and Chirwa 2011; Sanchez *et al.* 2007). Based on the same principles, NGOs have also been providing agricultural inputs to beneficiaries, as part of integrated rural livelihood programs, such as the Millennium Village Project (MVP) (Sanchez *et al.* 2007). In Kenya, Ethiopia, and Malawi, each household in the Millennium Villages received improved seed (primarily for maize) and fertilizer inputs for a typical smallholder farm size, as well as complementary extension training. In Kenya, the Sauri village experienced a 3.9 fold increase in maize production, enabling the village to satisfy 166 percent of its food needs from own production, compared to 43 percent before the intervention (Denning *et al.* 2009). Similarly, the so-called caloric food requirement index went from 0.13 to 1.10 in Ethiopia, and from 0.56 to 8.46 in Malawi (Sanchez *et al.* 2007).

The training component of the IMAGE program was found to have an estimated cost per DALY gained of $8,764 (2010) for the trial phase and $2,630 (2010) for the initial scale-up phase – but this only took into account DALY gain from reductions in intimate partner violence. Studies of the underlying economic interventions, such as the Millennium Village Project, found a benefit to cost ratio of between 2.3 and 3.5 in just six to nine months (Denning *et al.* 2009), while the external evaluation of Malawi's 2006–2007 farm input subsidy program estimated a modest benefit to cost ratio of 0.76 to 1.36 in terms of increased maize yields (Dorward and Chirwa 2011), excluding indirect benefits accrued through improved food security, health, or education outcomes.

Community mobilization and stigma reduction

Although still somewhat ill-defined, there is growing evidence that community mobilization and stigma reduction can be enablers of other core HIV-prevention interventions. Effective programs need to be conducted in partnership with the communities in which interventions are being implemented, and engage with those most affected by HIV. Indeed intervention delivery is highly dependent upon the support and involvement of community members and volunteers, and without these forms of partnership, services may struggle to reach key populations. For these reasons, community engagement and mobilization activities, aimed at creating a supportive, enabling, and empowering environment, are recognized by UNAIDS as an essential component of all HIV programs (Schwartländer et al. 2011). In addition, these forms of activity can support changes in community norms, that can change the environmental context in which people make decisions related to HIV risk (Khumalo-Sakutukwa et al. 2008).

Current evidence points towards this enabling virtue, particularly for interventions targeting youths and delivered through existing community-based organizations or centers that have been found to have more positive results (Maticka-Tyndale and Brouillard-Coylea 2006). Moreover, a study in Kenya found that individuals were four times more likely to report consistent condom use if living in areas with good engagement of CBOs (Schwartländer et al. 2011). Another multi-country study in Tanzania, Zimbabwe, and South Africa reported a four-fold increased uptake of voluntary counseling and testing (VCT), when provided at the community level, compared to facility-based VCT provision (Khumalo-Sakutukwa et al. 2008). In Ghana a significant negative interaction was found between risky sexual behaviors and community stigma (adjusted odds ratio (AOR) $= 0.44$; 95 percent confidence intervals $= 0.19$–0.67), indicating that the generally positive effect of risky sex on HIV testing is attenuated among women from communities with high levels of stigma (Koku 2011).

A review of the literature on stigma and HIV/AIDS by Mahajan et al. (2008) quotes studies from South Africa, China, and France, which reported increased unsafe sex and non-disclosure among PLHIV holding stigmatizing attitudes or experiencing HIV-related discrimination. Results from interventions to reduce stigma through community-, work-, and group-based approaches with information, peer education, and counseling activities in Uganda, Tanzania, and Zimbabwe documented increased HIV/AIDS knowledge and awareness increased reported desire to change behavior, better coping skills for PLHIV, reduced stigma and discrimination of PLHIV, participants were more empowered to negotiate safe sex, and increased demand for condoms and VCT (Brown et al. 2003). Hence, it is concluded that community mobilization intervention with a stigma reduction component can increase the uptake of VCT, adherence to ART, and help prevent mother-to-child transmission, as well as the effective targeting of social support to the most affected (Mahajan et al. 2008; Temin 2010).

Finally, the International HIV/AIDS Alliance piloted the participatory Social Return On Investment (SROI) methodology to determine the value for money of its community mobilization support in India and Zambia, as perceived and monetized by the beneficiaries themselves. The SROI study of the CHAHA program in the Maharashtra and Andhra Pradesh states in India reported that for every $1 invested, an additional $4 was generated in social, health, and financial value. This program targeted 64,000 children affected by HIV/AIDS through its outreach workers with nutritional, psycho-social, educational, and household support. It aimed to create an enabling environment through community mobilization in all settings (health, social, and legal) for stigma reduction. Most of the value created by the intervention was related to improved livelihoods (income), resulting from the decrease in stigma experienced by HIV-positive parents or caregivers, encouraging them to seek paid employment. The outcome area in which the second largest value was created according to stakeholders was improved health status, largely through improved child nutrition, which avoided considerable costs of travel, health support, and medicine (Biswas

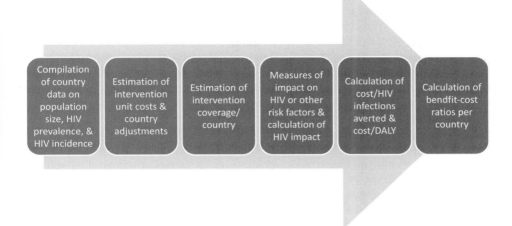

Figure 5.2 *Steps in analysis*

et al. 2010). A SROI study in Zambia also estimated similar benefits (International HIV/AIDS Alliance 2011).

Methodology

We present here both cost-effectiveness and cost-benefit analyses of the four interventions identified above based on the guidelines issued by *RethinkHIV*. To estimate cost-effectiveness, for each intervention option we calculate the incremental cost per disability adjusted life year (DALY) – which gives a measure that reflects the health-related benefits of each intervention considered. To conduct cost-benefit analysis, which evaluates the cost of an intervention relative to monetized outcomes, we represent both the health benefit in terms of monetized DALYs, additional economic benefits for those who are targeted by the intervention, and, in a very few cases, benefits from positive externalities associated with the intervention.

The time period for our analysis is the five-year period in which the intervention is carried out for the costs, with any benefits that derived from the five-year investment that accrued up until the target group dies included (although in some cases we only describe potential longer-term benefits as the data was not available to quantify them). Our broad approach can be seen in Figure 5.2.

It is important to note that for this analysis, wherever possible, we took a country by country approach, and disaggregated population-related data by sex. We only generalized across countries when there was no other option. We sought to incorporate this level of detail, as we recognize that a range of contextual factors will influence the relative benefit to cost ratios obtained. As well as there being substantial variability in the levels and distribution of HIV infection between countries in sub-Saharan Africa, there is also substantial variation in the size of the different sub-populations being targeted by each intervention, the costs of each intervention, and the degree to which the intervention is effective, both in the short and long term. While data constraints made it difficult to incorporate all these factors, we attempted to ensure our calculations were made and presented on a country by country basis, as can be seen in the Appendix to this report.

From the outset we recognized that our approach is limited in many ways. As well as the challenges of parameterization, in our modeling we focus on estimating the provider costs and the impacts on recipients of these specific interventions. This is a gross over-simplification of the potential value of social policy interventions, as using this perspective we fail to capture the potential longer-term and broader impact of achieving widespread societal change. It is now well recognized that HIV/AIDS is a long-wave event, and that resource decisions need to consider both the short- and long-term implications of different policy choices. Particularly, we were not able to model the potential longer-term social implications of reductions in levels of problematic alcohol use, shifts towards less inequitable gender roles and norms, and reductions in intimate partner violence; and the implications of achieving reductions in levels of stigma and discrimination against very marginalized groups and communities. A study by Brent (2009) for example shows that the longer-term impact of education on HIV is likely to be up to four fold its direct impact.[3] If this holds true (even to a lesser extent) for each of the strategies that we are considering, we would underestimate both the cost-effectiveness and benefit to cost ratios of these interventions considered by factors of four or more.

The first stage in our approach was to compile country data on population size and HIV epidemiology and use this to estimate intervention coverage. For several of the interventions this estimate took into account the existing coverage of complementary interventions and factors like those groups who are living below the poverty line. We then estimated the unit costs for each intervention, in some cases using a combination of the literature and a GDP adjustment, as recommended by *RethinkHIV*. Next, we estimated HIV infections and DALYs, taking into account the current degree of ART coverage. We also included cost savings from the prevention of future ART provision. Finally, we added in any additional economic benefits to arrive at our final benefit to cost ratios.

Detailed methods on costs, effectiveness, and benefit estimation for each intervention are presented below.

Determining coverage – compilation of country data on population size, HIV prevalence, and HIV incidence

A detailed spreadsheet was developed, compiling country-specific data on the size of the adolescent and adult population, and population HIV prevalence and incidence, for all countries in sub-Saharan Africa (listed in the Appendix). This data came largely from different UN agencies, including UNDESA, UNAIDS, and UNDP.

Broadly our modeling assumes an immediate scale-up of the interventions to the target coverage level, rather than a gradual one – in order to illustrate the costs and benefits of these interventions when "up and running." However, we have tried to remain conservative when setting coverage targets, i.e., 20 percent of microfinance and livelihood program beneficiaries per year; 30 percent increase in current coverage of community mobilization; and only schoolgirls living under the poverty line to be provided with conditional cash transfers. For alcohol taxation, we do not assume a high-end effect, but instead use conservative estimates of the prevalence of problematic alcohol use among men and women in each country, and then estimated how reductions in problematic use may lead to reductions in HIV incidence. When doing this, we recognize that the regulatory capacity of countries will vary widely, and so we correct our estimate of effect, using country-specific measures of the levels of unrecorded alcohol consumption. Details of the key literature used and the methods used for each intervention are provided below.

Alcohol taxation

Regulating the financial accessibility of alcohol through taxation is the most cost-effective, yet most politically sensitive, policy intervention to reduce problematic alcohol consumption (Chisholm *et al.* 2004; Wagenaar *et al.* 2009; WHO 2005). Increasing taxation is likely to meet strong resistance from the beverage industry, and in settings where there is a preponderance of homemade alcohol, there is the risk that consumers will switch their consumption to homemade alcohol.

Based on the approach adopted in a cost-effectiveness analysis undertaken by WHO's CHOICE (CHOosing Interventions that are Cost-Effective) exercise, we model a 25 percent increase

---

[3] However, we could not model this, as our definition of direct and indirect impact was different than in Brent (2009).

of the current alcohol excise tax for all alcoholic beverages per country (not a 25 percent increase in price). This includes excise taxes on all regulated alcohol sales of homebrewed alcohol, as well as larger commercially available brands of beers and spirits.

Target population

Given the nature of the intervention, we assumed the intervention will affect all consumers of regulated alcohol. However, through this blanket tax increase, we aim to reach our specific target, i.e., heavy drinkers, in order to curtail their hazardous drinking as a means of reducing their associated risky sexual behaviors and susceptibility to HIV infection. We extracted the most recent data on the prevalence of heavy episodic drinking among adult men and women per country from WHO's Global Information System on Alcohol and Health (2003–2008), which is defined as the proportion of adult men and women (15+ years) who have had at least 60 grams or more of pure alcohol on at least one occasion weekly. This allows us to estimate the number of male and female heavy drinkers to be reached, given the total adult population (15–49 years) per country.

Coverage

The cost-effectiveness analysis of interventions to prevent hazardous alcohol use determined that taxation was the most cost-effective in populations with moderate to high levels of drinking (above 5 percent prevalence) and lower unrecorded consumption (below 50 percent) (Chisholm *et al.* 2004). In SSA, this corresponds to countries in WHO's Africa sub-region E, characterized by their high child mortality and very high adult mortality. In countries with high amounts of unrecorded production and consumption, increasing the proportion of alcohol that is taxed could be a more effective way of influencing pricing than a simple increase in tax (Anderson *et al.* 2009). In some countries, prices may be at the top of the Laffer curve, and the focus may be on tax enforcement. However, as we were focusing on HIV, and this was not included in the previous analyses, in the first instance we estimated cost-effectiveness for all countries in SSA. More-

Table 5.1 Sources of data used on current coverage of interventions: increasing alcohol taxes

Intervention	Coverage / incidence	Source
Increasing alcohol taxes	Prevalence of heavy episodic drinking among men and women by country	WHO Global Information System on Alcohol and Health, most recent data from 2003–2008

over, in practice, given the country-specificity of the potential degree and severity of substitution, we did not feel we had sufficient data on this to justify excluding countries from our analysis in the first instance.

With a 25 percent tax increase, we assume a distortionary effect leading to a 10 percent increase in unrecorded consumption, as proposed in Chisholm *et al.* (2004), assuming that the proportion of unrecorded consumption is equivalent to the proportion of consumers drinking unregulated alcohol. We used country-specific estimates on the current unrecorded alcohol consumption levels from WHO's database, and thereby excluded unrecorded consumption, plus the 10 percent increase, from our effective coverage.

Keeping girls in secondary school

The World Bank cash transfer study was implemented in Malawi from 2008 to 2009 as an individually randomized controlled trial providing monthly cash transfers to 1,225 unmarried schoolgirls and young women, on the condition that they stay in (or return to) school. This trial was the first to evaluate and establish the impact of a cash transfer program on HIV prevalence and sexual behavior, based on detailed behavioral and STI biomarker data. Given its rigorous design and positive HIV outcomes, we chose to model this intervention for other countries in SSA.

Target population

The Malawi intervention targeted all unmarried girls aged between thirteen and twenty-two in the chosen geographical area, because it represents the period during which school dropout coincides with the onset of sexual activity. Due to data availability, with population data stratified by five-year age cohorts (10–14; 15–19; 20–24), we focus on girls between fifteen and nineteen. According to UNESCO data, this age group corresponds roughly to the normal secondary school age in most countries in the region, which is generally between twelve and eighteen (ranging from 10–17 in Angola to 14–20 in Tanzania). We choose to target girls already in secondary school, as the effectiveness of the intervention has only been demonstrated for this group, and not for girls who had already dropped out but were incentivized to return to school.

Coverage

In order to estimate the size of the target group, we consider net attendance ratios, defined as the percentage of girls of secondary school age attending secondary school or higher. Current ratios for each country were sourced from UNICEF's online database, containing the most recent figures from 2005 to 2009. In forty-four SSA countries, female net secondary school attendance ranges from 5 percent in Rwanda to 63 percent in Namibia, with a median of 22 percent. By default, these attendance ratios are used to determine the number of girls between 15 and 19 currently attending school. It is however clear that the total number of girls of secondary school age attending secondary school is likely to be higher than our estimates, given the wider age range in the definition (12–18 years). Nevertheless, we model a conditional cash transfer scheme that would target the poorest girls in these populations (living on under $1.25 a day), with a focus on keeping girls in secondary school for an additional two years. We do this as the evidence suggests that the income effect is most likely to drive the reduction in risk behavior amongst girls of this age – and thus assume that this group would benefit most from the intervention.

Adding HIV and gender training to livelihood programs

Target population

We target the adult population that is currently enrolled in ongoing microfinance and livelihood

Table 5.2 Sources of data used on current coverage of interventions: keeping girls in secondary school

Intervention	Coverage/incidence	Source
Keeping girls in secondary school	Levels of net secondary school attendance of girls by country	UNICEF, State of the World's Children 2011, most recent data from 2005–2009

programs with this incremental investment. We include women, as this is where the IMAGE intervention showed effect, as well as men, as the findings from the Stepping Stones Trial show that gender training activities with men can impact on their perpetration of violence, as well as on HSV-2.

Coverage

In order to estimate the size of this target population, we estimate current coverage levels of existing microfinance and livelihood schemes. In 2010, nearly 500 microfinance institutions reported providing services to over eight million people in SSA through the MIX MARKET platform.[4] Since not all institutions report, this is likely to be an underestimate, but we use the reported figures per country as current coverage levels. For countries without data, we assume a coverage equivalent to the regional mean of 1.7 percent of the adult population. The coverage of other livelihood interventions is estimated from the few documented experiences, i.e., the FFS and the Millennium Villages, based on the ratio of their total beneficiaries (Braun *et al.* 2006) to the total adult population. These average ratios for countries with data are then extrapolated to countries without data. For each country, we then determine a low estimate of coverage based on the intervention with the most beneficiaries. As a realistic scale-up plan, we target 20 percent of these current beneficiaries with an add-on training component.

---

[4] The MIX MARKET™ is a global, Web-based microfinance information platform that was launched by the UN Conference on Trade and Development and expanded by the Consultative Group to Assist the Poor (CGAP).

Table 5.3 Sources of data used on current coverage of interventions: participatory gender and HIV training

Intervention	Coverage / incidence	Source
Adding participatory gender and HIV training to existing microfinance and livelihood programs	Coverage of microfinance and livelihood programs	Microfinance Information eXchange (MIX MARKET) 2009 data Millennium Villages Project website Farmer Field Schools review (Braun *et al.* 2006)

Table 5.4 Sources of data used on current coverage of interventions: community mobilization

Intervention	Coverage / incidence	Source
Investing in community mobilization activities	Current coverage of community mobilization activities	Schwartländer *et al.* (2011)

Community mobilization

Community mobilization as an intervention is complex and wide-ranging, but can broadly be divided into three categories: outreach and engagement activities; support activities; and advocacy, transparency, and accountability activities. Activities such as peer education, group discussions, community forums, and establishing community networks come to mind (Schwartländer *et al.* 2011). It is particularly important to marginalized groups, who tend to be excluded from wider community processes, such as young people, women, sex workers, men who have sex with men, and people who inject drugs, as well as those affected by HIV. These groups are also particularly susceptible to HIV infection and stand to benefit from collectivization among themselves. Several have made use of community mobilization in the prevention and mitigation of HIV and AIDS, by means of peer outreach and the promotion of HIV testing. Support groups of sex workers, for example, have generally combined one-on-one or small group behavior change communication with access to commodities and services, including condoms, STI care, and VCT (Dandona *et al.* 2005; Schwartländer *et al.* 2011). We use the Futures Institute's online Goals Express[5] to model this intervention.

Target population

The modeled community mobilization intervention targets the general adult population (15–49).

Coverage

We model an increase of 30 percent from the current coverage of community mobilization for the nineteen SSA countries contained in the Goals Express model. Information on current levels of coverage of community mobilization is already programmed into the Goals Express model, and was also used for the investment framework presented in Schwartländer *et al.* (2011). This input came from information provided by national programs during UNAIDS resource needs workshops, and ranges from 0 percent in Burkina Faso to 60 percent in Benin. The Goals model assumes a relatively low coverage of 4 percent for countries where there were no specific data.

Estimation of total and unit costs

The costs of any social intervention are likely to be highly context specific. Due to data scarcity, our approach has been to source setting-specific costs and adjust them for other countries using GDP per capita, as recommended by *RethinkHIV*. Moreover, although we would have preferred to capture total societal costs per intervention, the data sources tended to concentrate on provider costs. This implies that the total costs of each intervention are likely to be underestimated in our analysis, as the various financial costs incurred by beneficiaries and their households to attend school, training sessions, or community mobilization events are largely omitted, as well as the associated opportunity costs. Finally, for most of the proposed interventions, economies of scale are likely to be achieved, even in the short to medium run, bringing unit costs

---

[5] http://policytools.futuresinstitute.org/goals.html.

Table 5.5 Unit costs used in calculation of policy interventions: increasing alcohol taxes

Intervention	Unit cost used	Key intervention activities	Range from other sources	Source
Increasing alcohol taxes	$0.17–$0.19	Policy/legislative change, tax collection, administration, and enforcement	$0.45 in US (Cohen *et al*. 2004)	Chisholm *et al*. (2004)

down. We have currently made no adjustment for scale-effect on costs. However, in order to partially take this into account, we have incorporated unit costs at scale rather than those incurred during the more capital-intensive start-up phases, where distinct cost data was available in the literature.

In general unit costs were extracted from peer-reviewed literature, publications from reliable development institutions, and the Futures Institute's online unit cost database, which was also utilized in the strategic investment framework proposed by Schwartländer *et al*. (2011). All costs are expressed in 2010 dollars, where necessary using OECD/DAC US $ deflators.

Alcohol taxation

Chisholm *et al*. (2004) estimate that the incremental costs of an increase in the excise tax on alcohol for a population of one million at $150,000 (2004 international dollars) in WHO Africa region E countries is equivalent to a unit cost of $0.17 in 2010 dollars. For Africa sub-region D, these unit costs were slightly higher, at $0.19. The costs relate to legislation activities, as well as the administration and enforcement of the tax policy once passed (Chisholm *et al*. 2004). The cost of the intervention is likely to be higher in the first year on account of the required change in legislation, followed by lower unit costs for the rest of the policy life. However, as we did not have data to inform this, we assume a flat cost function.

Keeping girls in school

The conditional cash transfer program in Malawi consisted of an average payment of $10 per girl per month (for 10 months of school a year), of which 30 percent on average went directly to the girl. Additional costs include the direct payment of secondary school fees, and program administration costs. It is

estimated that the average annual costs for each schoolgirl were approximately $100 in cash transfers, $20 in school fees, and $50 in administrative costs (Baird *et al*. 2010a, 2010b). The total financial cost per schoolgirl of $173 (adjusted to 2010 dollars) represents 56 percent of Malawi's GDP per capita.

The cash transfer of $10 per month represented around 15 percent of total monthly household consumption in the sample households at baseline, placing the program in the middle-to-high end of the range of relative transfer sizes for conditional cash transfer programs. For similar programs in Cambodia and Mexico, the cash transfers have ranged from as little as 2 percent to over 20 percent of total monthly household consumption (Baird *et al*. 2010). Relative to GDP per capita, however, Mexico's Progresa transfer was only about 6 percent, excluding administrative costs (King *et al*. 2007). In comparison, the more common unconditional cash transfer schemes in SSA represent between 24 percent and 52 percent of per capita income (Adato and Bassett 2008).

On the basis of this, we generalized the $20 and $50 for annual school fees and administrative costs to other settings adjusting by GDP per capita. However, since our target population were those living on less than $1.25 per day (and this is 74 percent of Malawi's population (WB figures)), we did not adjust the transfer amount by GDP per capita. Instead, we assumed that the $100 reported for Malawi would be sufficient in other countries to generate the same effect. In reality however this is likely to be highly context-specific, and therefore we conducted a sensitivity analysis for this.

Adding participatory gender and HIV training to livelihood programs

An economic evaluation was conducted for the IMAGE training component to determine its

Table 5.6 Unit costs used in calculation of policy interventions: keeping girls in secondary school

Intervention	Unit cost used	Key intervention activities	Range from other sources	Source
Keeping girls in secondary school	$173 (Malawi: 56% of GDP per capita)	Beneficiary identification, monitoring of school attendance, cash transfers, payment of school fees	$200–$1,662 (per household for unconditional cash transfers)	Baird *et al.* (2010a)

Table 5.7 Unit costs used in calculation of policy interventions: participatory gender and HIV training

Intervention	Unit cost used	Key intervention activities	Range from other sources	Source
Adding participatory gender and HIV training to existing microfinance and livelihood programs	$12.88 (South Africa: 1.1 percent of GDP per capita)	Development of materials, training of trainers, and training of beneficiaries	$0.4 (Stepping Stones training, Mozambique)	Jan *et al.* (2010) World Bank (2003)

incremental cost-effectiveness (Jan *et al.* 2010). The costing adopted a provider perspective, excluding costs to participants and families (e.g., travel and opportunity costs of attending meetings). During the two-year start-up phase, costs were estimated at $23.9 per participant per year (in 2010 dollars). The two-year scale-up phase registered an annual cost of $12.88 per participant. Old program cost data of a Stepping Stones intervention in Mozambique in the late nineties indicates an average cost per training participant of $0.40 (in 2010 dollars) (World Bank 2003). Although this is not rigorous costing data, it suggests that lower unit costs could be achieved, prompting us to model unit costs based on the IMAGE training in its scale-up phase. Moreover, as we source our effect data from the IMAGE study, we assumed the cost as reported by Jan *et al.* (2010) still to be the most relevant estimate. As these costs represent about 1.1 percent of the South African GDP per capita, we used this proportion to estimate costs for other SSA countries.

Community mobilization and stigma reduction

Costing studies were found for the Masaka intervention in Uganda and the "Mema kwa Vijana" youth intervention in Tanzania. For the Ugandan case, the average unit cost of the community IEC component of the intervention was $1.92 per person reached in 2010 dollars (Terris-Prestholt *et al.* 2006). For the Tanzanian case, the community mobilization component was estimated to account for 12.3 percent of total program cost, at an esti-

mated cost per targeted adolescent of $2.93 (Terris-Prestholt, Kumaranayake, Obasi *et al.* 2006).

The Futures Group presents additional unit cost data of community mobilization interventions for HIV in its online database, based on an unpublished analysis of the cost of PEPFAR-funded interventions in Ethiopia, South Africa, and Uganda, focusing on abstinence, "be faithful," and community mobilization approaches. These unit costs range from $0.40 to $12.90, with a median of $1.05. The remaining unit costs were sourced from the strategic investment framework model presented in Schwartländer *et al.* (2011), based on UNAIDS resource needs workshops. These estimates are based on data from community health worker programs in generalized epidemics. Here the median cost per person was slightly lower, at around $0.88 (mean: $2.06). Since community mobilization is not clearly defined as an intervention, we tried to adopt unit costs for different settings as far as possible. Where there was no country-specific data, the South African cost that was assumed in the Goals Express model (and Schwartländer *et al.* 2011) was adjusted by GDP.

Approach to modeling HIV infections averted/HIV impact

Estimating the potential benefits of each form of HIV intervention is complex, for several key reasons. First, as described above, there is limited effectiveness evidence available in the area of social

Table 5.8 Unit costs used in calculation of policy interventions: community mobilization

Intervention	Unit cost used	Key intervention activities	Range from other sources	Source
Investing in community mobilization	$0.33–$37.10 (South African cost then adjusted by GDP for countries with data gaps)	Outreach, support, advocacy	$0.40–$12.90 (Ethiopia, South Africa PEPFAR, and Terris-Presholt *et al.* 2006a and 2006b)	Schwartländer *et al.* (2011)

policy interventions on HIV impact, due to the relatively new interest in this area. Second, as with costs, even where evidence is available we face a particular problem in terms of estimating incremental effectiveness. For example, while we have good evidence on the combined cost-effectiveness of interventions that provide both community mobilization and HIV prevention services to high-risk groups, it is difficult to identify how much of this effectiveness is attributable to the community mobilization component alone.

In addition, ideally, for each intervention being considered, we would have used country-specific behavioral and epidemiological data, in combination with intervention-specific data about the effect of each intervention on patterns of sexual behavior and networking, to estimate the impact of the intervention on temporal trends in HIV transmission.

In practice, this form of evidence was not available. Because of this, we estimated the numbers of HIV infections averted by each form of intervention by first estimating the proportion of the sexually active population that could potentially be reached in each country, using national population and prevalence data to estimate the proportion of these people who are HIV uninfected, and then using evidence about the degree to which each factor is associated with HIV risk, to estimate how the annual incidence of HIV infection in this sub-group could potentially be reduced.

Mathematically, we adopted the following approach to estimate how reductions in risk may reduce HIV incidence:

If S people in a population of size N at need are not HIV infected at time t, if there is an annual incidence i, after 1 year $S(1 - i)$ will remain uninfected. Similarly, after t years $S(1 - i)^t$ will not be HIV infected, and $N - S(1 - i)^t$ will be HIV infected.

If an intervention leads to M HIV-uninfected people reducing their HIV risk behaviors, so that their annual risk of HIV infection is reduced by a factor a (<1), the annual HIV incidence will be $(1 - a)i$ rather than i, and after t years $M(1 - (1 - a)i)^t$ will not be HIV infected and $M(1 - (1 - (1 - a)i)^t)$ will be HIV infected.

Estimates of the cumulative number of HIV infections averted after time t can thus be obtained by subtracting the estimates of the cumulative numbers HIV infected with and without the intervention.

In each case, for each of these calculations the proportional reduction in the HIV incidence measure was estimated using available epidemiological evidence about either the effect size of the specific intervention on the prevalence of risk in the populations, and/or the strength of association between the exposure and HIV prevalence or incidence.

For the conditional cash transfer intervention we used the direct measure of the impact of the intervention on HIV incidence. For alcohol taxation we estimated how the levels of problematic alcohol use among women and men would decrease as a result of taxation, and the subsequent reduction in HIV incidence among these beneficiaries; for interventions to keep girls in secondary school we estimated the numbers of HIV infections averted by a 60 percent reduction in HIV incidence among the beneficiaries of this intervention; to model the effect of adding gender and HIV training to livelihood programs we estimated the effect of the intervention on ongoing levels of intimate partner violence, and then used data on the strength of association between exposures to violence and incident HIV to estimate the potential HIV benefits of this reduction. In practice for both the alcohol taxation and livelihoods training program we had to use measures of the strength of association between prevalent phenomena (e.g., intimate partner violence and problematic alcohol use and HIV) to estimate the potential reduction in incident risk. This estimation is likely to hold best in stable HIV epidemic settings.

The one exception to the modeling approach used was the community mobilization strategy. Here, we used the impact matrix developed as part of the Futures Institute's Goals Express model (Bollinger 2008), which specifies the forms of behavior change that result from exposure to community collectivization. These default parameters relate to a slight reduction in the age of first sex, and modest increases in condom use. The Goals Express model was then used to estimate how the reduction in the age of sexual debut and increases in the levels of condom use translate into reductions in HIV incidence.

Although our literature review suggested that in practice the benefits of community collectivization may be much broader than solely increasing condom use, it was not possible to adjust this parameterization in any way. Furthermore, as it was only possible to use the Goals Express model in a limited number of countries where there was data input, we used a very crude method to extrapolate the estimate of impact to other countries – by applying the median value of the ratio of the number of HIV infections averted/person reached across the countries modeled to the other countries.

Alcohol taxation

A global systematic review of 112 studies concluded that a 10 percent increase in alcohol prices resulted in a 5 percent reduction in drinking (Wagenaar et al. 2010). However, the price elasticity among heavy drinkers is expectedly lower, approximately -0.28 according to another review (Wagenaar et al. 2009). Chisholm et al. (2004) estimate that, in Africa sub-region E, a 25 percent increase in taxation, combined with a subsequent 10 percent increase in unrecorded consumption, would result in an 8.1 percent reduction in the incidence of hazardous alcohol use, considering the existing prevalence of three preferred beverages and their respective price elasticities.

Table 5.9 Key inputs used to estimate the impact of increases in taxation on HIV incidence

Policy intervention	Intermediate effects	Impact on HIV	Source
Increasing alcohol taxes	8.1% reduction in problem drinking, as a result of a 25% increase in alcohol taxation	77% reduction in annual HIV incidence among male and female problem drinkers who become non-problem drinkers	Chisholm et al. (2004) Fisher et al. (2007)

A systematic review and meta-analysis of African studies on the association between alcohol use and HIV infection found that, when compared to non-drinkers, problem drinkers had a 77 percent higher odds of being HIV-positive than non-problem drinkers (2.04 vs 1.57) (Fisher et al. 2007). Similarly, another global meta-analysis that restricted its selection criteria to incident HIV infection found that alcohol consumers were at 77 percent higher risk of HIV infection compared to non-drinkers (Baliunas et al. 2010). For our analysis we modeled a 77 percent reduction in annual HIV incidence for problem drinkers who become non-problem drinkers.

Given that alcohol affects the immune system and contributes to a worsened course of HIV/AIDS, there are more HIV-related benefits of reduced alcohol consumption through delayed disease progression, increased support-seeking behavior, and treatment adherence (Shuper et al. 2010). We model these additional benefits in terms of DALYs saved based on an estimation method that found that the percentage of AIDS deaths that can be attributed to alcohol consumption range from 0.03 percent to 0.34 percent for men and 0 percent to 0.17 percent for women (Gmel et al. 2011). Other morbidity and mortality benefits from reducing alcohol use through taxation were documented by Wagenaar et al. (2010), who find that doubling tax levels would reduce alcohol-related mortality by an average of 35 percent, traffic crash deaths by 11 percent, sexually transmitted disease by 6 percent, violence by 2 percent, and crime by 1.4 percent. These benefits were not included in our analysis.

Keeping girls in secondary school

We model a 60 percent annual reduction in HIV incidence among the target group, in line with the findings from the Malawi trial, that found that, eighteen months into the World Bank program, HIV prevalence was 60 percent lower and HSV-2 prevalence 75 percent lower among girls receiving the cash transfers who were already in school at the start of the intervention, compared to the control group. There is currently insufficient evidence to ascertain whether this short-term impact is likely to be sustained and therefore represent an infection averted for life, or to merely delay infection until after the intervention. Long-term post-intervention impact will be evaluated in 2012 (World Bank 2011).

At the intermediate level, the conditional cash transfer appears to have led to sexual behavior change, as evidenced by the delayed sexual debut, reduced number of sexual partners, and a lower frequency of sexual activity, but no effect on condom use. However, these reported changes in sexual behavior explain less than half of the program's impact on HIV prevalence. The change in the risk profiles of the girls' sexual partners accounts for the rest of the variation, with simulations revealing that the HIV prevalence among the male sexual partners of treatment girls was about 50 percent less than among partners of the control group girls. The causal pathway most supported by this intervention study is that girls in school are empowered to make safer choices of younger partners, resorting less to transactional and intergenerational sex. The study noted a dose response effect with payment size, suggesting that poverty was an important motivation for transactional sex (World Bank 2011).

The extent to which such an intervention is merely shifting the demand from older high-risk men towards the girls that are out-of-school, and thus increasing their susceptibility to HIV infection, remains to be determined. At the population level, this could mean a zero net benefit from the intervention. It would be important to determine what degree of coverage of keeping girls in school would be necessary to overcome this displacement effect and therefore alter the course of the epidemic.

Adding gender and HIV training to livelihood programs

The IMAGE program impact was assessed by comparing IMAGE clients in intervention communities with a control group of non-clients in matched non-intervention communities. The cluster randomized controlled trial showed a 55 percent decrease in past-year intimate partner violence within two years (Pronyk et al. 2006; Kim et al. 2007). A randomized trial of the Stepping Stones model found a 48 percent reduction in IPV perpetration by targeted men after two years (AOR = 0.48, 0.38 to 1.01) (Jewkes et al. 2008). Despite these impacts, over the relatively short durations of the trials neither IMAGE nor the Stepping Stones interventions were found to impact significantly on community levels of HIV incidence, although significant reductions in HSV-2 were documented among men in the Stepping Stones trial.

In our analysis, we model the potential influence of reductions in intimate partner violence (and the underlying issue of gender inequality) on subsequent HIV transmission. We focus on this link as a recent longitudinal analysis in South Africa found that HIV incidence was higher among women who reported more than one episode of intimate partner violence in the past year or who had low equity in their relationship. Gender inequalities and intimate partner violence are both associated with a 32–34 percent increased risk of incident HIV infection over two years (Jewkes et al. 2010).

Drawing upon these research findings, we model the impact of an intervention that leads to a 50 percent reduction in violence, assuming a conservative estimate of the past-year prevalence of IPV of 20 percent in all sub-Saharan countries (WHO 2008). We then estimate that among those who are in relationships where violence has ceased, the annual incidence of HIV infection would be reduced by 20 percent.

This approach to the modeling, where we consider the indirect benefits of gender training on levels of partner violence, may be conservative. Although initially there appeared to be no generalized impact of IMAGE on sexual behavior and HIV incidence (Pronyk et al. 2006), a

Table 5.10 Key inputs used to estimate the impact of adding HIV and gender training onto livelihood programs

Policy intervention	Intermediate effects	Impact on HIV	Source
Adding participatory gender and HIV training to existing microfinance and livelihood programs	55% reduction in incidence of intimate partner violence (IPV)	Assume 20% reduction in annual HIV incidence, given reduction in IPV	Pronyk et al. (2006)
Stepping Stones gender training for women and men	48% reduction in IPV perpetration by targeted men after 2 years		Jewkes et al. (2010)

Table 5.11 Key inputs used to estimate the impact of community mobilization

Policy intervention	Intermediate effects	Impact on HIV	Source
Investing in community mobilization	10% reduction in condom non-use for medium-risk groups 2.5% reduction in condom non-use for low-risk groups 0.3 reduction in age at first sex	Modeled effects by country using the Goals Express model	Bollinger (2008)

subsequent analysis focusing on a subset of young female beneficiaries (14–35 years) found that they were more likely to have accessed VCT and less likely to have had unprotected sex at last intercourse with a non-spousal partner (Pronyk et al. 2008).

The Stepping Stones intervention trial results found a 33 percent reduction in the incidence of HSV-2. Furthermore, it was found to significantly reduce certain risk behaviors in men, such as transactional sex and problem drinking. Interestingly, however, in the Stepping Stones trial women's sexual behavior and risk of violence did not change (Jewkes et al. 2008), underscoring the potentially critical role of the income effect from the microfinance component on women's sexual behavior and risk of violence.

Community mobilization

Few intervention studies to date have rigorously assessed the impact of community mobilization on HIV infection, but a number have determined its effects on intermediate indicators of sexual behavior, namely reported sexual debut and condom use. A review by Bollinger et al. estimated that community mobilization as an intervention has a negative effect, as it decreases age at first sex by 0.3 years, but also reduces condom non-use by 10 percent among medium-risk groups (i.e., men and women with more than one sexual partner in the previous year, excluding sex workers and their clients) and by 2.5 percent among low-risk groups (i.e., men and women with one partner only in the previous year) (Bollinger 2008). The consequent impact on HIV transmission is based on the Goals Express model discussed earlier.

It is worth noting, however, that the inputs used by Goals Express appear to underestimate the potential impact of this intervention, if evidence from other parts of the world can be considered applicable. Studies in India, for example, have found that female sex workers exposed to a community mobilization intervention were 41 to 109 percent more likely to report consistent condom use, than those receiving a standard care package (Blankenship et al. 2008; Halli et al. 2006; Swendeman et al. 2009). Additionally, those who were both exposed to the intervention and had high levels of collective agency were 2.5 times more likely to report consistent condom use than other female sex workers. Although this is specific to high-risk groups, it does suggest, at the very least, that community mobilization can have a more significant impact among these groups and in countries with more concentrated epidemics. Based upon our review, and emerging evidence on the potential importance of community mobilization activities as part of a targeted intervention approach, we feel that these effects are likely to severely underestimate the effects of community mobilization.

Estimating cost-effectiveness and benefit to cost ratios

Cost-effectiveness

We estimated the incremental cost per DALY of each intervention, but contained this to costs and DALYs directly related to HIV. The following broad formula was used: incremental cost per DALY = (incremental costs of the intervention – cost savings from reduced ART treatment)/DALYs from HIV infections averted.

Costs and HIV infections averted within the five-year period were included. We estimated DALYs averted from these HIV infections averted using standard formulae and disability weights. DALYs were calculated using the following assumptions. Those on ART have a longer life expectancy than those without, and require different disability weights. We assumed that the proportion of those on ART remained the same as in 2010 when estimating the overall DALYs averted. Our calculations were made for both a 3 percent and 5 percent discount rate, as recommended by *RethinkHIV*.

We estimated the incremental costs of each intervention by multiplying coverage with the unit costs described above. However, it is important to note that for the interventions of gender training and community mobilization activities, incremental costs related to HIV impact can be distinguished. In contrast, in the case of alcohol taxation and keeping girls in school, the separate costs that contribute to HIV reduction cannot be distinguished. In the latter case, we therefore had to include the entire cost of the intervention in the cost-effectiveness ratio.

We estimated cost savings from HIV infections averted assuming that the proportion of those who would get access to ART would remain similar to that in 2010 (WHO 2010). The estimate of lifetime cost was taken from Cleary *et al.* (2006). At a 3 percent discount rate this is estimated to be $9,426 and at a 5 percent discount rate $8,225 for South Africa (2010 dollars). Based on the detailed cost breakdown presented in Cleary *et al.* (2006) this was then adjusted to other countries assuming that the prices of drugs and other international supplies remain the same between countries (approximately 50 percent of expenditures), and the other

Table 5.12 DALY parameters

Parameters	Value	Source
Age weight	0.04	GBD 2004
Disability weight pre-AIDS	0.135	GBD 2004
Disability weight AIDS	0.505	GBD 2004
Disability weight ART	0.167	GBD 2004
Duration pre-AIDS	8 years	Creese *et al.* 2004
Duration ART	13 years	Cleary 2004
Duration AIDS (no ART)	3 years	Creese *et al.* 2004
Age-specific life expectancy	Country specific	WHO life tables
Age of onset of HIV:		
Keeping girls in school	17 years	
Alcohol taxation	20 years	
Economic empowerment and gender training	25 years	
Community mobilization	20 years	

50 percent was adjusted by GDP per capita (as recommended by *RethinkHIV*).

Benefit to cost ratios

For all interventions, we estimated the benefits of DALYs averted by converting DALYs using the amounts of $1,000 and $5,000 as recommended by *RethinkHIV*. For community mobilization and gender training, we conservatively assumed no additional DALY or further economic gain beyond those gained from reductions in HIV infections, due to the lack of data in this area. For keeping girls and alcohol taxation in school we made a number of adjustments for additional health benefits, economic benefit, and costs beyond those to HIV. These are described in detail below.

Keeping girls in school

Our literature review found a number of other health benefits of keeping girls in school including lower fertility, improved maternal health, and improved child nutrition. Moreover schooling has an economic benefit in terms of higher labor market productivity and future earnings. One conservative

Table 5.13 Benefit to cost ratio of keeping girls in school, excluding HIV impact

Scenario	B/C ratio of keeping girls in school, excluding HIV impact
Low discount, low DALY	6.9
Low discount, high DALY	18.28
High discount, low DALY	3.49
High discount, high DALY	9.24

estimate of these well-documented benefits suggests that a 1 percent increase in years of female schooling is associated with a 0.37 percent increase in per capita income (Knowles *et al.* 2002). We add both these non-HIV benefits into the model, by referring to previous work done for the Copenhagen Consensus Center (King *et al.* 2007). These estimate a benefit to cost ratio of conditional cash transfers for girls including the effect on income and on under-five mortality. We use here the most conservative estimates from that report. These assume that an extra 0.7 year of schooling is achieved for one year of CCT funding, but no direct mortality effect is included. It should however be noted that these effects are achieved at a lower cost than our estimates of the level of cost of conditional cash transfers required to achieve an HIV impact. However, for simplicity, we have conservatively assumed that any extra payment in the intervention will result in no additional benefits.

Alcohol taxation

A recent review of the effectiveness and cost-effectiveness of policies and programs to reduce the harm caused by alcohol highlights the complex interaction between alcohol and health (Anderson *et al.* 2009). Beyond this, there are likely to be a wide range of economic costs and benefits of changes in alcohol consumption. Given the complexity of these relationships, we consider only two issues here. The first is the additional benefits in terms of DALYs gained, as reported by Chisholm *et al.* (2004). These exclude the impact on HIV infection and only examine the direct impact on morbidity and mortality. As stated above, Chisholm *et al.* estimate that with a 25 percent increase in alcohol taxation it costs $92 to avert

a DALY in sub-region E in Africa. This reflects a gain of 1,589 DALYs averted per one million population per year. We applied this gain in DALYs averted to our model respectively, and then valued DALYs as *RethinkHIV* recommends, at $1,000 and $5,000.

We also included the deadweight (welfare) loss associated with tax distortions in our analysis. We estimate this using standard formula. We modeled the loss for 500ml discount beer, assuming a price elasticity of demand of -0.3. Retail prices and sales figures were sourced from WHO's global data repository. Where we had data gaps we filled them with regional averages. Table 5.14 shows the parameters used in our calculations below.

Other benefits that are excluded from our analysis

Apart from the specific issues above, there are two key types of benefits that are omitted from our analysis, reflecting our general approach, but need to be taken into account when interpreting our findings:

- Our findings exclude most externalities. For example, we do not account for any impact from those girls in school on other girls who may not receive conditional cash transfers. This could work in two ways. In a positive way, other girls may decide to also attend school, encouraged by their peers. On the other hand, men who are seeking young girls as partners may focus on other groups. We also do not include any consequences on orphans or others impacted by the loss of someone with HIV. Moreover, as stated above, our findings include only the short-term effect. This also applies to externalities. For example, a study by Brent *et al.* (2009) highlights the fact that in the longer run there may be additional externalities from education, such as other members in a household becoming educated and healthier, that may translate to longer-term productivity gains for all. For example, King *et al.* (2008) estimate that including these benefits may increase the low discount, low DALY B/C ratio of 6.90 to 8.45.
- We have applied no equity weight to our results. While there are those who argue that efficiency

Table 5.14 Parameters used in estimates of deadweight loss for alcohol tax

Location	500 ml discount beer					
	Current			With 25% increase in excise tax		
	Price ($)	Excise tax (as % of retail price)	Sales in 1,000 hectoliters	Sales in 500 ml (million)	New excise tax	Change in sales (PED = −0.3)	DWL ($)
Angola	1.5	0.22	5,695	1,139.0	0.28	−25,922,069	−1,494,541
Benin	0.8	0.1	622	124.4	0.13	−1,066,286	−12,491
Botswana	1.1	0.3	561	112.2	0.38	−4,039,200	−270,809
Burkina Faso	0.9	0.25	718	143.6	0.31	−3,916,364	−156,655
Burundi	0.5	0.35	1,348	269.6	0.44	−12,454,088	−450,662
Cameroon	0.7	0.22	5,054	1,010.8	0.28	−23,004,414	−645,710
Central African Republic	1.1	0.22	156	31.2	0.28	−710,069	−29,358
Chad	1.3	0.22	335	67.0	0.28	−1,524,828	−72,298
Comoros	2.9	0.22	1	0.2	0.28	−4,552	−502
Congo	0.9	0.22	1,324	264.8	0.28	−6,026,483	−212,589
Côte d'Ivoire	0.9	0.12	1,388	277.6	0.15	−3,026,127	−51,131
Democratic Republic of the Congo	1	0.1	3,476	695.2	0.13	−5,958,857	−85,127
Equatorial Guinea	1.3	0.22	205	41.0	0.28	−933,103	−46,012
Eritrea	3.3	0.2	3	0.6	0.25	−12,000	−1,332
Ethiopia	1	0.22	2,649	529.8	0.28	−12,057,517	−448,207
Gabon	1.1	0.22	1,131	226.2	0.28	−5,148,000	−218,197
Gambia	2.4	0.11	30	6.0	0.14	−59,214	−2,367
Ghana	1.1	0.2	2,046	409.2	0.25	−8,184,000	−304,832
Guinea	0.8	0.22	200	40.0	0.28	−910,345	−28,660
Guinea-Bissau	0.8	0.17	45	9.0	0.21	−142,464	−3,157
Kenya	0.8	0.22	4,682	936.4	0.28	−21,311,172	−622,433
Lesotho	1.2	0.18	328	65.6	0.23	−1,142,710	−38,152
Liberia	0.9	0.03	140	28.0	0.04	−65,455	−235
Madagascar	1.1	0.16	832	166.4	0.2	−2,457,121	−66,518
Malawi	1.1	0.22	191	38.2	0.28	−869,379	−36,849
Mali	0.2	0.22	103	20.6	0.28	−468,828	−3,912
Mauritius	1.1	0.22	298	59.6	0.28	−1,356,414	−57,491
Mozambique	0.6	0.4	1,461	292.2	0.5	−17,532,000	−1,086,984
Namibia	1.1	0.22	914	182.8	0.28	−4,160,276	−176,333
Niger	0.7	0.08	80	16.0	0.1	−106,667	−865
Nigeria	1.1	0.22	11,114	2,222.8	0.28	−50,587,862	−2,144,160
Rwanda	0.7	0.61	650	130.0	0.76	−25,042,105	−5,788,680

Table 5.14 (cont.)

Location	500 ml discount beer						
	Current				With 25% increase in excise tax		
	Price ($)	Excise tax (as % of retail price)	Sales in 1,000 hectoliters	Sales in 500 ml (million)	New excise tax	Change in sales (PED = −0.3)	DWL ($)
Senegal	1.6	0.22	242	48.4	0.28	−1,101,517	−65,179
Sierra Leone	1.6	0.03	276	55.2	0.03	−106,839	−538
South Africa	1.1	0.33	26,526	5,305.2	0.41	−223,495,660	−17,534,822
Swaziland	1.1	0.22	193	38.6	0.28	−878,483	−37,234
Togo	0.8	0.09	461	92.2	0.12	−718,847	−7,753
Uganda	0.8	0.22	1,735	347.0	0.28	−7,897,241	−230,654
United Republic of Tanzania	1.1	0.26	3,930	786.0	0.32	−22,577,523	−1,221,398
Zambia	0.3	0.6	639	127.8	0.75	−23,004,000	−2,139,372
Zimbabwe	1.1	0.4	523	104.6	0.5	−6,276,000	−701,292

analyses should include distributional weights, by excluding them we are assuming an equal value of welfare independent of income level. Yet, our interventions are primarily focused on those groups who may be more vulnerable and/or poorer than those who are recipients of alternative HIV interventions. For many, this provides additional value to the social interventions we consider.

Results

Table 5.15 shows the findings on the unit cost, annual cost, and total cost of each intervention modeled, using the coverage figures specified above.

The mean unit cost of the alcohol taxation was $0.17 per capita. At this cost, when summed, the total discounted costs of implementing the intervention across sub-Saharan Africa was around $343 million ($330 million using a 5 percent discount rate). For community mobilization, the mean unit cost was $3.60 per recipient, with a range of $0.33 to $37.10 between countries. When summed, the total discounted cost was $286 million using a 3 percent discount rate ($276 million using a 5 percent discount rate). The average unit costs for keeping girls in school was much higher – $434 per recipient, with a range of $161 to $2,867 between

countries. When summed, the total discounted cost was $8,850 million using a 3 percent discount rate ($8,859 million using a 5 percent discount rate). This reflects the high unit costs and high coverage assumptions used for this scenario. Gender/HIV training has a mean cost of $3.77 and the total costs would be around $21 million. In total, we estimate that these intervention scenarios would cost $9.5 billion (with a 3 percent discount rate) to implement – with keeping girls in school taking up the vast majority of the funding available.

Table 5.16 shows the infections and DALYs averted and the cost savings from reductions in ART costs from the infection averted. For the coverage scenarios considered in our analyses, the highest number of infections averted is generated from keeping girls in school (this covers all of those with an income under $1.25 per day), with alcohol tax also making a substantial contribution. As gender/HIV training and community mobilization have been constrained by the number of current participants in livelihood interventions, they make a relatively small contribution to overall infections averted. It is estimated that, over time, total ART cost savings from this package of intervention would amount to $263 million at a 3 percent discount rate ($224 million at a 5 percent discount rate).

Table 5.15 Unit cost (mean/min/max), annual cost, and total cost (3%/5% discount rates) (2010 dollars)

	Mean unit cost ($2010)	Min unit cost ($2010)	Max unit cost ($2010)	Annual coverage (million persons)	Annual cost ($2010)	Total cost (discounted 3%) ($2010)	Total cost (discounted 5%) ($2010)
Alcohol taxation	0.18	0.17	0.19	408.3	72,770,600	343,266,081	330,811,546
Keeping girls in school	434.01	161.62	2,867.71	5.8	1,876,176,436	8,850,108,871	8,529,005,216
Gender and HIV training on livelihood programs	3.77	0.36	34.27	1.7	4,508,099	21,265,144	20,493,593
Community mobilization	3.56	0.33	37.1	17.9	60,758,486	286,603,756	276,205,069

Table 5.16 Infections averted, DALYs averted, and cost savings (3%/5% discount rates) (2010 dollars)

	Cumulative infections averted by year 5	Cumulative DALYs averted by year 5 (3%)	Cumulative DALYs averted by year 5 (5%)	Cost savings ART from infections averted by year 5 (3%) ($2010)	Cost savings ART from infections averted by year 5 (5%) ($2010)
Alcohol taxation	29,764	361,945	348,958	88,820,287	76,932,062
Keeping girls in school	35,430	445,194	429,141	104,361,680	90,393,304
Gender and HIV training on livelihood programs	13,865	162,009	156,188	44,102,031	38,199,158
Community mobilization	7,086	87,756	84,572	26,307,689	19,084,100

Table 5.17 Total cost, cost savings, DALYs averted incremental cost per DALY (2010 dollars)

	Total cost (discounted 3%)	Total cost (discounted 5%)	Cost savings ART (3%)	Cost savings ART (5%)	Total DALYs averted (3%)	Total DALYs averted (5%)	Incremental cost per DALY (3%)	Incremental cost per DALY (5%)
Alcohol taxation	343,266,081	330,811,546	88,820,287	76,932,062	361,945	348,958	703	728
Keeping girls in school	8,850,108,871	8,529,005,216	104,361,680	90,393,304	445,194	429,141	19,645	19,664
Gender and HIV training on livelihood programs	21,265,144	20,493,593	44,102,031	38,199,158	162,009	156,188	−141	−113
Community mobilization	286,603,756	276,205,069	26,307,689	19,084,100	87,756	84,572	2,966	3,040

Table 5.17 shows our results for the incremental cost per DALY for each intervention. It should be noted that these costs include any cost savings from reductions in ART. The cost per DALY for all interventions, bar the training programs, appears high compared to other well-known health interventions. However, it should be noted that this is an artefact of the methods used. As we could not separate out the incremental costs of alcohol taxation and keeping girls in school in any meaningful way (the health impact would not be achieved without the full expenditure), the costs appear high when only compared to the DALY averted gain.

In the case of community mobilization and stigma reduction our estimates are also high. In practice our analyses rely heavily on the findings from the country-specific coverage and effect measured used for this analysis, that were drawn from previous modeling and resource projection activities on this issue, and the approach that we used to extrapolate the findings from the countries where we were able to use the Goals Express model to project impact on HIV, and the other countries.

Based upon our review of the literature we feel that it is very likely these modeled projections fail to adequately capture the benefits of community mobilization intervention activities focused on key vulnerable groups. However, using the Goals Express model we were not able to alter the community mobilization model inputs, to enable us to obtain estimates of these effects. Moreover, the approach that we used to extrapolate the country-specific modeled projections to other sub-Saharan African countries was also very limited. Our choice of applying the median ratio of the reduction in HIV incidence per beneficiary was pragmatic, chosen in the absence of other viable alternatives.

The low cost per DALY for gender and HIV programs is much lower than the work presented by Jan et al. (2010). This is because these previous estimates only took into account the DALY gain from the prevention of intimate partner violence. Adding the HIV impact, when dealing with such a low cost intervention, results in cost savings, due to long-term cost savings from ART treatment averted.

Table 5.18 illustrates how our results on incremental cost per DALY vary significantly by setting – here the mean, minimum, and maximum are provided (across countries). This illustrates that variation across settings is significant. For example, for alcohol taxation the incremental cost per DALY ranges from $262,874 to a negative value. The full results by country are presented in the Appendix.

Table 5.19 shows the average costs, benefits, and benefit to cost ratios at a 3 percent discount rate. The net health benefit includes both the benefit derived from DALYs averted and the cost savings from ART. Other benefits are added in the case of alcohol taxation and keeping girls in school.

It can be seen that in comparison to the cost-effectiveness figures presented above, both alcohol taxation and keeping girls in school start to fare better, once the additional economic benefits of each policy are added. As no additional benefits were added to community mobilization, and it had a relatively low cost-effectiveness result, this has the lowest benefit to cost ratio at around unity. Training as part of livelihood programs has the highest benefit to cost ratio. The economic benefits of alcohol taxation and keeping girls in school considerably outweigh the health benefit. In the case of keeping girls in school the broader economic benefits are so substantial that the added benefit from HIV infections averted makes little difference to the earlier results found by King et al. (2007).

Table 5.20 shows the same results, but for a 5 percent discount rate. This highlights the fact that the benefits from keeping girls in school are longer term and hence are highly sensitive to the discount rate being applied.

Given that our results vary substantially by country, we also present one example here (alcohol taxation) that illustrates how our results may be applied. Examining the drivers of our cost-effectiveness and benefit-cost ratios for alcohol taxation, as anticipated, cost-effectiveness is strongly influenced by the current levels of unrecorded consumption and HIV prevalence. As mentioned above, unrecorded consumption provides an indication of the probable levels of substitution from taxed to unrecorded consumption of alcohol, and as such will determine overall health and fiscal impact. Similarly, those countries with much higher levels of HIV prevalence will benefit considerably more than those

Table 5.18 Mean, minimum, and maximum incremental cost and cost per DALY per intervention (2010 dollars)

	Mean incremental cost per DALY (3%)	Min of incremental cost per DALY (3%)	Max of incremental cost per DALY (3%)	Mean incremental cost per DALY (5%)	Min of incremental cost per DALY (5%)	Max of incremental cost per DALY (5%)
Alcohol taxation	18,412	−603	262,874	18,435	−511	262,872
Keeping girls in school	113,627	3,695	1,142,031	113,647	3,724	1,142,050
Gender and HIV training on livelihood programs	461	−660	14,603	487	−561	14,615
Community mobilization	2,347	−817	22,982	2,489	−552	23,127

Table 5.19 Total cost, net health benefit, and benefit to cost ratio by intervention, using a 3% discount rate (2010 dollars)

	Total cost (discounted 3%)	Net benefit HIV only ($1,000) (3%)	Net benefit HIV only ($5,000) (3%)	Net benefit ($1,000) (3%)	Net benefit ($5,000) (3%)	B/C ratio ($1,000) (3%)	B/C ratio ($5,000) (3%)
Alcohol taxation	343,266,081	450,765,138	1,898,544,541	2,066,902,856	10,125,215,099	6.02	29.50
Keeping girls in school	8,850,108,871	549,555,902	2,330,332,791	61,615,307,110	162,329,546,058	6.96	18.34
Gender and HIV training on livelihood programs	21,265,144	206,110,555	854,144,652	206,110,555	854,144,652	9.69	40.17
Community mobilization	286,603,756	114,064,109	465,089,790	114,064,109	465,089,790	0.40	1.62

Table 5.20 Total cost, net health benefit, and benefit to cost ratio by intervention, 5% discount rate (2010 dollars)

	Total cost (discounted 5%)	Net benefit health only ($1,000) (5%)	Net benefit health only ($5,000) (5%)	Net benefit ($1,000) (5%)	Net benefit ($5,000) (5%)	B/C ratio ($1,000) (5%)	B/C ratio ($5,000) (5%)
Alcohol taxation	330,811,546	425,889,586	1,821,719,681	1,890,481,643	9,290,661,936	5.71	28.08
Keeping girls in school	8,529,005,216	519,534,677	2,236,100,168	31,436,435,861	82,324,561,867	3.69	9.65
Gender and HIV training on livelihood programs	20,493,593	194,386,888	819,137,806	194,386,888	819,137,806	9.49	39.97
Community mobilization	276,205,069	103,656,502	441,946,110	103,656,502	441,946,110	0.38	1.60

Table 5.21 List of countries where unrecorded consumption<50%, B/C ratio>1, and (HIV) CE threshold<3x GDP/cap

Country	Average of incremental cost per DALY	Sum of B/C ratio 1,000 (3%)	Unrecorded consumption	Prevalence of hazardous drinking (%)	GDP per capita	CE threshold (3 x GDP/cap)
Botswana	−603	14.6	38%	12.7	6,064	18,192
Gabon	796	1.19	21%	5.7	7,502	22,506
Malawi	902	1.48	29%	3.3	310	930
Mauritius	7,276	0.44	27%	4.0	6,735	20,205
Mozambique	−9	15.31	34%	18.6	428	1,284
Namibia	850	9.45	39%	7.3	4,267	12,801
Nigeria	559	1.96	20%	11.3	1,118	3,354
South Africa	−203	14.07	26%	11.2	5,786	17,358
Swaziland	33	11.11	0%	2.4	2,533	7,599
Uganda	147	12.21	8%	10.4	490	1,470
United Republic of Tanzania	1,031	9.45	30%	5.7	503	1,509
Zambia	173	10.42	39%	7.0	990	2,970
Zimbabwe	520	10.07	20%	5.4	449	1,347

with lower levels of HIV prevalence. Table 5.21 therefore provides a list of countries for which our analysis suggests alcohol taxation may be most beneficial in terms of reducing HIV, without substantially impeding taxation or creating other health concerns.

Sensitivity analyses

Although not presented here, we also explored the potential sensitivity of the findings to the various assumptions about the effect of the intervention on HIV incidence. Specifically, for alcohol taxation, we explored the effect of using the assumption of how moving from problematic to non-problematic alcohol use impacts on HIV incidence compared to more moderate drinkers (low 38.5 percent, high 90 percent). For community mobilization, we varied the method used to extrapolate the impact projections across settings, with the low estimate using the minimum value of the ratio of the infections averted per person reached across the settings modeled, and the high estimate coming from the maximum of these values. For interventions to keep girls

in school, the low estimate used an assumption of a 30 percent reduction in annual HIV incidence, and the high estimate used an assumption of a 90 percent reduction in annual HIV incidence per beneficiary. This upper range was used to capture the possible long-term benefits of education on HIV as reported in the study by Brent *et al.* (2009). For the gender/HIV training intervention, our low estimate considered a 25 percent reduction in intimate partner violence, with a 10 percent reduction in annual HIV incidence among beneficiaries. The high effect estimate was obtained using an estimate of a 75 percent reduction in intimate partner violence, and a resulting 30 percent reduction in risk of HIV infection.

The analyses highlighted that the findings that are most sensitive to changes in inputs are those that rely most on the estimates of HIV impact to generate benefit – i.e., community mobilization and training on livelihoods. As would be expected, the projected benefit to cost ratios are much higher for the higher effect assumptions, with increases in the effect assumptions near enough proportionally increasing the B/C ratio. Given the uncertainty around the input values used in our analyses, and in particular our concern over the robustness of our modeling of the impact of community mobilization, an important research priority is to generate better evidence of impact in different sub-Saharan African settings. However, for keeping girls in school and alcohol taxation, the impact of changing the HIV effect assumptions was more muted, as they contribute to such a small proportion of the overall benefits.

Discussion and conclusion

In our analyses we have sought to model, country by country, the benefit/cost ratios of four very varied forms of social policy intervention, drawing upon existing empirical cost and effects data, and linking this with country-specific economic, epidemiological, behavioral, and demographic data. This was challenging, both given the relative paucity of rigorous economic or impact evaluation data, and because we were forced to take an individual perspective on structural forms of interventions that may have much broader longer-term societal impact. A further limitation of our work has been the difficulty in distinguishing which costs to include and exclude. We were very pragmatic in our approach. If the HIV impact could be achieved by "piggy-backing," then we estimate the incremental cost of doing so. However, where this could not be achieved, we decided to fund the entire cost of the intervention. In reality HIV funds are unlikely to be used this way. A much higher cost-effectiveness and benefit to cost ratio is likely to be achieved by partnering with those involved in livelihoods improvement, community development, and education expansion.

Our findings suggest that alcohol taxation is potentially promising, even when we only include HIV-related consequences and have not factored in the broader economic and social effects. Although this form of intervention is potentially politically sensitive, we nevertheless sought to model its potential costs and benefits, given strong evidence on the price elasticity of alcohol consumption, good evidence of the relationship between problematic alcohol use and incident HIV infection, and demonstrated evidence of the impacts of alco-

hol taxation on levels of STI infection in the US. Although the practical and political challenges of such a policy should not be underestimated, we feel that it is important that HIV impact evidence is used to inform future policy discussions on this topic.

Our analyses of the potential benefit to cost ratios associated with paying girls to stay in secondary school support previous CCC analyses of the benefit of these forms of intervention. In practice we found that the lowest cost/HIV infection ratios were in low-GDP, high-HIV prevalence countries, with the HIV benefits generally improving already high B/C ratios. These findings suggest that in these settings it would be appropriate for HIV programs to finance some (albeit a percentage) of the total cost investments to keep girls in school.

Our modeling of the amounts of investments in community mobilization and gender and HIV training was limited by the scope of evidence available on each form of intervention. Our findings suggest that both forms of intervention are relatively low cost. Comparing the findings across countries, our B/C ratio estimates range from <1 to over 70, with the ratios being greatest in settings where HIV prevalence is high. These findings suggest that these forms of intervention are likely to be most cost-effective where the interventions are focused on targeted sub-populations or communities.

Although in our analyses we presented the findings from four specific intervention options, it is important to resist the temptation to devise a standard list of structural interventions across very different contexts and epidemic settings in SSA. Whilst, in this analysis, we have considered a relatively fixed intervention model, implemented in each sub-Saharan African country, in practice it is likely that specific adaptations to different settings would need to be made. For example, initiatives to keep girls in secondary school may or may not require a conditionality component, and community mobilization and stigma reduction interventions are likely to take different forms in different settings. Indeed, it has been strongly argued that structural approaches do not work the same way or have the same effect in all populations and settings. Specific details of both the people and the settings that make particular program or policy inputs relevant and effective must be established and analyzed (Gupta *et al.* 2008). These differences may have a fundamental impact on our results, both in terms of the effect size, but also which interventions are more cost-effective in which setting.

We must also caution, at this early stage in the field, of making too many direct comparisons between the four strategies considered, or between the evidence presented here and the more biomedical intervention options presented in other chapters. Whilst we have attempted to accurately incorporate the cost inputs and broad range of intervention benefits, the analysis of each of the interventions have their specific strengths and limitations. Although we were able to include many of the benefits of keeping girls in school, we were not able to adequately estimate the longer-term impact of income on HIV, nor many of the externalities that it may bring. Similarly, although we tried to estimate the benefits of reduced problematic alcohol use on HIV, we were not able to sufficiently value the other economic and well-being effects of this change. As discussed above, although we recognize that structural interventions – by their very nature – seek to achieve widespread societal change, in general we were not able to fully quantify the potential long-term or wider societal benefits of each of the interventions being modeled.

Finally, despite these challenges, our findings point to the untapped potential of each of these forms of intervention considered in different countries in sub-Saharan Africa. Unfortunately there is still much uncertainty in our analyses. Despite a growing body of program experience in each of the fields considered, we were able to draw upon only a handful of evaluation studies of a limited range of intervention options. This is a reflection on the research and donor priorities of the HIV/AIDS field. Whilst millions have been invested into the development and testing of new biomedical prevention options, limited resources have gone into structural intervention research. As part of *RethinkHIV*, the ambition is to promote innovative thinking on how to strengthen the HIV response in sub-Saharan Africa. Although it is too early to compare our findings with those from more researched areas of HIV intervention presented in other chapters, it would be wrong to conclude that a lack of evidence equates with a lack of effect. If anything, we hope that our findings demonstrate the potential value of moving beyond the more biomedical and health service intervention paradigms and that the current failure to invest in the implementation and evaluation of structural interventions is an important omission. We need to collect greater evidence on the costs of different social policy options, and to support rigorous evidence on the short- and long-term benefits of different social interventions.

Appendix – country-level results

Table 5.22 Coverage by country (persons)

	Alcohol taxation	Community mobilization	Keeping girls in school	Gender and HIV training on livelihood programs
Angola	8,868,000	177,360	112,292	3,547
Benin	4,336,000	780,480	60,918	28,695
Botswana	1,080,000	21,600	22,867	3,672
Burkina Faso	7,522,000	150,440	74,834	30,547
Burundi	4,437,000	88,740	23,805	2,822
Cameroon	9,706,000	194,120	42,842	41,023
Central African Republic	2,176,000	43,520	15,072	870
Chad	5,188,000	103,760	25,955	4,656
Comoros	356,000	7,120	1,724	1,210

(cont.)

Table 5.22 (*cont.*)

	Alcohol taxation	Community mobilization	Keeping girls in school	Gender and HIV training on livelihood programs
Congo	1,844,000	36,880	44,362	15,007
Côte d'Ivoire	10,307,000	206,140	56,339	9,482
Democratic Republic of the Congo	30,519,000	610,380	516,319	15,036
Djibouti	466,000	9,320	3,478	1,584
Equatorial Guinea	332,000	6,640	3,742	1,129
Eritrea	2,627,000	52,540	27,086	8,932
Ethiopia	39,765,000	4,771,800	431,995	462,482
Gabon	776,000	15,520	1,481	310
Gambia	827,000	16,540	11,079	2,658
Ghana	12,298,000	245,960	157,626	71,743
Guinea	4,829,000	96,580	38,645	14,163
Guinea-Bissau	754,000	15,080	2,767	332
Kenya	19,757,000	2,370,840	177,891	294,234
Lesotho	1,017,000	20,340	15,233	3,458
Liberia	1,940,000	38,800	30,584	5,694
Madagascar	9,577,000	191,540	160,747	13,119
Malawi	7,018,000	1,052,700	79,738	23,877
Mali	6,356,000	127,120	70,254	34,447
Mauritania		34,240	6,487	5,821
Mauritius	716,000	14,320	5,197	2,434
Mozambique	10,761,000	215,220	149,280	18,052
Namibia	1,155,000	23,100	38,099	646
Niger	6,663,000	133,260	31,342	9,779
Nigeria	75,181,000	1,503,620	2,224,221	100,639
Rwanda	5,026,000	100,520	20,621	9,114
Senegal	6,227,000	373,620	36,716	49,929
Sierra Leone	2,805,000	56,100	28,414	7,489
Somalia	4,262,000	85,240	11,032	14,491
South Africa	27,470,000	2,472,300	207,881	173,896
Sudan	21,534,000	430,680	234,075	73,216
Swaziland	611,000	12,220	19,600	909
Togo	3,368,000	67,360	41,115	19,249
Uganda	14,874,000	297,480	79,470	86,385
Tanzania	20,627,000	412,540	128,141	46,668
Zambia	5,940,000	118,800	157,085	6,268
Zimbabwe	6,368,000	127,360	165,370	2,555
Grand total	408,266,000	17,929,840	5,793,823	1,722,271

Table 5.23 Infections averted and DALYs by country (3% discount rate)

	Alcohol taxation		Community mobilization		Keeping girls in school		Gender and HIV training on livelihood programs	
	Cum inf avert yr5	Total DALYs (3%)	Cum inf avert yr5	Total DALYs (3%)	Sum of inf avert yr5	Sum of total DALYs (3%)	Sum of inf avert yr5	Sum of total DALYs (3%)
Angola	228	2,859	101	1,324	359	4,756	15	182
Benin	19	213	91	1,024	85	986	57	598
Botswana	300	2,899	51	499	536	5,406	83	743
Burkina Faso	15	178	86	1,013	120	1,443	6	67
Burundi	88	1,165	51	696	100	1,385	9	120
Cameroon	305	3,793	111	1,428	333	4,359	407	4,923
Central African Republic	31	396	25	334	66	900	3	35
Chad	13	148	59	714	130	1,593	13	151
Comoros	0	1	4	57	0	5	2	32
Congo	35	462	21	288	230	3,184	81	1,029
Côte d'Ivoire	111	1,420	55	744	169	2,306	20	251
Democratic Republic of the Congo	885	11,577	348	4,620	103	1,387	38	494
Djibouti	6	76	5	76	1	10	3	46
Equatorial Guinea	11	141	4	49	37	492	5	60
Eritrea	7	91	30	377	22	277	9	105
Ethiopia	131	1,775	343	4,832	86	1,226	1,933	25,790
Gabon	44	500	9	103	10	123	3	27
Gambia	21	286	9	131	53	744	11	143
Ghana	42	542	21	278	410	5,561	211	2,674
Guinea	29	345	55	672	70	864	28	320
Guinea-Bissau	19	230	9	107	11	140	1	16
Kenya	454	5,139	894	10,345	1,455	17,215	2,885	31,194
Lesotho	115	1,225	39	422	429	4,829	128	1,292
Liberia	23	324	22	321	43	624	11	154
Madagascar	68	1,011	109	1,699	32	501	26	388
Malawi	425	4,839	715	8,340	1,080	12,875	395	4,301
Mali	5	51	72	822	70	816	68	716
Mauritania	NA	NA	20	256	4	52	12	143
Mauritius	6	85	8	111	2	29	5	62
Mozambique	4,182	50,401	441	5,511	2,555	32,453	369	4,315
Namibia	59	577	13	130	441	4,492	5	44
Niger	31	402	76	1,021	31	425	0	2
Nigeria	7,653	97,762	203	2,708	12,880	173,677	731	9,145

(cont.)

Table 5.23 (*cont.*)

	Alcohol taxation		Community mobilization		Keeping girls in school		Gender and HIV training on livelihood programs	
	Cum inf avert yr5	Total DALYs (3%)	Cum inf avert yr5	Total DALYs (3%)	Sum of inf avert yr5	Sum of total DALYs (3%)	Sum of inf avert yr5	Sum of total DALYs (3%)
Rwanda	108	1,033	14	137	78	781	32	279
Senegal	3	32	67	750	51	588	99	1,027
Sierra Leone	47	611	32	431	85	1,158	21	260
Somalia	47	667	49	719	2	33	29	402
South Africa	8,329	97,374	1,748	21,017	5,610	68,779	4,110	46,220
Sudan	238	3,470	245	3,737	47	714	144	2,093
Swaziland	84	833	21	207	606	6,282	34	307
Togo	78	921	38	507	181	2,414	100	1,147
Uganda	3,001	37,506	209	2,555	761	9,483	1,174	14,282
United Republic of Tanzania	1,087	13,911	259	3,347	997	13,048	392	4,901
Zambia	772	7,619	185	1,848	2,782	28,828	123	1,127
Zimbabwe	607	7,057	120	1,449	2,273	27,952	36	404
Grand total	29,764	361,945	7,086	87,756	35,430	445,194	13,865	162,009

Table 5.24 Unit and total costs by country (2010 dollars)

	Alcohol taxation		Community mobilization		Keeping girls in school		Gender and HIV training on livelihood programs	
	Sum of unit cost	Sum of total cost (discounted 3%)	Sum of unit cost	Sum of total cost (discounted 3%)	Sum of unit cost	Sum of total cost (discounted 3%)	Sum of unit cost	Sum of total cost (discounted 3%)
Angola	0.19	7,947,933	9.83	8,225,865	858	454,470,082	9.08	152,007
Benin	0.19	3,886,134	1.62	5,951,922	266	76,296,106	1.66	224,475
Botswana	0.17	866,059	1.25	127,362	1,210	130,535,891	13.50	233,816
Burkina Faso	0.19	6,741,583	5.00	3,548,201	225	79,431,895	1.15	165,834
Burundi	0.17	3,558,060	0.39	161,361	162	18,147,671	0.36	4,742
Cameroon	0.19	8,698,990	1.62	1,480,354	335	67,691,040	2.53	489,353
Central African Republic	0.17	1,744,949	1.09	224,545	214	15,202,509	1.01	4,149
Chad	0.19	4,649,738	1.62	791,271	242	29,571,429	1.36	29,825
Comoros	0.17	285,479	1.96	65,705	277	2,256,168	1.81	10,320
Congo	0.17	1,478,716	9.00	1,565,699	595	124,538,446	2.46	174,288
Côte d'Ivoire	0.17	8,265,253	1.62	1,575,260	330	87,600,741	0.36	15,930
Democratic Republic of the Congo	0.17	24,473,391	0.39	1,109,889	162	393,620,004	5.79	410,657

Table 5.24 (*cont.*)

	Alcohol taxation		Community mobilization		Keeping girls in school		Gender and HIV training on livelihood programs	
	Sum of unit cost	Sum of total cost (discounted 3%)	Sum of unit cost	Sum of total cost (discounted 3%)	Sum of unit cost	Sum of total cost (discounted 3%)	Sum of unit cost	Sum of total cost (discounted 3%)
Djibouti	0.17	373,689	2.92	128,586	349	5,722,542	2.70	20,197
Equatorial Guinea	0.19	297,555	37.10	1,161,886	2,868	50,617,358	34.27	182,501
Eritrea	0.17	2,106,609	0.89	220,331	199	25,391,858	0.82	34,608
Ethiopia	0.17	31,887,821	0.33	7,427,987	194	395,926,108	0.77	1,670,572
Gabon	0.19	695,489	6.00	439,256	1,466	10,238,678	16.70	24,452
Gambia	0.19	741,198	1.04	80,828	210	10,952,078	0.96	12,001
Ghana	0.19	11,022,066	1.62	1,875,685	328	244,032,528	2.44	827,174
Guinea	0.19	4,327,985	1.62	736,517	205	37,458,241	0.91	60,531
Guinea-Bissau	0.19	675,772	1.25	88,946	225	2,941,592	1.16	1,812
Kenya	0.17	15,843,271	3.36	37,576,512	264	221,755,707	1.64	2,280,139
Lesotho	0.17	815,539	1.57	150,635	269	19,321,490	1.70	27,740
Liberia	0.19	1,738,722	0.53	97,891	173	24,904,519	0.49	13,274
Madagascar	0.19	8,583,374	1.62	1,460,679	211	159,984,264	0.98	60,338
Malawi	0.17	5,627,781	2.90	14,400,500	188	70,809,193	0.69	77,724
Mali	0.19	5,696,557	1.62	969,414	256	84,810,567	1.54	249,942
Mauritania			2.21	357,609	296	9,070,506	2.05	56,171
Mauritius	0.19	641,714	16.23	1,096,074	1,329	32,588,692	14.99	172,164
Mozambique	0.17	8,629,318	1.62	1,641,263	209	147,321,053	0.95	81,128
Namibia	0.17	926,202	4.49	489,085	891	160,131,609	9.50	28,954
Niger	0.19	5,971,705	1.62	1,016,238	196	28,935,476	0.78	36,144
Nigeria	0.19	67,380,873	1.62	11,466,570	332	3,480,749,682	2.49	1,181,466
Rwanda	0.17	4,030,383	1.62	766,563	226	21,974,071	1.16	49,958
Senegal	0.19	5,580,941	1.62	2,849,217	315	54,535,838	2.28	536,341
Sierra Leone	0.19	2,513,978	1.62	427,817	194	25,970,312	0.76	26,814
Somalia	0.17	3,417,726	0.53	215,058	173	8,983,294	0.49	33,780
South Africa	0.17	22,028,378	13.94	162,569,428	1,161	1,138,270,088	12.88	10,565,253
Sudan	0.17	17,268,259	1.62	3,284,355	173	190,607,409	0.49	170,675
Swaziland	0.17	489,965	1.62	93,382	583	53,905,971	5.64	24,172
Togo	0.19	3,018,566	1.04	329,943	210	40,678,677	1.09	99,040
Uganda	0.17	11,927,561	1.07	1,501,469	220	82,555,200	1.12	456,268
United Republic of Tanzania	0.17	16,540,930	1.62	3,152,507	223	134,510,650	0.96	211,208
Zambia	0.17	4,763,326	2.00	1,120,783	309	228,982,127	2.20	65,159
Zimbabwe	0.17	5,106,542	4.30	2,583,310	213	166,109,507	1.00	12,048
Grand total		343,266,081		286,603,756		8,850,108,871		21,265,144

Table 5.25 Incremental cost per DALY by country (2010 dollars)

	Alcohol taxation		Community mobilization		Keeping girls in school		Gender and HIV training on livelihood programs	
	Average of incremental cost per DALY	Sum of B/C ratio 1,000 (3%)	Average of incremental cost per DALY	Sum of B/C ratio 1,000 (3%)	Average of incremental cost per DALY	Sum of B/C ratio 1,000 (3%)	Average of incremental cost per DALY	Sum of B/C ratio 1,000 (3%)
Angola	2,567.00	0.60	5,968.00	0.20	95,349.00	6.91	618.00	1.46
Benin	17,882.00	0.43	5,426.00	0.24	77,101.00	6.92	31.00	3.58
Botswana	−603.00	14.60	−817.00	8.12	23,282.00	6.98	−660.00	6.27
Burkina Faso	37,652.00	0.37	0.00	0.00	54,813.00	6.92	2,225.00	0.51
Burundi	2,959.00	8.78	124.00	4.78	13,010.00	6.98	−56.00	27.69
Cameroon	2,117.00	0.80	834.00	1.16	15,361.00	6.98	−82.00	11.89
Central African Republic	4,302.00	8.78	552.00	1.67	16,790.00	6.97	10.00	9.46
Chad	31,209.00	0.38	849.00	1.14	18,345.00	6.97	−36.00	6.26
Comoros	262,874.00	8.55	1,024.00	0.98	461,126.00	6.90	209.00	3.48
Congo	3,067.00	8.76	5,290.00	0.21	38,998.00	6.93	31.00	6.72
Côte d'Ivoire	5,681.00	8.74	1,962.00	0.55	37,859.00	6.93	−80.00	17.99
Democratic Republic of the Congo	1,990.00	9.07	79.00	4.83	283,719.00	6.90	706.00	1.35
Djibouti	4,808.00	8.77	1,593.00	0.65	570,289.00	6.90	358.00	2.45
Equatorial Guinea	1,604.00	0.92	22,982.00	0.07	102,372.00	6.91	2,521.00	0.50
Eritrea	23,001.00	8.60	354.00	2.10	91,599.00	6.91	125.00	3.65
Ethiopia	17,874.00	8.59	1,437.00	0.72	322,862.00	6.90	−24.00	16.81
Gabon	796.00	1.19	3,566.00	0.40	82,566.00	6.92	272.00	1.81
Gambia	2,495.00	0.78	501.00	1.81	14,616.00	6.97	−19.00	13.16
Ghana	20,204.00	0.38	6,567.00	0.17	43,741.00	6.93	158.00	3.72
Guinea	12,329.00	0.45	833.00	1.15	43,127.00	6.93	−45.00	6.52
Guinea-Bissau	2,750.00	0.76	616.00	1.46	20,873.00	6.96	−78.00	10.36
Kenya	2,792.00	8.93	3,294.00	0.37	12,604.00	7.00	−231.00	17.84
Lesotho	342.00	10.49	−19.00	3.86	3,695.00	7.23	−321.00	62.53
Liberia	5,295.00	0.55	229.00	3.53	39,854.00	6.93	19.00	12.39
Madagascar	8,475.00	0.47	845.00	1.18	319,491.00	6.90	143.00	6.51
Malawi	902.00	1.48	1,422.00	0.76	5,250.00	7.13	−255.00	70.45
Mali	112,426.00	0.37	836.00	1.14	103,689.00	6.91	39.00	3.75
Mauritania	NA	NA	1,202.00	0.86	175,284.00	6.91	221.00	2.98
Mauritius	7,276.00	0.44	9,559.00	0.13	1,142,031.00	6.90	2,488.00	0.46
Mozambique	−9.00	15.31	91.00	4.05	4,369.00	7.16	−167.00	63.05
Namibia	850.00	9.45	2,878.00	0.50	34,924.00	6.95	−147.00	2.72
Niger	14,749.00	0.43	856.00	1.14	67,921.00	6.92	14,603.00	0.08
Nigeria	559.00	1.96	4,086.00	0.27	19,919.00	6.96	−3.00	8.76

Table 5.25 (cont.)

	Alcohol taxation		Community mobilization		Keeping girls in school		Gender and HIV training on livelihood programs	
	Average of incremental cost per DALY	Sum of B/C ratio 1,000 (3%)	Average of incremental cost per DALY	Sum of B/C ratio 1,000 (3%)	Average of incremental cost per DALY	Sum of B/C ratio 1,000 (3%)	Average of incremental cost per DALY	Sum of B/C ratio 1,000 (3%)
Rwanda	3,416.00	7.49	5,017.00	0.28	27,666.00	6.95	−349.00	8.53
Senegal	176,660.00	0.35	3,395.00	0.37	92,417.00	6.91	157.00	2.61
Sierra Leone	4,009.00	0.62	871.00	1.13	22,326.00	6.95	−6.00	10.74
Somalia	5,096.00	8.75	265.00	3.46	274,247.00	6.90	54.00	12.25
South Africa	−203.00	14.07	7,237.00	0.19	16,140.00	6.99	−218.00	6.33
Sudan	4,951.00	8.75	850.00	1.17	266,916.00	6.90	56.00	12.58
Swaziland	33.00	11.11	−203.00	3.67	8,053.00	7.08	−521.00	20.34
Togo	3,060.00	0.72	468.00	1.82	16,697.00	6.97	−138.00	14.18
Uganda	147.00	12.21	337.00	2.13	8,499.00	7.04	−144.00	36.82
United Republic of Tanzania	1,031.00	9.45	744.00	1.27	10,145.00	7.01	−119.00	26.96
Zambia	173.00	10.42	74.00	2.53	7,512.00	7.08	−431.00	25.75
Zimbabwe	520.00	10.07	1,549.00	0.69	5,750.00	7.10	−181.00	40.60

References

Adato, M. and Bassett, L. (2008). *What is the Potential of Cash Transfers to Strengthen Families Affected by HIV and AIDS? A Review of the Evidence on Impacts*. Boston: Joint Learning Initiative on Children and HIV/AIDS.

Adato, M. and Bassett, L. (2009). Social protection to support vulnerable children and families: the potential of cash transfers to protect education, health and nutrition. *AIDS Care* **21**: 60–75.

Anandajayasekeram, P., Davis, K. E. and Workneh, S. (2007). Farmer field schools: an alternative to existing extension systems? Experience from Eastern and Southern Africa. *Journal of International Agricultural and Extension Education* **14**: 81–93.

Anderson, P., Chisholm, D. and Fuhr, D. C. (2009). Effectiveness and cost-effectiveness of policies and programmes to reduce the harm caused by alcohol. *Lancet* **373**: 2234–46.

Baird, S., Chirwa, E., McIntosh, C. and Özler, B. (2010a). The short-term impacts of a schooling conditional cash transfer program on the sexual behavior of young women. *Health Economics* **19** Suppl.: 55–68.

Baird, S., McIntosh, C., Diego, S. and Özler, B. (2010b). Schooling, income, and HIV risk: experimental evidence from a cash transfer program. Presented at the World Bank and UNAIDS Economic Reference Group's Seventh Meeting.

Baliunas, D., Rehm, J., Irving, H. and Shuper, P. (2010). Alcohol consumption and risk of incident human immunodeficiency virus infection: a meta-analysis. *International Journal of Public Health* **55**: 159–66.

Barnes, C., Gaile, G. and Kibombo, R. (2001). *The Impact of Three Microfinance Programs in Uganda*. Washington, DC: US Agency for International Development.

Beegle, K. and Özler, B. (2006). *Young Women, Rich(er) Men, and the Spread of HIV*. Washington, DC: World Bank.

Bird, R. M. and Wallace, S. (2010). *Taxing Alcohol in Africa: Reflections and Updates*. International Studies Program Working Paper Series. International Studies Program, Andrew Young School of Policy Studies, Georgia State University.

Biswas, K., Kummarikunta, G., Biswas, A. and Tong, L. (2010). *Social Return on Investment: CHACHA Programme*. Hove: International HIV/AIDS Alliance.

Blankenship, K. M., Friedman, S. R., Dworkin, S. and Mantell, J. E. (2006). Structural interventions: concepts, challenges and opportunities for research. *Journal of Urban Health: Bulletin of the New York Academy of Medicine* **83**: 59–72.

Blankenship, K. M., West, B. S., Kershaw, T. S. and Biradavolu, M. R. (2008). Power, community mobilization, and condom use practices among female sex workers in Andhra Pradesh, India. *AIDS* **22** Suppl 5: S109–16.

Bollinger, L. (2008). How can we calculate the "E" in "CEA"? *AIDS* **22** Suppl 1: S51–7.

Braun, A., Jiggins, J., Röling, N., Berg, H. V. D. and Snijders, P. (2006). *A Global Survey and Review of Farmer Field School Experiences*. Wageningen: Endelea.

Brent, R. (2009). A cost-benefit analysis of female primary education as a means of reducing HIV/AIDS in Tanzania. *Applied Economics* **41**: 1731–43.

Budlender, D. (2009). *National and Provincial Government Spending and Revenue Related to Alcohol Abuse*. Cape Town: Community Agency for Social Inquiry.

Chisholm, D., Rehm, J., Van Ommeren, M. and Monteiro, M. (2004). Reducing the global burden of hazardous alcohol use: a comparative cost-effectiveness analysis. *Journal of Studies on Alcohol* **65**: 782–93.

Cleary, S. M., Mcintyre, D. and Boulle, A. M. (2008). Assessing efficiency and costs of scaling up HIV treatment. *AIDS* **22** Suppl 1: S35–42.

Cnossen, S. (2007). Alcohol taxation and regulation in the European Union. *International Tax and Public Finance* **14**: 699–732.

Cohen, D. A., Wu, S.-Y. and Farley, T. A. (2004). Comparing the cost-effectiveness of HIV prevention interventions. *Journal of Acquired Immune Deficiency Syndromes* **37**: 1404–14.

Cook, R. L. and Clark, D. B. (2005). Is there an association between alcohol consumption and sexually transmitted diseases? A systematic review. *Sexually Transmitted Diseases* **32**: 156–64.

Creese, A., Floyd, K., Alban, A. and Guinness, L. (2002). Cost-effectiveness of HIV/AIDS interventions in Africa: a systematic review of the evidence. *The Lancet* **359**: 1635–43.

Crowe, L. C. and George, W. H. (1989). Alcohol and human sexuality: review and integration. *Psychological Bulletin* **105**: 374–86.

Dandona, L., Sisodia, P., Kumar, S. P., Ramesh, Y., Kumar, A. A., Rao, M. C., Marseille, E., Someshwar, M., Marshall, N. and Kahn, J. G. (2005). HIV prevention programmes for female sex workers in Andhra Pradesh, India: outputs, cost and efficiency. *BMC Public Health* **5**: 98.

Davis, K., Nkonya, E., Kato, E., Mekonnen, D. A., Odendo, M., Miiro, R. and Nkuba, J. (2010). *Impact of Farmer Field Schools on Agricultural Productivity and Poverty in East Africa*. Discussion Paper 00992. Washington, DC: International Food Policy Research Institute (IFPRI).

De Walque, D. (2002). *How Does Educational Attainment Affect the Risk of Being Infected by HIV/AIDS? Evidence from a General Population Cohort in Rural Uganda*. University of Chicago.

De Walque, D. (2006). *Who Gets AIDS and How? The Determinants of HIV Infection and Sexual Behaviors in Burkina Faso, Cameroon, Ghana, Kenya, and Tanzania*. Policy Research Working Paper 3844. Washington, DC: World Bank.

Denning, G., Kabambe, P., Sanchez, P., Malik, A., Flor, R., Harawa, R., Nkhoma, P., Zamba, C., Banda, C., Magombo, C., Keating, M., Wangila, J. and Sachs, J. (2009). Input subsidies to improve smallholder maize productivity in Malawi: toward an African green revolution. *PLoS Biology* **7**: 9.

Dinkelman, T., Lam, D. and Leibbrandt, M. (2007). Household and community income, economic shocks and risky sexual behavior of young adults: evidence from the Cape Area Panel Study 2002 and 2005. *AIDS* **21**: S49.

Dorward, A. and Chirwa, E. (2011). The Malawi Agricultural Input Subsidy Programme: 2005–6 to 2008–9. *International Journal of Agricultural Sustainability* **9**: 232–47.

Duflo, E., Dupas, P., Kremer, M. and Sinei, S. (2006). *Education and HIV/AIDS Prevention: Evidence from a Randomized Evaluation in Western Kenya*. Policy Research Working Paper 4024. Washington, DC: World Bank.

Dunkle, K. L., Jewkes, R. K., Brown, H. C., Gray, G. E., Mcintyre, J. A. and Harlow, S. D. (2004). Gender-based violence, relationship power, and risk of HIV infection in women attending antenatal clinics in South Africa. *The Lancet* **363**: 1415–21.

FAO. (2010). *The State of Food Insecurity in the World: Addressing Food Insecurity in Protracted Crises.* Rome: Food and Agriculture Organization of the United Nations.

Fisher, J. C., Bang, H. and Kapiga, S. H. (2007). The association between HIV infection and alcohol use: a systematic review and meta-analysis of African studies. *Sexually Transmitted Diseases* **34**: 856–63.

Fritz, K., McFarland, W., Wyrod, R., Chasakara, C., Makumbe, K., Chirowodza, A., Mashoko, C., Kellogg, T. and Woelk, G. (2011). Evaluation of a peer network-based sexual risk reduction intervention for men in beer halls in Zimbabwe: results from a randomized controlled trial. *Aids and Behavior*.

Gil-Gonzalez, D., Vives-Cases, C., Alvarez-Dardet, C. and Latour-Pérez, J. (2006). Alcohol and intimate partner violence: do we have enough information to act? *The European Journal of Public Health* **16**: 278.

Gillespie, S., Kadiyala, S. and Greener, R. (2007). Is poverty or wealth driving HIV transmission? *AIDS* **21** Suppl 7: S5–16.

Gmel, G., Shield, K. D. and Rehm, J. (2011). Developing a method to derive alcohol-attributable fractions for HIV/AIDS mortality based on alcohol's impact on adherence to anti-retroviral medication. *Population Health Metrics* **9**: 5.

Greig, F. E. and Koopman, C. (2003). Multilevel analysis of women's empowerment and HIV prevention: quantitative survey results from a preliminary study in Botswana. *AIDS and Behavior* **7**: 195–208.

Gupta, G. R., Parkhurst, J. O., Ogden, J. A., Aggleton, P. and Mahal, A. (2008). Structural approaches to HIV prevention. *The Lancet* **372**: 764–75.

Hahn, J. A. and Woolf-King, S. E. (2011). Adding fuel to the fire: alcohol and its effect on the HIV epidemic in sub-Saharan Africa. *Current HIV/AIDS Reports*: 1–9.

Hallfors, D., Cho, H., Rusakaniko, S., Iritani, B., Mapfumo, J. and Halpern, C. (2011). Supporting adolescent orphan girls to stay in school as HIV risk prevention: evidence from a randomized controlled trial in Zimbabwe. *American Journal of Public Health* **101**: 1082–8.

Halli, S. S., Ramesh, B. M., O'Neil, J., Moses, S. and Blanchard, J. F. (2006). The role of collectives in STI and HIV/AIDS prevention among female sex workers in Karnataka, India. *AIDS Care* **18**: 739–49.

Halpern-Felsher, B. L., Millstein, S. G. and Ellen, J. M. (1996). Relationship of alcohol use and risky sexual behavior: a review and analysis of findings. *The Journal of Adolescent Health: Official Publication of the Society for Adolescent Medicine* **19**: 331–6.

Hargreaves, J. R., Bonell, C. P., Boler, T., Boccia, D., Birdthistle, I., Fletcher, A., Pronyk, P. M. and Glynn, J. R. (2008). Systematic review exploring time trends in the association between educational attainment and risk of HIV infection in sub-Saharan Africa. *AIDS* **22**: 403–14.

Hargreaves, J. R., Bonell, C. P., Morison, L. A., Kim, J. C., Phetla, G., Porter, J. D., Watts, C. and Pronyk, P. M. (2007). Explaining continued high HIV prevalence in South Africa: socioeconomic factors, HIV incidence and sexual behavior change among a rural cohort 2001–2004. *AIDS* **21** Suppl 7: S39–48.

Hargreaves, J. R., Hatcher, A., Strange, V., Phetla, G., Busza, J., Kim, J., Watts, C., Morison, L., Porter, J., Pronyk, P. and Bonell, C. (2010). Process evaluation of the Intervention with Microfinance for AIDS and Gender Equity (IMAGE) in rural South Africa. *Health Education Research* **25**: 27–40.

International HIV/AIDS Alliance. (2011). *The True Cost of Stigma.* Hove: International HIV/AIDS Alliance.

Jan, S., Ferrari, G., Watts, C. H., Hargreaves, J. R., Kim, J. C., Phetla, G., Morison, L. A., Porter, J. D., Barnett, T. and Pronyk, P. M. (2010). Economic evaluation of a combined microfinance and gender training intervention for the prevention of intimate partner violence in rural South Africa. *Health Policy and Planning* **26**: 366–72.

Jewkes, R. K., Dunkle, K., Nduna, M. and Shai, N. (2010). Intimate partner violence, relationship power inequity, and incidence of HIV infection in young women in South Africa: a cohort study. *The Lancet* **376**: 41–8.

Jewkes, R. K., Nduna, M., Levin, J., Jama, N., Dunkle, K., Puren, A. and Duvvury, N. (2008). Impact of Stepping Stones on incidence of HIV and HSV-2 and sexual behaviour in rural South Africa: cluster randomised controlled trial. *BMJ* **337**: a506–a506.

Jukes, M., Simmons, S. and Bundy, D. (2008). Education and vulnerability: the role of schools in protecting young women and girls from HIV in southern Africa. *AIDS* **22** Suppl 4: S41–56.

Kalichman, S. C., Simbayi, L., Jooste, S., Vermaak, R. and Cain, D. (2008). Sensation seeking and alcohol use predict HIV transmission risks: prospective study of sexually transmitted infection clinic patients, Cape Town, South Africa. *Addictive Behaviors* **33**: 1630–3.

Kalichman, S. C., Simbayi, L. C., Kaufman, M., Cain, D. and Jooste, S. (2007). Alcohol use and sexual risks for HIV/AIDS in sub-Saharan Africa: systematic review of empirical findings. *Prevention Science: The Official Journal of the Society for Prevention Research* **8**: 141–51.

Kalichman, S. C., Simbayi, L. C., Vermaak, R., Cain, D., Smith, G., Mthebu, J. and Jooste, S. (2008). Randomized trial of a community-based alcohol-related HIV risk-reduction intervention for men and women in Cape Town, South Africa. *Annals of Behavioral Medicine: A Publication of the Society of Behavioral Medicine* **36**: 270–9.

Khumalo-Sakutukwa, G., Morin, S. F., Fritz, K., Charlebois, E. D., Van Rooyen, H., Chingono, A., Modiba, P., Mrumbi, K., Visrutaratna, S., Singh, B., Sweat, M., Celentano, D. D. and Coates, T. J. (2008). Project Accept (HPTN 043): a community-based intervention to reduce HIV incidence in populations at risk for HIV in sub-Saharan Africa and Thailand. *Journal of Acquired Immune Deficiency Syndromes* **49**: 422–31.

Kim, J., Ferrari, G., Abramsky, T., Watts, C., Hargreaves, J., Morison, L., Phetla, G., Porter, J. and Pronyk, P. (2009). Assessing the incremental effects of combining economic and health interventions: the IMAGE study in South Africa. *Bulletin of the World Health Organization* **87**: 824–32.

Kim, J., Lutz, B., Dhaliwal, M. and O'Malley, J. (2011). The "AIDS and MDGs" approach: what is it, why does it matter, and how do we take it forward? *Third World Quarterly* **32**: 141–63.

Kim, J., Pronyk, P., Barnett, T. and Watts, C. (2008). Exploring the role of economic empowerment in HIV prevention. *AIDS* **22** Suppl 4: S57–71.

Kim, J. C., Watts, C. H., Hargreaves, J. R., Ndhlovu, L. X., Phetla, G., Morison, L. A., Busza, J., Porter, J. D. H. and Pronyk, P. (2007). Understanding the impact of a microfinance-based intervention on women's empowerment and the reduction of intimate partner violence in South Africa. *American Journal of Public Health* **97**: 1794–1802.

King, E. M., Klasen, S. and Porter, M. (2007). Women and development. *2008 Challenge Paper*. Copenhagen Consensus Center.

Knowles, S., Lorgelly, P. K. and Owen, P. D. (2002). Are educational gender gaps a brake on economic development? Some cross-country empirical evidence. *Oxford Economic Papers* **54**: 118.

Kohler, H.-P. and Thornton, R. (2010). Conditional Cash Transfers and HIV/AIDS Prevention: Unconditonally Promising? University of Michigan. Available: http://personal.umich.edu/~rebeccal/RebeccaLThornton/Home_files/KohlerThornton.CCTHIV.pdf (accessed August 15, 2011).

Koku, E. F. (2011). Stigma, sexual risk and desire for HIV tests in Ghana. *Sexual Health* **8**: 110–19.

Leigh, B. C. and Stall, R. (1993). Substance use and risky sexual behavior for exposure to HIV: issues in methodology, interpretation, and prevention. *American Psychologist* **48**: 1035.

Lopman, B., Lewis, J., Nyamukapa, C., Mushati, P., Chandiwana, S. and Gregson, S. (2007). HIV incidence and poverty in Manicaland, Zimbabwe: is HIV becoming a disease of the poor? *AIDS* **21**: S57.

Mahajan, A., Sayles, J. and Patel, V. (2008). Stigma in the HIV/AIDS epidemic: a review of the literature and recommendations for the way forward. *AIDS* **22**: 1–20.

Maticka-Tyndale, E. and Brouillard-Coylea, C. (2006). The effectiveness of community interventions targeting HIV and AIDS prevention at young people in developing countries. *World Health Organization Technical Report Series* **938**: 243–85; discussion 317–41.

Padian, N. S., McCoy, S. I., Karim, S. S. A., Hasen, N., Kim, J., Bartos, M., Katabira, E., Bertozzi, S. M., Schwartländer, B., Cohen, M. S. and Gates, M. (2011). HIV prevention transformed: the new prevention research agenda. *The Lancet* **378**: 269–78.

Parry, C. D. H. (2000). Alcohol problems in developing countries: challenges for the new millennium. *Suchtmed* **2**: 216–20.

Parry, C. D. H., Plüddemann, A., Steyn, K., Bradshaw, D., Norman, R. and Laubscher, R. (2005). Alcohol use in South Africa: findings from the first Demographic and Health Survey (1998). *Journal of Studies on Alcohol* **66**: 91–7.

Pettifor, A. E., Levandowski, B. A., Macphail, C., Padian, N. S., Cohen, M. S. and Rees, H. V. (2008). Keep them in school: the importance of education as a protective factor against HIV infection among young South African women. *International Journal of Epidemiology* **37**: 1266–73.

Piot, P., Bartos, M., Larson, H., Zewdie, D. and Mane, P. (2008). Coming to terms with complexity: a call to action for HIV prevention. *The Lancet* **372**: 845–59.

Pronyk, P. M., Hargreaves, J. R., Kim, J. C., Morison, L. A., Phetla, G., Watts, C., Busza, J. and Porter, J. D. H. (2006). Effect of a structural intervention for the prevention of intimate-partner violence and HIV in rural South Africa: a cluster randomised trial. *The Lancet* **368**: 1973–83.

Pronyk, P. M., Hargreaves, J. R. and Morduch, J. (2007). Microfinance programs and better health: prospects for sub-Saharan Africa. *JAMA: the Journal of the American Medical Association* **298**: 1925–7.

Pronyk, P. M., Harpham, T., Busza, J., Phetla, G., Morison, L. A., Hargreaves, J. R., Kim, J. C., Watts, C. H. and Porter, J. D. (2008). Can social capital be intentionally generated? A randomized trial from rural South Africa. *Social Science and Medicine* **67**: 1559–70.

Pronyk, P. M., Harpham, T., Morison, L. A., Hargreaves, J. R., Kim, J. C., Phetla, G., Watts, C. H. and Porter, J. D. (2008). Is social capital associated with HIV risk in rural South Africa? *Social Science and Medicine* **66**: 1999–2010.

Pronyk, P. M., Kim, J. C., Abramsky, T., Phetla, G., Hargreaves, J. R., Morison, L. A., Watts, C., Busza, J. and Porter, J. D. (2008). A combined microfinance and training intervention can reduce HIV risk behavior in young female participants. *AIDS* **22**: 1659–65.

Rashad, I. and Kaestner, R. (2004). Teenage sex, drugs and alcohol use: problems identifying the cause of risky behaviors. *Journal of Health Economics* **23**: 493–503.

Sanchez, P., Palm, C., Sachs, J., Denning, G., Flor, R., Harawa, R., Jama, B., Kiflemariam, T., Konecky, B., Kozar, R., Lelerai, E., Malik, A., Modi, V., Mutuo, P., Niang, A., Okoth, H., Place, F., Sachs, S. E., Said, A., Siriri, D., Teklehaimanot, A., Wang, K., Wangila, J. and Zamba, C. (2007). The African Millennium Villages. *Proceedings of the National Academy of Sciences of the United States of America* **104**: 16775–80.

Schwartländer, B., Stover, J., Hallett, T., Atun, R., Avila, C., Gouws, E., Bartos, M., Ghys, P. D., Opuni, M., Barr, D., Alsallaq, R., Bollinger, L., De Freitas, M., Garnett, G., Holmes, C., Legins, K., Pillay, Y., Stanciole, A. E., McClure, C., Hirnschall, G., Laga, M. and Padian, N. (2011). Towards an improved investment approach for an effective response to HIV/AIDS. *The Lancet* **377**: 2031–41.

Shuper, P. A., Neuman, M., Kanteres, F., Baliunas, D., Joharchi, N. and Rehm, J. (2010). Causal considerations on alcohol and HIV/AIDS – a systematic review. *Alcohol and Alcoholism* **45**: 159–66.

Steele, C. M. and Josephs, R. A. (1990). Alcohol myopia: its prized and dangerous effects. *The American Psychologist* **45**: 921–33.

Swendeman, D., Basu, I., Das, S., Jana, S. and Rotheram-Borus, M. J. (2009). Empowering sex workers in India to reduce vulnerability to HIV and sexually transmitted diseases. *Social Science and Medicine* **69**: 1157–66.

Terris-Prestholt, F., Kumaranayake, L., Foster, S., Kamali, A., Kinsman, J., Basajja, V., Nalweyso, N., Quigley, M., Kengeya-Kayondo, J. and Whitworth, J. (2006). The role of community acceptance over time for costs of HIV and STI prevention interventions: analysis of the Masaka Intervention Trial, Uganda 1996–1999. *Sexually Transmitted Diseases* **33**: S111–6.

Terris-Prestholt, F., Kumaranayake, L., Obasi, A. I. N., Cleophas-Mazige, B., Makokha, M., Todd, J., Ross, D. A. and Hayes, R. J. (2006). From trial intervention to scale-up: costs of an adolescent sexual health program in Mwanza,

Tanzania. *Sexually Transmitted Diseases* **33**: S133–9.

Thomas, G. and Lungu, E. (2010). A two-sex model for the influence of heavy alcohol consumption on the spread of HIV/AIDS. *Mathematical Biosciences and Engineering: MBE* **7**: 871.

Townsend, L., Rosenthal, S. R., Parry, C. D. H., Zembe, Y., Mathews, C. and Flisher, A. J. (2010). Associations between alcohol misuse and risks for HIV infection among men who have multiple female sexual partners in Cape Town, South Africa. *AIDS Care* **22**: 1544–54.

UNAIDS (2010a). *HIV-Sensitive Social Protection: What Does the Evidence Say?* Geneva: UNAIDS.

UNAIDS. (2010b). *Report on the Global AIDS Epidemic*. Geneva: UNAIDS.

Volkerink, B. (2009). *Tax Policy in Sub-Saharan Africa: A Survey of Issues for a Number of Countries*. Working Paper Series. Utrecht: Centre for Taxation and Public Governance.

Wagenaar, A. C., Salois, M. J. and Komro, K. A. (2009). Effects of beverage alcohol price and tax levels on drinking: a meta-analysis of 1003 estimates from 112 studies. *Addiction* **104**: 179–90.

Wagenaar, A. C., Tobler, A. L. and Komro, K. A. (2010). Effects of alcohol tax and price policies on morbidity and mortality: a systematic review. *American Journal of Public Health* **100**: 2270–8.

Weinhardt, L. S. and Carey, M. P. (2000). Does alcohol lead to sexual risk behavior? Findings from event-level research. *Annual Review of Sex Research* **11**: 125.

Weiser, S. D., Leiter, K., Bangsberg, D. R., Butler, L. M., Percy-De Korte, F., Hlanze, Z., Phaladze, N., Iacopino, V. and Heisler, M. (2007). Food insufficiency is associated with high-risk sexual behavior among women in Botswana and Swaziland. *PLoS Medicine* **4**: 10.

Weiser, S. D., Leiter, K., Heisler, M., McFarland, W., Percy-De Korte, F., Demonner, S. M., Tlou, S., Phaladze, N., Iacopino, V. and Bangsberg, D. R. (2006). A population-based study on alcohol and high-risk sexual behaviors in Botswana. *PLoS Medicine* **3**: e392.

WHO (2005). *Alcohol Use and Sexual Risk Behaviour: A Cross-Cultural Study in Eight Countries*. Geneva: World Health Organization.

WHO and London School of Hygiene and Tropical Medicine. (2010). *Preventing Intimate Partner and Sexual Violence Against Women: Taking Action and Generating Evidence*. Geneva: World Health Organization.

Woolf-King, S. E. and Maisto, S. A. (2011). Alcohol use and high-risk sexual behavior in sub-Saharan Africa: a narrative review. *Archives of Sexual Behavior* **40**: 17–42.

World Bank. (2003). *Education and HIV/AIDS: A Sourcebook of HIV/AIDS Prevention Programs*. Washington, DC: World Bank.

World Bank. (2011). A Cash Transfer Program Reduces HIV Infections among Adolescent Girls. Available: http://siteresources. worldbank.org/DEC/Resources/ HIVExeSummary(Malawi).pdf (accessed July 14, 2011).

5.1 Social policy interventions to enhance the HIV/AIDS response in sub-Saharan Africa

Sets, metaphors, and hope

TONY BARNETT

Introduction

The social and economic aspects of the HIV/AIDS epidemics have often been framed in metaphorical language. These metaphors frame the way that people think about epidemics and thus social policy interventions designed to prevent, mitigate, or slow them down. Inattentive subscription to unexamined metaphors may have substantial implications for choosing between possible social policy interventions. If socio-economies[1] affected by HIV/AIDS are mis-specified in this way, when cost-benefit analysis (CBA) and cost-effectiveness analysis (CEA) are used to choose between competing proposals for social policy interventions, mis-specification, sometimes indeed homogenization, of the object for intervention, may lead to inappropriate choices as interventions inappropriate to the particularities of socio-economies are applied: the wrong medicine is prescribed for the patient. Unrecognized metaphors at the early stages of scientific conceptualization and later analysis may obscure the true nature of the problem and lead to incorrect analysis, conclusions, and policy prescriptions.

The first part of this paper examines three key metaphors which are often used in framing the problem of social policy interventions in HIV/AIDS epidemics. This discussion reveals the dangers of homogenizing socio-economies. It points to the complex relationship between cultural, social, and economic structures in influencing behaviors and choices which may expose people to infection and the dangers of assuming that people act similarly independent of their social and economic situation. This points to a very considerable problem at the root of prescriptive social policy, the problem of arriving at a way of capturing the interaction of social and economic structures and individual agency. The second part of this paper introduces a way of resolving this problem in a way which is theoretically defensible, pragmatically applicable, and likely to provide a diagnostic instrument for identifying and prioritizing areas for social policy interventions appropriate to the particular circumstances of a specific epidemic.

Section 1: unexamined metaphors

Natural languages contain metaphors. We use these metaphors so easily and often as part of our everyday thinking and speaking that we may fail to see them as such (Lakoff and Johnson 1980). Metaphors often use the image of the tangible and known to represent something which is less known and tangible.

Metaphorical usage is all too easily and carelessly transferred from the realm of everyday discourse to the world of scientific endeavor. In this context it is more precisely described as a "conceptual metaphor."

Metaphors work on the basis that the characteristics of one thing are shared by another. This is the essence of the metaphor when it is used as a

---

[1] This shorthand term is used to include culture and politics as well as social and economic structures.

component of rhetoric. In scientific language, we aim to arrive at conceptual clarity which leads to specification and operationalization of variables. It is almost inevitable that metaphors are used in the early stages of specification of scientific problems. Closer examination and reflection may reveal that chosen conceptual metaphors are inappropriate and misleading. This is because they do not adequately describe the object to which the metaphorical comparison is being made.

We often use metaphors in scientific work and we do so without considering them as metaphors – they are "dead metaphors." With regard to the description of the origins of an HIV/AIDS epidemic and its effects, the terms "upstream" and "downstream" are dead metaphors. As the basis for scientific work their unconsidered introduction at the stage of conceptualization, model construction, and data selection may have unforeseen consequences and lead to erroneous conclusions. Against this background, we should not omit to notice that even models which are elegantly constructed mathematical artefacts may contain metaphorical thinking, the implications of which have not been considered prior to the writing of the mathematical argument.[2]

Leaving metaphors unexamined can have significant negative effects for the scientific status of argument and for the conclusions and recommendations drawn from that argument. Some of the ways in which this has apparently occurred in Watts *et al.* (2011), *Going Upstream: A Cost-Benefit Analysis of Social Policy Interventions to Enhance the HIV/AIDS Response in Sub-Saharan Africa*, are considered below. In section 3, some modest suggestions are made for an approach based less on metaphor and more on indicators of underlying empirical variables.

The idea of "going upstream": unexamined metaphor 1

The key metaphor in the Watts *et al.* paper is in its title: "Going upstream." It is dependent upon an unexamined metaphor, that of a river. While not venturing into junior school geography, it is useful to consider some of the implications and difficulties of deploying this metaphor in the context of under-standing the structural drivers of an HIV/AIDS epidemic.

Rivers differ one from another: they rise in different geological, climatic, and watershed environments; their rates of fall differ; they differ in volume of water; they may have many different tributary streams; as Heraclitus famously noted, rivers flow and change, and therefore you can never step into the same river twice. Indeed, "you" are never the same person from one minute to the next.[3]

Insofar as we are concerned with the "upstream" of rivers, which is a metaphor for the "structural drivers" of HIV epidemics, we should pay particular attention to the effects of different upstream characteristics of real rivers on their later course as a way of thinking about the diversity of drivers and their effects. In their introduction to a recent publication on AIDS and rural livelihoods, Niehoff *et al.* note the complexity and dynamically changing characteristics of the epidemic stream (Niehof, Rugalema *et al.* 2010).

Thus, numbers of tributaries, initial water volume, altitude of watersheds of origin, steepness of descent, mineral and chemical load, all of these affect the midstream and ultimately the downstream of a real river. So it is with an HIV epidemic considered as a river. Epidemics and their structural drivers cannot be assumed to be one river. They should instead be thought of as a large number of different rivers, sometimes quite distinct from each other, sometimes having a "family relationship" (Wittgenstein 1953) in their source and therefore in their structural drivers. This idea will be expanded and discussed further when we come to the misplacement of the metaphor of the body. However, it is helpful to note the significance of Wittgenstein's point about "family resemblances." It is that objects which may be thought of as connected by one essential common feature may in fact be connected by *a series of overlapping similarities, where no one feature is common to all*. Games, which

---

[2] Although some mathematical modelers report that they think directly into mathematical statements. I am grateful to Roy Anderson and Mark Woolhouse for this explanation.

[3] Ποταμοῖς τοῖς αὐτοῖς ἐμβαίνομέν τε καὶ οὐκ ἐμβαίνομεν, εἶμέν τε καὶ οὐκ εἶμεν. This may be translated as: "We both step and do not step in the same rivers. We are and are not."

Wittgenstein used to explain the notion, have become the paradigmatic example of a group that is related by family resemblances. The same point may be made about real rivers and also, in this context, epidemics. On closer examination this turns out to be an aspect of set theory. Furthermore the use of CEA and CBA rest on the idea of choosing between sets of objects. But allocation of choice objects to inappropriate sets will result in inappropriate choices. This is the fundamental problem with which we are concerned here.

And of course, the geomorphology and other characteristics of real rivers are altered by their own action over time. Thus, to continue the parallel, over a period an epidemic has an effect on its environment. This will be most pronounced in hyperepidemic environments. In addition, other changes in the environment of an epidemic, for example changes in crop prices, in political regimes, in local climatic conditions, and a multitude of other environmental alterations, all of these will ensure that the epidemic and its environment are in a process of interacting and dynamic change over the characteristically long wave of an HIV epidemic, a wave which may be 120 years long (Barnett and Blaikie 1992; Barnett 2006).

These observations have many implications for thinking about the idea of upstream interventions in the processes of the HIV/AIDS epidemic. Among these are: HIV/AIDS epidemic events are very variable and disaggregation of gross statistics often reveals great diversity within one country or one area of a country. For example, in 2008 Tanzania had a national HIV prevalence rate of 6 percent of the adult population, with regional prevalence ranging from 0.3 percent in Pemba to 15.7 percent in Iringa (Tanzania Commission for AIDS (TACAIDS), Zanzibar AIDS Commission (ZAC) et al. 2008; Nombo 2010). Such data suggest that the "Tanzanian epidemic" as constructed in official sources has many tributaries and headwaters. Given the long period in which HIV has been present in Tanzania, it may be concluded that "upstream" in Iringa may be rather different from "upstream" in Pemba. Indeed, while they may form part of the same epidemiological river system, they are perhaps better considered to be discrete

rivers with their own watersheds, river basins, and "upstreams."

The same is true for many other "national epidemics" and, in the quest for apt and effective policy interventions, the different nature of these "upstreams" must be considered in describing the "structural drivers" of each constituent epidemic. Recognition of empirical heterogeneity is probably a more rigorous approach than the premature and incorrect homogenization of structural drivers in relation to diverse sub-national, national, and even regional HIV/AIDS epidemics.[4] The assumption of homogeneity has deep roots (another metaphor!) and these can be identified in for example (a) the uniform short- and medium-term intervention programs prescribed for all countries with epidemics during the 1990s by the Global Programme on AIDS (precursor to UNAIDS); (b) the assumption that behavioral change interventions should be the same from one context to another in the same period of the global response to the epidemic. While these were good *emergency* responses to a new and growing epidemic, they were not cost-effective given the diversity of situations into which they were inserted. In particular, they tended to view "sexual behavior" as one thing when in fact it may mean many things depending on context (Barnett and Parkhurst 2005).

The metaphor of a body undergoing treatment: unexamined metaphor 2

The second metaphor is that of the body to be treated by the intervention. It implies the question whether all patients are the same and require the same medicine. In other words, policy interventions may not be directly transferable from one sociocultural-economic situation to another because, for example, what works in Pemba may not work in Iringa, and is even less likely to work in Limpopo or

---

[4] Here one may think of the annual slide sets which used to be produced by UNAIDS showing the countries of Africa as blocs with shading or coloring according to their supposed "national" seroprevalence. The more recent UNAIDS epidemiological slide sets no longer do this and indeed have for the last few years indicated the range around reported regional prevalence figures. See: www.unaids.org/documents/20101123_epislides_core_en.pdf.

Juba, because these are in important respects quite different entities: the patients waiting to receive the proposed intervention are markedly different from each other.

Discussions of social policy intervention where the intervention is of a very specific type, for example conditional cash transfers, invite us to think about the notion of dose-response, thus taking further our exploration of the unstated metaphor. At first sight, dose-response may appear simply a statistical term describing a gradient relationship between a cause and an effect. Most typically the term describes the change in effect on an organism caused by differing levels of exposure (dose) to a stressor (usually a chemical – often a medication) after a certain exposure time. The term may be used to describe the effect on individual human beings or organisms or populations of human beings or other organisms. Here we find ourselves embroiled in a tussle with an unstated metaphor which obscures the true nature of the problem.

Generalizations about dose-response derive from the known effects of a stressor on a known body or organism. Where medications are concerned, the assumption is that doses will elicit the same range of responses in the receiving bodies because of the high level of homogeneity between those bodies. This has been a safe assumption for many medications for many years, although the distribution of responses to doses in any population is of course normally distributed, for human bodies are not identical, and some adverse responses are linked to presence or absence of particular genetic markers in certain individuals, for example as in the differential intolerance response to the anti-retroviral Abacavir between patients with different genetic inheritances (Mallal, Nolan *et al.* 2002; Michel, LeVan *et al.* 2003). If there are distinct differences in dose-response between apparently phenotypically similar human beings, how much greater will be the difference in dose-response when, in the social policy arena, the same social policy is applied to extremely different social/cultural/economic entities such as countries, regions, sub-regions, culturally distinct areas of countries, different social groups within a community, etc. To put the point very clearly indeed and to pose it as a question: if we provide conditional cash transfers to keep young women and girls in school in place A, will

they respond the same as young women and girls in place B?

The assumption that evidence of apparent social policy effectiveness taken from one environment will indicate the same dose-response in another is heroic.[5] It is heavily dependent upon the strength of the body metaphor used in relation to a society/economy/culture. In such circumstances, this metaphor error is likely to deepen the analytical problem rather than facilitate a policy solution to a real world problem. Fortunately, there is some evidence that the importance of heterogeneity versus assumptions of homogeneity is taking its place in mainstream policy deliberations. Thus, Schwartländer *et al.* recognize, in relation to financing responses to HIV/AIDS, the need for "a nuanced understanding of country epidemiology and context" (Schwartländer, Stover *et al.* 2011).

If the two preceding metaphors did not give rise to sufficient confusion, the final metaphor, that of "structural drivers," certainly adds to the problem. This metaphor states that there are structures which "drive" epidemics. The use of the term "drive" appears to indicate that it is not clear how the supposed "driver" is related to the phenomenon it is supposed to drive, usually acquisition of HIV by an individual. In other words, how the driver relates to the infection is not clear: neither is it clear that the term means "cause" or, indeed, how the term "driver" does or does not relate to the idea of cause.

Risk behaviors versus structural drivers: unexamined metaphor 3

The idea of "drivers" is the third metaphor in the conceptual set which frames the analysis of social policy interventions. Its key metaphorical content is the idea of a motive source transmitting power through a transmission unit to produce a final effect.

---

[5] In a recent paper, Mead Over notes that: "Real world prevention interventions, such as the Avahan initiative in India, take for granted that they must pass through the appropriate channel to access their clients. However, prevention organizations have typically focused on a single channel, thus failing to provide financiers with evidence of the effectiveness of various channels, or of different channel mixes, at achieving prevention goals in a given target population" (Over 2010).

The structural driver approach has the following advantage: it displaces analytical focus from risk behaviors (characteristics of individuals are all too easily assimilated to various forms of rational choice theory) (Ajzen and Fishbein 1980; Nelkin 1989; Taylor 1991; Slovic 1992; Wynne 1992; Singleton and Hoyden 1994; Chin 2006) toward attempts to understand the genesis of those behaviors from within a specific matrix of social, economic, and cultural conditions. These matrices of social, cultural, and economic conditions may be described as "risk environments," environments wherein risk comes into being via the niches the environment establishes in which virus and human host can come into contact with each other. Such a broad definition accommodates all kinds of transmission, from blood-borne to sexual (Barnett and Blaikie 1992).

The idea of a risk environment leads to that of an *ecology of risk* (Barnett and Blaikie 1992) where risk is thought of as differentially distributed across a social or geographical space depending on the coming together of specific factors which made a particular activity "risky" in a specific environment. The idea of a risk *environment* in relation to risk *behaviors* may perhaps be elucidated by altering the title of a once popular song written by Sy Oliver and Trummy Young and sung by Ella Fitzgerald: "It ain't what you do but it *is* where you do it." Thus, given the periodicity of HIV infection and associated variations in levels of viremia, concurrent sexual partnerships may present a greater or lesser risk in different risk environments, and interventions to prevent them will be more or less cost-effective in these different settings. In other words, *behavior* is not intrinsically more or less risky, but a particular environment will alter the probability of disease acquisition. The idea of risk environment has recently been developed quantitatively and found analytically useful in relation to drug use and HIV risk (Strathdee, Hallett *et al.* 2010). It is in these different risk environments that "drivers" come into existence and are reproduced. Reproduction of such drivers may consist of cultural attitudes and practices (dry sex, which can result in genital lesions), economic conditions (labor migration with the increased possibility of concurrent partnering), and forms of social relations (polygyny and patriarchy). But while such

components of a risk environment may be common from one environment to another, it is not at all clear that they operate in the same way *across* diverse environments.

There are some distinct disadvantages with the vague term "driver." These include the ways that vagueness can suggest causality where it is not present, eliciting interventions based on observations of correlation or the even vaguer, and scientifically discredited, idea of "elective affinity." Associated with this are the manifold ways in which conceptual vagueness can spoil a useful conceptualization by permitting the importation of ideologically acceptable rather than rigorously determined variables as drivers. An example of this is to be found on the website of the Tanzanian AIDS Commission. Here we find a list of "drivers" of the epidemic, and also of "contextual factors" which illustrate some of the practical and ideological difficulties with the terms. Thus:

Drivers of the epidemic

1. Promiscuous sexual behaviour
2. Intergerational [*sic*] sex
3. Concurrent sexual partners
4. Presence of other sexually transmitted infections such as herpes simplex x 2 virus.
5. Lack of knowledge of HIV transmission

Contextual factors shaping the epidemic in the country

1. Poverty and transactional sex with increasing numbers of commercial sex workers
2. Men's irresponsible sexual behaviour due to cultural patterns of virility
3. Social, economic and political gender inequalities including violence against women
4. Substance abuse such as alcohol consumption
5. Local cultural practices e.g. widow cleansing
6. Mobility in all its forms which leads to separation of spouses and increased establishment of temporary sexual relationships
7. Lack of male circumcision.[6]

Formulations of the problem can be found in several places (Görgens-Albino, Mohammad *et al.* 2007; Gupta, Parkhurst *et al.* 2008). Recurring themes

---

[6] www.tacaids.go.tz/hiv-and-aids-information/current-status-of-hiv-and-aids.html, accessed September 7, 2011.

include: the nature of sexual cultures in framing sexual risk and risk-taking, and the differential influence of distal and proximal factors, for example the major structural factor of the role of differential wealth and income inequality as contributory factors to the epidemiology of HIV (Barnett and Whiteside 1999).

Geeta Rao Gupta and her co-authors provide a useful overview of the problem and experience with structural interventions. They comment significantly that: "Mapping the way in which each of these factors increases individual HIV vulnerability is essential to determine the most appropriate type and level of response . . . Taking a structural approach . . . begins by understanding the causal pathways in order to identify the points of maximum effect for any given intervention or agency" (Gupta, Parkhurst *et al.* 2008).

These are important but challenging insights. They may be insights which we would rather not know for they point to a constantly recurring problem. This is the conflict between cost-effective interventions and the growing knowledge that where social policy is concerned, while dose-response frames of thought and funding constraints may point to cost-effectiveness and cost-benefit analysis as *the* starting point, interventions dependent upon these perspectives are unlikely to be cost-effective because the objects for treatment are more heterogeneous than homogeneous. Such an idea is of course hardly welcome to funding agencies whose political constituencies and financial contributors naturally demand generalizability of solutions through cost-effectiveness, sometimes, it seems, with the emphasis on the administrative benefit of controlling cost and being seen to spend budgets rather than on the quality or quantity of social outcome effectiveness or benefit.

Section 2: if the metaphors are inappropriate, what is to be done?

If this is the case then what should we do? The answers are that we should: (a) take each situation on its merits and design structural interventions specific to that situation; (b) recognize that structural approaches can be more or less distal;

(c) understand that the more distal structural factors are the most intractable and challenging and that therefore we should identify the most proximal level at which to intervene; (d) not assume that structural interventions are the sole valid type of interventions but that they can and should be combined with more individual interventions. If this is to be done, careful contextual analysis of social, economic, and cultural contexts would seem necessary.

Such contextual analyses are likely to be expensive, time-consuming, and subject to suspicion from policy-makers and politicians because of their very specific recommendations and probable use of qualitative as well as quantitative (including participatory) techniques. The challenge is to deploy such detailed information pragmatically together with insights from understanding the *ecology of risk*. The building blocks for such a pragmatic engagement rest on two foundations: first, recognition of the links between individual risk behaviors and the environments in which these occur; second, clarity about the ways in which different environments permit differing degrees of hope for the future and thus longer or shorter decision horizons for individuals.

Hope seems to offer the possibility of being a fundamental and measurable concept for linking individual behavior to the characteristics of the surrounding risk environment (Snyder 1994; Snyder, Sympson *et al.* 1996). In other words, it offers a way of measuring the role of both structure and agency without having to understand or conceptualize them separately. The next section proposes that the concept of hope is a missing piece of the jigsaw linking the individual to the environment.

The environment is best thought of as a *regulator* of individual behavioral decisions, imposing constraints and opportunities that shape behavioral risk factors (Glass and McAtee 2006). Whereas some environments permit hope for a future, thus enabling individuals to take a long-term perspective on their current behaviors, other environments have the opposite effect, resulting in harmful *sequelae* for individuals and societies. A growing body of research links aspects of the social environment to risk behavior and health inequality (Marmot 2003, 2005). Indeed, with recent developments in epigenetics, we are now able to understand far more about the complex relationship between individual genetic inheritance and its interaction within the environment prior to and after birth. The detailed mechanisms whereby nature and nurture interact are becoming so clear that what Richard Sennett once described as *The Hidden Injuries of Class* (Random House 1988) are no longer so opaque and are increasingly revealed as embodied in the cells of individuals; see Nessa Carey, *The Epigenetic Revolution* (Icon Books 2011).

Important here is the idea of the *embodiment of social conditions*. It seems very likely that this is no longer merely a rhetorical descriptive term; rather it is an explanation of how social structures are written into individual bodies, a process whereby wider social forces shaping health opportunity and inequality are internalized over time by individuals, quite literally *embodying* their social, economic, and cultural experience. In this sense, the term "embodiment" is in the process of changing from mere description to explanation. Evidence exploring health inequalities shows links between the environments people occupy and perceptions of stress, autonomy, and self-efficacy, which in turn shape the self-regulation of risk behavior (Siegrist 2000). Some characterize this process as a kind of *oppression illness* in its effects among the socially excluded, including populations vulnerable to HIV. In short, environments are regulators of hope, and hope shapes risk decisions and thus the epidemiology of some infectious diseases, notably, in this context, HIV.

The approach outlined above offers a way into the conundrum about the relationship between HIV and poverty. A direct relationship has often been claimed, more frequently seemingly for purposes of advocacy simplification rather than in the pursuit of scientific understanding. However, careful attention to this question suggests that the causal relationships are more complex, depending in part on the stage of the epidemic; for example, it is well established that in African circumstances, in the early stages, the wealthier have been more likely to become infected than the poorer, and that only later did the inverse relationship develop between high prevalence and low socio-economic class. For a long time, however, and more convincingly, it

has been hypothesized that the degree of income inequality, perhaps as a proxy for social cohesion, is an important link in the complex chain of causation between poverty and transmission susceptibility (Cohen 1993, 1998; Hargreaves and Glynn 2002; Hargreaves, Morison *et al.* 2002; Boerma, Gregson *et al.* 2003; Lurie, Williams *et al.* 2003; Nguyen and Peschard 2003; Drain, Smith *et al.* 2004; Gregson, Garnett *et al.* 2006; Johnson and Way 2006; Mishra 2006; Mishra, Vaessen *et al.* 2006; Tladi 2006; Gillespie, Kadiyala *et al.* 2007; Hargreaves, Bonell *et al.* 2007; Hargreaves, Morison, Bonnell *et al.* 2007; Hargreaves, Morison, Kim *et al.* 2007; Helleringer and Kohler 2007; Lachaud 2007; Masanjala 2007; Mmbaga, Hussain *et al.* 2007; Nombo 2007).

To put the matter very simply and distinctly: where the distribution of wealth and income results in social structures and hierarchies where people feel powerless, where insecurity is the normal condition of existence, then people will be less able to have realistic hope for the future. Rather they are constantly pressed back into situations where only short-term decisions are realistic responses to the conditions they endure. Thus it is that a low security, unpredictable risk environment is related to short-term decisions, which include decisions about sexual behavior, with a marked gender aspect where women may be forced to use transactional sex as an element in their livelihood or survival strategy. A starting point for engaging with the difficult questions associated with developing social policies for structural interventions is to recognize that the question is incorrectly formulated. It is not solely about "structural" interventions. A more proper formulation is to see that at the center of the "structural intervention problem" lies the meeting point of agency and structure – a long-standing and familiar theoretical problem in the social sciences. Once we have reformulated the problem in these terms, we can move our analysis logically into one of the two following alternative positions: (a) each situation must be analyzed in its own terms, with no attempt to generalize from the findings; (b) we can try to develop and deploy a pragmatic and practical diagnostic tool which summarizes and gives access to the key point where structure and agency come together and which in so doing enables us to identify locations where effective interventions can be made which, because they have taken agency into account, engage with the subjective experience of those people who are to be the likely recipients of the medicinal dose of social policy intervention.

Section 3: hope as a diagnostic tool: steps toward social policy interventions

The key question is how we might identify what alters the possibilities for people to be able to make rational choices *within the context of their particular socio-economic and cultural situation.* With regard to infectious diseases, we also need to understand the links between individual susceptibility to infection and epidemiological observations of the social distribution of patterns of infection. Finally, we need to reach conclusions about workable social policy interventions. The answer, for at least a large proportion of heterosexually acquired HIV infections, may lie in the concept of hope. This argument can certainly be made in relation to evidence that in some circumstances young people ignore prevention messages because they cannot think beyond the present, and have little or no hope for the future (Rotheram-Borus, Kracker *et al.* 2000; Cambell and MacPhail 2002). Thus, we need a conceptual approach which captures the following: (a) individual decision matrices; (b) the situations within which they make their decisions. The concept of hope may be one practical way of capturing these complexities by means of a single variable. In other words, we can use the concept of hope – both theoretically for thinking purposes and also practically as part of intervention programs. Hope links structure and individual behavior and has the potential advantage of being measurable using validated psychological instruments at the individual and possibly at the aggregate level. It has the additional advantages of being part of the everyday lexicon of ordinary people, researchers, policy-makers, and politicians.

There has been surprisingly little work on hope (J. Braithwaite 2004a, b, c; V. Braithwaite 2004d, e; Drahos 2004; McGeer 2004; Pettit 2004; Bernays,

Rhodes and Barnett 2007). However, some of the most useful was done by the psychologist Richard Snyder. This work defined hope in a very specific way: as a way of thinking about the future which takes into account *both* a vision of that future, and pragmatic ways of achieving envisioned goals. Thus hope is to be distinguished from mere optimism, which lacks pragmatic engagement. In contrast, hope can be nominally defined as:

- "a cognitive set that is comprised of a reciprocally derived sense of successful (1) agency (goal-directed determination), and (2) pathways (planning of ways to meet goals)" (Snyder 1995); or
- "goal-directed thinking in which people appraise their capability to produce workable routes to goals (pathway thinking), along with their potential to initiate and sustain movement via the pathway(s) (agency thinking)" (Snyder 1998); or
- "goal-directed thinking in which the person appraises his or her perceived capability to produce workable routes to goals (pathways thinking), as well as the potential to initiate and sustain movement along the pathways (agentic thinking)" (Snyder 1996).

Each of these overlapping definitions emphasizes a mental attitude ("cognitive set"), appraisal of the future ("goal directed"), and practical engagement with the future via consideration of agency (individual or communal action) and pathways (pragmatic consideration of how to act).

The concept of hope is of interest as a possible composite explanatory variable in relation both to individual and communal regulation of infection pathways. It may account for a number of observed characteristics of the HIV epidemic which do not fit neatly into either the simple individual rational choice model or into the structural poverty and disempowerment causes HIV infection model. In particular it may serve as a way of focusing the complex relationships of various kinds of inequality – gender, income, wealth, ethnic – which are components in the risk environments within which individual infections occur.

Hope can be seen as a conceptually distinct and operationalizable variable which provides a possibility for measuring, via individuals and groups of individuals, ways in which ecologies of risk regulate and reveal risk to individuals and thus influence their decisions. Thus hope concentrates and summarizes the individual behavior and characteristics of the risk environment as experienced by individuals and provides a framework for understanding differing potentials for behavior change (Snyder, Harris *et al.* 1991; Snyder 1998; Snyder, Cheavens *et al.* 1999; Snyder 2000; Snyder, Sympson *et al.* 2000). The concept of hope may lead us to a better understanding of the pathways between individual perspectives on the world, social, cultural, and economic conditions, and risk-taking behaviors.

Deployed in this way, surveys of relative hope levels within and between communities could help in identification not only of low- and high-risk environments, but also of changes in communities over time in response to wider system changes, including changes resulting from distal phenomena such as changes in global commodity prices affecting a particular country or region. The next step would then be location of communities on a scale of hope–hopelessness, an approach which would be particularly appropriate in poor countries where more general background socio-economic data are not available. Such a strategy could facilitate pinpointing geographical areas and social segments in which further exploration of the social and economic conditions leading to hopelessness could expose leads into effective policy and program responses. This style of developing and designing intervention studies would of course not meet the criteria for a randomized controlled trial (RCT). RCT designs are all but impossible to achieve in circumstances of contextual heterogeneity. However, studies could be designed in ways which meet the kinds of plausibility criteria it has been cogently argued are more appropriate to public health interventions (Victora, Habicht *et al.* 2004).

Because the ideas of hope and hopelessness are probably translatable into most languages the concept lends itself to deployment in techniques such as surveys, focus groups, and other methods of data collection whereby members of such communities could themselves be directly involved in dialogue (and even diagnosis) intended to identify ways in which the existing situation could be improved. A very early example of such a structural inter-vention based on local diagnosis was encountered by this author in 1989 in Rakai, Uganda where village elders had banned Saturday night discos, thus reducing the opportunities for young men and women to go off into the bush together.

Hope has not been deployed as a concept in relation to infectious diseases. Indeed, it has not been the focus of any significant research in relation to health issues other than in relation to palliative care (Snyder 1996, 1998). However, transposed to a different field, as a link between the pathogen, the individual, and social and economic structures which form a risk environment, hope offers the following analytical advantages:

(a) it is measurable using fairly straightforward scales (Snyder, Harris *et al.* 1991; Babyak, Snyder *et al.* 1993; Snyder, Sympson *et al.* 1996; Snyder, Hoza *et al.* 1997);
(b) it is easily understood by politicians and others in a position to allocate resources;
(c) it is understood by ordinary people who may be able to tell us directly what is required to restore hope and therefore directly inform policy.

Furthermore, it may turn out that levels of individual hope are not directly related only to income (Diener and Oishi 2000), although up to a certain point this is undoubtedly the case, but that thereafter other factors such as the nature of government and of civil society become of considerable importance (Oswald 1997; Diener and Oishi 2000; Frey and Stutzer 2002; Nettle 2005). The evidence from studies of happiness certainly lead to this kind of conclusion (Frey and Stutzer 2003).

As a diagnostic tool for understanding the agency-structure points where social policy interventions may be possible, hope may offer some clear pointers towards policy interventions which are effective, community driven, specific, and cost saving. It is certainly *not* being argued here that *all* HIV infections reflect relative hopelessness, and it probably does not help us very much as a concept for explaining men who have sex with men (MSM) epidemics in Western Europe and North America. There it has often been the highly articulate, educated, and relatively prosperous who have become infected. Notably in North America, the *individual* behavior change model has been most effective, but never alone; it has always been accompanied by attention to structural factors, which include collective action, solid funding support, and, in some cases, government leadership. But, it is this latter case which really suggests the power of hope as an addition to our analytical – and possibly preventive – armory. Where there is hope (and this requires structures and other resources if it is to be effective), individual behavior change in response to rational argument is possible. Where hope and resources are absent, behavior change messages are less likely to be effective on their own. Social policy interventions in the HIV epidemic which are based on diagnosis of the structural conditions which make people hopeless may be the way forward and ultimately these policy interventions may be both cost-effective and cost beneficial. Regardless of the technical sophistication of the cost-benefit or cost-effectiveness analysis deployed in choosing between one policy intervention and another, choosing between structural interventions which have not been linked to and designed in relation to their particular "upstreams" may turn out to be neither cost-effective nor cost beneficial.

References

Ajzen, I. and Fishbein, M. (1980). *Understanding Attitudes and Predicting Social Behavior*. Englewood Cliffs, NJ: Prentice Hall.

Babyak, M., Snyder, C. R. *et al.* (1993). Psychometric properties of the Hope Scale: a confirmatory factor analysis. *Journal of Research in Personality* **27**: 154–69.

Barnett, T. (2006). A long-wave event: HIV/AIDS, politics, governance and "security": sundering the intergenerational bond? *International Affairs* **82**(2): 297–301.

Barnett, T. and Blaikie. (1992). *AIDS in Africa: Its Present and Future Impact*. New York: Belhaven Press, London and Guildford Press.

Barnett, T. and Parkhurst, J. (2005). HIV/AIDS: sex, abstinence, and behaviour change. *The Lancet Infectious Diseases* **5**(9): 590–3.

Barnett, T. and Whiteside, A. (1999). HIV/AIDS and development: case studies and a conceptual framework. *Eur J Dev Res* **11**: 220–34.

Bernays, S., Rhodes, T. and Barnett, T. (2007) Hope, prevention and treatment: a new way to look at the HIV epidemic. *AIDS* **21** (Suppl 5): S5–S11.

Boerma, J., Gregson, S. *et al.* (2003). Understanding the uneven spread of HIV within Africa: comparative study of biologic, behavioral, and contextual factors in rural populations in Tanzania and Zimbabwe. *Sexually Transmitted Infections Diseases* **30**(10): 779–87.

Braithwaite, J. (2004a). Emancipation and hope. *The Annals of the American Academy of Political and Social Science* **592**: 79–98.

Braithwaite, J. (2004b) Collective hope. *The Annals of the American Academy of Political and Social Science* **592**: 6–15.

Braithwaite, V. (2004c). The hope process and social inclusion. *The Annals of the American Academy of Political and Social Science* **592**: 128–51.

Cambell, C. and MacPhail, C. (2002). Peer education, gender and the development of critical consciousness: participatory HIV prevention by South African youth. *Social Science and Medicine* **55**: 331–45.

Chin, J. (2006). *The AIDS Pandemic: The Collision of Epidemiology with Political Correctness*. Oxford and Seattle: Radcliffe Publishing.

Cohen, D. (1993). *Poverty and HIV/AIDS in Sub-Saharan Africa*. Issues paper. Geneva: UNDP.

Cohen, D. (1998). *Socio-Economic Causes and Consequences of the HIV Epidemic in Southern Africa: A Case Study of Namibia*. Geneva: UNDP.

Diener, E. and Oishi, S. (2000). Money and happiness: income and subjective well-being. In Diener and Suh (eds.) *Culture and Subjective Well-Being*. Cambridge, MA: MIT Press.

Drahos, P. (2004). Trading in public hope. *The Annals of the American Academy of Political and Social Science* **592**: 18–38.

Drain, P. K., Smith, J. S. *et al.* (2004). Correlates of national HIV seroprevalence: an ecologic analysis of 122 developing countries. *J Acquir Immune Defic Syndr* **35**(4): 407–20.

Frey, B. and Stutzer, A. (2002). *Happiness and Economics: How the Economy and Institutions Affect Well-Being*. Princeton University Press.

Frey, B. and Stutzer, A. (2003). *The Economics of Happiness*. Princeton University Press.

Gillespie, S., Kadiyala, S. *et al.* (2007). Is poverty or wealth driving HIV transmission? *AIDS* **21**(Suppl 7): S5–S16.

Glass, T. and McAtee, M. (2006). Behavioral science at the cross roads in public health: extending the horizons, envisioning the future. *Social Science and Medicine* **62**: 650–71.

Görgens-Albino, M., Mohammad, N. *et al.* (2007). *Results of the World Bank's Response to a Development Crisis: The Africa Multi-Country AIDS Program 2000–2006*. Washington DC: The World Bank.

Gregson, S., Garnett, G. P. *et al.* (2006). HIV decline associated with behavior change in eastern Zimbabwe. *Science* **311**: 664–6.

Gupta, G. R., Parkhurst, J. O. *et al.* (2008). Structural approaches to HIV prevention. *The Lancet* **372**(9640): 764–75.

Hargreaves, J. R., Bonell, C. P. *et al.* (2007). Systematic review exploring time-trends in the association between educational attainment and risk of HIV infection in sub-Saharan Africa. *AIDS*: in press.

Hargreaves, J. R. and Glynn, J. R. (2002). Educational attainment and HIV infection in developing countries: a systematic review. *Tropical Medicine and International Health* **76**: 489–98.

Hargreaves, J. R., Morison, L. A. *et al.* (2002). Socioeconomic status and risk of HIV infection in an urban population in Kenya. *Tropical Medicine and International Health* **7**(8): 1–10.

Hargreaves, J. R., Morison, L. A., Bonnell, C. *et al.* (2007). Explaining persistently high HIV incidence in rural South Africa: a cohort study 2001–2004. *AIDS* **27**: s39–s48.

Hargreaves, J. R., Morison, L. A., Kim, J. C. *et al.* (2007). The association between school attendance, HIV infection and sexual behaviour among young people in rural South Africa. *Journal of Epidemiology and Community Health* **662**: 113–19.

Helleringer, S. and Kohler, H.-P. (2007). Sexual network structure and the spread of HIV in Africa: evidence from Likoma Island, Malawi. *AIDS* **21**(17): 2323–32.

Johnson, K. and Way, A. (2006). Risk factors for HIV infection in a national adult population: evidence from the 2003 Kenya Demographic and Health Survey. *J Acquir Immune Defic Syndr* **42**(5): 627–36.

Lachaud, J. P. (2007). HIV prevalence and poverty in Africa: micro- and macro-econometric evidences applied to Burkina Faso. *J Health Econ* **26**(3): 483–504.

Lakoff, G. and Johnson, M. (1980). *Metaphors We Live By*. University of Chicago Press.

Lurie, M., Williams, B. G. *et al.* (2003). Who infects whom? HIV-1 concordance and discordance among migrant and non-migrant couples in South Africa. *AIDS* **17**(15): 2245–52.

Mallal, S., Nolan, D. *et al.* (2002). Association between presence of HLA-B*5701, HLA-DR7, and HLA-DQ3 and hypersensitivity to HIV-1 reverse-transcriptase inhibitor abacavir. *Lancet* **359**: 727–32.

Marmot, M. (2003). Self esteem and health. *British Medical Journal* **327**: 574–5.

Marmot, M. (2005). Social determinants of health inequalities. *The Lancet* **365**: 1099–104.

Masanjala, W. (2007). The poverty-HIV/AIDS nexus in Africa: a livelihood approach. *Soc Sci Med* **64**(5): 1032–41.

McGeer, V. (2004). The art of good hope. *The Annals of the American Academy of Political and Social Science* **592**: 100–27.

Michel, O., LeVan, T. D. *et al.* (2003). Systemic responsiveness to lipopolysaccharide and polymorphisms in the toll-like receptor 4 gene in human beings. *The Journal of Allergy and Clinical Immunology* **112**(5): 923–9.

Mishra, V. (2006). *Patterns of HIV Seroprevalence and Associated Risk Factors: Evidence from the Demographic and Health Surveys and AIDS Indicator Surveys. Abstract 48*. The 2006 HIV/AIDS Implementers Meeting of the President's Emergency Plan for AIDS Relief, Durban, South Africa.

Mishra, V., Vaessen, M. *et al.* (2006). HIV testing in national population-based surveys: experience from the Demographic and Health Surveys. *Bull World Health Organ* **84**(7): 537–45.

Mmbaga, E. J., Hussain, A. *et al.* (2007). Prevalence and risk factors for HIV-1 infection in rural Kilimanjaro region of Tanzania: implications for prevention and treatment. *BMC Public Health* **7**(58).

Nelkin, D. (1989). Communicating technological risk: the social construction of risk perception. *Annual Review of Public Health* **10**: 95–113.

Nettle, D. (2005). *Happiness: The Science Behind Your Smile*. Oxford University Press.

Nguyen, V.-K. and Peschard, K. (2003). Anthropology inequality and disease: a review. *Annu. Rev. Anthropol* 447–74(32).

Niehof, A., Rugalema, G. *et al.* (eds.) (2010). *AIDS and Rural Livelihoods: Dynamics and Diversity in Sub-Saharan Africa*. London and Washington DC: Earthscan.

Nombo, C. I. (2007). *When AIDS Meets Poverty: Implications for Social Capital in a Village in Tanzania*. Wageningen Academic Publishers.

Nombo, C. I. (2010). Sweet cane, bitter realities: the complex realities of AIDS in Mkamba, Kilombero District, Tanzania. In A. Niehof, G. Rugalema and S. Gillespie (eds.) *AIDS and Rural Livelihoods: Dynamics and Diversity in Sub-Saharan Africa*. London and Washington DC: Earthscan, 61–76.

Oswald, A. J. (1997). Happiness and economic performance. *Economic Journal* **107**: 1815–31.

Over, M. (2010). *Using Incentives to Prevent HIV Infections*. Washington DC: Center for Global Development.

Rotheram-Borus, M. J., Kracker, Z. O. K. R. *et al.* (2000). Prevention of HIV among adolescents. *Prevention Science* **1**(1): 15–30.

Schwartländer, B., Stover, J. *et al.* (2011). Towards an improved investment approach for an effective response to HIV/AIDS. *The Lancet* **377**(9782): 2031–41.

Siegrist, J. (2000). Place, social exchange and health: proposed sociological framework. *Social Science and Medicine* **51**: 1283–93.

Singleton, W. T. and Hoyden, J. (1994). *Risk and Decisions*. Chichester: Wiley.

Slovic, J. (1992). Perception of risk: reflections on the psychometric paradigm. In S. Krimsky and D. Golding (eds.) *Social Theories of Risk*. Westport, CT: Praeger.

Snyder, C. R. (1994). Hope and optimism. In V. S. Ramachandran (ed.) *Encyclopedia of Human Behavior*. San Diego, CA: Academic Press, 535–42.

Snyder, C. R. (1995). Conceptualizing, measuring, and nurturing hope. "Current Trends" Focus Article. *Journal of Counseling and Development* **73**: 355.

Snyder, C. R. (1996). To hope, to lose, and hope again. *Journal of Personal and Interpersonal Loss* **1**: 1–16.

Snyder, C. R. (1998a). A case for hope in pain, loss and suffering. In J. H. Harvey (ed.) *Perspectives on Loss: A Sourcebook*. Washington DC: Taylor and Francis Ltd.

Snyder, C. R. (1998b). Hope. In H. S. Friedman (ed.) *Encyclopedia of Mental Health*. San Diego, CA: Academic Press, 421–31.

Snyder, C. R. (ed.) (2000). *Handbook of Hope: Theory, Measurement, and Interventions*. San Diego, CA: Academic Press.

Snyder, C. R., Cheavens, J. *et al.* (1999). Hoping. In C. R. Snyder (ed.) *Coping: The Psychology of What Works*. Oxford University Press, 205–31.

Snyder, C. R., Harris, C. *et al.* (1991). The will and the ways: development and validation of an individual differences measure of hope. *Journal of Personality and Social Psychology* **60**: 570–85.

Snyder, C. R., Hoza, B. *et al.* (1997). The development and validation of the Children's Hope Scale. *Journal of Pediatric Psychology* **22**: 399–421.

Snyder, C. R., Sympson, S. C. *et al.* (1996). Development and validation of the State Hope Scale. *Journal of Personality and Social Psychology* **2**: 321–35.

Snyder, C. R., Sympson, S. C. *et al.* (2000). The optimism and hope constructs: variants on a positive expectancy theme. In E. C. Chang (ed.) *Optimism and Pessimism*. Washington DC: American Psychological Association.

Strathdee, S. A., Hallett, T. B. *et al.* (2010). HIV and risk environment for injecting drug users: the past, present, and future. *The Lancet* **376**(9737): 268–84.

Tanzania Commission for AIDS (TACAIDS), Zanzibar AIDS Commission (ZAC) *et al.* (2008). Tanzania HIV/AIDS and Malaria Indicator Survey 2007–08. Dar es Salaam, Tanzania.

Taylor, S. E. (1991). *Health Psychology*. New York: McGraw-Hill.

Tladi L. S. (2006). Poverty and HIV/AIDS in South Africa: an empirical contribution. *SAHARA* **3**(1): 369–81.

Victora, C. G., Habicht, J.-P. *et al.* (2004). Evidence-based public health: moving beyond randomized trials. *Am J Public Health* **94**(3): 400–05.

Wittgenstein, L. (1953). *Philosophical Investigations*. Oxford: Blackwell.

Wynne, B. (1992). Risk and social learning: reification to engagement. In S. Krimsky and D. Golding (eds.) *Social Theories of Risk*. Westport, CT: Praeger.

Social policy

Perspective paper

HAROUNAN KAZIANGA

In the assessment paper, Vassall, Remme, and Watts (VRW) present cost-benefit analyses of four interventions aimed at enhancing the response to HIV/AIDS in sub-Saharan Africa (SSA). The interventions they identified are: i) cash transfers to keep girls in secondary schools, ii) increasing alcohol taxation, iii) adding gender training to existing microfinance and livelihood programs, and iv) community mobilization. They identified these solutions based on a detailed review of the literature and on consultations with HIV experts.

VRW selected these four interventions based on their assessment of the empirical literature which points to several structural interventions that have the potential to mitigate some of the structural HIV risks through economic empowerment, social protection, financial incentives, and transformative processes. VRW stress that evidence on the effectiveness of these interventions on HIV prevention is limited, presumably because HIV prevention *per se* is not often the primary objective for many of these interventions.

The authors show that the benefit to cost ratios they obtained are sensitive to critical assumptions related to the net benefits of each intervention, the discount rate, and the costs of the interventions. Under the assumptions that VRW make, the benefit to cost ratios for these interventions are quite large, hence justifying public investments. Overall the interventions considered are promising. Cost-effectiveness and benefit to cost ratios, however, vary greatly across countries presumably because epidemiological and socio-economic factors are country-specific.

The assessment paper by VRW is selective in the choice of the interventions considered. The analysis is very well executed and the exposition is clear. Their selection of four interventions is largely justified based on the existing evidence. In this perspective paper, I use the assessment paper as a starting point to propose a discussion of the findings and offer further perspectives on the topic, on the basis of existing studies.

This perspective paper will start by discussing the issues policy-makers are likely to be confronted with when they attempt to scale up promising pilot studies. Next, it will argue that cost-effectiveness calculations should better integrate how unit costs are likely to vary when pilot studies are scaled up. It will argue in particular that varying average costs will determine in part the size of the full-scale project. Further, it will discuss some implications of increasing alcohol taxation that are not sufficiently addressed in the assessment paper. Finally, it will propose a possible intervention – offering life insurance to adults to stay HIV-free. Calibration exercises by Araujo and Murray (2010) suggest that this intervention can reduce HIV transmission significantly, but randomized controlled trials would provide more credible evidence.

From pilots to scaled-up interventions

Three of the interventions reviewed in this assessment paper were based on pilot studies and/or randomized controlled trials. Since *RethinkHIV* is aiming at identifying the most promising prevention interventions, two issues would need to be addressed. First, it is important to stress the difference between efficacy and efficiency studies. In particular, interventions which have demonstrated impact under closely managed conditions may not necessarily be as successful under normal conditions. Second, the cost structure could change when moving from a pilot to a scale-up, and therefore modifying the cost-benefit ratios.

External validity

The first concern is related to the external validity of pilot studies. In other words, will a promising randomized controlled trial produce the same outcome in a different context? Are there any steps that can be taken to ensure that results obtained at a pilot stage can be replicated either at a larger scale or in different settings? One way to overcome this critique has been to repeat similar experiments in different contexts. The rationale is that by testing hypotheses in different places, with enough contextual variety, we can confidently state that a theory holds and therefore can be used to inform policy decisions in other places. For instance, the effects of conditional cash transfers on education and child health have been replicated in many contexts (e.g., Baird *et al.* 2011; Fiszbein and Schady 2009; Gertler 2004; Paxson and Schady 2008). As a result, a consensus has formed on the effectiveness of conditional cash transfers at improving educational and health outcomes. Their effects on sexual behavior, however, are still less researched. Therefore, it is hard to argue that the results observed in one location in Malawi will hold in different contexts. For example, Baird *et al.* (2010) stress that their sample is representative of never-married adolescent girls in Southern Africa, a region with a high HIV/AIDS prevalence rate[1] compared to – let's say – West Africa. It is not clear whether the estimated impacts will remain the same if regions with a lower HIV prevalence rate were considered.

It is notable that three of the four interventions considered have another purpose in addition to HIV/AIDS prevention. Let us consider the conditional cash transfers intervention, for example. It was intended also to keep girls in school. It is not clear whether education or HIV prevention was the primary purpose, or these two important development goals received an equal weight. The participatory gender intervention was piggybacked to a microfinance program. Finally, governments may choose to pursue different objectives with alcohol taxation, including increasing tax revenues. Obviously, this underscores the need for a multi-sectoral approach of HIV/AIDS prevention programs.

This type of approach raises the question, however, of how pilot studies can be replicated. In particular, understanding how different elements of the intervention work could provide useful insights when assessing the cost-effectiveness of alternative interventions. For example, the study considered has demonstrated that conditional cash transfers for keeping girls in school reduce HIV/AIDS transmission. The reduction of HIV/AIDS transmission could have operated through two channels. First, when girls' income increases, they are less likely to engage in transactional sexual intercourse with older men, thereby reducing intergenerational HIV transmission. Second, as argued by Baird *et al.* (2010), it is the desire to stay in school that leads to reduced sexual activity, and hence reduced HIV transmission.

If decreased sexual activity is driven essentially by income, then any cash transfers could be equally good. In fact, unconditional cash transfers, if they are less costly to administer, may be more cost-effective than conditional cash transfers. Social safety nets could also be as effective in reducing HIV transmission. If, on the other hand, the observed impact is driven by girls' desire to stay in school, any policy that increased girls' marginal benefits from attending school (everything else being constant) would be as just as effective. Disentangling the underlying mechanisms which drive the impact can help decide among alternative interventions.

Varying average costs

Basic microeconomic theory suggests that the average cost curve is U-shaped. Under ordinary circumstances, the average cost curve slopes downward, flattens out, and eventually turns up. While the concept of diseconomies of scale easily relates to the theory of the firm, the causes of scale diseconomies also affect public interventions such as the ones discussed in the assessment paper (Marseille *et al.* 2007; Over 1986). For instance, increasing costs of communication, bureaucratic inertia, and duplication of effort could contribute to increasing costs. Some inputs may become more costly as well. In the

---

[1] It is estimated that about 24.6 percent of women aged 15 to 49 are HIV-positive in the study area (Baird *et al.* 2010, p. 58).

short run, an intervention may exhaust the available supply of lower-wage but adequately trained staff in the area. The intervention may be forced then to hire staff that are more expensive or less well trained and this would translate actually into an increase in average costs. It is apparent that successfully scaling up pilot interventions would require information concerning the threshold beyond which average costs increase (Over 1986).

VRW assume constant unit costs when calculating the benefit to cost ratios. The unit costs for the interventions analyzed by VRW vary by a factor of 1.12 (for alcohol taxation) to 46.47 (for community mobilization). In addition to differences between countries (and possibly between different sites within countries), such variations may reflect differences in economies of scale as well (Preya and Pink 2006).

When conducting sensitivity analysis, it would be informative to allow unit costs to vary with the size of the intervention. A more formalized approach which utilizes regression analysis can also be considered if the number of experiments is large enough. With enough observations on experiments, one could estimate a regression which relates program unit costs to program size (e.g., Guinness *et al.* 2005; Marseille *et al.* 2007). Even if crude, these estimates could provide useful information on how to project the costs of full-scale programs from the costs of pilot studies.

How big should an intervention be? Conditional on identifying a promising pilot and deciding to scale up, policy-makers would eventually have to decide on the size of the full-scale project. Let us say the objective is to maximize the reduction of HIV transmission among poor girls in Malawi. Given a fixed budget, should the full-scale project target all girls who are below the poverty line, or would the objective be maximized by spending the available budget on a portfolio of interventions, for example?

Brandeau and Zaric (2009) propose using an economic framework to address these types of questions. The authors propose a model which has two main building blocks. The first part of the model uses a production function which captures the relationship between expenditure in prevention and the HIV sufficient contact rate. The second part

of the model uses an epidemic model to describe the impact of changes in the sufficient contact rate on the spread of HIV. Instead of using simulation methods as in previous studies, Brandeau and Zaric use an economic framework that employs the concepts of cost-effectiveness analysis in order to determine the optimal level of expenditure, i.e., the level of expenditures that equalize marginal costs to marginal benefits. They identify two special cases: i) spend the entire budget on a given intervention if the marginal benefits are always greater than the marginal costs, and ii) spend nothing if marginal costs always exceed marginal benefits. Brandeau and Zaric further assume that alternative HIV prevention programs exist so that funds not invested in the given HIV prevention program can be used to fund alternative programs. As more pilot studies become available, this type of study has the potential of helping policy-makers allocate their limited resources more efficiently.

Alcohol taxation

VRW motivate this intervention by arguing that alcohol drinkers are more likely to be infected by HIV than non-alcohol drinkers (Fisher *et al.* 2007). Let us accept that drinking alcohol increases risky sexual behaviors and HIV transmission.[2] Following Chisholm *et al.* (2004), VRW estimate that a 25 percent increase in alcohol taxation will result in an 8.1 percent reduction in hazardous alcohol consumption, after accounting for a 10 percent increase in unrecorded consumption. VRW re-state Chisholm *et al.*'s (2004) argument that the hypothesized reduction in hazardous alcohol consumption will hold as long as unrecorded alcohol is between 5 percent and 50 percent. Countries in WHO's Africa sub-region E are in this category. Moreover, the conclusions hinge on Chisholm *et al.*'s assumption of an increase in unrecorded alcohol consumption, which in turn depends on the elasticities of substitution between legal alcoholic beverages and unrecorded ones. Unfortunately, the

---

[2] VRW provide useful references on the potential causal effect of alcohol consumption on risky sexual behaviors and on HIV/AIDS. Whether or not there is a causal relation between alcohol consumption and risky sexual behaviors is not central to the discussion in this perspective paper.

elasticities of substitutions are not discussed in Chisholm *et al.*

Estimates of price elasticity for alcohol in Africa are hard to come by. However, for Tanzania (which is part of the WHO's Africa sub-region E), Osoro, Mpango, and Mwinyimvua (2001) estimated an own-price elasticity of −0.3 for a local market beer.[3] The authors also found a relatively high cross-price elasticity of demand, 2.7, between Tanzania's local brew chibuki and market beer.[4] Based on these estimates, if the price of beer increases by 10 percent, the demand for beer will decrease by 3 percent and the demand for the local chibuki will increase by 27 percent. It is apparent that consumers may substitute local brews, or even worse illegal beverages, for taxed beverages (Bird and Wallace 2010). Depending on the actual alcohol content of the unrecorded illegal beverages, hazardous drinking might not decrease. If there are substantial health hazards associated with unrecorded alcoholic beverages, then raising tax on "legal" alcoholic beverages such as beer could impose nonnegligible costs in terms of public health.[5]

It is undeniable that alcohol taxation could potentially reduce HIV transmission. However, whether taxing alcohol actually ends up reducing hazardous drinking (and thereby HIV transmission) will require thorough understanding of the local demand for alcoholic beverages. In particular, the prevalent own-price elasticity of "taxable" alcoholic beverages, and the elasticity of substitution between "taxable" alcoholic beverages and potential substitutes, especially home-brewed and/or smuggled alcohols that carry other health risks. Hence, without relatively robust measures of these unintended consequences, it is hard to ascertain the effectiveness of raising taxes on alcoholic beverages as policy interventions to reduce risky sexual behaviors. Fortunately, microeconomic surveys with detailed consumption data are becoming increasingly available in Africa. The availability of these types of data makes the estimation of more elaborated demand systems possible and even a low-cost exercise. The potential role that alcohol taxation could have on reducing HIV transmission suggests that it is worth investing the necessary efforts to uncover robust estimates of elasticities.

Incentivizing adults

A well-established fact is that heterosexual intercourse is the dominant mode of HIV transmission in sub-Saharan Africa. The Global HIV/AIDS Program (2008) provides a summary of the pathways of HIV transmission in the sub-Saharan African context. In many instances, female sex workers (FSWs) form the dominant core group in sub-Saharan Africa. Male clients of FSWs form the bridge between sex workers and the general population.

Given these pathways of HIV transmission, analysts and decision-makers should be specific about which group(s) they want to target. For example, conditional cash transfers for keeping girls in school aimed at reducing the number of sexual contacts between adolescent girls and older adult males, among whom the HIV prevalence rate might be high. A complementary approach would be to target older adult males directly, incentivizing them to remain HIV-free. For example, a randomized controlled trial in Tanzania uses conditional cash transfers in Tanzania to remain free of sexually transmitted infection and HIV (de Walque *et al.* 2010). The pilot requires that participants be screened periodically for STI, which serves as a proxy for risky sexual behavior.

Recently, Araujo and Murray (2010) have proposed using a life insurance scheme to incentivize adult males to stay HIV-free. In their model, agents can collect the life insurance benefits if their death is not the result of AIDS. They argue that excessive risky behavior results from low life expectancy and low levels of income, and illustrate the conditions

---

[3] Note that VRW assume a price elasticity of −0.3 to estimate the dead weight loss associated with the tax increase.

[4] The authors use aggregate time series data, and estimate one equation at a time.

[5] Although rigorous analyses are rare, there are numerous anecdotes on the consequences of adulterated alcoholic beverages across sub-Saharan Africa. Deaths attributed to adulterated alcohol have been reported in Cote d'Ivoire (www. panapress.com/19-die-from-adulterated-alcohol-in-Cote-d-ivoire-13-447060-17-lang2-index.html), or in Uganda (www.news24.com/Africa/News/Uganda-Illegal-alcohol-kills-30-20100408), for example. Bird and Wallace (2010) mention also several instances of death and illness arising from the use of illicit alcoholic beverages in South Africa.

for which the life insurance benefit can replicate the effects of higher income and life expectancy, thereby deterring risky sexual behavior and reducing the spread of HIV/AIDS. The life insurance policy can be made available to female sex workers as well. There is some evidence that some sexual workers are willing to engage in risky sexual intercourse with clients who are willing to pay more to avoid using condoms (e.g., Gertler *et al.* 2005; Rao *et al.* 2003). This type of life insurance contract can provide enough incentives to sexual workers to take the test, and if they are HIV-negative to abstain from risky sex.

Araujo and Murray use calibration techniques to explore the model implications for Zambia, Kenya, Tanzania, Ethiopia, and Rwanda. With a life insurance of $20,000, the annual costs per person range from $19.81 for Kenya to $38.40 for Zambia. Their results suggest a reduction in HIV prevalence by 6.4 percent in Kenya, to 24.4 percent in Ethiopia. Although the simulated results appear promising, randomized controlled trials could provide more credible evidence.

Conclusion

Building on the assessment paper, this paper offers further perspectives on the potential challenges that policy-makers are likely to be confronted with when they desire to scale up promising pilot studies. The perspective paper stresses the need for providing policy-makers with the tools and the information to move from promising pilot studies to full-scale projects. It also argues that cost-effectiveness calculations should better integrate changes in average costs that are likely to occur when going from a pilot study to full-scale project. Furthermore, it recommends devoting more efforts to understanding the underlying mechanisms that explain how specific interventions work. Finally, it proposes offering life insurance to adult individuals to stay HIV-free as a means for reducing risky sexual behavior and hence HIV transmission. Calibration exercises have suggested promising results, but randomized controlled trials would provide more credible evidence on the effectiveness of this policy.

References

Baird, S., McIntosh, C. and Özler, B. (2010). The short-term impacts of a schooling conditional cash transfer program on the sexual behavior of young women. *Health Economics* **19** Suppl: 55–68.

Baird, S., McIntosh, C. and Özler, B. (2011). Cash or condition? Evidence from a cash transfer experiment. *Quarterly Journal of Economics*, forthcoming.

Bird, R. M. and Wallace, S. (2010). *Taxing Alcohol in Africa: Reflections and Updates.* International Studies Program Working Paper Series. International Studies Program, Andrew Young School of Policy Studies, Georgia State University.

Brandeau, M. L. and Zaric, G. S. (2009). Optimal investment in HIV prevention programs: more is not always better. *Health Care Management Science* **12**: 27–37.

Chisholm, D. *et al.* (2004). Reducing the global burden of hazardous alcohol use: a comparative cost-effectiveness analysis. *Journal of Studies on Alcohol* **65**: 782–93.

de Araujo, P. and Murray, J. (2010). A life insurance deterrent to risky behavior in Africa. Department of Economics, University of Wisconsin – La Crosse.

de Walque, D., Dow, W. H., Nathan, R. *et al.* (2012). Incentivizing safe sex: a randomized trial of conditional cash transfers (CCTs) for HIV/STI prevention in rural Tanzania. *BMJ Open* **2**: e000747. doi:10.1136/ bmjopen-2011-000747.

Fisher, J. C., Bang, H. and Kapiga, S. H. (2007). The association between HIV infection and alcohol use: a systematic review and meta-analysis of African studies. *Sexually Transmitted Diseases* **34**: 856–63.

Fiszbein, A. and Schady, N. (2009). *Conditional Cash Transfers: Reducing Present and Future Poverty.* World Bank Policy Research Report. Washington, DC: World Bank.

Galarraga, O. M., Colchero, A., Wamai, R. and Bertozzi, S. (2009). HIV prevention cost-effectiveness: a systematic review. *BMC Public Health* **9** (Suppl 1): S5. doi:1186/ 1471-2458-9-S1-S5.

Gertler, P. (2004). Do conditional cash transfers improve child health? Evidence from Progresa's control randomized experiment. *American Economic Review* **94**(2): 332–41.

Gertler, P., Shah, M. and Bertozzi, S. M. (2005). Risky business: the market for unprotected sex. *Journal of Political Economy* **113**: 518–50.

Guinness, L., Kumaranayake, L., Rajaraman, B., Sankaranarayanan, G., Vannela, G., Raghupathi, P. and George, A. (2005). Does scale matter? The costs of HIV-prevention interventions for commercial sex workers in India. *Bulletin of the World Health Organization* **83**: 747–55.

Kumaranayake, L. (2008). The economics of scaling up: cost estimation for HIV/AIDS interventions. *AIDS* **22** (Suppl. 1): S23–S33.

Marseille, E., Dandona, L., Marshall, N. *et al.* (2007). HIV prevention costs and program scale: data from the PANCEA project in five low and middle-income countries. *BMC Health Services Research* **7**: 108.

Osoro, N., Mpango, P. and Mwinyimvua, H. (2001). *An Analysis of Excise Taxation in Tanzania.* African Economic Policy Discussion Paper No. 72, September 2001.

Over, M. (1986). The effect of scale on cost projections for a primary health care program in a developing country. *Social Science and Medicine* **22**(3): 351–60.

Paxson, C. and Schady, N. (2008). *Does Money Matter? The Effects of Cash Transfers on Child Health and Development in Rural Ecuador.* World Bank Policy Research Working Paper 4226.

Pierani, P. and Tiezzi, S. (2009). Addiction and interaction between alcohol and tobacco consumption. *Empirical Economics* **37**: 1–23.

Preyra, C. and Pink, C. (2006). Scale and scope efficiencies through hospital consolidations. *Journal of Health Economics* **25**: 1049–68.

Rao, V., Gupta, I., Lokshin, M. and Jana, S. (2003). Sex workers and the cost of safe sex: the compensating differential for condom use among Calcutta prostitutes. *Journal of Development Economics* **71**: 585–603.

The Global HIV/AIDS Program. (2008). *West Africa HIV/AIDS Epidemiology and Response Synthesis: Implications for Prevention.* World Bank Report.

Vassall, A., Remme, M. and Watts, C. (2011). Social Policy. Assessment paper: *RethinkHIV.*

Walker, D. (2003). Cost and cost-effectiveness of HIV/AIDS prevention strategies in developing countries: is there an evidence base? *Health Policy and Planning* **18**: 4–17.

Vaccine research and development

Assessment paper

ROBERT HECHT AND DEAN T. JAMISON, WITH
JARED AUGENSTEIN, GABRIELLE PARTRIDGE,
AND KIRA THORIEN

Thirty years have passed since the recognition of the infectious disease now named acquired immune deficiency syndrome (AIDS). In that relatively short time AIDS has killed over 30 million individuals, and an additional 33.3 million people are now living with the infection. Africa shoulders the burden of the epidemic: UNAIDS estimates that in 2009 1.3 million people died from AIDS in Africa, 22.5 million were living with HIV, and a further 1.5 million acquired the infection during the year. Even though prevention and treatment programs are expanding, the epidemic is holding its ground. Only two out of every five people requiring antiretroviral therapy currently have access to treatment – and this number is threatened by financial pressures of the global recession. Though universal access to treatment is a morally compelling goal, the high costs associated with treatment argue for a strategy that emphasizes prevention.

An AIDS vaccine[1] is the ultimate goal of prevention – vaccination would provide a manageable and affordable way to confer protection against HIV infection. When fully developed and licensed, an AIDS vaccine could have a powerful and immediate impact; the International AIDS Vaccine Initiative (IAVI) estimates that an AIDS vaccine of 50 percent efficacy given to just 30 percent of the population could reduce the number of new infections in the developing world by 24 percent in fifteen years (IAVI 2009a). Yet AIDS vaccine development is proving to be enormously expensive. Is the perhaps $15–20 billion of additional resources that it may cost the world to develop an AIDS vaccine worth it?

Other *RethinkHIV* papers assess the benefits of further application of available technologies for controlling AIDS in Africa, and weigh these benefits against the costs. This paper addresses the potential returns to expanding the technological base through the development, manufacture and utilization of a vaccine to prevent HIV infection. The paper does not argue for investment in vaccine development at the expense of ongoing HIV prevention or treatment interventions. Rather, its main purpose is to evaluate the extent to which maintaining and slightly expanding investment in AIDS vaccine development would have high

The authors thank each of the following reviewers for their helpful comments and insight: Kasper Anderskov, Dr Steven Forsythe, Dr Stephen Resch, and Dr Joshua Salomon. John Stover of the Futures Institute provided critical assistance with data and advice. We also thank participants in the June 2011 *RethinkHIV* preliminary review meeting, which was hosted by the Department of Global Health, University of Washington. Each of the meeting participants and fellow paper authors provided helpful comments which contributed to the shaping of this paper. We held phone conversations with three scientists actively working on development of an AIDS vaccine to get their sense of the likelihood of success, obstacles to success, probable timing of licensing and probable operating characteristics of possible AIDS vaccines. We very much appreciate the time afforded us by Dr Wayne Koff (International AIDS Vaccine Initiative), Dr Gary Nabel (NIH) and Dr Bruce Walker (Harvard University). While acknowledging with gratitude the advice we have received, we alone take responsibility for interpretations (and potential errors) in the paper.

[1] We use the term "AIDS vaccine" to denote the probable set of vaccines that could emerge from ongoing development efforts. Hypothetical values of vaccine cost and efficacy in this paper are for the best (mix) to emerge over time, and in a more extended assessment the sensitivity of the cost-benefit results presented in this paper to these parameters would be evaluated. We limit our discussion in this paper to vaccines that prevent infection, but it is important to note that efforts are also under way to develop vaccines that strengthen the immune system's response to established disease. Recent animal trials have generated hope for the prospects of this type of vaccine (Maurice 2011).

benefit relative to cost – and hence justify continuing the high rate of product development expenditures.

The secondary purpose of this paper is to address the question of whether spending more to advance the time of availability of a vaccine would be worth the associated cost. We explore the implications of assuming that a $100 million per year increase in the level of investment would advance vaccine availability by either about 0.4 years or 1 year. It is clear that even rough estimates of time sensitivity are speculative. It further appears improbable – according to experts – that increasing current rates of expenditure could speed the progress of a single vaccine candidate through trials. The question, instead, is whether additional expenditures could constructively broaden the portfolio of candidates being developed. This seems plausible, but is subject to debate. What our results show is that even very modest decreases in the time to product availability would have high benefits.

The current and likely future sources of funding for vaccine development are parts of the public sector that differ from those that fund AIDS control. Private sector product development funds likewise do not come at the cost of control money. Only in foundations is there likely to be genuine fungibility between product development resources and control resources. In this environment, the *RethinkHIV* role is thus justifiably not one of trading off vaccine development resources with resources for attractive control options. Rather, a conclusion that the economic attractiveness of a continued vaccine development effort is high relative to control would be *signaled* by perhaps modest allocation of control resources to vaccine development by the *RethinkHIV* Panel. That new products such as potential AIDS vaccines constitute international public goods – unlikely to be domestically financed by developing countries – is an additional factor relevant to judgments of the *RethinkHIV* Panel. This paper aims to help inform these judgments.

We begin by pointing to the great successes to date of R&D efforts on AIDS and to the range of potentially attractive areas for further scientific investment. We next discuss ongoing efforts and potential for developing an AIDS vaccine. The final main section turns to our benefit:cost assessment by sketching several alternative scenarios for the evolution of the AIDS epidemic; these scenarios constitute the "status quos" that determine the attractiveness of an AIDS vaccine investment. While we emphasize benefits to Africa, we also discuss the larger global context. As a first approximation, given the scale of the global AIDS pandemic, one can think of global benefits as being roughly 150 percent of benefits in sub-Saharan Africa.

AIDS R&D: accomplishments and the future agenda

The world's scientific establishment has committed extraordinary resources and talent to understanding all aspects of HIV/AIDS, and to creating a range of products and algorithms for dealing with it. This section begins by reviewing scientific progress, and then turns to an outlined agenda for further R&D. It concludes with a brief overview of the history, including cost history, of AIDS vaccine development efforts, in order to set the stage for the subsequent benefit:cost assessment.

Accomplishments of AIDS R&D to date

The enormous accomplishments of the AIDS R&D community to date include the following:

- Demonstration that a hitherto unidentified retrovirus (Human Immunodeficiency Virus, or HIV) causes AIDS and that the principal routes of transmission are sexual.
- Development of diagnostic tests for antibodies to AIDS, and for extent of disease progression.
- Development of drugs to control the level of HIV in the body. These drugs, like the diagnostics, have become ever cheaper and now include a single pill coformulation for daily use. Clinical researchers have evolved more effective ways of combining drugs to slow the progression of resistance, encouraging adherence and managing opportunistic infections.
- Identification of a broad range of potential methods to reduce the probability of infection for a given level of exposure – these methods

include treatment of other sexually transmitted infections, male circumcision, treatment of HIV-positive individuals to reduce viral load and hence probability of infecting someone else, and pre- and post-exposure prophylaxis of HIV-negative individuals to increase the probability that they remain that way.

- Generation of substantial knowledge of the epidemiology of AIDS and of what works (and fails to work) in terms of control measures (Aral and Holmes 2008).

It is worth highlighting several of the more important results from recent clinical trials on new prevention tools that could have a significant impact on slowing the epidemic. These results also show that progress in R&D continues today, with potential for further gains in other areas such as a vaccine. Male circumcision and pre-exposure prophylaxis are two such advancements. Studies suggest that male circumcision has a strong impact on heterosexual transmission of HIV, reducing men's risk of acquiring HIV as much as 60 percent (Auvert *et al.* 2005; Bailey *et al.* 2007; UNAIDS 2010). Though male circumcision does not benefit women directly, it gradually reduces HIV incidence and therefore the risk of a woman having an HIV-positive partner. Use of oral and topical anti-retrovirals may also act as effective prevention – studies suggest that oral pre-exposure prophylaxis may reduce HIV acquisition and transmission among men and transgendered women by as much as 42 percent (UNAIDS 2011). Similarly, a new microbicide currently in clinical trials was found to reduce new infections in women by 39 percent (Karim *et al.* 2010). These interventions, when combined, may prove to be powerful tools in the fight against AIDS – tools that an eventual vaccine will complement but is unlikely to replace.

These advances in knowledge have enabled a marked slowing of the epidemic. In high-income parts of the world, resources have flowed to implement the products of this knowledge with good (but far from complete) results. In Africa, substantial resources have begun to flow only recently, but, again, with encouraging effects. In high prevalence countries, infection rates have dropped about a quarter from their earlier peak levels. As a result

of the reduction in new infections, prevalence in Zimbabwe dropped from 26 percent to 14 percent between 1997 and 2009 (UNAIDS 2010b). And according to UNAIDS, Zimbabwe is only one of the 22 countries that have reduced the rate of new infections by more than a quarter between 2001 and 2009.

Yet while the current base of science and resource commitment has succeeded in slowing the epidemic, huge problems remain. The fact that 1.8 million persons in Africa were newly infected with HIV in 2009, roughly double the number that started treatment in that year, is a testimony to the large remaining gaps and challenges.

Elements of the agenda for future research

The ingenuity of the scientific community has ensured that there is a range of potentially attractive investment areas for increasing the base of knowledge and scope of other new products for controlling AIDS. The productivity of AIDS-related science in recent decades suggests the possibility that continuing with such investments will have high pay-off, and underscores the importance of continuing to spend vigorously on AIDS R&D over the coming decade. To provide a suggestive overview of potential directions for AIDS research and development, we indicate a number of broad areas of promise below. This provides the context for our more detailed discussion of AIDS vaccine development.

On the product development side there are two very high pay-off items:

1. an AIDS vaccine; and
2. a drug to clear the body of HIV.[2]

There are several classes of other product development efforts possible:

3. less expensive, more effective, and safer ARVs;
4. better therapies for treating or preventing opportunistic infections;

---

[2] Leading AIDS research and development experts suggest that item 2, a drug to clear the body of HIV, has a low probability of success in the next 25 years. That said, research is being and should continue to be undertaken to develop such a drug.

5. better diagnostics; and
6. better barrier devices for transmission interruption.

Finally there is development, testing, and evaluation of new operational protocols, e.g.:

7. treatment as prevention protocols;
8. pre-exposure prophylaxis protocols;
9. improved counseling and testing protocols;
10. improved clinical management protocols (earlier initiation of treatment, or of higher quality drugs); and
11. mechanisms for lowering the financial and time costs to patients of access to prevention or treatment services.

As evidenced by the list above, the R&D agenda is broad, promising, and highly significant. Most of the R&D investments listed involve incremental, rather than quantum, breakthroughs in terms of additional benefits from infections averted or healthy life years gained via improved therapeutics and thus longer survival for HIV-positive individuals. These incremental gains are likely to outweigh the additional investment and delivery costs involved, and may thus be quite attractive. We would urge more benefit-cost analysis to inform priorities on investments among them. We have not attempted such analysis in this paper, in part because of time constraints, and in part because the magnitude of the impact on the AIDS epidemic from these other technological gains would not be as large as in the case of a successful vaccine.

We focus on vaccine development partially to make the topic tractable and partially because a vaccine is the holy grail of disease control efforts, potentially conferring enormous health benefits at relatively low implementation cost. Although the analysis that follows looks only at benefits and costs of vaccine development, we are *not* arguing for vaccine development expenditures at the expense of other AIDS-related R&D. Indeed our conclusion that vaccine investments have high benefit:cost ratios despite their attendant uncertainty leads us to feel that R&D investments more generally are likely to have high pay-off. Financing should be found in transfer from currently low-yield parts of development assistance budgets.

To have an effective HIV/AIDS vaccine available for introduction by 2030 could cost as much as twenty times the $1 billion typically required to develop a new drug (Adams *et al.* 2010). This expensive development cost makes a benefit-cost analysis of AIDS vaccine relevant, particularly in the face of other competing priorities and options to control AIDS. This note is intended to suggest, in broad strokes and by example, where such an analysis might lead.

AIDS vaccine development: history and prospects

The world has spent approximately $9 billion dollars to date toward development of an AIDS vaccine, and the recent rate of expenditure is on the order of $800–900 million per year, slightly lower than the peak rate of expenditure in 2007 of just over a billion dollars (Table 6.1). A published estimate for 2010 (Resource Tracking Working Group 2011) suggests continuation in 2010 at about the same rate of expenditure as 2008 and 2009, i.e., $859 million. R&D spending on vaginal microbicides in 2010 was also substantial, about $247 million. R&D on adult male circumcision and treatment as prevention were funded at about $20 million each.

The search for the AIDS vaccine has had both success and setbacks. The failed Merck vaccine of 2007, which used an engineered adenovirus to deliver select HIV genetic material and seemed promising until the trial was terminated for failing to show efficacy, was a great disappointment to the international community.

By contrast, 2009 was a year of encouraging developments in AIDS vaccine research (Maurice 2011). These included the discovery of new broadly neutralizing antibodies, which recognize a broad range of HIV variants, bind to the surface of the virus so that it cannot infect other cells, and are highly potent. Furthermore, the antibodies target the virus's weakness – a location on the surface of the virus that does not mutate as the rapidly changing virus takes on new forms. These broadly neutralizing antibodies offer a new route of attack for scientists seeking an AIDS vaccine – one that may be successful in the near future (IAVI 2011).

Table 6.1 Annual investment in HIV vaccine R&D, 2000–2009 (US millions, expressed in 2010 dollars)

	2000	2001	2002	2003	2004	2005	2006	2007	2008	2009	2000–2009 total
Public-sector											
US	344	386	455	548	595	640	707	707	627	659	5,668
Europe	29	39	47	52	65	77	88	88	69	66	620
Other	12	14	25	25	32	30	41	51	41	31	302
Multilateral	2	2	2	2	2	2	2	2	2	1	19
Total public	387	441	529	627	694	749	838	848	739	757	6,609
Philanthropic sector	25	8	135	17	13	13	88	92	105	93	589
Commercial sector	...	...	...	...	78	83	85	92	33	30	401
Total global investment	412	449	664	644	785	845	1,011	1,032	877	880	7,599

Source: Resource Tracking Working Group (2010).

Also in 2009, the Thai RV144 vaccine proved 30 percent effective against heterosexual HIV transmission in Phase III clinical trials. Albeit only moderately effective, the vaccine offers encouragement and opportunity for further study. Additional trials will be conducted on the vaccine's ability to protect against HIV infection among high-risk populations. The Appendix to this paper provides an overview of recent and ongoing research and trials (IAVI 2010).

Despite this progress, the world remains perhaps twenty years away from having an effective, licensed vaccine and attendant capacity for mass production. Interviews with a selection of leading AIDS vaccine scientists[3] conducted specifically for this *RethinkHIV* process suggest that a prototype vaccine with moderately good levels of protection against acquiring infection (50 percent or greater) could achieve proof of efficacy (Phase IIb) by 2020–2025. After this, the prototype could be licensed, scaled for manufacturing, and available for large-volume introduction within a further five years, i.e., by 2025–2030. While this may seem a long way into the future, the potential benefits of having such a vaccine are so large that a compellingly high rate of return may still be achievable. Calculating such a rate of return is the task we have set for ourselves in this paper.

Blockbuster drugs (e.g., some of the statins for high cholesterol and drugs for arthritis and other pain medications) generate revenues of several billion dollars a year for many years. For these drugs

the benefit-cost ratio to the company, for that drug considered by itself, can easily exceed 10:1 in net present value terms. Revenues from vaccine sales, however, have rarely reached the blockbuster level, even though the recently launched vaccines against childhood pneumonia, rotavirus diarrhea, and cervical cancer are beginning to generate annual sales for manufacturers that approach or exceed a billion dollars a year.

Would an AIDS vaccine have benefits on the order of those accruing to blockbuster drugs? This would be necessary to justify its extraordinarily high development costs. By "benefits" we refer, in this case, not to the present value of a revenue stream potentially accruing from vaccine sales – though an AIDS vaccine would enjoy commercial sales in rich-country markets – but to the present value of benefits to society, expressed in monetary terms or HIV infections averted. Averted HIV infections generate a number of benefits, including increased life expectancy, averted ART and other healthcare costs, and increased productivity and other social gains from obtaining core healthy adult years.

This paper now turns to a simple example of an approach to answering the question: excluding the past investments on AIDS vaccine development (totaling about $8 billion), but assuming continued expenditure at about the current rate of

---

[3] Interviews were conducted with leading AIDS vaccine scientists named in our acknowledgements.

$900 million/year would lead to a successful product, would the additional $18 billion or more spent have been worth it, particularly given the state of the epidemic at the time of introduction? Further, if additional resources could advance the time of availability of a vaccine, how valuable would that be?

Cost-benefit analysis of AIDS vaccine development

The value of an AIDS vaccine will depend on the future state of the epidemic, available prevention and treatment options, the projected rate of uptake of the AIDS vaccine in groups at risk, and the characteristics of the vaccine itself.

For the purposes of our paper, we make a number of important assumptions about the characteristics of the AIDS vaccine. As stated previously, these assumptions are based on interviews conducted with expert AIDS scientists and researchers. First, we assume that the vaccine is 50 percent effective by 2030. This is a conservative estimate – experts suggest a more efficacious vaccine will be available by at least 2040, if not 2030. Second, we assign cost values of both $60 and $150 for full individual immunization. Experts suggest that a first generation vaccine will likely require several booster shots and these two cost estimates, one more realistic and the other conservative, seek to account for the range of possible vaccine characteristics (IAVI 2007). Lastly, we assume that the vaccine is given to the general population, targeting men and women ages ten through forty-nine.

Our approach is to assess the value of this vaccine if introduced in 2030, under three alternative scenarios. The following three scenarios project what the AIDS epidemic may look like in the world in 2030, dependent on the state of AIDS prevention and treatment, political will, and science and technology. All benefit-cost analyses are incremental to an indicated status quo, and these three scenarios provide alternative visions for the status quo at the likely time of vaccine availability. After establishing these scenarios, following subsections discuss costs, benefits, and probable benefit to cost ratios.

Alternative scenarios for the AIDS epidemic in 2030

Scenario I: an effective curative drug has become available

The drug would be simple to use, is assumed to already have cured half of the then prevalent HIV infections, and is on track to cure the rest within a decade at most. The epidemic is all but over. The added benefit of a vaccine would in this case be minimal, even though very large costs will have been incurred to produce such a vaccine.

Scenarios II and III below are ones in which there will be major pay-off to an AIDS vaccine. The scenarios are drawn directly from work of the aids2031 Financing Task Force – see aids2031 (2010a) and Hecht *et al.* (2010). The outcomes of these scenarios stress the substantial uncertainty in projections like these. The numbers nonetheless provide reasonable first approximations.

Scenario II: rapid scale-up

Political will to achieve universal access is strong and resource availability continues to grow rapidly. The focus is on scaling up direct approaches to preventing HIV transmission and providing care and support. All countries achieve universal access (defined as 80 percent coverage) to all key prevention and treatment interventions, and remain at those levels through to 2031. This rapid scale-up has a great benefit for sub-Saharan Africa; by 2030, 9.8 million of the 21.9 million HIV-positives in sub-Saharan Africa (SSA) are being effectively managed at a total cost of $500 per year per patient. Incidence of HIV infection is 1.1 million new cases per year in SSA, reflecting moderate success with concomitant preventive interventions, including newly available ones such as those discussed earlier in this paper. In 2030 there would be around 1.0 million AIDS deaths per year in SSA.

Scenario III: current trends

This scenario assumes that current trends in the AIDS epidemic will prevail for the next five years, based on moderate political support and a slight increase in funding that flattens out in 2015. Coverage of key interventions continues to expand

Table 6.2 Two scenarios for 2030 in sub-Saharan Africa (and globally) – numbers in millions

Scenario	Number of HIV+ individuals	Number of new infections per year	Number of AIDS deaths per year	Number of people on ART
Scenario II (rapid scale-up)	21.9 (32.9)	1.1 (1.6)	1.0 (1.4)	9.8 (12.4)
Scenario III (current trends)	25.7 (38.6)	1.9 (2.6)	1.5 (2.0)	7.6 (10.1)

Note: Global numbers appear in parentheses after the African numbers.

to 2015 as it has in the past years. Some countries achieve universal access to some services, but not others. All interventions reach approximately two-thirds of universal access by 2015, and remain at those levels until 2031. In Scenario III, there are 25.7 million HIV-positives in sub-Saharan Africa, but only 7.6 million people are on drugs effectively controlling viral load at $500 per year per patient. Incidence of HIV infection is 1.9 million/year, higher than where it is today. In 2030 this would entail 1.5 million HIV deaths per year, and this number would be growing.

Table 6.2 summarizes the two scenarios in which AIDS is a continuing problem and provides Africa-specific as well as global estimates of the numbers.

What, then, would be the value of having an AIDS vaccine (i.e., a vaccine to prevent infection) become available in 2030? The value depends on the scenario.

In Scenario I (perfect cure available), there would be minimal value to having a vaccine. In Scenario II (rapid scale-up), a sufficiently inexpensive and easy to use vaccine would both save on ARV (drug) and treatment costs for opportunistic infections, and save many years of healthy life as compared to the situation without such a vaccine (that is, healthy years for the minority who become infected and do not obtain treatment, plus the extra healthy years for the majority who do benefit from treatment but still die somewhat earlier than those who are not HIV infected). In Scenario III (current trends) the vaccine would pay off handsomely, mostly by saving large numbers of lives of individuals who would die quite prematurely because of infection and lack of access to ARV treatment. Under this more pessimistic scenario, the vaccine would pay off dramatically, particularly in sub-Saharan Africa. It would be a powerful health impact tool, with the ability to fight the epidemic and save many numbers of

lives and potentially even generate wider benefits by preserving the social fabric in high prevalence country settings.

For the sake of discussion we assign probabilities to these scenarios for 2030 as shown below. We have given the lowest probability to Scenario I, given the scientific challenges of developing a drug that clears the HIV virus completely once established in the body and integrated into the genome of bone marrow cells. We give nearly equal probabilities to Scenarios II and III to reflect the recent efforts to sustain political support and domestic and external funding for the AIDS programs in Africa and other low and middle income countries, with a slightly higher chance assigned to the more optimistic picture in which there are expanded resources for mainstream prevention and treatment.

Scenario I: 0.10
Scenario II: 0.50
Scenario III: 0.40

The paragraphs below sketch out our preliminary benefit-cost analysis (BCA) for such AIDS vaccine development. The discussion is structured around the scenarios just described. We model the costs and benefits 24 years after vaccine introduction. For introduction in 2030, our most probable case, we model the costs and benefits until the end of 2054. For our more pessimistic case, vaccination in 2040, we model the costs and benefits until the year 2064.

The cost of an AIDS vaccine

We take 2011 as the base year for calculation of present values of future (and past) expenditures. We apply discount rates of 3 percent and 5 percent per year to calculate present values, as suggested by *RethinkHIV* (and, for reference, we also use a 0 rate of discounting). As indicated above, we note the value of all AIDS vaccine development expenditures over the period 2000–2009 to be $8.7 billion, and assume $900 million was expended in 2010.[4] An increment of $900 million per year over the 19 year period 2011 to 2030 would add $17.1 billion in total, or roughly $13.9 billion discounted at 3 percent.

For purposes of this paper we assume that the additional $17.1 billion in development effort results in an efficacious vaccine that is licensed and ready for large-scale manufacturing by 2030. For our analysis, we run calculations using both a minimum of $60 and a maximum of $150 per full vaccination. These values are intended to account for the cost of the marginal cost of production (so-called "cost of goods" for vaccine companies), production profit margin, packaging, distribution, and administration. As IAVI suggests, we assume that this first generation vaccine will require three doses throughout a person's lifetime. The lower $60 cost per full course is consistent with studies on HIV vaccine demand, as well as past vaccine development costs (IAVI 2007). The upper bound of $150 per course is arguably high, and is likely to be much lower, as both the private and public sector are expected to intervene to reduce cost and improve affordability. Yet the first generation vaccine may be complex to produce and deliver, and the costs may be higher. To remain conservative, analyze the full range of possibilities, and account for uncertainty, we chose to include the higher estimate.

These conservative estimates attempt to make up, in part, for the other obstacles which are more difficult to quantify, such as liability. Vaccine development faces a number of challenges, even beyond science – the liability of the vaccine and uncertainty of the investment are two factors which factor into the total development cost of the vaccine.

The benefits of preventing 1,000 HIV infections

What about benefits? Bloom, Canning, and Jamison (2004) provide an overview of measuring the economic impact of better health. This literature, drawing on the early work of Schelling (1968) and Usher (1973), was at one point controversial but is increas-

Table 6.3 Costs of AIDS vaccine program for sub-Saharan Africa ($ billions)

Panel A: total vaccine cost $60				
	Present value of costs if AIDS vaccine becomes available in:			
Discount rate, per year	2030		2040	
	Development	Delivery	Development	Delivery
0	$17.1	$87.6	$26.1	$100.5
3%	$13.9	$39.3	$18.3	$33.8
5%	$11.9	$23.8	$14.7	$17.0
Panel B: total vaccine cost $150				
	Present value of costs if AIDS vaccine becomes available in:			
Discount rate, per year	2030		2040	
	Development	Delivery	Development	Delivery
0	$17.1	$218.8	$26.1	$251.3
3%	$13.9	$98.1	$18.3	$84.5
5%	$11.9	$59.3	$14.7	$42.3

ingly accepted – give or take a factor of 2 – by economists. McGreevey *et al.* (2004) also suggest using this literature for evaluation of AIDS vaccine development. This line of work can be summarized by saying that evidence on actual willingness to pay to avoid risk of death suggests that the value of averting a death is on the order of 100 to 200 times GDP per person (Viscusi and Aldy 2003). The point estimate is around 135 for low and middle income countries.[5] The World Bank estimates an average per capita income in sub-Saharan Africa of $1,127 in 2009 (World Bank WDI Online), a reasonable number for us to use for this exercise. Multiplying this by 135 gives a defensible estimate of the value of averting a death in SSA of about $150,000. This is an estimate derived, albeit circuitously, from what people in those countries themselves appear willing to pay to alter their annual risk of death.

It is worth noting that the above estimates do not in any direct way deal with the value of

---

[4] An estimate of $859 million was published as we completed this paper (Resource Tracking Group 2011).
[5] Alternatively the value of an extra year of life is about two to four times per capita GDP. The main point about the two to four range is that it definitely excludes one.

averting an AIDS death, much less of the value to an individual of receiving an effective AIDS vaccine. Estimates of the value of an AIDS vaccine derived, as above, from the value of life literature should therefore be viewed as indirect. More direct estimates do exist in empirical studies by Ainsworth, Whittington, and their colleagues (Whittington *et al.* 2002; Bishai *et al.* 2004; Suratdecha *et al.* 2005) of stated willingness to pay for an AIDS vaccine, if one existed, in communities in Mexico, Thailand, and Uganda. The congruence of studies of the willingness to pay for a vaccine with the value of life studies needs to be explored.

Based on the above theories, one could assume a figure of $150,000 for an AIDS death averted or, more or less the same, a value of $3,800 for avoiding the loss of a year of life from AIDS. For consistency we adopted values of $1,000 and $5,000 per life year according to *RethinkHIV* guidelines.

In our calculations, we assume that the vaccine's benefits would broadly lie in the reduction of expenditure on ARVs, OI (opportunistic infection) treatment costs averted, and healthy life years saved. The sum of these three simplified vaccine benefits depends on the state of the epidemic at the time of vaccine introduction. The different scenarios sketched above, Scenarios II and III, differ in the extent to which vaccine benefits accrue to deaths averted or to treatment costs avoided.

As discussed above, the first step to quantifying benefits of averted HIV infections is to find the value of life years gained. We make a number of important assumptions in our calculations. First, we assume that the average infection occurs at twenty-five years of age, as evidenced by a study recently conducted in Uganda (Mills *et al.* 2011). Second, we assume that an HIV-positive individual on anti-retroviral therapy lives twenty-five years after infection. This contrasts to an HIV-negative person of the same age, who roughly lives about forty additional years. Lastly, we assume that an HIV-positive person not receiving treatment will live roughly eleven years post-infection (ALPHA Network 2011).

Following these assumptions, we assign values of $1,000 or $5,000 per statistical life year, per

RethinkHIV guidelines. For example, the value of life years gained under Scenario II would be, for the people successfully treated with ARVs, fifteen years per person (40 − 25). For the untreated people the gain would be twenty-nine years each (40 − 11). Valuing these life years at $1,000 (or $5,000) each and discounting back to the present gives the present value per life years saved. It is worth noting that the benefits derived from vaccination will occur far into the future, when the value of life may be higher than it is today. If current predictions for an accelerated growth path (and associated GDP growth) in sub-Saharan Africa hold true, the value of life in the future could arguably be much higher than the present value. Given this growth, our calculated benefits are likely conservative.

The other primary benefit of averting an HIV infection is the averted health care cost. This includes both averted ART costs and averted (or diminished) OI treatment costs. These costs are significant and together account for a large portion of the benefits incurred from vaccination. For purposes of our analysis, we assume a constant $500/per patient per year cost for anti-retroviral therapy. While ART costs in sub-Saharan Africa range from $500 to $1,000 per patient per year,[6] for the purposes of our study we assume the lower bound. Since we are conservative in assuming $500 in ART treatment per person per year, we assume that this cost estimate remains constant through to 2030 and 2040.

Opportunistic infections include a range of skin infections, severe pneumonia and diarrhea, and various exotic and dangerous forms of cancer, all of which can be expensive to treat. If all HIV-positives were effectively treated with ARVs, the treatment costs for opportunistic infections would greatly diminish, at least until the point of treatment failure. To remain conservative in our analysis, we assume that all patients on ARVs do not have OI treatment costs – only the minority of people with HIV who do not have access to treatment incur these costs.

---

[6] This range on average ART costs was supplied by *RethinkHIV*. It is reflective of the work produced by other paper authors participating in this exercise.

Table 6.4 Benefits of averting 1,000 infections: estimates by year and scenario (in $ millions)

Panel A.1: Scenario II (rapid scale-up); vaccine introduction in 2030			
Benefits incurred in year:	Value of life years gained (VSLY= $1,000)	Value of life years gained (VSLY= $5,000)	OI treatment costs averted	ART treatment costs averted
2030	10.2	51.2	0.4	2.5
2042	7.2	35.9	0.3	1.8
2054	5.0	25.2	0.2	1.2

Panel A.2: Scenario II (rapid scale-up); vaccine introduction in 2040			
Benefits incurred in year:	Value of life years gained (VSLY= $1,000)	Value of life years gained (VSLY= $5,000)	OI treatment costs averted	ART treatment costs averted
2040	7.5	37.3	0.3	2.0
2052	5.2	26.1	0.2	1.4
2064	3.7	18.3	0.1	0.9

Panel B.1: Scenario III (current trends); vaccine introduction in 2030			
Benefits incurred in year:	Value of life years gained (VSLY= $1,000)	Value of life years gained (VSLY= $5,000)	OI treatment costs averted	ART treatment costs averted
2030	11.2	56	0.1	1.7
2042	7.9	39.3	0.2	1.2
2054	5.5	27.5	0.3	0.8

Panel B.2: Scenario III (current trends); vaccine introduction in 2040			
Benefits incurred in year:	Value of life years gained (VSLY= $1,000)	Value of life years gained (VSLY= $5,000)	OI treatment costs averted	ART treatment costs averted
2040	8.3	41.4	0.2	1.3
2052	5.8	29.0	0.1	0.9
2064	4.1	20.3	0.7	0.6

Note: Values above are given at a 3% discount rate.

Using these assumptions, Table 6.4 shows the benefits from averting 1,000 HIV infections in Scenarios II and III in a given year. The value of averting 1,000 infections is dependent upon the charac-

teristics of the year, and thus the value of averting 1,000 infections changes by the year. In Table 6.4, we offer snapshots of the first year of vaccine introduction (2030 or 2040); the median year (2042 or 2052); and the final year modeled (2054 or 2064).

As evidenced by Table 6.4, the benefits remain significant despite the 10-year lag between vaccine introduction in 2030 and 2040. The greatest benefit in averted ART drug costs occurs under Scenario II (rapid scale-up), at $2.6 billion dollars in treatment costs averted for 1,000 infections in 2030 alone. Although Scenario III (current trends) does not avert such a great number of treatment costs, it saves many healthy life years.

Table 6.5 shows the cumulative number of vaccines administered and infections averted. These numbers are dependent upon the vaccine characteristics and state of the epidemic, as previously explained. Though the numbers differ slightly depending upon the year of introduction, approximately 1.4–1.6 billion people receive the vaccine, and as a result, 7 to 16 million people avert infections.

Table 6.6 shows the cumulative benefits to introducing the vaccine in both 2030 and 2040. Panel A details the benefits of vaccination in Scenario II, while Panel B details the benefits of vaccination under Scenario III. For sensitivity analysis, discount rates of 0, 3 percent, and 5 percent are used, as well as a value per statistical life ranging from $1,000 to $5,000 per year.

Benefit-cost calculations

1. Continued investment

How would the cost of the vaccine play out against its ultimate benefit of preventing infections? Assuming the vast majority of infections will occur through adolescence and adulthood, vaccination will likely occur at preadolescence, approximately at age ten. We took the estimated population of sub-Saharan Africa between the ages of 10–49 (842 million people) as our initial cohort to be immunized over ten years at 80 percent coverage (a base cohort of approximately 674 million). In addition we aim for 80 percent coverage of the continent's annual "turning-10" cohort, estimated to be 35 million

Table 6.5 Vaccine beneficiaries and infections averted (in a 25-year period after vaccine becomes available) in millions

| | AIDS vaccine becomes available in | | | |
| | 2030 | | 2040 | |
Scenario	Beneficiaries	Infections averted	Beneficiaries	Infections averted
II	1,460	8.0	1,660	7.1
III	1,460	16.0	1,660	15.9

in 2030. If it were to take ten years to immunize 80 percent of the base cohort, then the number immunized in fifteen years would be 1.2 billion (= 35.2 million (base cohort) + 35.2 million (annual birth cohort) multiplied by 15, plus 674 million "catch-up" individuals aged ten to forty-nine at the time of the first immunization).

The next step is to calculate benefit-cost ratios of the entire AIDS vaccine program through 2065, including the discounted development costs. Table 6.4 shows the costs under each scenario, and Table 6.5 shows the benefits modeled through to 2054 and 2064 (twenty-five years past vaccine introduction) with the vaccine assumed to be introduced in both 2030 (as suggested by experts) and 2040 (to remain conservative). All of the benefits and costs are presented with the assigned *RethinkHIV* discount rates.

Given the probabilities for the scenarios, and the numbers in Tables 6.4 and 6.5 that were hypothesized earlier, it is reasonable to expect a net present value (NPV) for the program of the order of $2 trillion and the benefit-cost ratio to range from approximately 2 to 67, depending on the cost of the vaccine, the value of a statistical life year (VSLY), the discount rate, and the scenario for the epidemic. Table 6.7 summarizes the benefit to cost ratios through each of the scenarios. Though there is a significant range in these ratios, it is evident that the investment is cost-effective, even in the most conservative and pessimistic scenarios. The ratios in Table 6.7 weigh the benefits of an eventual vaccine against all development costs from the present on. We also address the question of the value of having a vaccine sooner: what would it be worth in terms of higher vaccine development costs to have a vaccine in 2030 rather than

Table 6.6 Total benefit of AIDS vaccine introduction in Africa ($ billion)

| Panel A: Scenario II (rapid scale-up) | | | |
| | | AIDS vaccine becomes available in | |
Value of statistical life year (VSLY)	Discount rate, per year	2030 Total benefit	2040 Total benefit
$1,000	0	$1,300	$1,100
	3%	$473	$303
	5%	$247	$131
$5,000	0	$6,000	$4,600
	3%	$1,900	$1,200
	5%	$1,000	$530

| Panel B: Scenario III (current trends) | | | |
| | | AIDS vaccine becomes available in | |
Value of statistical life year (VSLY)	Discount rate, per year	2030 Total benefit	2040 Total benefit
$1,000	0	$2,300	$2,200
	3%	$812	$565
	5%	$426	$245
$5,000	0	$10,000	$9,400
	3%	$3,500	$2,500
	5%	$1,900	$1,100

2040? Table 6.6 provides answers to this question under a range of assumptions. In no case would the present value of that benefit be less than $115 billion. This provides the basis for a (tentative) evaluation of the attractiveness of additional expenditures directed toward advancing the time of vaccine availability.

2. Accelerating vaccine development

What would be the consequences if we could scale up funding and reduce the amount of time it takes

Table 6.7 Benefit-cost ratios for AIDS vaccine development

		Panel A: total vaccine cost $60							
		B:C if AIDS vaccine becomes available in							
		2030				2040			
Value of statistical life year (VSLY)	Discount rate, per year	Scenario				Scenario			
		I	II	III	Weighted	I	II	III	Weighted
$1,000	0	0.0	12.8	22.4	15.4	0.0	9.0	17.1	11.3
	3%	0.0	8.9	15.3	10.6	0.0	5.8	10.8	7.2
	5%	0.0	6.9	11.9	8.2	0.0	4.2	7.6	5.1
$5,000	0	0.0	52.4	97.3	65.1	0.0	36.4	74.0	47.8
	3%	0.0	36.4	67.3	45.1	0.0	23.5	47.5	30.8
	5%	0.0	28.4	52.5	35.2	0.0	16.8	33.9	22.0
		Panel B: total vaccine cost $150							
		B:C if AIDS vaccine becomes available in							
		2030				2040			
Value of statistical life year (VSLY)	Discount rate, per year	Scenario				Scenario			
		I	II	III	Weighted	I	II	III	Weighted
$1,000	0	0.0	5.6	9.9	6.8	0.0	4.1	7.8	5.2
	3%	0.0	4.2	7.3	5.0	0.0	3.0	5.5	3.7
	5%	0.0	3.5	6.0	4.2	0.0	2.3	4.3	2.9
$5,000	0	0.0	23.3	43.2	28.9	0.0	16.6	33.8	21.8
	3%	0.0	19.8	32.0	22.7	0.0	11.9	24.1	15.6
	5%	0.0	17.1	26.3	19.1	0.0	9.3	18.8	12.2

Note: Calculations are based on assumptions indicated in the text.

to develop an AIDS vaccine? We undertake a hypothetical exercise assuming modest but real time savings from an additional $100 million expenditure per year. The $100 million figure is again based on our interviews with vaccine experts, who argued that the award of five to ten packages of $10–20 million a year over a decade to carefully selected research consortia would substantially accelerate progress.

In particular we conservatively assume elasticities of accelerated time-to-product with respect to R&D spending of 0.5 and 0.2 – that is, for a 1 percent increase in R&D, the time to a vaccine would be reduced by 0.5 percent or 0.2 percent. Over the nineteen-year period to the launch of a successful AIDS vaccine, this 11 percent increase in vaccine R&D ($100 million more each year) corresponds to a shortened time to product launch of 1.05 or 0.42 years. Assuming first a 1.05-

year gain, the time to vaccine approval would be 17.95 years as opposed to 19 years. Further, we estimate that an additional $100 million expenditure per year would increase the total discounted funding requirement from $13.9 billion to $15.4 billion. However, shortening the time to approval would also decrease proportionally the number of years in which one would have to pay development costs. Because of this shortened period of expenditure, we expect that the (discounted) funding requirement would result in a net increase to $14.6 billion. The calculation of discounted R&D financing for accelerating vaccine development by 0.42 of a year follows the same steps as the ones outlined above.

What would be the benefits of such accelerated vaccine development? To calculate this, we use the estimated benefits from receiving the vaccine in 2030 (or in 2040, under alternative assumptions

Table 6.8 Hypothetical benefit-cost ratios from advancing time of vaccine availability

Value of statistical life year (VSLY)	Discount rate, per year	Years sooner that vaccine is available	
		1.05	0.42
$1,000	3%	26:1	6:1
$1,000	5%	18:1	4:1
$5,000	3%	106:1	22:1
$5,000	5%	71:1	16:1

Note: Entries in the table are benefit-cost ratios.

about product launch), then calculate the incremental benefit associated with accelerating the time to vaccine development by 1.05 and 0.42 years. We find that for a $5,000 VSLY and a 4 percent discount rate, the benefits of advancing the approval time by 1.05 years is $73.5 billion (or $29.3 billion when the time gain is 0.42 years). From there, we estimate the benefit-cost ratio with sensitivity analyses around the VSLY and the discount rate. Even in the most conservative case of a $1,000 VSL, a 3 percent discount rate, and a 0.42-year advance, the benefit-cost ratio exceeds 6:1.

Table 6.8 displays the significant benefit-cost ratio of accelerating vaccine development. These findings make a strong case for increased funding to AIDS vaccine research and development.

Assumptions and limitations

Further refinements can be made to enhance the precision of our analysis. We chose to run a conservative estimate, though a more detailed study may yield a slightly higher benefit to cost ratio. For example, we chose not to quantify the smaller health care costs associated with infection or averted orphan care costs. Neither did we quantify the benefits of maintaining the productivity of healthy adults, in part because the VSLY is intended to capture these benefits. These benefits are important in themselves, though, and are discussed qualitatively below.

In our model, we did not account for orphan care costs averted. In 2009, approximately 16.6 million children were orphaned by AIDS, 90 percent of whom are located in sub-Saharan Africa (UNAIDS

2010b). Community programs and foster households must absorb the urgent costs of caring for these orphans, including food, clothing, education, and health care costs (Foster and Williamson 2000; Stover *et al.* 2007). While we did not quantitatively include these averted costs, they are considerable and can be used to strengthen the benefits of the vaccine.

Similarly, we chose not to account for the effect of the HIV vaccine on productivity levels. Since most men and women acquire HIV during their prime working years, averting infection would save healthy, productive years of life. As the HIV infection progresses, patients are often in ill health and cannot maintain their previous levels of productivity (Haacker 2004). The vaccine would avert infection and maintain productivity, thereby benefitting all of society as a whole.

Though we account for averted treatment costs, we assume that a patient on ART never incurs costs due to opportunistic infections. This simplifying assumption does not account for the costs of opportunistic infections at the point of treatment failure, costs that will be incurred both at the end of life and during the switch between first-line and second-line treatment. Neither did we account for the health care costs which are incurred during treatment initiation.

As noted at the outset, our calculations are for sub-Saharan Africa which indeed will account for perhaps two-thirds of the benefits. That said, a vaccine for Africa is likely (but not certain) to be of value to the rest of the world.

Lastly, we do not account for secondary infections averted, although they would certainly occur. To be conservative, we assume that the vaccine only averted at most one infection (the person that got the vaccine that would have gotten another person infected). However, each averted, infection decreases the risk of passing on the virus to someone else, thereby increasing the value of the vaccine by lowering general prevalence and reducing risk of infection. Though we do not account for these secondary infections averted they are an important benefit of an AIDS vaccine, at least while vaccine coverage remains low, and should be considered.

While we chose to model universal coverage, a strategy targeting at-risk groups is worth further examination. Targeting at-risk groups would yield a higher benefit-cost value, since the direct vaccination costs would be less, while both the direct and secondary benefits of averting infections would be higher. Ultimately, we chose to model universal coverage because of the high general prevalence throughout much of Africa, the substantial risk that even individuals in stable sexual partnerships are facing, and the likely political pressures to provide the vaccine to all adults even in countries with moderate levels of infection. Lengthy research conducted by IAVI has indicated that governments would promote universal coverage for a vaccine of at least 50 percent efficacy. Universal vaccination may also be the right course of action, both from a financial and public health standpoint.

An interesting point pending further study is the question of spill-over benefits from AIDS vaccine research and development. Although we did not attempt to incorporate this element into our analysis, a study of the economic impact of medical research by Murphy and Topel (2003) found that the social and monetary benefits of new medical knowledge are enormous. A recent UK study reaches similar conclusions. We did not include these benefits in our analysis, but it should be noted that such spillover benefits are likely to be substantial.

Conclusions

Despite progress in the fight against AIDS, the disease continues to impose a high human and financial toll, especially in Africa. Though prevalence and incidence rates are decreasing, they are still high enough to ensure that the epidemic will remain a huge social and financial burden in the coming decades. In this environment, a moderately effective vaccine could play a critical role in reversing the epidemic, complementing the arsenal of other effective tools becoming available.

A vaccine would be a game-changing technology that could finally break the epidemic,

providing long-term protection against HIV, averting treatment and health care costs, and saving healthy, productive lives. Our main benefit-cost analysis, of the value of continuing current vaccine investments, generates a benefit to cost ratio estimated conservatively at 2:67. Thus continued AIDS vaccine development appears to be an attractive investment, despite exceptionally high development costs and a long lead time to success. Our model is conservative – we assume a high cost per vaccination, a non-targeted immunization strategy, and do not account for any secondary infections prevented.

We further find a vaccine to be cost-effective, even with a ten-year lag (to 2040) in vaccine introduction. Whether the vaccine is introduced in 2030 (as experts suggest) or in 2040 (a pessimistic case), the investment appears to be compelling. That it would be worth, on our calculations, well over $100 billion more to have the vaccine in 2030 rather than 2040 points to the potential value of increasing the rate of expenditure on vaccine development above its current level of $900 million per year. Our secondary benefit-cost analysis draws on this hypothesis, generating estimates based on assumed reductions in time to vaccine availability that could materialize as a result of a $100 million per year increase in the rate of R&D expenditure. Under alternative (and hypothetical) assumptions that the vaccine becomes available either about 0.42 or 1.05 years earlier as a result of this additional expenditure, our estimates point to high potential benefits relative to costs.

Appendix: research developments and clinical trials

Table 6.9 provides an outline of recent developments in research principally in the Phase 1 stage.

Table 6.10 details all ongoing and completed Phase II and Phase III trials, as listed in IAVI's Vaccine Trials Database. Although many studies are initiated, only studies that show promise progress to Phase II and Phase III. Each of the vaccine trials – even those that eventually failed to show efficacy – have added to the knowledge base.

Table 6.9 Recent research advances

Protocol G	IAVI	The discovery of two broadly neutralizing antibodies (PG9 and PG16) against HIV and the identification of a potentially vulnerable point on the virus. The antibodies: (1) target the point on the HIV spike that infects other cells, a spot that cannot mutate, (2) are highly potent, and (3) recognize and attack many HIV subtypes. Research suggests that if the antibodies can be "reverse engineered" into a vaccine immunogen that elicits the antibody reaction, then an effective HIV vaccine may be produced.
Cytomegalovirus clinical development program	IAVI, MedImmune/ Astrazeneca, Oregon Health and Sciences University	A vaccine prototype based on a cytomegalovirus vector has been the most effective thus far in controlling SIV among monkeys. This vector is attractive because it persists in the body and may incur long-term immunity. In the study, half of the monkeys given the cytomegalovirus-based SIV vaccine remained protected against HIV for a year, and others held the virus at undetectable levels in the blood. This is the first time such a result was viewed in a viral vector-based model.
Canine distemper	IAVI	Scientists are investigating this virus as a way to deliver a vaccine because it targets immune cells in the guts, where early HIV infection becomes established. This could be a vital location to control HIV before it spreads.
Chimeric Venezuelan equine encephalitis	IAVI, Non-Profit Global Vaccines, Inc	The Chimeric VEE targets the cells in which HIV replicates, making this a good candidate for future study in primates. In this experiment, researchers insert several HIV genes into the Venezuelan equine encephalitis virus, which is similar to a live vaccine used to vaccine horses in some countries and is being tested by the US military as a human vaccine against encephalitis.
Vesicular stomatitis virus	IAVI	This is also a viral vector study, in which HIV genes are inserted into the vesicular stomatitis virus – which naturally infects pigs and horses, but does not make humans sick. In research, the virus becomes very weak yet is able to selectively target lymphoid tissue.
Sendai virus	IAVI, DNAVEC of Japan	Research is looking into a vector-based vaccine candidate using the Sendai virus, in which HIV genes are inserted.

Source: IAVI (2011).

Table 6.10 Ongoing and completed Phase II and Phase III AIDS trials

Phase III

Trial name: RV 144

Trial detail:	A Phase III trial of Sanofi Pasteur Live Recombinant ALVAC-HIV (vCP1521) Priming with VaxGen gp120 B/E (AIDSVAX B/E) Boosting in HIV-uninfected Thai adults
Study status:	Completed
Start date:	10/2/2003
Sponsor:	USG, Thailand MOPH, NIAID, TAVEG, Sanofi, VaxGen
Project site:	Phan Tong District Hospital, Phan Tong District, Chon Buri, Thailand; Ao Udom Hospital, Sri Racha District, Chon Buri, Thailand; Ban Lamung District Hospital, Ban Lamung District, Chon Buri, Thailand; Sattahip District Hospital, Sattahip District, Chon Buri, Thailand
Number of volunteers:	16,403
Design:	Prevention, Randomized, Double Blind (Subject, Caregiver, Investigator), Placebo Control, Parallel Assignment, Efficacy Study

Trial name: VAX 003

Study detail:	A Phase III trial to determine the efficacy of AIDSVAX B/E vaccine in intravenous drug users in Bangkok, Thailand
Study status:	Completed
Start date:	3/1/1999
Sponsor:	VaxGen
Project site:	17 clinics in Bangkok, Thailand
Number of volunteers:	2,500
Design:	The purpose of this study is to determine whether immunization with AIDSVAX B/E vaccine protects intravenous drug users from HIV-1 infection. HIV-1 infection will be defined as having a positive antibody test by commercial HIV-1 ELISA and confirmatory immunoblot. Volunteers are immunized and followed for a minimum of 2 years. Any volunteer that becomes infected with HIV-1 is followed every 4 months post infection for up to 36 months. Behavior effects associated with study participation are assessed.

Trial name: VAX 004

Study detail:	A Phase III trial to determine the efficacy of bivalent AIDSVAX B/B vaccine in adults at risk of sexually transmitted HIV-1 infection in North America
Study status:	Completed
Start date:	6/1/1998
Sponsor:	VaxGen
Project site:	56 clinics in US; 3 in Canada; 1 in Puerto Rico; 1 in Netherlands
Number of volunteers:	5,400
Design:	The purpose of this study is to determine whether immunization with AIDSVAX B/B vaccine protects at-risk persons from acquiring HIV-1 infection. To determine whether prior immunization with AIDSVAX B/B (bivalent) vaccine reduces viral load and protects against persistent viremia in HIV-1-infected patients. To evaluate the safety of AIDSVAX B/B vaccine in persons who have become infected with HIV-1 after receiving one or more vaccinations. To evaluate the immunologic response in patients who have received a vaccine and have become infected with HIV-1 compared to those patients who have received a vaccine but remain uninfected. Volunteers receive 7 blinded, intramuscular vaccinations (at Months 0, 1, 6, 12, 18, 24, 30) containing either the AIDSVAX B/B vaccine or a placebo (aluminum adjuvant only). Volunteers are randomized in a 2 to 1 vaccine-to-placebo ratio. HIV-uninfected persons are followed for a total of 16 visits beginning at screening and continuing until Month 36. Patients who become HIV infected during study are followed every 4 months for at least 24 months.

Table 6.10 *(cont.)*

Phase II

Trial name: HVTN 205

Study detail:	Phase IIa trial testing the safety and immunogenicity of GeoVax's HIV-1 DNA prime followed by GeoVax's HIV-1 MVA (Modified Vaccinia Virus) boost
Study status:	Ongoing
Start date:	1/12/2009
Sponsor:	GeoVax, HVTN
Project site:	Atlanta, Georgia; Birmingham, Alabama; Boston, Massachusetts; Nashville, Tennessee; New York, New York; Rochester, New York; Seattle, Washington; San Francisco, California; Iquitos, Peru; and Lima, Peru
Number of volunteers:	225
Design:	Prevention, Randomized, Double Blind (Subject, Caregiver), Placebo Control, Parallel Assignment, Safety/Efficacy Study

Trial name: HVTN 505

Study detail:	Safety and effectiveness of HIV-1 DNA Plasmid Vaccine and HIV-1 Recombinant Adenoviral Vector Vaccine in HIV-uninfected, circumcised men
Study status:	Ongoing
Start date:	7/6/2009
Sponsor:	NIAD, HVTN
Project site:	Alabama Vaccine, Birmingham, Alabama, United States 35294-2050; San Francisco Vaccine and Prevention, San Francisco, California, United States 94102-6033; Hope Clinic of the Emory Vaccine Center, Decatur, Georgia, United States 30030; VRC Clinical Trials Core, Bethesda, Maryland, United States 20816; Fenway Community Health Clinical Research Site (FCHCRS), Boston, Massachusetts, United States 02115; Univ. of Rochester HVTN, Rochester, New York, United States 14642-0001; HIV Prevention and Treatment, New York, New York, United States 10032; 3535 Market Street, Philadelphia, Pennsylvania, United States 19104-3309; FHCRC/UW Vaccine, Seattle, Washington, United States 98104
Number of volunteers:	2,200
Design:	Participants will receive a recombinant DNA plasmid vaccine injection at study entry and on Days 28, and 56, followed by a recombinant adenoviral serotype vector vaccine injection on Day 168

Trial name: ANRS VAC 18

Study detail:	Randomized double blinded phase II AIDS vaccine study comparing immunogenicity and safety of 3 doses of lipopeptide (LIPO-5) versus placebo in non-infected HIV volunteers (ANRS liVAC 18)
Study status:	Completed
Start date:	9/1/2004
Sponsor:	ANRS, Sanofi Pasteur
Project site:	Cochin hospital, Paris, France; European Georges Pompidou hospital, Paris, France; Tenon hospital, Paris, France; Saint Marguerite hospital, Marseille, France; Purpan hospital, Toulouse, France; Nantes hospital, Nantes, France
Number of volunteers:	156
Design:	Prevention, Randomized, Double-Blind, Placebo Control, Parallel Assignment, Safety/Immunogenicity Study

(cont.)

Table 6.10 (*cont.*)

Trial name: AVEG 201

Study detail:	A Phase II clinical trial to evaluate the immunogenicity and reactogenicity of the Recombinant Subunit HIV-1 Envelope Vaccines SF-2 RGP120 in MF59 (Biocine) and MN rgp120 in alum (Genentech)
Study status:	Completed
Start date:	12/9/1992
Sponsor:	NIAID
Project site:	Sites within the USA
Number of volunteers:	296
Design:	The purpose of this study is to evaluate the safety and immunogenicity of SF-2 rgp120 vaccine in MF59 versus MN gp120 vaccine in alum in volunteers who are seronegative for HIV-1. AS PER AMENDMENT 07/02/97: To determine the ability of immunization with MN rgp120/HIV-1 in combination with alum or SF-2 rgp120 in combination with MF59 to induce an HIV-1 envelope-specific delayed-type hypersensitivity (DTH) response in volunteers who receive rsgp120/MN skin testing. HIV-seronegative volunteers (including four populations at higher risk for HIV infection and two populations at lower risk) receive one of four regimens. Two treatment groups receive 50 mcg SF-2 rgp 120 (BIOCINE) in MF59 adjuvant or 600 mcg MN rgp120 (Genentech) in alum. Two control groups receive vehicle (placebo) in MF59 adjuvant alone or alum adjuvant alone. Immunizations are given at Months 0, 1, and 6. AS PER AMENDMENT 10/93: patients enrolled by June 15, 1993, receive a fourth immunization at Month 12 or 18 (50 percent of patients for each schedule). Patients are followed until 2 years after the first injection. AS PER AMENDMENT 05/10/94: a special study of vaccine acceptability and HIV-related risk behavior will be conducted at some time between Months 12 and 18. AS PER AMENDMENT 07/02/97: a special DTH study will be conducted in consenting volunteers who have received three or four immunizations. The injections will be given at the end of the study (on or after Day 1, and 56). Follow-up is extended to 56 days after administration of the intradermal injection.

Trial name: AVEG 202/HIVNET 014

Study detail:	A Phase II safety and immunogenicity trial of Live Recombinant Canarypox ALVAC-HIV vCP205 with or without HIV-1 SF-2 RGP-120 in HIV-1 uninfected adults
Study status:	Completed
Start date:	5/22/1997
Sponsor:	NIAID
Project site:	Sites within USA
Number of volunteers:	420
Design:	

Trial name: HIVNET 026

Study detail:	A multisite Phase II clinical trial to evaluate the immunogenicity and safety of ALVAC-HIV vCP1452 alone and combined with MN rgp120
Study status:	Completed
Start date:	6/1/2000
Sponsor:	NIAID
Project site:	Brazil, Haiti, Peru, Trinidad and Tobago
Number of volunteers:	200

Table 6.10 (cont.)

Design:	The purpose of this study is to evaluate the immunogenicity and confirm the safety of 2 vaccine regimens: ALVAC-HIV vCP1452 combined with MN rgp120, and ALVAC-HIV vCP1452 given alone. The primary objectives related to immunogenicity include: 1) evaluation of the net CD8+ CTL response rate for each active treatment arm and 2) comparisons of mean titers of neutralizing antibodies to HIV-1 MN between each active treatment arm and the placebo arm. The primary objectives related to evaluation of safety are: comparison of the rates of severe systemic and rates of severe local reactions for each of the active treatment arms to the placebo arm. PA = Placebo ALVAC MN = MN rgp120 (300mcg/ml MN rgp120 in 0.6mg alum adjuvant) P: Alum placebo Part 2: A = ALVAC-HIV vCP1452 107.26 TCID50 PA = Placebo ALVAC MN = MN rgp120 (300mcg/ml MN rgp120 in 0.6mg alum adjuvant) P: Alum placebo. Blood and urine samples are collected for immunologic assays, virologic determinations, pregnancy testing, and safety assessments. Risk behavior and social harms are assessed every 6 months during follow-up. At all clinic visits volunteers receive counseling on avoidance of HIV infection and pregnancy. Participants are tested for HIV-1 every 3 to 6 months. Counseling and follow-up for any needed medical care are provided.

Trial name: HTVN 068

Study detail:	A Phase I clinical trial to evaluate immune response kinetics and safety of two different primes, Adenoviral Vector Vaccine (VRC-HIVADV014-00-VP) and DNA Vaccine (VRC-HIVDNA009-00-VP), each followed by Adenoviral Vector Boost in healthy, HIV-1 uninfected adults
Study status:	Completed
Start date:	2/3/2006
Sponsor:	NIAID
Project site:	Univ of Alabama-Birmingham, AL; San Francisco Dept. of Public Health, CA; Mt. Zion Hospital – GCRC, CA; New York Blood Center – Union Square, NY; New York Blood Center – NY; Univ of Rochester, NY; Columbia Univ, NY; Vanderbilt Univ, TN; FHCRC/UW-VTU, WA
Number of volunteers:	66
Design:	Prevention, Randomized, Double Blind (Subject, Caregiver, Investigator), Placebo Control, Parallel Assignment, Safety Study

Trial name: HTVN 203

Study detail:	A Phase II clinical trial to evaluate the immunogenicity and safety of a combined regimen using ALVAC vCP1452 and AIDSVAX B/B
Study status:	Completed
Start date:	12/14/2000
Sponsor:	NIAID
Project site:	USA
Number of volunteers:	330

Trial name: IAVI 010

Study detail:	This trial tests the safety and immunogenicity of a clade A HIV-DNA/MVA prime-boost combination, in HIV-uninfected healthy volunteers at low risk for HIV infection. In addition, the effect of the route of administration of the MVA boost will be studied.
Study status:	Completed
Start date:	4/19/2003
Sponsor:	IAVI

(cont.)

Table 6.10 (cont.)

Project site:	Dept. of Medical Microbiology, Univ. of Nairobi, Kenya; St Thomas' Hospital, London
Number of volunteers:	115
Design:	This trial tests the safety and immunogenicity of a clade A HIV-DNA/MVA prime-boost combination, in HIV-uninfected healthy volunteers at low risk for HIV infection. In addition, the effect of the route of administration of the MVA boost will be studied.
Trial name: IAVI A002	
Study detail:	A Phase II, placebo controlled, double blind trial to evaluate the safety and immunogenicity of tgAAC09, an HIV vaccine containing clade C DNA in an adeno-associated virus capsid, administered twice, and three dosage levels and two dosing intervals
Study status:	Completed
Start date:	11/1/2005
Sponsor:	IAVI
Project site:	South Africa, Uganda, Zambia
Number of volunteers:	84
Design:	

Source: IAVI Vaccine trials database 2011. www.iavireport.org/trials-db/Pages/default.aspx.

References

Adams, C. P. and Brantner, V. (2010). Spending on new drug development. *Health Economics* **19**(2): 130–41.

aids2031 Costs and Financing Working Group. (2010a). *Costs and Choices: Financing the Long-Term Fight against AIDS.* Washington, DC: Results for Development Institute.

aids2031 Costs and Financing Working Group. (2010b). *The Long-Term Costs of HIV/AIDS in South Africa.* Washington, DC: Results for Development Institute.

ALPHA Network. (2011). Phase 1 Summary. London School of Hygiene and Tropical Medicine, University of London. Available from: www.lshtm.ac.uk/eph/psd/alpha/phase1/ (accessed August 15, 2011).

Aral, S. O. and Holmes, K. K. (2008). The epidemiology of STIs and their social and behavioral determinants: industrialized and developing countries. In K. K. Holmes, P. Sparling, W. Stamm, P. Piot, J. Wasserheit, L. Corey, and M. Cohen (eds.) *Sexually Transmitted Diseases, 4th edn.* New York: McGraw-Hill.

Auvert, B., Taljaard, D., Lagarde, E., Sobngwi-Tambekou, J., Sitta, R. and Puren, A. (2005). Randomized, controlled intervention trial of male circumcision for reduction of HIV infection risk: the ANRS 1265 Trial. *PLoS Medicine* **2**(11): 1112–22. doi:10.1371/journal.pmed.0020298.

Bailey, R. C., Moses, S., Parker, C. B., Agot, K., Maclean, I., Krieger, J. N., Williams, C. F. M., Campbell, R. T. and Ndinya-Achola, J. O. (2007). Male circumcision for HIV prevention in young men in Kisumu, Kenya: a randomised controlled trial. *The Lancet* **369**(9562): 643–56. doi:10.1016/S0140-6736(07)60312-2.

Bertozzi, S., Guitierrez, J. P., Opuni, M., Bollinger, L., McGreevey, W. and Stover, J. (2002). *Resource Requirements to Fight HIV/AIDS in Latin America and the Caribbean.* Washington, DC: Inter-American Development Bank.

Bishai, D., Pariyo, G., Ainsworth, M. and Hill, K. (2004). Determinants of personal demand for an AIDS vaccine in Uganda: contingent valuation survey. *Bulletin of the World Health Organization* **82**: 652–60.

Bloom, D. E., Canning, D. and Jamison, D. T. (2004). Health, wealth, and welfare. *Finance and Development* **40**(1): 10–15.

Foster, G. and Williamson, J. (2000). A review of current literature on the impact of HIV/AIDS on children in sub-Saharan Africa. *AIDS* **14**(3): S275–84.

Haacker, M. (2004). *HIV/AIDS: The Impact on the Social Fabric and the Economy, in The*

Macroeconomics of HIV/AIDS. Geneva: International Monetary Fund.

Hammitt, J. K. and Robinson, L.A. (2011). The income elasticity of the value per statistical life: transferring estimates between high and low income populations. *Journal of Benefit-Cost Analysis* **2**(1). Available from www.bepress.com/jbca/vol2/iss1/1/ (accessed May 5, 2011).

Health Economics Research Group. (2008). *Medical Research: What's It Worth? Estimating the Economic Benefits from Medical Research in the UK*. London: UK Evaluation Forum.

Hecht, R., Stover, J., Bollinger, L., Muhib, F., Case, K. and De Ferranti, D. (2010). Financing of HIV/AIDS programme scale-up in low-income and middle-income countries 2009–2031. *The Lancet* **376**(9748): 1254–60.

International AIDS Vaccine Initiative. (2007). Forecasting the gobal demand for preventative HIV vaccines, IAVI. Available from www.bcg.com/documents/file27442.pdf (accessed August 3, 2011).

International AIDS Vaccine Initiative. (2009a). Estimating the potential impact of an AIDS vaccine in developing countries. Available from www.iavi.org/Lists/IAVIPublications/attachments/2c678572-e031-4fc2-b4120794e04c9409/IAVI_Policy_Notes_Estimating_the_Potential_Impact_of_an_AIDS_Vaccine_in_Developing_Countries_2010_ENG.pdf (accessed April 22, 2011).

International AIDS Vaccine Initiative. (2009b). Uganda: estimating the potential impact of an AIDS vaccine. Available from www.iavi.org/Lists/IAVIPublications/attachments/454d7f8e-f58a-4bf0-969436447fa52211/IAVI_Uganda_Estimating_the_Potential_Impact_of_an_AIDS_Vaccine_2009_ENG.pdf (accessed April 22, 2011).

International AIDS Vaccine Initiative. (2010a). Brazil: estimating the potential impact of an AIDS vaccine. Available from www.iavi.org/Lists/IAVIPublications/attachments/59b6940e-e617-4287-b225a22611ede716/IAVI_Brazil_Estimating_the_Potential_Impact_of_an_AIDS_Vaccine_2010_ENG.pdf (accessed April 22, 2011).

International AIDS Vaccine Initiative. (2010b). Kenya: estimating the potential impact of an AIDS vaccine. Available from www.iavi.org/Lists/IAVIPublications/attachments/3f762fb5-38f1-4e84-b1ea61eacc257417/IAVI_Kenya_Estimating_the_Potential_Impact_of_an_AIDS_Vaccine_2009_ENG.pdf (accessed April 22, 2011).

International AIDS Vaccine Initiative. (2010c). *2009 Annual Progress Report: Promise, Progress, Partners*. Available from www.iavi.org/about-IAVI/Documents/IAVI_APR_2009.pdf (accessed August 15, 2011).

International AIDS Vaccine Initiative. (2011). *2010 Annual Progress Report: Innovation, Flexibility, Impact*. Available from www.iavi.org/Lists/IAVIPublications/attachments/e7c3fa54-ed10-4dd4-b22b-0294202c8807/IAVI_Annual_Report_2010_ENG.pdf (accessed August 15, 2011).

Jamison, D. T., Jha, P. and Bloom, D. E. (2008). Disease control. In B. Lomborg (ed.) *Global Crises, Global Solutions: Costs and Benefits*. Cambridge University Press, 3.

Jamison, D. T., Sachs, J. D. and Wang, J. (2001). The effect of the AIDS epidemic on economic welfare in sub-Saharan Africa. *CMH Working Paper Series No 13*. Geneva: World Health Organization.

Karim, A. Q. *et al.* (2010). Effectiveness and safety of Tenofovir gel, an anti-retroviral microbicide, for the prevention of HIV infection in women. *Science* **329**(5996): 1168–74.

Leelahavarong, P. *et al.* (2011). Is a HIV vaccine a viable option and at what price? An economic evaluation of adding HIV vaccination into existing prevention programs in Thailand. *BMC Public Health* **11**(534).

Maurice, J. (2011). Quest for an effective AIDS vaccine takes a new tack. *The Lancet* **378**: 213–14.

McGreevey, W. *et al.* (2004). Literature Review of HIV and Other Vaccine Costs. Futures Group. Draft report.

Mills, E. J. *et al.* (2011). Life expectancy of persons receiving combination antiretroviral therapy in low-income countries: a cohort analysis from Uganda. *Annals of Internal Medicine* **155**(4).

Murphy, K. M. and Topel, R. (2003). *Measuring the Gains from Medical Research: An Economic Approach*. University of Chicago Press.

Nordhaus, W. (2003). The health of nations: the contributions of improved health to living standards. In K. M. Murphy and R. H. Topel (eds.) *Measuring the Gains from Medical Research: An Economic Approach*. University of Chicago Press.

Policy Cures. (2010). *Neglected Disease Research and Development: Is the Global Financial Crisis Changing R&D?* London International Development Centre.

Resource Tracking Working Group (for HIV Vaccines and Microbicides). (2011). Capitalizing on Scientific Progress: Investment in HIV Prevention R&D in 2010. www.hivresourcetracking.org.

Schelling, T. (1968). The life you save may be your own. In S. B. Chase (ed.) *Problems in Public Expenditure Analysis.* Washington, DC: Brookings Institution.

Stover, J. *et al.* (2007). Resource needs to support orphans and vulnerable children in sub-Saharan Africa. *Health Policy Plan* **22**(1): 21–7.

Suraratdecha, C., Ainsworth, M., Tangcharoensathien, V. and Whittington, D. (2005). The private demand for an AIDS vaccine in Thailand. *Health Policy* **71**(3): 271–87.

UNAIDS. (2010a). Press statement: UNAIDS and WHO welcome new findings that could provide an additional tool for HIV prevention for men who have sex with men. Available from www.unaids.org/en/media/unaids/contentassets/documents/pressstatement/2010/20101123_PS_iprex_en.pdf (accessed August 3, 2011).

UNAIDS. (2010b). Report on the global AIDS epidemic. Available from www.unaids.org/globalreport/global_report.htm (accessed August 3, 2011).

UNAIDS. (2010c). Unite for Universal Access 2011 High Level Meeting on AIDS. Geneva: UNAIDS.

UNAIDS. (2011). Press statement: UNAIDS and WHO hail new results showing that a once-daily pill for HIV-negative people can prevent them from aquiring HIV. Geneva: UNAIDS.

Usher, D. (1973). An imputation to the measure of economic growth for changes in life expectancy. In M. Moss (ed.) *The Measurement of Economic and Social Performance.* New York: National Bureau of Economic Research. Available from www.nber.org/chapters/c3616.pdf (accessed April 22, 2011).

Viscusi, W. K. and Aldy, J. E. (2003). The value of a statistical life: a critical review of market estimates throughout the world. *Journal of Risk and Uncertainty* **27**(1): 5–76.

Whittington, D., Matsui-Santana, O., Freiberger, J. J., Van Houtven, G. and Pattanayak, S. (2002). Private demand for a HIV/AIDS vaccine: evidence from Guadalajara, Mexico. *Vaccine* **20**(19/20): 2585–91.

6.1 Vaccine research and development

Perspective paper

STEVEN S. FORSYTHE

RethinkHIV has posed the question of how an additional $2 billion per year over the next five years should be allocated to best address HIV and AIDS in sub-Saharan Africa. The paper by Hecht and Jamison (Hecht and Jamison 2011) makes a compelling argument for why investing in AIDS vaccine research and development (and subsequent production) should consume a disproportionately large proportion of any new resources. Specifically Hecht and Jamison argue that $900 million per year should be allocated to vaccine research and development (approximately double current expenditures), or 45 percent of the hypothetical $2 billion of incremental resources. This compares to estimates that only approximately 5 percent of all global resources are currently being spent on an AIDS vaccine ($900 million/$15.9 billion). Given the large request for funds, it becomes necessary to convincingly justify that such a significant proportion of new funds be allocated in this way.

The following perspective paper is designed to assess if the assumptions and conclusions in the Hecht and Jamison paper are supported by evidence. In other words, is there data which can lead policy-makers to reasonably conclude that a doubling of the current budget for an AIDS vaccine would be reasonable and advisable based on this analysis?

In addition to a brief analysis of the assumptions contained in the Hecht and Jamison paper, the following paper also introduces a number of additional issues which might be considered for further analysis and consideration.

Furthermore, Hecht and Jamison introduce a number of alternative scenarios under which a vaccine might be introduced. The following perspective paper will attempt to determine if these scenarios are appropriate, and/or whether alternative scenarios might need to be considered.

Results

Hecht and Jamison lay out their rationale for their argument that the societal benefits of an AIDS vaccine could be between four and twenty times greater than the costs associated with the development and subsequent production of an AIDS vaccine. Despite the potential risks involved in the development of an AIDS vaccine (including the potential that such a vaccine would be dominated by other interventions, including a cure), such a high benefit to cost ratio would appear to justify the risks associated with such an investment (particularly if the vaccine is highly effective, has few side-effects, is available by 2030, and can be produced at a relatively low cost). The calculation of this high benefit to cost ratio is determined by using a number of assumptions, some of which seem quite reasonable or even conservative while others may be viewed as being too optimistic. The following sections focus on some key issues which the author of this perspective paper believes to be critical in concluding whether the benefits of an AIDS vaccine would substantially exceed the costs.

There are eight discussion themes that the author of this perspective paper would recommend for further consideration that could potentially modify the conclusions of Hecht and Jamison and could cause a reconsideration of the recommendation that a large proportion of any new HIV and AIDS resources should be allocated to AIDS vaccine research and development. The following issues will be addressed below:

- What will an AIDS vaccine really cost?
- What additional costs should be considered?
- How effective will an AIDS vaccine be?
- What should be assumed about the future course of Africa's epidemic?

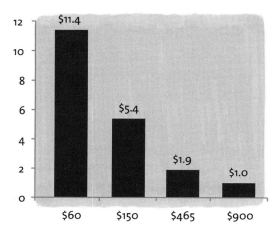

Figure 6.1.1 *Benefit to cost ratio based on variations in the unit cost of an AIDS vaccine* Note: *Figures based on an assumed 3 percent discount rate, 50 percent effectiveness, $3,000 per statistical life year, initiation in 2030, and Scenario 2.*

- How should the issue of disinhibition be addressed?
- What other benefits should be considered?
- Who should receive an AIDS vaccine?
- Who should pay for an AIDS vaccine?
- Is an AIDS vaccine better than alternative "vaccines"?

What will an AIDS vaccine really cost?

One critical assumption regarding the costs and benefits of an AIDS vaccine will be "what will it cost?" The assessment paper specifically addresses two potential cost values for any AIDS vaccines which would be available for sub-Saharan Africa: $60 and $150 per full vaccination. Both of these assumptions may in fact be overly optimistic, as it is conceivable that any vaccine might in fact be more expensive than $150. In the case of the HPV vaccine, Gardasil, for example, the initial international median price was $155/dose or $465/patient (based on a three-dose combination).[1] If $465 was used rather than the proposed unit cost of $150, the benefit to cost ratio declines from 5.4 to 1.9 (assuming that the vaccine became available in 2030, the discount rate was 3 percent, and the value of life year was $3,000). However, as long as the cost of

the vaccine remains below $900, the benefit to cost ratio still remains positive, so the conclusions about an AIDS vaccine being cost-saving remain valid.

Perhaps a more key assumption concerns the cost of the research and development required to develop the AIDS vaccine. In the Hecht and Jamison paper, the description of resources required for vaccine development ($8 to $12 billion over fourteen years) is not well explained. It appears that this figure is obtained by multiplying the cost of developing a new drug ($800 million) ten- to fifteenfold in order to obtain this estimate. This justification could be strengthened by designing something more tenable, including a description of the types of trials that would be funded if resources for the development of an AIDS vaccine were increased by the amounts recommended by Hecht and Jamison. In addition, it would be useful to investigate the historical cost of developing similar vaccines, in order to determine whether $8 to $12 billion is a reasonable estimate. At the very least, the authors should explain why the existing resources are unlikely to produce results by 2030, but with the additional resources the vaccine would be achievable.

What additional costs should be considered?

In addition to the development costs and the delivery costs, it is valuable to recognize that there will be other costs which need to be included. One factor would include the number of doses required to assure a sustained response. The larger the number of doses that are required, the more resources will be required (not only for the product itself, but also for the follow-up required to assure that the clients complete their full course of vaccinations). In addition, the frequency of booster shots should be considered (assuming that a vaccine does not provide lifetime protection). A realistic assumption might be that the effectiveness of a vaccine would wane and eventually require booster shots.

There are also other critical costs which need to be considered. Hecht and Jamison have included the

[1] www.pmprb-cepmb.gc.ca/english/View.asp?x=924&mp= 572.

cost of production, profit, packaging, distribution, and administration in their estimate of $60–$150 per full vaccination. However, a key cost not included is demand creation. Lessons learned from the delivery of the HPV vaccine, Gardasil, indicate that a vaccine for a sexually transmitted infection may not produce either the desired uptake or the expected revenues (DuBois 2010). Similar experience from male circumcision interventions in Africa indicate that unless there are sufficient resources, there is unlikely to be the required uptake (Bertrand, Njeuhmeli *et al.* 2011). It would not be unreasonable to assume that demand creation would cost millions of dollars per African country per year. If resources are not allocated to demand creation, it is conceivable that any AIDS vaccine could be plagued by slow uptake and misinformation about the real value of the vaccine being distributed.

Other factors which might need to be considered in any benefit to cost ratio include liability, supply chain management, and waste management. Liability costs could be significant, whether this liability is taken on by the manufacturers or donors (Boffey 1984). Furthermore the supply chain and waste management costs could be significant, particularly if the vaccine requires constant refrigeration and/or special handling.

Finally, it should be noted that economies of scale will be essential to keeping the unit cost of any vaccine as reasonable as possible. If manufacturers are only able to produce small quantities, or there is insufficient demand coming from sub-Saharan Africa, the cost of a vaccine is likely to remain high. However, if sufficient supply and demand exist from the initial stages of the vaccine manufacture, it is likely that the unit cost of the vaccine will decline significantly.

How effective will an AIDS vaccine be?

One of the key assumptions about the benefits of a vaccine concerns the effectiveness of the vaccine. Hecht and Jamison assume that an AIDS vaccine will be 50 percent effective, which is comparable to the efficacy of a cholera vaccine (Sinclair, Abba *et al.* 2011). The authors recognize that the

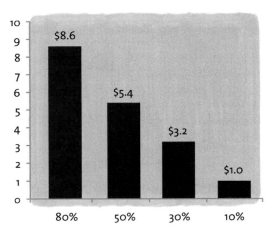

Figure 6.1.2 *Benefit to cost ratio based on variations in the effectiveness of an AIDS vaccine*
Note: *Figures based on an assumed 3 percent discount rate, $150/patient vaccinated, $3,000 per statistical life year, initiation in 2030, and Scenario 2.*

most promising vaccine trial (Thai RV144) to date demonstrated an effectiveness of only 31 percent (Rerks-Ngarm, Pitisuttithum *et al.* 2009). A key question then becomes at what point an AIDS vaccine would be deemed sufficiently effective such that scale-up would be warranted. From a purely economic point of view, a 30 percent effective vaccine would produce benefits that are 3.2 times greater than the costs, while an 80 percent effective vaccine would produce a benefit to cost ratio of 8.6. In fact a vaccine with an efficacy above 10 percent would still produce greater benefits than the costs. This again indicates that the conclusions made by Hecht and Jamison would still be valid, even with much more conservative assumptions.

Another key assumption concerns when a vaccine becomes available. Hecht and Jamison present two different scenarios for this: a vaccine becomes available in 2030 or 2040. These differing assumptions indicate that producing a vaccine in 2030 (5.4 benefit to cost ratio) would clearly be preferred to one which began manufacturing in 2040 (3.7 benefit to cost ratio). Yet the conclusion is still arrived at that benefits will far exceed costs regardless of which of these two years are assumed to be the year of manufacture.

It should be noted, however, that Hecht and Jamison assume a twenty-four-year lifespan regardless of when manufacture of an AIDS vaccine begins. In other words, a vaccine initiated in 2030 would be dominated by something better by 2054, whereas a vaccine initiated in 2040 would be dominated by something better by 2064. A more reasonable assumption would be to assume that an AIDS vaccine would be dominated in one specific year, regardless of when the AIDS vaccine was itself first produced. This would potentially create a much higher benefit to initiating development in 2030 as opposed to 2040.

What should be assumed about the future course of Africa's epidemic?

By setting up three plausible scenarios about what the world will look like in fifteen years – (1) a cure becomes available before an AIDS vaccine becomes available, (2) universal access to prevention and treatment services have been achieved before an AIDS vaccine becomes available, or (3) current trends towards scale-up are maintained, reaching two-thirds of universal access by 2015 and being maintained thereafter – Hecht and Jamison have avoided the temptation to simply assume that every other intervention (e.g., ARV treatment) will remain stagnant for the next twenty years. By including a scenario in which a cure is found before a vaccine is developed (Scenario 1), the authors recognize that a twenty-year investment in an AIDS vaccine might produce no benefits because the vaccine has been replaced by something better. Whether the 10 percent weight assigned to this potential scenario is reasonable can be debated, but it nonetheless is important to recognize that this could occur.

However, Hecht and Jamison do not explicitly discuss the uncertainty regarding the course of the HIV and AIDS pandemic in sub-Saharan Africa. In Scenario 2 (rapid scale-up), it is assumed that there will be 21.9 million persons living with HIV in 2030 and 1.1 million new HIV infections. In Scenario 3 (current trends), the number of people living with HIV is assumed to be 25.7 million and the annual number of new infections is

assumed to be 1.9 million. These numbers do not significantly vary from the current estimates that 22.5 million are living with HIV in sub-Saharan Africa and that 1.5 million people per year are becoming infected. The reality, however, is that there is much greater uncertainty than these data suggest about what the status of the epidemic will look like twenty years into the future. For example, data from Uganda and more recent estimates from Zimbabwe indicate that a significant drop in incidence has occurred (Kirby 2008; Halperin, Mugurungi et al. 2011). In the case of Zimbabwe, HIV prevalence dropped from 26 percent in 1997 to 14 percent in 2009. Furthermore, as cited by Hecht and Jamison, UNAIDS reports that twenty-two sub-Saharan African countries have reduced the number of new HIV infections by more than 25 percent (UNAIDS 2010).

The reason why the course of the pandemic in sub-Saharan Africa is relevant to a discussion on the costs and benefits of an AIDS vaccine is that the benefits of an AIDS vaccine rely heavily on the assumed number of new HIV infections to be averted when that AIDS vaccine becomes available. If the number of new HIV infections is much lower than what is projected by Hecht and Jamison, then the number of new HIV infections that can be averted by 2030 (or 2040) would be much less (and thus the benefits of an AIDS vaccine would be much less).

Furthermore, as shown by the article by Venkatesh et al. (Venkatesh, Flanigan et al. 2011) and from research on the benefits of early treatment as a prevention strategy, access to treatment may have a much more significant effect on the number of new HIV infections than was previously assumed. If this is the case, access to treatment would result in fewer new HIV infections by 2030 (and in turn, fewer new HIV infections that could be averted by an AIDS vaccine).

How should the issue of disinhibition be addressed?

There are a number of factors which are likely to affect the ultimate costs and benefits of an AIDS vaccine, but which are difficult to predict.

One of these factors is disinhibition. In the context of an AIDS vaccine, disinhibition might occur if those vaccinated assume that they are immune from infection (rather than being only partially protected) and take risks that they would not otherwise take, thus offsetting the benefits of a vaccine. This could particularly be a problem in lower incidence countries, since vaccine-related disinhibition might ultimately cause new HIV infections to rise rather than decrease. An upcoming analysis of male circumcision, for example, has indicated that, in Rwanda, male circumcision may increase new HIV infections if there is 30 percent disinhibition (Njeuhmeli, Forsythe *et al.* 2011). Similarly, an analysis of an AIDS vaccine in Brazil concluded that a partially effective vaccine that produced an immediate 50 percent disinhibition would actually increase the number of new HIV infections in that country (Fonseca, Forsythe *et al.* 2010). If this is the case in Africa with an AIDS vaccine, then the number of new HIV infections averted may be significantly overstated by the analysis by Hecht and Jamison.

What other benefits should be considered?

There are a number of ways in which an AIDS vaccine program could be anticipated to produce synergistic benefits which might not be fully evaluated in Hecht and Jamison's benefit to cost ratio. One could anticipate, for example, that those who would choose to get vaccinated would first be encouraged to be tested for HIV and, if they were found to already be infected, to then pursue early treatment (assuming that any vaccine would have no benefits for an individual who is already infected). The synergistic benefits of an AIDS vaccine (for those uninfected), combined with early treatment (for those infected), would potentially be substantial.[2]

There could also be synergistic benefits to those who are HIV-negative, receive an AIDS vaccine, and simultaneously receive other preventative services. For example, an AIDS vaccine campaign could potentially provide counseling, STI treatment, male circumcision, condom distribution, etc. Provided in unison, it is possible that a 50 percent

effective vaccine, in combination with these other interventions, could provide much more than 50 percent protection (given the potential for disinhibition, providing services such as counseling would be particularly critical).

Who should receive an AIDS vaccine?

A key question not addressed by Hecht and Jamison concerns whether it makes sense to target an AIDS vaccine at particular subpopulations. Ideally an effective AIDS vaccine would be affordable and available enough that it could be given to anyone at risk of becoming infected. However, vaccines such as Gardasil are recommended only for girls between the ages of nine and twenty-six, even though the vaccine can be of benefit for women or men of any age. For HIV prevention strategies such as male circumcision, different countries target males at different ages, in order to best focus resources on those populations which are likely to most benefit from the intervention. In the case of an AIDS vaccine, it may be preferable to target all males and females of reproductive age, or to prioritize those who are just about to become sexually active. Alternatively an AIDS vaccination campaign might target those in Africa who are at a particularly high risk of becoming infected, including truck drivers, sex workers, miners, etc. The selection of the population that is to be targeted can have a significant impact on both the costs and the benefits of an AIDS vaccine. In Brazil, for example, an analysis of a potential AIDS vaccine indicated that it would be much more cost-effective to target a vaccine to high-risk subpopulations, rather than to provide the vaccine to a general cross-section of the population (Fonseca, Forsythe *et al.* 2010).

Who should pay for an AIDS vaccine?

Hecht and Jamison do not address the issue of possible private benefits which are not included in the valuation of societal benefits. The development of

---

[2] Conversely, a partially effective vaccine could potentially produce disinhibition by decreasing the demand for condoms, male circumcision, STI treatment, etc.

an AIDS vaccine for use in sub-Saharan Africa could produce significant financial benefits outside of the continent (e.g., there may be a significant private market for an effective AIDS vaccine in Europe, Asia, and the Americas). This in turn leads back to the question of "who should pay?" Hecht and Jamison appear to assume that the $0.9 billion should be paid for by taxpayers in developed countries as an international public good. However, it might be argued that if the benefits are really external to Africa, then perhaps the payer should be the private sector? On the other hand, if the vaccine were to be piloted in Africa but the economic benefits would be derived outside of the region, perhaps governments in Africa should be able to derive some of the economic benefits of the vaccine (e.g., perhaps the manufacturing of the ultimate vaccine should be conducted by African companies)?

Is an AIDS vaccine better than alternative "vaccines"?

Finally, while Hecht and Jamison might wish to assume that there is no competition going on for funds, in reality there are limited new resources, and an argument needs to be made for allocating resources to an AIDS vaccine over other alternatives. Therefore perhaps the most significant issue that was left unaddressed in Hecht and Jamison was why policy-makers should wait for a vaccine which "might" be 50 percent effective twenty years from today, when "vaccines" already exist with an efficacy of 39 percent (microbicide gel) (Abdool Karim, Abdool Karim *et al.* 2010), 76 percent (male circumcision) (Auvert, Rech *et al.* 2011), or even 96 percent (treatment as prevention). Given the potential value of these demonstrated tools, why should policy-makers delay action and instead invest in a longer-term technology which has not yet been proven?[3]

It is useful, for example, to evaluate an AIDS vaccine relative to other strategies. Modeling efforts for male circumcision have estimated that $2 billion spent between 2011 and 2025 would prevent 3.4 million new HIV infections in sub-Saharan African countries by 2025 (Njeuhmeli, Forsythe *et al.* 2011). Over that same time period, spending on an AIDS vaccine would cost $13.5 billion, with

an actual AIDS vaccine not being introduced until 2030. This type of comparison indicates that over $13 billion could be spent on research and development associated with an AIDS vaccine with the potential for no new HIV infections being averted (and even in the most optimistic assumption, producing an AIDS vaccine with 50 percent effectiveness no sooner than 2030). Alternatively $2 billion could be spent on the actual intervention of male circumcision, with more than three million HIV infections being averted in sub-Saharan Africa.

Conclusions and recommendations

Benefit to cost ratios provide useful information to national and international policy-makers about the return on their investment. Benefit to cost ratios can help to prioritize alternative strategies for allocating additional resources and they should therefore not be ignored.

However, economists must also recognize that the decision to produce and manufacture an AIDS vaccine will not be made based purely on benefit to cost ratios (if they did, then Thai RV144 would have already been scaled up, even with an effectiveness of only 30 percent). There are many qualitative and non-economic issues which will need to be addressed by national and international policy-makers as they consider doubling the current investment in an AIDS vaccine. Economists are unlikely to be able to provide information about such things as the likelihood of producing an effective AIDS vaccine, the potential side-effects of a vaccine, etc.

Economic analyses often struggle with the issue of risk. In the case of an AIDS vaccine, economists must recognize that there is tremendous uncertainty about the characteristics of an AIDS vaccine. At present, economists don't know what an AIDS vaccine will cost, either for research and development

---

[3] One potential response to this question can be addressed by identifying the potential size of the population reached with each intervention. A vaccine, for example, could presumably be given to any adult, whereas male circumcision would only be appropriate for males, predominantly only of a certain age. Early treatment would similarly only be relevant for populations of fairly limited size.

or for manufacture. The effectiveness of this hypothetical AIDS vaccine is unknown, as well as the year in which it might be available. Will those who receive the vaccine in turn stop using condoms? How many new HIV infections will there be in 2030 or 2040 to avert? Who will receive the vaccine? Finally, and perhaps most importantly, should an AIDS vaccine be prioritized over alternative approaches to HIV and AIDS prevention?

Based on the paper by Hecht and Jamison, there appears to be a strong case for developing an AIDS vaccine. However, it is important to recognize that resources are limited and therefore funds allocated to an AIDS vaccine will not be available for other interventions, such as the scale-up of male circumcision, an expanded distribution of condoms, increased treatment, etc. As previously indicated, policy-makers face the choice of spending over $13 billion on an AIDS vaccine that might not avert one HIV infection until 2030, vs. spending $2 billion on male circumcision which could prevent more than three million new HIV infections by 2025 in sub-Saharan Africa.

References

Abdool Karim, Q., Abdool Karim, S. S. *et al.* (2010). Effectiveness and safety of tenofovir gel, an antiretroviral microbicide, for the prevention of HIV infection in women. *Science* **329**(5996): 1168–74.

Auvert, B. D., Rech, D. *et al.* (2011). Effect of the Orange Farm (South Africa) Male Circumcision Roll-Out (ANRS-12126) on the Spread of HIV. 6th IAS Conference on HIV Pathogenesis, Treatment and Prevention. Rome.

Bertrand, J., Njeuhmeli, E. *et al.* (2011). The challenges of costing demand creation for male circumcision in Eastern and Southern Africa. *PLoS One* Upcoming.

Boffey, P. (1984). Vaccine Liability Threatens Supplies. *The New York Times*.

DuBois, S. (2010). What Went Wrong with Gardasil? *CNN Money*.

Fonseca, M. G., Forsythe, S. *et al.* (2010). Modeling HIV vaccines in Brazil: assessing the impact of a future HIV vaccine on reducing new infections, mortality and number of people receiving ARV. *PLoS One* **5**(7): e11736.

Halperin, D. T., Mugurungi, O. *et al.* (2011). A surprising prevention success: why did the HIV epidemic decline in Zimbabwe? *PLoS Med* **8**(2): e1000414.

Hecht, R. and Jamison, D. (2011). Cost-Benefit Analysis of Developing an AIDS Vaccine for Sub-Saharan Africa.

Kirby, D. (2008). Changes in sexual behaviour leading to the decline in the prevalence of HIV in Uganda: confirmation from multiple sources of evidence. *Sex Transm Infect* **84** Suppl 2: ii35–41.

Njeuhmeli, E., Forsythe, S. *et al.* (2011). Voluntary medical male circumcision: modeling the impact and cost of expanding male circumcision for HIV prevention in Eastern and Southern Africa. *PLoS Medicine* **8**(11): e1001132.

Rerks-Ngarm, S., Pitisuttithum, P. *et al.* (2009). Vaccination with ALVAC and AIDSVAX to prevent HIV-1 infection in Thailand. *N Engl J Med* **361**(23): 2209–20.

Sinclair, D., Abba, K. *et al.* (2011). Oral vaccines for preventing cholera. Cochrane Database Syst Rev(3): CD008603.

UNAIDS. (2010). MDG6: Six Things You Need to Know About the AIDS Response Today.

Venkatesh, K. K., Flanigan, T. P. *et al.* (2011). Is expanded HIV treatment preventing new infections? Impact of antiretroviral therapy on sexual risk behaviors in the developing world. *AIDS*.

Vaccine research and development

Perspective paper

JOSHUA A. SALOMON

The aim of *RethinkHIV* is to assess the expected costs and benefits associated with a range of different alternatives for addressing the HIV/AIDS pandemic. The specific charge is to consider how an additional $2 billion per year over the next five years could "best be spent . . . given some reasonable assumptions about sensible policies in subsequent decades."[1] The assessment paper by Hecht, Jamison *et al.*[2] focuses on development and future deployment of a new preventive HIV vaccine (Hecht *et al.* 2011). This perspective paper takes the assessment paper as a starting point, and proceeds in three main sections. The first offers some reflections on the general enterprise of priority-setting for investments in research and development toward future health technologies. The second provides a summary and brief critique of the assessment paper with the aim of drawing out some of the most significant findings from the analysis, and highlighting the implications of these findings and their sensitivity to key assumptions and modeling choices. This second section includes additional figures based on the Hecht and Jamison results in order to emphasize some of these points. The third presents some modest extrapolations of the analyses in the assessment paper to note other important considerations and trade-offs that might be relevant to evaluating the economic attractiveness of investments for development of HIV vaccines. In this final section I offer a brief sketch of how vaccines might be compared to other options for research and development on new tools against HIV/AIDS.

On priority setting for investments in new technologies

The overall objective in this enterprise, to assess the costs and benefits of alternative decisions regarding competing "solutions" (in the vocabulary of *RethinkHIV*) to the HIV/AIDS pandemic, presents a number of formidable challenges in general. Data limitations are considerable, uncertainty is ubiquitous, and comparability across possible solutions demands standardization of methods and social value choices. With respect to the assessment, in particular, of putative new technologies that may or may not actually emerge at some time in the future, these challenges are amplified in several important ways. First, there are additional uncertainties that derive from the fact that the assessment must necessarily be based on some postulated characteristics of a technology and associated strategies for delivering this technology, none of which yet exist. Will the technology indeed be attained, and if so, when will it be ready for deployment? How will it be formulated, and how efficacious will this formulation be? What will be the costs of producing the technology and delivering it to the target population? Resolution of these uncertainties is essential to understanding the potential returns to investments in research and development on new tools, but at the time of the investment decision, such resolution can only be speculative. Second, and on a related note, research and development decisions typically are made before strategies for delivering the new technology are fully specified, whereas most of the economic evaluation is preoccupied with trade-offs between alternatives that are already available, evaluated in their current specifications. This means that economic evaluation of an investment in research and development requires

[1] This language derives from the *RethinkHIV* guidance to authors.
[2] Hereafter "Hecht and Jamison" for brevity, although credit is due to co-authors Jared Augenstein, Gabrielle Partridge, and Kira Thorien.

consideration of a branching decision, with at least two stages separated by a significant time lag. Should we invest now in a technology that may be ready at a certain date and have a certain efficacy and cost? This choice depends on anticipating the resolution of a later decision: once a technology is available, how should it be deployed? (And, for that matter, will it be worth deploying compared to other competing alternatives that may also be available at that future time?) The qualifier in the mandate for *RethinkHIV* quoted at the beginning of this paper (to identify optimal choices at present "given some reasonable assumptions about sensible policies in subsequent decades") is significant, and nowhere more so than for the vaccine case.

At this juncture, it is useful to pause and draw an important distinction that is not always clearly articulated, between *technologies, interventions*, and *strategies*. Health *technologies*, broadly defined, include such things as devices and diagnostic assays, but also drugs, vaccines, and surgical procedures. *Interventions* may be understood as processes and standards for administering technologies to individuals, for example characterized by specific indications, target populations, and dosing schedules in the cases of drugs or vaccines. *Strategies* (or policies) may be defined as particular adoptable decisions and operational plans aimed at delivering interventions to defined populations, which require contextualization of intervention delivery within existing (or planned) systems and constraints on available resources. Taking the example of a preventive HIV vaccine, a particular vaccine formulation would be a technology, an associated intervention might be a three-dose immunization schedule for those ten years and older, and a strategy might be a national school-based program to immunize ten-year-olds, in combination with a catch-up campaign focusing on national HIV immunization days targeting the baseline population of 10–49-year-olds who were not exposed to the school-based program in the past.

This distinction between technologies, interventions, and strategies has some bearing on how we locate the evaluation of vaccine development within the context of *RethinkHIV*. Scanning across the options presented in the assessment papers, we see that the other solutions being considered are predominantly strategies based on current technologies. For technologies that already exist, economic evaluation of the technology itself has limited meaning. Only a specific strategy accommodates an interpretable assessment of costs and benefits. For a future technology, on the other hand, evaluating the investment required to successfully develop one technology vs. another does make sense. Such an evaluation, as noted above, is complicated by the need to know – or to speculate – about the decisions that will be taken once the technology is available for deployment.

Another relevant issue concerns the source of financing for vaccine development, in relation to financing of other current strategies. Hecht and Jamison argue that the analysis of investments in HIV vaccines should not be viewed as competing with spending on today's efforts at treatment and prevention. However, it seems to me that this argument is only partially correct. Continuing with the distinction drawn above, while it is true that financing for development of the technology itself is not likely to draw from the same resources as ongoing treatment and prevention strategies, it is also the case that once a vaccine is developed, any strategy for scaling up delivery of this vaccine will indeed compete with other HIV control strategies for a severely constrained resource pool, derived mostly from domestic HIV/AIDS budgets and official development assistance. Later in this perspective paper I will highlight the relative contributions of different cost components to the overall cost of developing and deploying a new vaccine, as quantified in Hecht and Jamison. For now, suffice it to say that the development cost evidently represents a rather small minority of the total costs of vaccine-based solutions, and this observation has important implications for weighing the costs and benefits of investing in vaccines vs. alternative uses of scarce resources.

Assessment paper summary and critique

The authors of the assessment paper have produced a thoughtful and thorough examination of the range

of considerations relevant to decisions on investment in a preventive HIV vaccine. Overall, they
make a convincing case that further funding for
vaccine development will likely yield high social
value over the several decades after a vaccine is
introduced, assuming that it has at least moderate
efficacy. The assessment paper includes a review of
the array of other research and development options
that is clear and concise, and the authors' justification for focusing on vaccines amidst these other
options seems reasonable. The information on past
financing for AIDS vaccine research is also very
useful, and the thorough review of past and ongoing vaccine trials in the Appendix will be a valuable
resource for those interested in this topic. Assessment of the costs and benefits of a future vaccine
is complicated by some of the added uncertainties
about the future course of the epidemic, vaccine
characteristics, and deployment strategies, as discussed above, so it required some effort to try to
understand all of the computations at the heart of
the Hecht and Jamison analysis, and to navigate
through the many different variants of the analyses.
As not all of the calculations were fully described
in the paper, it was not possible to replicate the
analysis, so I will focus my comments on the main
assumptions and results as reported, with a view
toward identifying the key findings that stand out
amidst the extensive array of results reported in
the paper.[3] Overall, I found appealing the approach
of basing the analysis on a relatively simple set of
computations rather than developing a complex and
inscrutable model, although there are inevitable pitfalls that result from simplifying assumptions and
computational shortcuts, and I will try to identify
some of the most important of these.

Hecht and Jamison present a wide span of benefit
to cost ratios, ranging between 2 and 97 in Table
6.7. In Figure 6.2.1 below, I have summarized the
results from Tables 6.4, 6.5, and 6.6 in terms of the
components of costs and benefits across an array
of analytic variants that differ in terms of baseline
epidemiologic scenarios, discount rates, valuations
for a year of life, assumed costs per fully immunized
person, and assumed year of introduction of a new
vaccine.

The purpose of Figure 6.2.1 is to unpack the
estimates of benefits and costs across the different

scenarios and sets of assumptions so that we may
focus on two key observations that were not emphasized in the assessment paper. The first observation
is that the major component of costs is not the
development cost but the delivery cost, across all
epidemiologic scenarios and values for discount
rates, vaccine prices, and valuations of life years.
This is important to highlight because it offers a
counterpoint to the argument that vaccine development does not necessitate trade-offs against preventive or curative interventions. Certainly, once
a vaccine is developed, widespread delivery will
demand a great deal of resources from both domestic budgets and bilateral and multilateral channels
for development assistance, and there will surely
be an opportunity cost in the form of other forgone
options for intervening against HIV/AIDS.

The second observation, on the benefits side, is
that only a small fraction of the expected benefits from a new vaccine with high coverage would
be from averted costs of anti-retroviral therapy
or (smaller still) treatment for opportunistic infections. The largest component of benefits, by a wide
margin, is the social value of healthy life years.
This observation further underscores the point that
delivery of a vaccine would demand a vast scale-
up of new resources, as the cost of producing and
delivering the vaccine is unlikely to be recovered
fully from savings due to other expenditures on
HIV/AIDS. We return to this point in the final
section below.

Another way to distill the findings across the
many different variants presented in the assessment
paper is to construct a set of one-way sensitivity
analyses on each of the key assumptions and value
choices that parameterize the array of results in
the paper. Figure 6.2.2 presents the results from
such an exercise, defining a base-case through relatively straightforward manipulation of the reported

---

[3] I also confine my remarks to the analysis of investment in
AIDS vaccine development at continued high levels, rather
than to expanded investment to speed the availability of a
vaccine. The latter was added to the analysis during the
RethinkHIV expert panel meeting, after the completion of
this paper. Because the additional analysis is described par-
simoniously in the revised assessment paper, I found it difficult to evaluate the assumptions and computations behind
this addition.

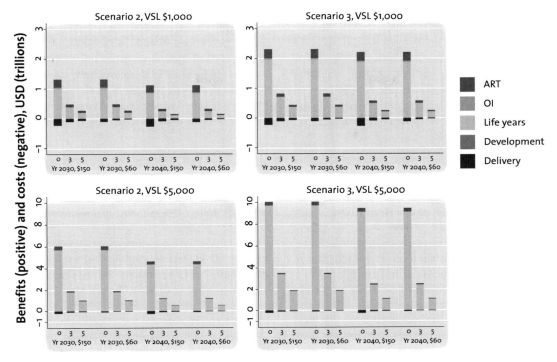

Figure 6.2.1 *Components of costs and benefits for a new preventive HIV vaccine*

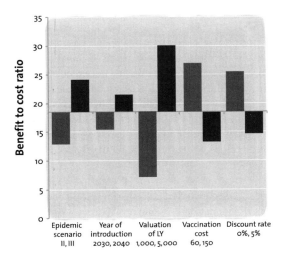

Figure 6.2.2 *One-way sensitivity analyses on key assumptions and value choices*

results, and characterized by the following assumptions: (1) discount rate of 3 percent per year; (2) vaccine cost of $100 per complete dose; (3)

valuation of a year of life at $3,000; (4) baseline epidemiologic circumstances between Scenarios II and III (approximated by averaging results computed separately for each of these two scenarios); and (5) vaccine introduction in 2035 (approximated by averaging results computed separately for 2030 and 2040).[4]

For the base-case analysis, the benefit to cost ratio was around 18.5. Figure 6.2.2 shows clearly that the most influential assumption was that regarding the valuation of a year of life. Among the remaining parameters considered, the next most influential was the cost of vaccination, and the least consequential assumption pertained to the year of vaccine introduction.

[4] An earlier version of the assessment paper in fact defined a base-case using the first three of these assumptions, but the revised paper has focused instead on examining scenarios based on the high and low range values for each parameter. For the purpose of conducting one-way sensitivity analyses, it is useful to define a base-case using intermediate values, so we adopted the values from the earlier version.

Extensions and concluding remarks

I would like to conclude this perspective paper by elaborating somewhat on the previously mentioned concern for financing, and considering what this implies for the evaluation of vaccines relative to other options under consideration. In comparing the expected benefits and expected costs of developing and delivering a new HIV vaccine, an element that is missing is an analysis of the financial (as opposed to "economic") implications of vaccination. Specifically, there is a question of the totality of the resources that will be required to implement the ambitious coverage targets analyzed in the assessment paper. One point to note is that by reporting on the sum of outcomes in the first twenty-five years after a vaccine is introduced, important issues around the timing of costs (for delivery) and cost offsets (from averted treatment of AIDS with antiretrovirals or treatment of opportunistic infections) are obscured. Putting those timing issues aside for a moment, we may begin by comparing the net financial costs of implementing vaccination, computed as the costs of delivery minus the averted costs for ART and treatment of opportunistic infections. The range in these values across the scenarios is substantial, from a net cost of around $56 billion to a net saving of around $190 billion. Of note, it is not the case that vaccination would under all circumstances be expected to produce cost savings. In twenty of the forty-eight scenarios examined, vaccination would actually increase the costs of treatment and prevention over this period (assuming all else were equal apart from the captured ART and OI costs).

As noted above, consideration only of the total cost misses the important lag between expenditures on vaccination and subsequent recovery of these costs through averted treatment, which means that even if a vaccine appears cost-saving, based on the present value of expenditures in all years, that does not necessarily mean that it will be cost-saving in terms of the financial resources required in all specific budget periods. Based on the assumptions in the assessment paper, the lag between vaccination and averted treatment is not trivial. In equilibrium, the assessment paper envisions an adolescent vaccination strategy, assuming the first dose would

be administered around age ten. The assessment paper further assumes that the average age at infection is twenty-five. A reasonable estimate for the delay from infection to the need for ART (based on current eligibility criteria, the push for earlier treatment as prevention notwithstanding) is around eight years. Thus, in the early period of vaccine scale-up, the expectation of cost savings would not be realized for an average of twenty-three years, so virtually all resources for vaccination would need to be incremental on all other expenditures for HIV/AIDS at that time.

What, then, would be the order of magnitude for these expenditures? Again, taking the figures in the assessment paper as the point of reference, we may estimate that to attain a coverage of 80 percent for new cohorts of persons turning ten, while at the same time scaling up among the baseline population over a ten-year period (implying additional vaccination of approximately 10 percent of 674 million people), the required number of vaccinations administered during the first year of the program would be around 100 million. Maintaining the two values of either $60 or $150 for administering a full course of vaccination (including a first dose and two later boosters), we may assume a cost of at least $20 or $50 for the first dose; if the full-course estimates include some fixed costs associated with developing infrastructure and systems for vaccination then this single-dose estimate will be biased downward. Based on these assumptions the total cost in the first several years of the program would be on the order of at least $2 to $5 billion per year. This cost would presumably multiply a few years later as the early vaccination cohorts began to require boosters.

There have several recent attempts to characterize current expenditures on HIV/AIDS from different sources, including overseas development assistance and national country resources. The latest report on global health financing from the Institute for Health Metrics and Evaluation estimated that in the year 2008 a total of around $6 billion was spent on HIV/AIDS through bilateral and multilateral assistance, which likely constituted the minority of all spending on HIV/AIDS when combined with domestic resources (IHME 2010). Similar figures on development assistance were reported by Hecht and colleagues (2009), who estimated

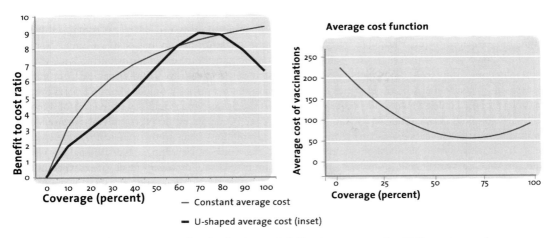

Figure 6.2.3 *Benefit to cost ratios for developing and delivering a preventive HIV vaccine under alternative assumptions about vaccination coverage*

the total spending for AIDS in developing countries, including public and private domestic spending, to be more than $15 billion in 2008. Following a number of prior efforts to project resource needs for HIV/AIDS, Hecht and colleagues have also developed forecasts of HIV/AIDS financing needs through 2031, and estimated that the total need would be on the order of approximately $35 billion in that year (Hecht *et al.* 2010). Assuming, as argued above, that the resources needed for vaccination would be largely additive to the needs expressed in these estimates (i.e., for prevention efforts, delivery of treatment, etc.), an estimate of approximately $5 billion per year for vaccination alone constitutes a sizeable increment to the baseline estimate of resource need.

In light of concerns about possible affordability of a scale-up strategy with high coverage targets, it is worth considering how different assumptions about attainable coverage targets would impact on the benefit to cost ratios reported in the assessment paper. All vaccination scenarios in the paper assumed coverage of 80 percent. Figure 6.2.3 shows how the benefit-to-cost ratio for one variant reported in the paper (assuming a discount rate of 3 percent, a vaccine arriving in 2030 at an average cost of $60, and a valuation of $1,000 for a year of healthy life) would vary as a function of the assumed vaccination coverage rate. The shape of the curve depends only on the combination of

a fixed development cost with delivery costs and benefits that vary linearly with respect to coverage. The general shape of the curve is preserved across the different variants of the analysis. Figure 6.2.3 also presents an alternative set of estimates for benefit to cost ratios in relation to coverage, under the assumption of a U-shaped average cost function. The particular function chosen (shown in the inset) was arbitrary, in order to serve as an illustrative example, but the level of the curve was deliberately adjusted so that the average cost at a coverage level of 80 percent was $60, to match the value in the constant average cost function base-case.

As the figure illustrates, assuming that benefits scale linearly with coverage but that only delivery (and not development) costs scale linearly with coverage implies that benefit-to-cost ratios will be increasing in coverage. If we further assume that the average cost function is not flat but U-shaped, then the decline in the benefit to cost ratio as coverage declines is sharpened, with the ratio falling by approximately half as the coverage is halved from 80 percent to 40 percent. Compared to the sensitivity analyses shown previously in Figure 6.2.2, this simple example suggests that coverage assumptions could be more influential than any of the other parameter values that were varied in this analysis, apart from the valuation assigned to a year of life.

Finally, let me offer a few brief thoughts regarding how investments in developing a new vaccine might be compared to other possible investments in new technologies. Taking the other potentially game-changing future technology mentioned in the assessment paper, which would be a drug to clear the body of HIV, under what circumstances might such a technology present an equally attractive option for increased investment as a preventive vaccine? To begin to answer this question, we may consider the total costs and benefits of these alternatives at the time that they become available. For the vaccine, based on Table 6.5, we may first compute the "number needed to treat" to prevent one infection through vaccination; this number ranges between around 90 and 230 across scenarios, with an average value around 150. At an average cost of $60 per vaccinated person this implies a total cost of around $9,000 to prevent one infection. At an average cost of $150 per vaccinated person, the cost per infection averted would be $22,500. Turning to benefits, if the averted infection were immediately following vaccination, the present value at the incremental life years gained would be between seven and ten years at a discount rate of 3 percent. If the lag between vaccination and the averted infection were fifteen years (as for a vaccinated ten-year-old expected to be infected at age twenty-five), then the gains drop to 5–6 years. Locating a value around the middle of these ranges, assume seven years gained per vaccination, which then combines with the cost estimate to yield a cost per life year gained – at the time of vaccination – of around $1,300 or $3,000, depending on the cost of the vaccination.

Following a similar logic for a curative drug, let us imagine that treatment eligibility occurs around eight years after infection, so that treated patients enjoy a remaining life expectancy of seventeen years vs. only three years for untreated patients. This might be a conservative assumption, as it is based on the premise that a curative drug would produce similar overall benefits as lifetime treatment with current therapies, as opposed to restoring infected people to the same life expectancy as uninfected people. Even under this conservative assumption the present value of the gain,

discounted at 3 percent, would be around ten years. Equating the value of the gains through vaccination or cure, this implies that we might be willing to substitute one cure for one vaccine even if the cure cost up to $13,000 or $30,000, assuming the beneficiary would otherwise be untreated. If the beneficiary would have been treated anyway, there is no gain in life years under the conservative assumptions here, so the trade-off for the curative drug would be only the net reduction (if any) in the lifetime cost of treatment. In any case, it seems safe to say that a curative drug, priced at a reasonable level, would compare quite favorably to a vaccine that were available at the same time. Extending this comparison to the present-day decision about investments in research and development requires some quantification of the likelihood that further research toward each technology will bear fruit over the coming decades. Pending such an assessment, an acknowledgment of the timing differences in the realization of benefits from vaccines and drugs, and the complementarity in the populations of beneficiaries, points at least to the modest conclusion that further investments toward curative drugs are worth pursuing alongside continued funding for research on preventive vaccines.

References

Hecht, R., Bollinger, L., Stover, J., McGreevey, W., Muhib, F., Madavo, C. E. and De Ferranti, D. (2009). Critical choices in financing the response to the global HIV/AIDS pandemic. *Health Affairs* **28**(6): 1591–605.

Hecht, R., Jamison, D. T., Augenstein, J., Partridge, G. and Thorien, K. Cost-benefit analysis of developing an AIDS vaccine for sub-Saharan Africa. [This volume.]

Hecht, R., Stover, J., Bollinger, L., Muhib, F., Case, K. and De Ferranti, D. (2010). Financing of HIV/AIDS programme scale-up in low-income and middle-income countries 2009–31. *Lancet* **376**: 1254–60.

Institute for Health Metrics and Evaluation. (2010). *Financing Global Health 2010: Development Assistance and Country Spending in Economic Uncertainty*. Seattle, WA: IHME.

PART II
Ranking the opportunities

Findings of the Nobel laureate economist expert panel

ERNEST ARYEETEY, PAUL COLLIER, EDWARD C.
PRESCOTT, THOMAS C. SCHELLING, AND
VERNON L. SMITH

In September 2011, a panel of economic experts, comprising five of the world's most distinguished economists, convened at Georgetown University to interview the authors of the eighteen research chapters presented in *RethinkHIV*. The members of the Georgetown University Expert Panel were:

- Professor Ernest Aryeetey, Vice Chancellor, University of Ghana;
- Professor Paul Collier, Director, Centre for the Study of African Economies, Oxford University;
- Professor Edward Prescott, Arizona State University (Nobel laureate);
- Professor Thomas Schelling, University of Maryland (Nobel laureate);
- Professor Vernon L. Smith, Chapman University (Nobel laureate).

During the roundtable meeting, the panel appraised the research and engaged with the eighteen sets of authors. This built on the panel's experience over the course of 2011 of examining and reviewing draft versions of the research papers.

The panel was tasked with answering the question:

> If we successfully raised an additional $10 billion over the next five years to combat HIV/AIDS in sub-Saharan Africa, how could it best be spent?

In ordering the proposals, the panel was guided predominantly by consideration of economic costs and benefits. The panel agreed that the cost-benefit approach was an indispensable organizing method. In setting priorities, the panel took account of the strengths and weaknesses of the specific cost-benefit appraisals under review, and gave weight both to the institutional preconditions for success and to the demands of ethical or humanitarian urgency.

As a general point, the panel concluded that there is a clear and urgent need for more high-quality analysis of the costs and benefits of many responses to the HIV/AIDS epidemic. Considering the toll of the epidemic, and the amount of money that is being allocated, the panel found the lack of evaluation of interventions alarming. The panel found an overwhelming need for policy-makers to be better informed when making decisions among competing HIV/AIDS priorities.

Each panel member assigned his own ranking to the proposals. The panel jointly endorses the priority list shown overleaf as representing their agreed, consensus view on priorities.

On specific interventions, the panel offers the following comments, sorted by chapter.

Vaccine research and development

Unlike every other investment option examined, the proposal to increase vaccine research spending (Chapter 6) has, at the upper-end of possible outcomes, the opportunity of achieving potential long-term eradication of HIV.

Even using extremely cautious assumptions and focusing on lower-end possible outcomes, it is likely that spending an extra $100 million per year on vaccine research outside the prevailing funding channels will meaningfully shorten the time in which a vaccine is developed. This represents around a 10 percent increase in current funding

Table 7.1 Expert economist panel outcome

Intervention	Chapter
1 Accelerate AIDS vaccine development by scaling up funding for innovative vaccine research by 10 percent or $100 million per year	Vaccine research and development
2 Introduce and scale up medical infant male circumcision to reach 50 percent coverage	Prevention of sexual transmission
3 Prevent mother-to-child transmission by scaling up Option A treatment of pregnant women and breastfeeding infants to 90 percent coverage in all countries	Prevention of non-sexual transmission
4 Make blood transfusions safe by achieving 100 percent coverage of quality-assured HIV testing of donated blood	Prevention of non-sexual transmission
5 Scale up antiretroviral treatment starting with the most sick and most infectious patients first	Treatment
6 Make 95 percent of medical injections safe by providing adequate supply of auto-disposable syringes and training of health staff in medical equipment disposal	Prevention of non-sexual transmission
7 Scale-up male circumcision for young adults in high HIV prevalence countries	Prevention of sexual transmission
8 One-time innovative information campaign using mass media and peer group counseling in high HIV prevalence countries	Prevention of sexual transmission
9 Large-scale home- and clinic-based HIV testing and counseling focusing on young adults in high HIV prevalence countries	Prevention of sexual transmission
10 Create incentive for less risky sexual behavior by offering conditional cash transfers for all girls from impoverished families to keep girls in secondary school	Social Policy
11 Reduce risky injecting drug user behavior in Kenya, South Africa and Tanzania by increasing coverage rate to 60 percent for outreach, information and education campaigns, needle and syringe exchange programs and opioid substitution therapy	Prevention of non-sexual transmission
12 Focused treatment of HIV patients to reduce the opportunistic infection of Cryptococcal Meningitis	Strengthening health systems
13 Add gender and HIV training to micro-finance and livelihood programs to reach 1.7 million adults or 20 percent of the adult population currently enrolled	Social Policy
14 Introduce 25 percent increase in alcohol tax in countries with moderate-to-high levels of drinking and high adult mortality	Social Policy
15 Increase coverage of community mobilization and stigma reduction programs by 30 percent or 18 million adults	Social Policy
16 Create incentive for universal testing, information and counseling with a conditional cash transfer of US$5 to all 400 million adults	Strengthening health systems
17 Enhance numbers, training and skill-development of community health workers to strengthen basic health services for the rural population	Strengthening health systems
18 Create an Abuja Goals Fund offering a 'cash-on-delivery' incentive to nations that meet Abuja Declaration target of spending 15 percent of public revenues on public health	Strengthening health systems

levels. This spending could accelerate the number of years to the introduction of a vaccine by at least half to one-and-a-half years, even using conservative assumptions.

Another important consideration is that the bulk of the overall costs of this investment will come not from developing but from distribution of the vaccine, which is a future cost.

Based on these considerations, the panel found vaccine research to be a compelling investment.

Prevention of sexual transmission

The panel found that, in general, male circumcision offers considerable opportunities to reduce the scale of the epidemic.

The research (Chapter 1) found a strong benefit to cost ratio for adult male circumcision (not as high as blood transfusions or mother-to-child transmission, but very high). The panel noted that scaling up adult male circumcision (with accompanying campaigns) could well be more costly than is typically assumed in order to generate significant demand on the population level, causing a lower benefit to cost ratio.

The panel also observed that although disinhibition effects are documented to be small or non-existent in pilot studies, these are based on small, typically voluntary samples, and that when scaled up the disinhibition effect could likely escalate, further lowering the benefit to cost ratio. The key incentive for adult males to be circumcised would undoubtedly be that unprotected multi-partner sexual intercourse would become less risky. This could potentially change behavior, inducing more unprotected sexual encounters. Evidently, in societies where circumcision as an infant is a social norm, the net effect is to reduce AIDS. But one could only safely extrapolate from this to the effect of adult circumcision as a choice were everybody always fully aware of the objective risks they run in a sexual encounter. In fact, it is known that misunderstandings and misperceptions of risks are fundamental to the spread of AIDS.

In highlighting circumcision, they focused on infant male circumcision, where the surgical procedure cost is significantly lower, the demand generation cost likely to be considerably lower, and the risk of disinhibition very low. The drawback, of course, is that it will only work 15–20 years from now. With discounting, the cost to benefit ratio is comparable with AMC, but without the attendant behavioral risk factors.

The lower rankings assigned to mass media information campaigns and large-scale testing and counseling reflected the lack of reliable data and analysis showing where and how these campaigns work, despite the fact that anecdotally some of these campaigns have clearly had some impact.

Prevention of non-sexual infection

The panel found scaling up the prevention of mother-to-child transmission (Chapter 2) to be a compelling investment not just for ethical reasons, but also because of the considerable benefit-to-cost ratios, very low costs, and strong evidence of its effectiveness.

Making blood transfusions safer was also considered a compelling investment. Apart from the number of lives saved, the panel found value in the increase in public trust of health systems should transfusions be made safer.

The other two investment options considered by the panel under this topic, making medical injections safer, and reducing risky injecting drug-user behavior, were given a lower but still fair ranking based on their lower benefit to cost ratios.

Treatment

The panel gave a high ranking to the proposal of scaling up ART enrollment (Chapter 3), focusing on extending coverage to patients with low CD4 counts. Despite its high costs, the preventative effect of ART means that the benefits of scaling up ART are considerable. Moreover the ethical imperative to continue treatment was deemed to be overwhelming and best informed by a decision to treat where most cost-beneficial first.

Social policy

The panel endorses using social policy levers (Chapter 5) in an effort to reduce the economic and social factors that fuel HIV risk behaviors and undermine proven HIV interventions.

While the panel believes that the use of cash transfers to keep girls in schooling is a sound policy choice, they formed the view that the benefits relating to HIV/AIDS were a small element of its overall effects.

They gave a lower ranking to the use of an alcohol tax, reflecting concerns about its implementation given the possibility it could reduce overall revenue for developing nations and encourage substitution of licensed beverages with more alcoholic and toxic "home brews."

Adding gender and HIV training to livelihood programs and community mobilization investment show promise, and the panel find a need for further analysis and research into these.

Strengthening health systems

The panel found the prevention of cryptococcal meningitis (Chapter 4) an overlooked policy with merit.

In examining the cash transfer for counseling and testing, the panel noted that while cash transfers can be used successfully, design is very important. There is a significant risk that this intervention could ruin natural incentives for knowledge about one's own health status. They did not find that the proposed cash transfer structure had an optimal set-up, and ranked this as a lower priority policy option.

While recognizing the potential benefits of deploying community health workers, the panel found that the costs could be considerably higher than those identified.

The panel feared that the set-up of an Abuja Goals Fund, as proposed, would lead to indiscriminate spending on health with little measure of whether or not the spending was optimal.

Findings from African civil society

BACTRIN KILLINGO, NDUKU KILONZO, CHRISTIANA LANIYAN, RETTA MENBERU, AND KEN ODUMBE

On December 4, 2011, delegates at the International Conference on AIDS and STIs in Africa (ICASA) held in Addis Ababa were invited by the Rush Foundation and the Copenhagen Consensus Center to attend a pre-conference satellite meeting to learn about the research papers published in *RethinkHIV*.

A panel of civil society representatives led a discussion about HIV/AIDS priorities. A similar discussion took place at a youth forum organized for Addis Ababa University Public Health School students. The panel comprised:

- Bactrin Killingo;
- Nduku Kilonzo;
- Christiana Laniyan;
- Retta Menberu;
- Ken Odumbe.

Two members of this panel, Bactrin Killingo and Ken Odumbe, had also attended the Nobel laureate meeting at Georgetown University in September 2011, and were part of the project's planning and dialogue process.

All of the civil society panel members examined the draft research papers in advance of the conferences in Addis Ababa.

The events in Addis Ababa in December were designed to provide a framework for African civil society and youth to review key recommendations generated by the research presented in this volume, and to agree on a set of bold, new, actionable priorities for HIV and AIDS spending in Africa.

In this chapter, the members of the civil society panel set out their perspectives regarding the project's goals, achievements, and specific findings.

The panel stresses that HIV and AIDS remain major challenges to the development of sub-Saharan Africa (SSA). Mortality and morbidity caused by the epidemic contribute significantly to

Table 7.1.1 ICASA civil society outcome

	Intervention	Chapter
1	Prevent mother-to-child transmission by scaling up Option A treatment of pregnant women and breastfeeding infants to 90 percent coverage in all countries	Prevention of sexual transmission
2	Scale up anti-retroviral treatment starting with the most sick and most infectious patients first	Treatment
3	Create incentive for less risky sexual behavior by offering conditional cash transfers for all girls from impoverished families to keep girls in secondary school	Social policy
4	Create an Abuja Goals Fund offering a "cash-on-delivery" incentive to nations that meet the Abuja Declaration target of spending 15 percent of public revenues on public health	Strengthening health systems
5	Make blood transfusions safe by achieving 100 percent coverage of quality-assured HIV testing of donated blood	Prevention of non-sexual transmission
6	Accelerate AIDS vaccine development by scaling up funding for innovative vaccine research by 10 percent or $100 million per year	Vaccine research and development
7	Scale up male circumcision for young adults in high HIV prevalence countries	Prevention of sexual transmission
8	Introduce 25 percent increase in alcohol tax in countries with moderate-to-high levels of drinking and high adult mortality	Social policy

the failure to attain the Millennium Development Goals in Africa, and have impacts on all sectors of development.

The project's theme of "redefining priorities" is deemed particularly timely in the wake of the global economic crisis which is already having negative impacts in Africa. Funding shortfalls, donor fatigue, and competing global priorities such as the food crisis, climate change, and fuel crisis make it likely that there will be less money for AIDS programs in Africa.

Ken Odumbe highlights that with African nations relying, on average, on foreign assistance for about 80 percent of HIV/AIDS funding, any interruptions to resource flows have serious implications. HIV programs are vulnerable.

Panelists stress that addressing the issue of the sustainability and predictability of long-term AIDS funding is critical for African governments. It is imperative that the region confronts not only the realities of how to raise additional resources to fight the epidemic but also considers more effective and efficient ways to deploy available resources. Establishing how to prioritize interventions – doing more with less and making difficult choices between competing interventions – was deemed crucial.

"The research project *RethinkHIV* demonstrates the importance of adopting evidence-based, scientific prioritization processes that should help to guide decision-making at all levels," underlines Bactrin Killingo.

Furthermore, he observes that the prioritization exercises that have been held as part of the project – at Georgetown University and in Addis Ababa – have revealed the different perspectives of stakeholders. It is important that these different points of view are brought together to make decisions on the basis of evidence.

The project demonstrated how different interest groups can interpret the same evidence differently and prioritize various interventions accordingly. One example of this is the way that male circumcision was prioritized. This intervention was ranked high by both the Nobel laureates and the Global Fund Forum, yet received a much lower ranking by African civil society and Addis Ababa public health students.

Differences could exemplify the fact that, historically, decisions have been made "top-down" even when they might be perceived to be less relevant by certain communities on the ground. The *RethinkHIV* process was able to draw attention to such differences, and to stress the importance of starting at the level where services are actually provided and then move upwards.

On the top four-ranked specific interventions, the civil society panel offers the following comments.

Prevent mother to child transmission (PMTCT)

The panel members agree that this intervention ought to be a top priority. Shifts in the HIV/AIDS epidemic that have been witnessed over the last decade suggest progress in the prevention of transmission of the virus, yet vertical transmission still counts for a significant proportion of new HIV infections.

Christiana Laniyan outlines the importance of this investment:

> Given the number of women and children who benefit from this intervention and the fact that the resources required to achieve these targets are not large, as well as the cost-benefit ratio, this intervention ought to be the number one focus. Furthermore, additional benefits of PMTCT interventions include increased family planning uptake and its effect in improving maternal health, reduced child and infant mortality and morbidity, as well as health systems strengthening.

She also notes the data presented by Lori Bollinger (Chapter 2) indicating that there was a 24 percent decrease in infections among new infants between 2001 and 2009, yet one-third of this reduction occurred in 2009 alone due to increased resource allocation and effective programming. Thus, it can be argued that with a strategy that targets reduction of MTCT, it is possible within a very short timeframe to effectively eliminate this mode of transmission and to see a generation of African children born without the virus.

Nduku Kilonzo points out that the high median benefit to cost ratio of PMTCT was based on effects on the child only:

> Drawing on prior discussions of the interconnectedness of policy and interventions, prioritizing PMTCT must take into cognizance that not saving the mother's life may have a primary cost to the life of the child and incremental costs in other life areas that are not currently calculated. Further, evidence demonstrates that children cared

for by mothers have lower levels of mortality and morbidity and are more likely to be productive adults.

Therefore, Nduku Kilonzo concludes, a policy decision on this basis would posit additional cost-benefit-related questions such as: what is the value of a child with a live, healthy mother versus that of a child without a live, healthy mother? And what is the benefit to cost ratio of PMTCT when the child's mother is on/not on long-term ART?

Scale up ART enrollment

The panel notes that the median benefit to cost ratio of scaling up ART (Chapter 3) is low compared to other interventions; however, evidence on ART as prevention and the moral imperative for treatment necessitate that scale-up of ART remains a priority. Retta Menberu feels strongly that ART needs to be scaled up, yet he acknowledges that:

> Given the current financing shortfalls and general climate of donor fatigue, efforts to scale up ART enrollment face formidable challenges and resources for policy-makers are limited.

Furthermore, Nduku Kilonzo observes that scaling up ART has the potential to absorb most, if not all, of the financing presently available for HIV:

> However, in view of the high incidence, with 3 new infections for every 2 people put on treatment, ART scale-up without prevention interventions to reduce incidence is unsustainable. Thus, policy priorities will need to establish trade-offs between: 1) offering ART and making tough prioritization decisions based on the highest impact and need. For instance, in generalized epidemics, sero-discordant couples or women of reproductive health age (to attain PMTCT goals) may be prioritized; and 2) retaining funds for delivering optimal mix of HIV prevention interventions.

She points out that the impact and cost-benefit of delivering different combinations of proven prevention interventions for different populations is currently unknown, yet is essential:

> Logically therefore, the investment in ART scale-up will only reduce in cost and increase benefits

accrued over time if delivered alongside effective prevention where incidence is reduced, making investment in combination prevention an imperative for ART scale-up.

Bactrin Killingo underscores the need for a gradual scale-up of ART to eventually reach everyone:

> Although we cannot treat everyone now, there shouldn't be a flat-lining of treatment. Treatment needs to be extended to those most critically ill first, then consider all those patients with CD4 counts of between 250 and 350. It would be great to also put those with higher CD4 counts but are well on treatment for preventative purposes depending on available resources.

He further notes that resources are needed to deal with the obstacles that relate to testing and treatment; people still don't want to get tested because they are not sure if and where they will get treated.

Cash transfers to keep girls in schooling

The panel underlines the importance of investment in girls' education (Chapter 5), especially in relation to its benefits that extend beyond HIV prevention. This intervention contributes to a broader range of national goals and priorities. Christiana Laniyan expands on these benefits:

> These types of investments in girls' education not only help reduce HIV and AIDS but also have other benefits and important development gains including family planning uptake, reduced reproductive health mortality and morbidity, to name a few.

Nduku Kilonzo underscores this point by pointing out that policy decisions are not made in isolation: "They are informed by inter-connectedness of sector plans, resource envelopes, and operational guidance by government, a factor that may often be not considered in cost-benefit analysis of specific interventions." She notes that most sub-Saharan African governments do not have dedicated HIV resource envelopes within the national budgets:

> Those that provide HIV financing make allocations primarily through health and also other sector

budgets premised on a multi-sectoral response. With less HIV financing internationally, prioritization and innovation in financing must take into consideration interventions that accrue benefits beyond HIV in order to influence investments from other sectors. Cash transfers for keeping girls in school could be funded by the education sector with benefits for HIV prevention. The effects of conditionality of cash transfers require further research. These interventions provide a framework against which gender and HIV training can be adapted into cash transfer programs, based on the assumption that this would enhance women's and girls' empowerment, and reduce risk behavior and intimate partner violence at marginal costs.

Create an Abuja Fund

The creation of an Abuja Goals Fund (Chapter 4) is based on a "cash-on-delivery" incentive to nations that meet the Abuja Declaration target of 15 percent of public revenues on public health spending.

Christiana Laniyan observes that most SSA countries are not allocating enough resources to health and the development sector or even matching spending with allocation, which will be required if HIV and AIDS programs are to be sustained for benefits to accrue over time:

> While I recognize the challenges most countries face in raising needed resources for development, the disproportionately high security budgets of the many countries only illustrates the priority given to human development.

> Considering the vicious cycle that exists between low educational attainment, unemployment, and poverty on the one hand with insecurity on the other hand, African nations must stop the inadequate budgeting to the social-sector of the economy and any incentives to get them to do this will be most appreciated.

However, the panel expresses some skepticism about the design of the Abuja Fund as proposed in the research paper. Christiana Laniyan explains: "The question is: Are the incentives provided adequate to cause the desired change? I very much doubt this."

HIV testing and counseling (HTC)

Owing to time pressures, this was not considered as one of the eight priorities deliberated on and discussed within the African civil society prioritization exercises in Addis Ababa. However, the panel notes the centrality of HTC as a primary enabler to the HIV response. Therefore, this merits discussion as a priority within the fight against HIV in Africa. Nduku Kilonzo elaborates:

> From a policy and practice perspective, the reality of implementation therefore would be:
>
> (1) each of the different interventions has its own sinking costs and operational costs associated with HTC (training providers, supervision, tools, and data collection);
> (2) each program tests to screen the populations they need to reach and everyone else is "wasted" as they are not channeled to other services in order to optimize on the benefits of the range of post-test services.
>
> In the long run, people will get re-tested by different programs, increasing the overall costs of HTC without a concomitant increase in the benefits accrued from each test.

She concludes that scaling up HIV testing and counseling as a priority for any country, designed to act as a funnel and filter for all programs, would potentially reduce the HTC costs associated with each program prioritized, while optimizing referrals (an important element of the benefit calculation for HTC) to different post-test services.

Discussion

The panel members agree that while this ranking exercise has considered sub-Saharan Africa as a whole, there are distinct differences between various sub-regions of the continent and indeed variations within many countries.

Christiana Laniyan highlights this point: "In the application of cost-benefit analysis as a resource allocation decision-making tool, it is imperative that the analysis be adapted to suit the specific circumstances of nations within the continent."

Nduku Kilonzo points out that policy decisions will need to be approached differently as the need to prioritize HIV interventions becomes increasingly pressing:

> Choices regarding interventions will include letting go of what provides least value for money, is least effective, or is least likely to be achieved. The idea of evaluating the return on investment for each intervention, as provided by these benefit-cost ratios, provides one of the compelling perspectives to be utilized regarding what interventions to continue funding, and/or bring to scale. It is important to recognize that, in addition, there are additional essential and complementary policy and practical considerations required in each setting that would ideally inform prioritization processes.

The process of designing the studies is as important as the outcomes. Ken Odumbe notes that the researchers have relied heavily on desktop research. He proposes that a mix of primary data through key informant interviews would have added to the robustness of the studies, and suggests that targeting key government officials (preferably from the ministries of health) in select countries in Africa as key respondents would have helped in injecting legitimacy and managing the politics of ownership by African governments since these are studies about Africa.

> The studies' recommendations, although very useful and clear on what Africa should prioritize, may stand the risk of remaining academic because governments were not involved in the design. In case similar studies are planned in future to inform government policy, I highly recommend that the researchers work with National Technical Teams (NTTs) in select countries to provide strategic and technical inputs. I know this may present bureaucratic challenges but it comes with big benefits depending on how it is managed.
>
> Some of the roles of the NTTs could include: advising on the overall technical design of the studies;

ensuring the study protocols align with national research standards; maintaining liaison between the lead researcher and other relevant national agencies and stakeholders; technical review, etc. The value of this approach lies in the politics of national ownership, which may be a more strategic way to influence government policy.

Ken Odumbe also outlines a potential path forward for the project. Noting that the studies have undergone multi-stage reviews (prioritization exercises with the Nobel laureate economists, Global Fund-hosted AIDS stakeholders, civil society panelists, and youth forums in Georgetown University and Addis Ababa), he highly recommends "that the next level of review be done with the Africa Ministers of Finance and Health Forums convened under the auspices of the African Union."

He also outlines an area where future research is needed: the benefit-cost analysis of family unit-based interventions, so that the costs and benefits of combining PMTCT, ART, and cash transfer interventions can be explored as a comprehensive approach.

The panel concludes that the project's theme and approach is particularly timely. Retta Menberu finds that the project's approach could be useful in other areas:

> It is not only this topic, HIV/AIDS, that can benefit from utilizing the lessons of cost-benefit analysis, but also other spending and development-related areas, for instance in order to increase government accountability, especially in a time of decreased budgets.

The panel recommends that the project's research be built on and expanded, to increase the relevance in specific contexts and to allow countries to better allocate their scarce resources. It finds that the approach of cost-benefit analysis provides a useful new tool for decision-making, and the new research offers an additional resource and a helpful, fresh perspective.

Conclusion

BJØRN LOMBORG

In Part II of *RethinkHIV*, we have seen how two informed groups interpreted the research and formed views about which investments should be given precedence.

Before we consider some of the implications from the findings of the Georgetown University panel of expert economists and the African civil society panel, it is helpful to add two more prioritization outcomes to the mix for discussion.

The first of these took place at Georgetown University in September 2011. An event co-hosted by the Global Fund to Fight AIDS, Tuberculosis and Malaria attracted more than twenty senior representatives from funding bodies, NGOs, and other organizations engaged in the fight against HIV/AIDS in Africa. Among those represented were the United Nations Development Programme (UNAIDS), the Joint United Nations Programme on HIV/AIDS (UNDP), the World Health Organization (WHO), the World Bank, US administration officials, and the embassies of Denmark and Australia.

Over a morning, this group considered presentations from each of the primary chapter authors, and voted on priorities from among eight leading initiatives that were chosen by the authors themselves for prioritization. (The same eight initiatives were subsequently used for other prioritizations.)

The results of this short prioritization exercise are summarized in Table 7.2.1.

In December 2011, at the same time as the International Conference on AIDS and STIs in Africa (ICASA) in Addis Ababa, more than 100 university students (most of whom were from the Addis Ababa University School of Public Health) were convened to take part in a prioritization considering the *RethinkHIV* research. Most were post-graduate students of public health or related fields.

Table 7.2.1 Global Fund-hosted event prioritization

	Intervention	Chapter
1	Scale up male circumcision for young adults in high HIV prevalence countries	Prevention of sexual transmission
2	Scale up anti-retroviral treatment starting with the most sick and most infectious patients first	Treatment
3	Prevent mother-to-child transmission by scaling up Option A treatment of pregnant women and breastfeeding infants to 90 percent coverage in all countries	Prevention of non-sexual transmission
4	Accelerate AIDS vaccine development by scaling up funding for innovative vaccine research by 10 percent or $100 million per year	Vaccine research and development
5	Create incentive for less risky sexual behavior by offering conditional cash transfers for all girls from impoverished families to keep girls in secondary school	Social policy
6	Make blood transfusions safe by achieving 100 percent coverage of quality-assured HIV testing of donated blood	Prevention of non-sexual transmission
7	Introduce 25 percent increase in alcohol tax in countries with moderate-to-high levels of drinking and high adult mortality	Social policy
8	Create an Abuja Goals Fund offering a "cash-on-delivery" incentive to nations that meet the Abuja Declaration target of spending 15 percent of public revenues on public health	Strengthening health systems

Over an afternoon, the five members of the African civil society panel led the students through a discussion of the evidence. The Addis Ababa University Public Health School co-hosted the event. Students were challenged to come up with their own view on priorities. Table 7.2.2 represents their findings.

Table 7.2.2 Addis Ababa youth forum prioritization

	Intervention	Chapter
1	Prevent mother-to-child transmission by scaling up Option A treatment of pregnant women and breastfeeding infants to 90 percent coverage in all countries	Prevention of non-sexual transmission
2	Create an Abuja Goals Fund offering a "cash-on-delivery" incentive to nations that meet the Abuja Declaration target of spending 15 percent of public revenues on public health	Strengthening health systems
3	Scale up anti-retroviral treatment starting with the most sick and most infectious patients first	Treatment
4	Create incentive for less risky sexual behavior by offering conditional cash transfers for all girls from impoverished families to keep girls in secondary school	Social policy
5	Make blood transfusions safe by achieving 100 percent coverage of quality-assured HIV testing of donated blood	Prevention of non-sexual transmission
6	Accelerate AIDS vaccine development by scaling up funding for innovative vaccine research by 10 percent or $100 million per year	Vaccine research and development
7	Introduce 25 percent increase in alcohol tax in countries with moderate-to-high levels of drinking and high adult mortality	Social policy
8	Scale up male circumcision for young adults in high HIV prevalence countries	Prevention of sexual transmission

Table 7.2.3 contrasts each of the prioritization forums, and specifically how they treated the eight initiatives that were selected by authors.

As I outlined in the Introduction, both the civil society panel and the economist expert panel found that further evaluation analysis is needed, to better establish the costs and benefits of many initiatives.

In particular, evaluation of cross-intervention benefits is deemed by all to provide far greater clarity into the real costs and benefits in specific contexts.

Even for some mainstays of the HIV response, there is simply insufficient data to support the evaluation of benefit to cost ratios. It would be troublesome to place undue weight on benefit-cost estimates that are unreliable; likewise it would be foolhardy to dismiss outright interventions for which data is not yet available. But as things stand today, there is simply insufficient data to support robust decision-making.

It is impossible to overstate the need for further location-specific and Africa-wide analysis of intervention effectiveness, costs, and benefits.

But there is also evidence that some investments can be highly effective.

As we look across the differing views of priorities from within and outside Africa, we can see that there is considerable agreement – among economists, African civil society, tomorrow's African health leaders, and western organizations focused on HIV – that scaling up prevention of mother-to-child transmission should be a top priority.

This reflects the evidence presented in Chapter 2 by Lori Bollinger.

In 2010, around 390,000 children under fifteen became infected with HIV, mainly through mother-to-child transmission (UNAIDS 2011). This type of infection can occur through pregnancy, labor, delivery, or breastfeeding.

The number of new infections declined by a quarter between 2001 and 2009 (UNAIDS 2010): this positive development shows that the tools that we have at our disposal do work.

Bollinger argued that programs that prevent mother-to-child transmission are among the most cost-effective interventions available in the HIV/AIDS arsenal. Strong benefit to cost ratios show us that this investment offers considerable returns to society.

As Bollinger noted, however, these depend on establishing effective ways to increase clinic attendance and hospital deliveries, as well as reducing the considerable stigma associated with an HIV-positive diagnosis.

Similarly, we can see broad agreement that a scale up in ART enrollment for the most vulnerable is a commendable investment. It should be pointed out that the treatment scale-up that has been ranked is the specific option laid out in Chapter 3 by Mead Over and Geoffrey Garnett, rather than endorsing a more generic desire "to increase treatment." As Over and Garnett's research made clear – and the civil society panel expanded upon in Part II – policy-makers face challenging decisions

Table 7.2.3 Overview of prioritizations

	Economist expert panel	Global fund-hosted event	ICASA civil society	Addis ababa youth forum
1	Scale up vaccine funding by $100 million per year	Scale up male circumcision	Prevent mother-to-child transmission	Prevent mother-to-child transmission
2	Prevent mother-to-child transmission	Scale up ART enrollment	Scale up ART enrollment	Create an Abuja Goals Fund
3	Make blood transfusions safe	Prevent mother-to-child transmission	Cash transfer to keep girls in schooling	Scale up ART enrollment
4	Scale up ART enrollment	Scale up vaccine funding by $100 million per year	Create an Abuja Goals Fund	Cash transfer to keep girls in schooling
5	Scale up male circumcision	Cash transfer to keep girls in schooling	Make blood transfusions safe	Make blood transfusions safe
6	Cash transfer to keep girls in schooling	Make blood transfusions safe	Scale up vaccine funding by $100 million per year	Scale up vaccine funding by $100 million per year
7	Introduce alcohol taxation	Introduce alcohol taxation	Scale up male circumcision	Introduce alcohol taxation
8	Create an Abuja Goals Fund	Create an Abuja Goals Fund	Introduce alcohol taxation	Scale up male circumcision

in attempting to continue to gradually and sustainably expand treatment coverage.

We also see, across the four groups that prioritized investments, that certain investment options were consistently ranked lowly.

Alcohol taxation, for example, was given a fourteenth place ranking out of the eighteen investments considered by the Georgetown University expert economist panel group, and was given the lowest or second-lowest ranking out of the eight investments considered by the other three groups.

This does not mean that some form of alcohol taxation, *per se*, is a poor investment. Each of the options examined in *RethinkHIV* has a benefit to cost ratio above one, meaning that the spin-offs to society are estimated to be higher than the costs.

However, the economists of the Georgetown University expert panel expressed concerns about its implementation, given the possibility it could reduce overall revenue for developing nations. In the forums in Addis Ababa, similar concerns were expressed by civil society and university students, including around the substitution of market-bought alcohol with home-brew products. Both groups adopted a skeptical note in ranking it lowly.

There are also clearly points of difference between the stakeholders.

In Washington DC, the major organizations including donors and NGOs gave adult male circumcision (AMC) the highest ranking: they believe

that this should be a top priority in the fight against HIV/AIDS. This should not surprise us, because increasing AMC coverage is indeed one of the strongest focuses of donors and decision-makers today.

However, we can see that, in Addis Ababa, both civil society representatives from across Africa and local youths who considered the research expressed more skepticism about the strong benefit to cost ratios for this initiative, in particular with regard to generating uptake in non-research settings. They gave it a very low ranking. The difference in perspective draws once again attention to the varied profile of the epidemic in sub-Saharan Africa and highlights the need to remain sensitive to the local context and to the challenges of implementation. The expert economist panel offered a different take on this issue when they suggested that infant male circumcision could be seen as a longer-term strategy against this disease, with fewer of the behavioral challenges of AMC such as demand-generation and potential disinhibition.

The differences in the prioritizations conducted for *RethinkHIV* show that, while economic arguments about costs and benefits can take us so far, room remains for additional, non-economic arguments. Economic arguments should not be the only inputs used for policy decisions – but they will be especially important at a time of declining resources.

Using cost-benefit analysis – as opposed to other measures – provides a framework of equivalence, in which different interventions can reliably be measured against each other. We can capture and compare all of the costs and benefits to society, and make decisions accordingly.

This is a different approach than that predominantly used today. In Chapter 1, Jere Behrman and Hans-Peter Kohler included a useful comparison of the differences between cost-benefit analysis (used in this book) and cost-effectiveness analysis. They point out that cost-effectiveness analyses have been more commonly applied to HIV prevention programs than cost-benefit analyses.

Yet cost-effectiveness cannot reliably inform a choice between interventions. It can only validate the viability of any one intervention. Cost-effectiveness identifies the effectiveness of using a given amount of resources to achieve a set goal, often using summary measures such as the quality- or disability-adjusted life years (QALYs/DALYs) gained or averted. The sparse cost-effectiveness evidence is not easily comparable due to a lack of uniform reporting of costs and outcomes and the lack of comparability makes it less useful for broader decision-making. *RethinkHIV*, therefore, has offered us a different prism through which we can view the epidemic. It is important to recognize that researchers have provided a marginal analysis. Each chapter looked at what could be achieved with a limited increase in spending on specific initiatives, on top of the status quo.

Wherever possible, authors have used the same set of broad assumptions and analytical tools to examine different interventions. This was the first comprehensive attempt at using cost-benefit analysis by teams of authors in this way. It is to be expected that future projects and critiques will find ways to create stronger harmony and comparability between papers.

The project also endeavored to ensure that authors would identify where specific implementation issues exist for any specific intervention. This is one reason why three research papers were commissioned for each topic: to ensure a range of expert perspectives on what works, where, and why.

However, by necessity, this remains primarily a broad analysis. A natural next step is to focus more specifically on national and cultural-specific issues that modify the general findings of research papers and to look at cross-intervention benefits.

The African civil society panel made some very constructive recommendations for the project, suggesting that researchers work in future with national technical teams (NTTs) to provide strategic and technical inputs, leading to national ownership, and a more strategic way to influence government policy.

The panel also made the excellent recommendation that another prioritization project take place with the Africa Ministers of Finance and Health Forums convened under the auspices of the African Union, in order to engage Africa's political leadership with the research presented here.

African political leadership is a vital ingredient to stepping up the fight against HIV/AIDS in a sustainable way. But we must not leave important decisions about the prioritization of scarce resources to governments. The response to HIV/AIDS in Africa is at a crucial juncture. At a time when there is a risk of further declining funding, we all have a responsibility to ensure that HIV/AIDS resources achieve the most impact possible.

This volume of research has presented the reader with the evidence to make your own decisions about the most effective ways to step up the fight against this epidemic. The challenge now is to use the economic arguments in this volume to press for further funding and sustained attention, and to ensure that the best and most effective interventions are enacted, so that we can eventually foresee the end of HIV in Africa.

References

UNAIDS. (2010). *Global Report: UNAIDS Report on the Global AIDS Epidemic 2010*. Geneva: Joint United Nations Programme on HIV/AIDS (UNAIDS).

UNAIDS. (2011). *UNAIDS World AIDS Day Report 2011*. Geneva: Joint United Nations Programme on HIV/AIDS (UNAIDS).

Index

ABCE models 18
Abuja Goals Fund *see* AGF
AD (auto-disposable syringes) 81, 83
  transmission probability 83
Addis Ababa conference *see* Civil Society Panel
Addis Ababa Youth Forum Prioritization 347
adolescent sexual activity 239, 241, 245, 251–2, 254, 258,
  260–1, 269–70, *see also* keeping girls in school
Afrobarometer project 227, 230–1, 232
age factors 20–1
AGF (Abuja Goals Fund) 6, 183, 184, 186, 201–5, 206,
  222, 229–33, 344, 346, 347
AIDS
  deaths averted costs 306–7
  denial by politicians 234, 235
  epidemiology 301
  funding 342
  future scenarios 304–5
  R&D *see* vaccine research and development
  retro-virus discovered 61, *see also* ART
  trials 314–18
  vaccine 7
*AIDS in the Twenty-First Century: Disease and
  Globalisation* 68
AIDS: Taking a Long-Term View 2
AIDS vaccine
  accelerating development 309–12, 346, 347
  access to 325
  alternatives to 326
  benefit-cost ratios 310, 321, 326
  benefits 309
  costs 305–6, 321, 322–3
    in sub-Saharan Africa 306
  disinhibition 146, 324–5
  effectiveness 323–4
  and epidemic future 324
  paying for 325–6
  research 330
  societal benefits 321
  synergistic benefits 325
aids2031 Consortium xx, 2
  Modeling Working Group xix
AIDSCost projection program 128, 147
AIM (AIDS Impact Model) 78–9, 89–90, 96–7
alcohol
  abuse as HIV epidemic driver 285

Laffer Curve 244
  problematic use of 239, 242–5
  substitution 244
  taxation 241, 243, 247, 250–1, 254, 257, 261, 262–3,
    267, 268, 269–70, 293, 295–6, 346, 347, 348
Angola
  alcohol tax 262–3
  blood supply testing 86
  HIV epidemic scale 65–6
  HIV incidence/prevalence 13
  key indicators 115–16
anthropometric outcomes 55
Appel, Jacob 191
ART (anti-retroviral treatment)
  access to treatment 125, 140–1, 181, 185, 233–4
  AIDSCost projection program 128, 147
  anti-retroviral prophylaxis options 109–10, 122
  at-risk groups targeting strategy 312
  and behavioral responses 50–1
  benefit-cost analyses
    for successful infection prevention treatment 159–60
    for unsuccessful infection prevention treatment 156
  benefit-cost ratios 76, 77–8, 137, 138–9, 143, 145,
    178–82
  benefit-cost results 141–2, 146–8
  best treatment stage 125–6
  CD4 cells 110–12, 125–6, 127–30, 136, 137–9, 141–2,
    143–4, 156, 160, 178
  CD4 counts and eligibility 181
  cost-effectiveness 141–2
  costs 32, 77, 126–7, 145, 169, 178
  coverage 128
    and family planning 222
  drug costs 308
  and dynamics of HIV infection 103–4
  eligibility guidelines 213–14
  extension of 15
  feedback effects 219–20
  future cost per patient 178–9
  historical counterfactual 135
  HIV transmission models 79–81, 131–3
  incremental spending 140
  infections reduction incremental benefits 194
  life years gained 179–81, 184
  lifelong treatment 109–10, 112
  mother-to-child infections 75

national uptake rate 128
Nobel Laureate Economist Expert Panel findings on 339
non-AIDS mortality rate 180
numbers treated by 1
oral 301
patient life expectancy 138–9
and prevention techniques 70
primary infection prevention 159
scaling-up benefits 181, 346, 347
scaling-up enrollment 343, 347–8
secondary infection prevention 159
simulated scenarios 135–7
spillover benefits 145
statistics provision 79
in sub-Saharan Africa xix
sufficient damage factor 127
survival years 180–1
TDF/FTC combination 54
test-and-treat strategy 12–14, 18, 19–20, 22–3, 25, 53–4, 58, 112, 192
topical 301
topical microbicides 238
treatment cost per person/year 135, 173–4
treatment criteria 128
treatment dynamics modeling 127–30
treatment eligibility 334
treatment emergence 125
treatment impact modeling 130–3, 142–5
treatment unit costs 133–5
treatment uptake rate modeling 128–30
    impact of 135
uptake projection 139–40
value of lives saved 78
zero uptake 135, 136
    and benefit-cost ratios 151
    simulation results 139
ARV (anti-retroviral prophylaxis regimen) 109–10, 135, 160–3, 172–3, 175–6
adverse side effects 174
and AIDS vaccine 305
benefit-cost ratio 173
cost decline 179
deployment of 146
potential cost reduction 179
Aryeetey, Ernest 337–8
at-risk groups targeting strategy 312
AVERT model 79–81
AZT (Zidovudine) program 162

B/C ratios, naive estimates of 155
Baltussen, Rob 5
Banerjee, Abhijit 191
Barnett, Tony 6
Bärnighausen, Till 6
BCC (behavioral change communication) 16
BCR see benefit-cost ratios
behavioral prevention programs 14–15

Behrman, Jere 4, 349
benefit estimates 103–4
benefit-cost analyses 21, 23
continued investment 308–9
DALYs (disability-adjusted life years) 20, 22, 26–9, 32–3, 34–40, 41–2, 49, 62, 226
decline in World Bank 190
dynamic framework time representation 155–60
HC (Human Capital) approach 170
HIV treatment pre-pregnancy 164–6
information campaigns (IC) 25–6
and interventions 108
life-cycle perspective 26, 30, 62
Nobel Laureate Economist Expert Panel findings on 337
for policy interventions 26–32
    discounting 31
    estimation challenges 31–2
    general considerations 26–30
    interaction among solutions 31
    prices 30
    range of costs 31
    range of impacts 30
    scale 31
pregnant women 167–8
and sets of objects 283
for successful infection prevention treatment 159–60
and unrecognized metaphors 281
for unsuccessful infection prevention treatment 156
vaccine research and development 304–9
WTP (willingness to pay) 170–1
benefit-cost ratios 5, 36–7, 40–1, 181–2, 189
AIDS vaccine development 310
ART 32, 76, 77–8, 137, 138–9, 143, 145, 146–8, 178–82
and ARV provision 173
CCTs 220–2
CD4 cell count 158–60
community health 198
cross-country variations 293
discounted/undiscounted 156, 175
health system strengthening 208
HIV reduction interventions 34–7, 41–2, 63–4, 174, 293
infections averted 32
interventions 260–3
male circumcision 36–7, 40–1, 63–4, 339
pMTCT in sub-Saharan Africa 160–1, 163, 174–5
procedures summary 32–3
treatment costs 32
treatment as prevention 151
unit costs 294–5
varying average costs 294–5
VSL (Value of a Statistical Life) approach 170–1
Benin
    alcohol tax 262–3
    blood supply testing 86
    HIV incidence/prevalence 13, 114–17
    key indicators 115–16
    problems faced by government (Afrobarometer) 232

blockbuster drugs 303
blood safety intervention 186
blood transfusions 4, 74, 86–8, 89, 102–3, 346, 347
Bloom, David 5–6
BMGF (Bill and Melinda Gates Foundation) 213
body undergoing treatment metaphor 283–4
Bollinger, Lori 4, 102, 105, 121, 169–70, 171, 259,
    347–8
Botswana
  alcohol tax 262–3
  health priority survey 230–1
  HIV epidemic scale 65–6
  HIV incidence/prevalence 12, 13, 29, 30, 34, 39–40
  key indicators 115–16
  life expectancy with/without AIDS 162
  male circumcision 25, 40–1
  problems faced by government (Afrobarometer) 232
  resources allocated to 15–17
  unmet need for family planning 165
Brandeau, M. L. 295
Brazil, AIDS vaccine 325
Brent, Robert 5
British Columbia Center for Excellence on HIV/AIDS
    69–70
Burkina Faso
  Abuja target 202
  alcohol tax 262–3
  HIV incidence/prevalence 13, 114–17
  key indicators 115–16
  life expectancy with/without AIDS 162
  unmet need for family planning 165
Burundi
  alcohol tax 262–3
  HIV incidence/prevalence 13
  key indicators 115–16
  life expectancy with/without AIDS 162
  unmet need for family planning 165
bush circumcisions 52

Cambodia, conditional cash transfers 254
Cameroon
  alcohol tax 262–3
  HIV incidence/prevalence 13
  key indicators 115–16
  life expectancy with/without AIDS 162
  unmet need for family planning 165
Campbell Collaboration 65
cancer as investment priority 189
canine distemper, and vaccine research and development
    313
Cape Verde, problems faced by government
    (Afrobarometer) 232
CAPRISA (Centre for the AIDS Programme of Research in
    South Africa) 64
CAPRISA Study 54
cash incentive programs see CCT
CBA (cost-benefit analysis) see benefit-cost analyses

CCT (conditional cash transfer) 21, 23, 31, 53, 54–8,
    191–3, 218
  benefit-cost ratios 220–2
  conceptual foundations of 56
  current evidence on 57–8
  female education 245
  and HIV awareness 192
  and HIV testing 228–9
  and infection reduction 222
  and joint objectives 184
  keeping girls in school see keeping girls in school
  potential impacts of 186
  rationale for 54–7
  RESPECT study 193
CD4 cells 110–12, 125–6, 127–30, 136, 137–9, 141–2,
    143–4, 156, 160, 172, 173, 178, 199
  cell count and ART eligibility 181
  cell count benefit-cost ratios 158–60
  and death probability 180–1
  point of care dipsticks 179
  screening 161
CEA see cost-effectiveness analyses
Central African Republic
  alcohol tax 262–3
  health worker shortage 196
  HIV incidence/prevalence 13, 196
  key indicators 115–16
  life expectancy with/without AIDS 162
Chad
  alcohol tax 262–3
  HIV incidence/prevalence 13
  key indicators 115–16
  unmet need for family planning 165
CHAHA program 248–9
childhood diseases, as investment priority 189
Chimeric Venezuelan Equine Encephalitis 313
China, conditional cash transfers (one-child policy) 191
CHWs (community health workers)
  deployment 216, 218
  Technical Task Force 186, 196, 197–9
  training costs/benefits 220–2
circumcision see MC
Civil Society Panel 341, 349
  Abuja Goals Fund 344
  AIDS funding 342
  ART (anti-retroviral treatment) scaled-up enrollment 343
  CCT (conditional cash transfer) and keeping girls in
    school 343–4
  keeping girls in school 343–4, see also keeping girls in
    school
  mother-to-child transmission prevention (pMTCT)
    342–3, 347–8
  redefining priorities theme 341
CM (contingency management) 55–6
CMH (Commission on Macroeconomics and Health) 104,
    195, 203
COD (cash on delivery)

and Abuja Goals Fund (AGF) 201–5, 206, 229–33
   donor assistance 184
   to governments 218
Collier, Paul 337–8
combination prevention 145
commodity approach to strategies 15
community health workers 183, 184, 206, 207, 228
community mobilization 248–9, 253, 255, 259, 265, 267, 268, 269–70, 293
Community Systems Strengthening Framework 235
Comoros
   alcohol tax 262–3
   HIV incidence/prevalence 13, 114–17
   key indicators 115–16
concurrent sexual partners, as HIV epidemic driver 285
condoms 11, 19, 51, 56, 68, 170, 248
Congo
   Abuja target 202
   alcohol tax 262–3
   HIV incidence/prevalence 13, 114–17
   key indicators 115–16
   life expectancy with/without AIDS 162
   unmet need for family planning 165
contraception, unmet need for 164
   see also condoms; family planning
Copenhagen Consensus 2–3, 7, 8, 71
Copenhagen Consensus Center, global development project (2008) 2
Copenhagen Consensus Challenge paper 245
Copenhagen Consensus project (2004) 2
cost-effectiveness xx, 11, 17–23, 37–9, 49, 58
   blood transfusions 74, 86–8
   ICER (incremental cost-effectiveness ratio) 75–6
   injecting drug users 92–5
   interventions 17–23, 242–5, 260
   medical injections 74, 81–6
   mother-to-child transmission 74, 121
   in sub-Saharan Africa 11, 20, 104
cost-effectiveness analyses 22, 283
   and unrecognized metaphors 281
cost estimates 103
cost per death 194, 198
cost per infection 104
Cote d'Ivoire
   alcohol tax 262–3
   HIV incidence/prevalence 13, 114–17
   key indicators 115–16
   life expectancy with/without AIDS 162
   OIs (opportunistic infections) 76–7, 78
   unmet need for family planning 165
cotrimoxazole prophylaxis 161
couple-based HIV testing 20
CRAG (cryptococcal antigen)
   costs and benefits 186, 200–1, 208
   testing 199–200, 201, 228
critical enablers 188–9
cross-intervention benefits 347

cryptococcal meningitis (CM) 183, 200–1, 206, 216, 218, 220, 340
Cryptococcosis neoformans 184, 199–201
cultural practices, as HIV epidemic driver 285
Cytomegalovirus Clinical Development Program 313

DALYs (disability-adjusted life years) 20, 22, 26–9, 34–40, 41–2, 49, 62, 63–4, 75–6, 104, 170–1, 175–6, 189–90, 197, 200, 203, 205, 206, 207, 226, 243, 260, 263–5, 349
   by country 271–2
      incremental cost 274–5
   parameters 260–1
DCP2 190–1
de Walque, Damien 4
dead metaphors 282
deaths averted 188–9, 194, 202, 203, 204, 306–7, 308
DemProj software tool 78
diagnostic tests 300
discounting 171–2, 173, 175, 189–90, 200, 263, 333
disinhibition 146, 324–5, 339
Djibouti
   Abuja target 202
   key indicators 115–16
DMPTT see Male Circumcision: Decision Makers' Program Planning Tool
donor support flat-lining 213–14
dose-response 284
drug costs 126–7, 308
drug development 300
drug supply systems intervention 186
drug users, injecting 92–5
Duflo, Esther 191

Earth Institute Technical Taskforce 195
ecology of risk 285, 286
The Economist, end of AIDS? 12
Efavirenz 111, 126
effectiveness estimates 103–4
efficiency solution 188
embodiment of social conditions 287–8
emergency rescue intervention 186
epidemic model 295
EPP (Estimation and Projection Package) 78
Equatorial Guinea
   alcohol tax 262–3
   HIV incidence/prevalence 13
   key indicators 115–16
Eritrea
   alcohol tax 262–3
   HIV incidence/prevalence 13, 114–17
   infant mortality 204
   key indicators 115–16
   life expectancy with/without AIDS 162
Ethiopia
   alcohol tax 262–3
   HIV prevalence 12, 114–17, 296–7

Ethiopia (*cont.*)
    key indicators 115–16
    life expectancy with/without AIDS 162
    life insurance incentivization 296–7
    Millennium Village Project (MVP) 247
    PEPFAR-funded interventions 255
    unmet need for family planning 165
    Voices of the Poor project 196
evidence-based allocation strategy 17–18
external validity of interventions 294

faith-based abstinence 68
family planning 97, 117, 161, 163–4, 197, 198, 202,
        222
    cost-effectiveness of 164, 198–9
    social benefits 164
    unmet need for in sub-Saharan Africa 165
Farm Input Subsidy Programme 247
FDA, and microbicide 64
FEM-PrEP trial 54
female education 245
female sex workers 296–7
FFS (Farmer Field School) 247, 252
first-line treatment benefits/costs 157
flat-lining donor support 213–14
Forsythe, Stephen 7
funding 1
    alternative use for 214–15
    competing demands 213–14

G8 (Gleneagles 2005) 185
Gabon
    alcohol tax 262–3
    HIV incidence/prevalence 13
    key indicators 115–16
    life expectancy with/without AIDS 162
Gambia
    alcohol tax 262–3
    HIV incidence/prevalence 13
    key indicators 115–16
Gardasil 322, 323, 325
Garnett, Geoffrey 5, 173–4, 178–82, 347–8
GAVI Alliance 184–6
gender inequalities, as HIV epidemic driver 285
gender role perceptions/training 239, 240, 246–7, 248–9,
        252, 254–5, 258–9, 263, 267, 269–70, 293
general structure (GS) interventions 216–18, 221
genital lesions 285
Georgetown University Expert Panel *see* Nobel Laureate
        Economist Expert Panel
GFATM *see* Global Fund to Fight AIDS, Tuberculosis and
        Malaria
Ghana
    alcohol tax 262–3
    health priority survey 230–1
    HIV incidence/prevalence 13, 114–17
    HIV/AIDS stigma 248–9

key indicators 115–16
    problems faced by government (Afrobarometer) 232
    sexually transmitted HIV 11
    unmet need for family planning 165
    Voices of the Poor project 196
girls in school 239, 241, 245, 251–2, 254, 258, 260–1, 267,
        268, 269–70, 284, 343–4
Gleneagles Summit (2006) 125
Global Crises, Global Solutions 184–5, 190
Global Fund Forum 342
Global Fund to Fight AIDS, Tuberculosis and Malaria
        (GFATM) 61, 182, 184–6, 189, 202–3, 213, 214–15,
        230, 233–6, 346
Global Fund-hosted Event Prioritization 346
global political commitment, to fighting HIV 213
Global Programme on AIDS 283
GNI per capita statistical life value 189–90
goal-directed thinking 288
Goals and Allocation by Cost-Effectiveness (ABCE)
        models 18
Goals Model/Goals Express 79–81, 93, 96–7, 259, 265
*Going Upstream: A Cost-Benefit Analysis of Social Policy
        Interventions to Enhance the HIV/AIDS Response in
        Sub-Saharan Africa* 282–3
going upstream metaphor 282–3
Granich, Reuben M. 69–70, 191–2
GS (general structure) interventions 216–18, 221
Guinea
    alcohol tax 262–3
    HIV incidence/prevalence 13, 114–17
    key indicators 115–16
Guinea-Bissau
    alcohol tax 262–3
    HIV incidence/prevalence 13
    key indicators 115–16
    life expectancy with/without AIDS 162
Gupta, Geeta Rao 286

Halperin, D. T. 19
HCT *see* HTC
health benefits, advances in estimating 190–1
health care costs, and HIV prevention 307
health care reform, political legitimacy of 231–3
health center upgrade/construction intervention 186
health inequalities and environments 287
health priority survey 230–1
health services strengthening, in rural areas 196–7
health services upgrade 195–9
health spending ratios 187
health system capacity 226–8
health system infrastructure and pMTCT 117–18
health system intervention evaluation 215–17
    benefits evaluation 216–17
    costs 217
    feasibility 215
    flexibility 215
    intervention level/scope 216

technical efficiency 215
time lags/certainty levels 217–18
health system strengthening 213–23, 226–36
    access improvement 228
    benefit evaluation 216–18
    challenges
    cost-benefit ratio 208
    cost evaluation 217–18
    feasibility 215
    flexibility 215
    intervention evaluation 215–16, 217
    intervention scope 216
    life year value monetization 226
    methodological issues 226–33
    Nobel Laureate Economist Expert Panel findings on 340
    structures 214–15
health workers
    shortage 196
    skills upgrade 195–9
    staff expansion 197–9
heart attacks, as investment priority 189
Hecht, Robert 7
herpes
    as epidemic driver 285
    and Stepping Stones 246
heterosexual HIV transmission 303
HIA (HIV infection averted) 63–4
high-risk groups 153, 155
HIPC (highly indebted poor countries) initiative 202–3
historical counterfactual 135
HIV
    and alcohol consumption 242
    in couples 126, 159
    deaths statistics xix, 153, 299
    dynamic models of effect on 152–5
    epidemic drivers 285
    epidemic scale 65–6
    fatality rate 125
    global political commitment to fighting 213
    hope and social intervention 288–90
    impact modeling 255–9
    incidence (of infection) 131
    incidence/prevalence ratio 146–8, 213, 226–8
    infections averted 255–9, 271–2
    modes of transmission 66–7
    POC (point-of-care) diagnostic tests 119–21
    in women in sub-Saharan Africa 172–3
    see also vaccine research and development
HIV counseling, universal 183
HIV information, universal 183
HIV prevention, as investment priority 189
HIV programs, demand side 218
HIV testing
    monetization 229
    universal 183, 228–9
HIV transmission
    heterosexual 303

models 79–81, 131–3
rate estimation 151
in sub-Saharan Africa 238
susceptibility and income inequality 287
HIV treatment
    for all women 164–6
    benefits of prevention 306–8
    costs 70
    efficiency 215
    immediacy 70
    individual effects 70
    population effects 70
    programs' integration with primary health care 214–15
    selective expansion 214–15
    selective integration 214–15
    stand-alone programs 215
    see also ART (anti-retroviral treatment); HSS (health system strengthening)
HIV vulnerability, social drivers 239
HIV-infected children, survival rate 77
HIV/AIDS
    disease statistics 200
    R&D see vaccine research and development
    social policy interventions 281–90
    spending and health systems strengthening 186–7
HIVNS (HIV-focused non-structural) interventions 216–18, 221
HLT (High Level Taskforce on International Innovative Financing for Health Systems) 185, 195, 202–3
Hontelez, Jan 5
hope
    analytical advantages 289
    as diagnostic tool 289–90
    and income 289
    and optimism 288
    and palliative care 289
    and social intervention 288–90
HSS (health systems strengthening) 184, 186–7, 204–5
    expansion of 214–15
    and health worker skills upgrade 195–9
    intervention scale 219
    interventions implementation time 219
    potential of 215
    priority setting 220
    targeting vulnerable populations 220
    unintended consequences 218–19
HTC (HIV testing and counseling) 14–15, 19–20, 22–3, 25, 41–2
    benefits of 49–50, 62–3
    and Civil Society Panel 344
    cost-benefit ratio 63–4
    cost-effectiveness 37
    costs of 33–4
    and HIV incidence 33–4
    as prevention 69–70, 192–3
    treatment as prevention 166–8
    uptake at community level 248

Humair, Sal 6
human resources training intervention 186
human rights and conditional cash transfers 191
hyperbolic discounting 190

IAVI (International AIDS Vaccine Initiative) 299, 305–6
    research developments source 313
IC (information campaigns) 20, 25–6, 34, 41–2, 49–50,
    52–3, 62, 63–4, 70–1
ICASA 341, 346
ICD (infectious and communicable diseases) 188
ICER (incremental cost-effectiveness ratio) 75–6
IDU (injecting drug use) interventions 92–5, 96, 102–3,
    104, 105
IeDEA Consortium 180
IHP+ (International Health Partnerships) 184–5, 195,
    202–3, 204–5
IMAGE (Intervention with Microfinance for AIDS and
    Gender Equity) 21, 246, 247, 252, 254–5, 258–9
immunodeficiency virus 20–1
impact evaluations 50
inappropriate metaphors 281–8
income inequality and poverty/transmission susceptibility
    287
incremental benefits 194
incremental spending results 140
India, conditional cash transfers (vasectomy grants) 191
individual behavior
    environment as regulator of 286–7
    and risk environments 286
infant HIV exposure diagnosis 161
infant infections 188, 198
infant lives saved 207
infant mortality 203, 204
infants, as most valued lives 190
infection probability model 79–81
information technology intervention 186
initiation schools 52
injecting drug users 75, 92–5
Institute for Health Metrics and Evaluation 332
intergenerational sexual behavior as HIV epidemic driver
    285
intergenerational transmission of disease 33, 285
International Conference on AIDS (ICASA) 341, 346
International Group on Analysis of Trends in HIV
    Prevalence and Behaviors in Young People in
    Countries most Affected by HIV (2010) 19
International HIV/AIDS Alliance 248–9
interventions
    adolescent sexual activity 239, 241, 245, 247, see also
        keeping girls in school
    AGF (Abuja Goals Fund) see AGF
    alcohol
        problematic use of 239, 242–5
        taxation see alcohol taxation
    anthropometric outcomes 55
    beneficiaries of 105

benefit-cost ratios 260–3
and CBA (cost-benefit analysis) 108, 242–5
CCT (conditional cash transfer) see CCT (conditional
    cash transfer)
community mobilization see community mobilization
cost-effectiveness 17–23, 242–5, 260
criteria for 61–2
cross-intervention benefits 347
demand-side 55, 245
effectiveness 17–23, 242–5
evidence-based allocation strategy 17–18
external validity of 294
gender role perceptions/training see gender roles
    perception/training
GS (general structure) 216–18
HIV infection reduction 34–9, 255–9
HIV reduction benefit-cost ratios 34–7, 41–2, 63–4,
    174
HIV treatment issues 70
and HIV vulnerability social drivers 239
HIVNS (HIV-focused non-structural) 216–18, 221
and hope 288–90
HSS (health systems strengthening)
    and cost-benefit analyses 221
    objectives 186
    scale 219
IDU 92–5
IMAGE see IMAGE
impact evaluations 50
implementation time 219
investment priorities 189
keeping girls in school see keeping girls in school
local diagnosis 289
location-specific 15–17
long-lasting 222
and MSM 53
Nobel Laureate Economist Expert Panel findings 337–8
and orphan care costs 311
pMTCT (mother-to-child transmission) 109–13, 118,
    121, 151, 160–6
and population size 17
potential behavioral responses 50–2
potential beneficiaries 39–41
pre-exposure chemoprophylaxis 53, 54
preventative vs treatment 104–5
prevention efficiency 52–3
priority setting 220
sexually transmitted infections 50
Stepping Stones 246, 258–9
stigma of HIV/AIDS 1, 4, 6, 20, 97, 238, 239, 240, 242,
    255, 265
structural interventions 286
target populations 220, 247, 248–9
targeted approaches 53
and technologies/strategies 329
total costs per country 272–3
transferable social policy 283–4

treatment for prevention (test-and-treat) 12–14, 18, 19–20, 22–3, 25, 53–4, 166–8
trusted interventions 19
unit costs per country 272–3
vulnerable populations 220
investment approach to strategies 15, 17, 21
six program components 15
iPrEx study 54
IPV (intimate partner violence) 265
irresponsible sexual behavior as HIV epidemic driver 285

Jamison, Dean 7, 189
Johri, Mira 5

Karlan, Dean 191
Kazianga, Harounan 6–7
keeping girls in school 245, 251–2, 254, 258, 260–1, 267, 268, 269–70, 284, 293, 294, 343–4, 346, 347
Kemron 51
Kenya
    alcohol tax 262–3
    alcohol taxation 244
    ART cures 51
    development indicators 227
    family planning unmet needs 165
    health priority survey 230–1
    HIV epidemic scale 65–6
    HIV incidence/prevalence 12, 13, 66–7, 296–7
    IDU (injecting drug use) interventions 92–5, 96–7
    key indicators 115–16
    life expectancy with/without AIDS 162
    life insurance incentivization 296–7
    male circumcision 23–5
    Millennium Village Project (MVP) 247
    needle-sharing infections 74
    problems faced by government (Afrobarometer) 232
    sexually transmitted HIV 11
    unsafe medical injections 74
Killingo, Bactrin 341, 342, 343
Kilonzo, Nduku 341, 342–4, 345
Kohler, Hans-Peter 4, 349

labor ward screening 118–19
laboratory infrastructure improvement intervention 186
lack of knowledge as HIV epidemic driver 285
Laniyan, Christiana 341, 342, 343, 344
Lesotho
    alcohol tax 262–3
    blood transfusion infections 74
    bush circumcisions 52
    health worker shortage 196
    HIV epidemic scale 65–6
    HIV incidence/prevalence 12, 13, 29, 30, 34, 66–7, 196
    key indicators 115–16
    life expectancy with/without AIDS 162
    needle-sharing infections 74
    problems faced by government (Afrobarometer) 232

sexually transmitted HIV 11
    unmet need for family planning 165
liability and cost ratio 323
Liberia
    Abuja target 202
    alcohol tax 262–3
    HIV incidence/prevalence 13
    key indicators 115–16
    life expectancy with/without AIDS 162
life expectancy 161, 169
life insurance 6–7
    incentivization 296–7
life-cycle perspective 26, 30, 62
life-year costs 145
life-year values 137, 164, 170–1, 188–9
    monetization 226
life-years gained 179–81, 188, 200, 307
LiST software tool 78
location-specific interventions 15–17
LoveLife campaign 70

McGreevey, William 5–6
Madagascar
    alcohol tax 262–3
    health priority survey 230–1
    HIV incidence/prevalence 13
    key indicators 115–16
    problems faced by government (Afrobarometer) 232
Makhwapheni Campaign 70–1
Making Services Work for Poor People 233
malaria, as investment priority 189
Malawi
    alcohol tax 262–3
    cash incentive programs 21, 57–8
    CCTs (conditional cash transfers) 192–3, 245
        keeping girls in school 245, 254, 258
    development indicators 227
    donor money corruption 231
    family planning 197
    Farm Input Subsidy Programme 247
    GNI per capita 226–8
    health priority survey 230–1
    health workers 196, 228
    HIV epidemic scale 65–6
    HIV incidence/prevalence 13, 34, 196
    HIV and sexual contact 14
    key indicators 115–16
    life expectancy 226–8
        with/without AIDS 162
    male circumcision 23–5
    Millennium Village Project (MVP) 247
    PBI (performance-based incentive) 192
    problems faced by government (Afrobarometer) 232
    SIHR (Schooling, Income, and HIV Risk) study 193
    unmet need for family planning 165
    Voices of the Poor project 196
male circumcision see MC

Mali
    alcohol tax 262–3
    HIV incidence/prevalence 13, 114–17
    key indicators 115–16
    problems faced by government (Afrobarometer) 232
mass media IC (information campaigns) 25–6, 34, 41–2,
        49–50, 52–3, 62, 63, 70–1
maternal health and child survival 111
maternal mortality 197, 198, 202
Mauritania
    HIV incidence/prevalence 13, 114–17
    key indicators 115–16
Mauritius
    alcohol tax 262–3
    HIV incidence/prevalence 13, 114–17
    IDU (injecting drug use) infection 92–5
    key indicators 115–16
MBB (marginal budgeting for bottlenecks) 185, 203
Mbeki, President Thabo 234, 235
MC (male circumcision) 4, 12, 15, 18, 21, 22–5, 41–2,
        49–50, 300, 301, 346
    benefit-cost ratios 36–7, 40–1, 63–4, 339
    bush circumcisions 52
    cost-effectiveness of 58, 62
    costs of 33
    as high priority 348
    infant 339, 348
    and infection prevention 326
    intervention efficiency 52–3
    intervention requirements 39–41
    key issues 69
    lack of as HIV epidemic driver 285
    long-term benefits 25–6, 62, 66, 68–9
    Male Circumcision: Decision Makers' Program Planning
        Tool (DMPPT) 18
    neonatal 25, 52
    uptake and resources 323
MDGs see Millennium Development Goals
Medecins Sans Frontiers 159
medical injections 4, 74, 81–5, 86, 102–3
medical male circumcision see MC
Mema wa Vijana intervention 255
men who have sex with men see MSM
Menberu, Retta 341, 343, 345
Merck vaccine failure 302
metaphorical language in social policy interventions
        281–90
metaphors
    and cost-effective analyses 281
    inappropriate 281–8
    risk behavior 284–6
    structural drivers 284–6
    unexamined 281–6
    unrecognized 281
Mexico, conditional cash transfers 191, 254
microbicides and HIV risk 64, 71
microfinance schemes 21, 246, 247

Millennium Development Goals
    failure to achieve 341
    Goal 4 (reduce child mortality) 121–2
    Goal 5 (improve maternal health) 121–2
    Goal 6 (combat HIV/AIDS) 121–2, 242
Millennium Village Project (MVP) 247, 252
Mills, Anne 185
Mix Market platform 252
modes of transmission 66–7
Montaner, J. S. G. 69–70
moral hazard 146
More than good intentions 191
most-valued persons 189–90
MOT (Modes of Transmission) model 81, 102, 103–4
mother-to-child transmission 4, 5, 74, 75, 77, 88–92, 160–6
    anti-retroviral prophylaxis options 109–10, 121
    AP (assessment paper) analysis 107, 108, 110–12
    CBA (cost-benefit analysis) 108
    CD4 screening 161
    contraception 164
    family planning 117, 161, 163–4
        cost-effectiveness of 164
    infant HIV exposure diagnosis 161
    labor ward screening 118–19
    maternal health and child survival 111
    maternal mortality 197
    multiplex POC (point-of-care) diagnostic tests 119–21
    non-health facility births 119
    pMTCT cascade 107, 117, 118, 122
    potential HIV rates in sub-Saharan Africa 163
    prevention (pMTCT) 77, 78, 79, 91–2, 97, 103, 105, 107,
        108, 169–70, 347–8
        analytic timeframe 111–12
        benefit-cost reduction 174–5, 342–3
        CD4 cell count 110–12, 172
        and Civil Society Panel 342–3
        comprehensive vs narrow approach to 108–9
        costs
            and health system infrastructure 113
            and HIV prevalence 113
        emerging technology 122
        forward transmission impact 107, 112
        full benefits definition 161
        and health system infrastructure 117–18
        intervention options 109–12, 113, 151
        key challenges 113–18
        Nobel Laureate Economist Expert Panel findings
            342–3
        pre-pregnancy 164–6
        scaling up 346, 347
        services increase requirements 121–2
        solutions 118–21
        therapeutic options 111, 112, 121
        treatment evaluation 172
        treatment targets 156
        treatment vs family planning 163–4
    primary prevention 164

screening tests 161
in sub-Saharan Africa 74, 107, 163
testing and counseling 161
treatment for prevention (test-and-treat) 12–14, 18,
    19–20, 22–3, 25, 53–4, 166–8
WHO Option A strategies 107–8
Mozambique
    alcohol tax 262–3
    development indicators 227
    health worker shortage 196
    HIV epidemic scale 65–6
    HIV incidence/prevalence 13, 34, 39–40, 196
    key indicators 115–16
    life expectancy with/without AIDS 162
    male circumcision 40–1
    problems faced by government (Afrobarometer) 232
    unmet need for family planning 165
MSM (men who have sex with men) 4, 53, 66–7, 69, 238
MTCT *see* mother-to-child transmission
multiple partners 126, 159
multiplex POC (point-of-care) diagnostic tests 119–21

Namibia
    alcohol tax 262–3
    health priority survey 230–1
    HIV incidence/prevalence 13, 34
    key indicators 115–16
    life expectancy with/without AIDS 162
    male circumcision 23–5
    problems faced by government (Afrobarometer) 232
    unmet need for family planning 165
NAT (nucleic acid amplification testing) 86
national epidemics 283
national strategies xx
National Technical Teams (NTTs) 345
Nattrass, Nicoli 6
needle-exchange 105
neonatal circumcision 25, 52
Nevaprine 126, 161–2
Niger
    alcohol tax 262–3
    blood supply testing 86
    HIV incidence/prevalence 13, 114–17
    key indicators 115–16
Nigeria
    alcohol tax 262–3
    development indicators 227
    health system capacity 226–8
    HIV epidemic scale 65–6
    HIV incidence/prevalence 13
    key indicators 115–16
    life expectancy with/without AIDS 162
    problems faced by government (Afrobarometer) 232
    unmet need for family planning 165
Nobel Laureate Economist Expert Panel 337–8
non-sexual HIV transmission prevention
    AIDS impact model 78–9

analysis methods 102, 103–4
benefits calculation 76–8
benefits summary 96
blood transfusions 74, 86–8, 102–3
Goals Model/Goals Express 79–81
HIV infections averted model 78
injecting drug users 92–5
medical injections 4, 74, 81–5, 86, 102–3
mother-to-child transmission 4, 5, 74, 88–92, 169–70
multi-country analysis options/limitations 102–3
recommendations 96–7
resource allocation equity 105
NVP (Nevirapine) program 126, 161–2

O&G model of infections 152–3
    and high-risk groups 155
    infection flows 155
    with interventions 153–4
    transmission mechanism specification 154–5
Odumbe, Ken 341, 342, 345
OIs (opportunistic infections) 76–7, 78, 89, 307, 311
One Million Community Health Workers 195
operations research intervention 186
opiate substitute therapies 105
oppression illness 287
oral anti-retrovirals 301
oral prophylaxis 238
orphan care costs 311
OST (opioid substitution therapy) 75, 105
Over, Mead 5, 173–4, 178–82, 347–8

Padian, N. S. 2
patient transport intervention 186
PBI (performance-based incentive) 192
Pearl Omega 51
Peer Group IC (information campaigns) 25–6, 34, 41–2,
    49–50, 52–3, 62, 63
PEPFAR (Presidential Emergency Plan for AIDS Relief)
    61, 67, 92–5, 179, 182, 184–6, 189, 213, 214–15,
    217, 255
pilot studies, external validity of 294
Piot, Peter xx
Platform for Health System Strengthening 195
pMTCT *see* mother-to-child transmission
POC (point-of-care) diagnostic tests 119–21
*Poor Economics, a Radical Rethinking of the Way to Fight
    Global Poverty* 191
poverty as HIV epidemic driver 285, 287
pre-exposure prophylaxis 154, 301
    chemoprophylaxis 53, 54, 58
Prescott, Edward C. 337–8
preventative interventions 104–5
Prevention of Non-sexual Transmission Assessment Paper
    169–70
primary health care, HIV treatment integration with 214–15
primary infection prevention 159
production function model 295

program enablers 194–5
promiscuous sexual behavior as HIV epidemic driver 285
Protocol G 313

QALYs (quality-adjusted life years) 21–2, 75, 175–6,
    349

RAPID software tool 78
Rasmussen, Prime Minister Anders Fogh 2
RBF (results-based financing) 184
RBF (results-based funding) programs 202–3
RCTs (randomized controlled trials) 18–19, 24, 69
    hope and intervention studies 289
    role of 64–5
    and spillover benefits 145–6
Remme, Michelle 6
research intervention 186
RESPECT study 57, 193
RethinkHIV project 11, 21–2, 23, 25–6, 41, 52, 61–2, 65,
    74, 76, 77, 104, 108–9, 121–2, 137, 151, 155, 163,
    164, 170–1, 174, 175–6, 218, 233, 238, 299, 300,
    328, 342
risk behavior 284–6
risk compensation 146
risk ecology 285, 286
risk environments 285
    and individual behavior 286
risk-taking behavior patterns 130–1, 133, 146
risk-taking behavior research 56
RNM (Resource Needs Model) 18
Rome International AIDS Conference 238
RP (revealed preference) approach 170
Rush Foundation 2, 7, 8
Rwanda
    Abuja target 202
    alcohol tax 262–3
    HIV awareness 192
    HIV incidence/prevalence 13
    key indicators 115–16
    life expectancy with/without AIDS 162
    life insurance incentivization 296–7
    male circumcision 23–5, 325
    OIs (opportunistic infections) 76–7, 78
    unmet need for family planning 165

S-I (susceptible-infection) transmission system 152–5
safe blood transfusions *see* blood transfusions
safe medical injections 81–6
    precautions intervention 186
Salomon, Joshua 7
Schelling, Thomas C. 337–8
schistosomiasis 97
schoolgirls *see* keeping girls in school
secondary infection prevention 159, 311
Sendai virus 313
Senegal
    alcohol tax 262–3
    HIV incidence/prevalence 13, 114–17

key indicators 115–16
    problems faced by government (Afrobarometer) 232
sexual abstinence 68, 255
sexual abstinence month 4, 71
sexual behavior, different contexts 283
sexual health, and CM (contingency management)
    55–6
sexual infections 11, 41–2, 49
sexual practices, cultural 285
sexual relations
    frequency 193
    and HIV prevention 11–17, 20, 33, 34–7, 41–2
    risk-taking behavior 56–7
    see also keeping girls in school
sexually transmitted diseases (STDs)
    and alcohol 243
    HIV 11, 18, 32, 50–2, 63–4, 66–7, 74, 169–70, 238, 300,
        339
        prevention basics 67–8
    see also non-sexual HIV transmission
sexually transmitted infections (STIs) 11, 41–2, 49, 50, 65,
    300, 339
    as HIV epidemic drivers 285
Sierra Leone
    alcohol tax 262–3
    HIV incidence/prevalence 13
    key indicators 115–16
SIHR (Schooling, Income, and HIV Risk) study 193
simulated scenarios in ART (anti-retroviral treatment)
    135–7
Smith, Vernon L. 337–8
Snyder, Richard 288
social conditions, embodiment of 287–8
social intervention, and hope 288–90
social policy interventions 281–90
    Nobel Laureate Economist Expert Panel findings on
        339–40
Somalia, key indicators 115–16
Somaliland, *Voices of the Poor* project 196
South Africa
    alcohol tax 262–3
    alcohol taxation 243
    ART program 217
    development indicators 227
    GNI per capita 226–8
    health system capacity 226–8
    HIV epidemic scale 65–6
    HIV incidence/prevalence 12, 13
    HIV testing 195
    HIV/AIDS disease statistics 200
    HIV/AIDS stigma 248–9
    IDU (injecting drug use) intervention 92–5, 96–7
    IMAGE (Intervention with Microfinance for AIDS and
        Gender Equity) 21, 246, 247
    key indicators 115–16
    life expectancy 226–8
        with/without AIDS 162
    male circumcision 23–5

Medecins Sans Frontiers project 159
microfinance schemes 247
PEPFAR-funded interventions 255
problematic alcohol use 242
problems faced by government (Afrobarometer) 232
TAC (Treatment Action Campaign) 234–5
unmet need for family planning 165
voluntary HIV testing and counseling uptake at
    community level 248
Spectrum policy models 78–9, 89–90, 93, 96–7, 102, 103–4
spillover benefits 145
SROI (Social Return on Investment) 248–9
SSA see sub-Saharan Africa
stand-alone HIV programs 215
standard dynamic model of infections 152
    with interventions 153–4
statistical life value 189–90
Stavudine 126, 174
STDs see sexually transmitted diseases
Stein, Zena 64
Steinberg, Jonny 234
Stepping Stones 246, 258–9
stigma of HIV/AIDS 1, 4, 6, 20, 97, 238, 239, 240, 242,
    248–9, 255, 265
STIs (sexually transmitted infections) 50, 65, 66–7
Stover, John 5
strategies 329
Strengthening Health Systems 5–6
stressors 284
structural drivers metaphor 284–6
structural interventions 286, 287
sub-Saharan Africa
    Abuja Goals Fund (AGF) see AGF
    age-specific survival 29, 30
    AIDS funding 342
    AIDS spending and health systems strengthening (HSS)
        186–7
    AIDS vaccine
        costs 306, 322–3
        and epidemic future 324
    ART (anti-retroviral treatment) xix
        benefits 184
        coverage 77–8
    BCC (behavioral change communication) 16
    behavioral strategies 14–15
    benefit-cost ratios for ARV 178–82
    benefits of HIV prevention 306–8
    blood supply testing 86
    CCT programs
        effectiveness 55
        and keeping girls in school 220–2, 245, 251–2, 254,
            258, 293, 294, 343–4
    Civil Society Panel see Civil Society Panel
    community health workers
        costs of 196–7
        deployment 183
    community mobilization programs 34
    cost-effectiveness 11, 20, 104

cryptococcal antigen (CRAG) test 199–201
cryptococcal meningitis 183, 199–201
death avertion 188–9, 194, 203, 204
development indicators 227
family planning see family planning
female sex workers 296–7
financial incentives for 5–6
gender role perceptions 239, 240, 246–7
GNI per capita 75–6
HIV incidence in xix, 1, 12, 19, 29, 30, 34, 39–41, 181,
    238
HIV transmission 238
    models 79–81, 131–3
HIV in women 172–3
HIV/AIDS disease statistics 200
HIV/AIDS social policy interventions 281–90
HIV/AIDS solutions 41–2
HTC, home-based 25
ICD (infectious and communicable diseases) 188
incentivizing adults 296–7
income per capita 306
increased health spending 188
infant infections 198
infections and injections 83
interventions see interventions
keeping girls in school see keeping girls in school
key indicators 115–16
labor ward screening 118–19
life expectancy 162, 184
life-year values 137
male circumcision 12, 23–5, 62
maternal mortality 197, 198
modes of transmission 66–7
mother-to-child transmission 74, 107
Nobel Laureate Economist Expert Panel findings
    337–8
OIs (opportunistic infections) 76–7, 78
pMTCT benefit-cost ratios 160–1
pMTCT options 112–13
pMTCT services increase requirements 121–2
potential beneficiaries of intervention 39–41
potential HIV rates 163
pre-exposure chemoprophylaxis 53, 54, 58
RethinkHIV project 11
safe blood transfusions 86–8
screening tests 161
sexual relations and HIV prevention 11–17
sexually transmitted HIV 11
Strengthening Health Systems 5–6
testing and counseling 161
treatment cost per person/year 135
UNAIDS spending proposal 205
universal testing, informing, and counseling 183
unmet need for family planning 165
women and HIV 172–3
substance abuse, as HIV epidemic driver 285
Sudan, unmet need for family planning 165
supply chain management 323

Swaziland
  alcohol tax 262–3
  ARV requirement 174
  blood transfusion infections 74
  HIV epidemic scale 65–6
  HIV incidence/prevalence 12, 13, 29, 30, 34, 66–7,
      114–17
  key indicators 115–16
  life expectancy with/without AIDS 162
  male circumcision 23–5
  resources allocated to 15–17
  sexually transmitted HIV 11
  unmet need for family planning 165
  unsafe medical injections 74
synergies with development sectors 188–9

TAC (Treatment Action Campaign) 234–5
Tanzania
  Abuja target 202
  alcohol taxation 244, 262–3, 296
  blood supply testing 86
  cash incentive programs 57–8
    CCTs (conditional cash transfers) 245, 296
  condoms 170
  cost-effectiveness of HIV prevention 5, 73
  development indicators 227
  HIV epidemic scale 65–6
  HIV incidence/prevalence 13, 283
  HIV/AIDS stigma 248–9
  IDU (injecting drug use) intervention 92–5, 96–7
  intervention studies 170–1
  key indicators 115–16
  life expectancy with/without AIDS 162
  life insurance incentivization 296–7
  listed HIV epidemic drivers 285
  Mema kwa Vijana intervention 255
  problems faced by government (Afrobarometer) 232
  RESPECT study 193
  sexually transmitted infections 50
  unmet need for family planning 165
  voluntary HIV testing and counseling uptake at
      community level 248
  VSL (Value of a Statistical Life) approach 170–1
Tanzanian AIDS Commission 285
Tanzanian epidemic 283
targeting strategy 312
TASO (AIDS Support Organization) 234–5
technologies 329
temporary sexual relationships as HIV epidemic driver 285
tenofovir 126
test-and-treat strategy see ART
Thai RV144 vaccine 303, 326
Thematic Panel Discussion 214
Togo
  alcohol tax 262–3
  blood supply testing 86
  HIV incidence/prevalence 13

key indicators 115–16
  life expectancy with/without AIDS 162
topical anti-retrovirals 301
topical microbicides 238
transferable social policy interventions 283–4
transmission susceptibility and income inequality 287
Treatment 2.0 Initiative 5, 174, 179
treatment interventions 104–5
treatment as prevention 166–8, 171–2
treatment resources vs stated goals 213–14
treatment unit costs 133–5
TRIPS (Trade-Related Intellectual Property Rights)
    agreements 168
Tshabalala-Msimang, Manto 234
tuberculosis as investment priority 189

Uganda
  and Abuja Goals Fund (AGF) 207
  alcohol tax 262–3
  blood transfusion infections 74
  CCTs (conditional cash transfers) 245
  development indicators 227
  HIV in couples 126
  HIV epidemic scale 65–6
  HIV incidence/prevalence 13, 66–7, 81, 324
  HIV/AIDS stigma 248–9
  infection age 307
  injection infections 81
  interventions, local diagnosis of 289
  key indicators 115–16
  life expectancy with/without AIDS 162, 307
  Masaka intervention 255
  microfinance schemes 247
  OIs (opportunistic infections) 76–7, 78
  PEPFAR-funded interventions 255
  problems faced by government (Afrobarometer) 232
  sexually transmitted HIV 11
  sexually transmitted infections 50
  TASO (AIDS Support Organization) 234–5
  unmet need for family planning 165
UNAIDS 185–6, 188–9, 205, 235–6, 346
  cost of saving life 205–6
  founding of 61
  improved investment approach 194–5
  International Group on Analysis of Trends in HIV
      Prevalence and Behaviors in Young People in
      Countries most Affected by HIV (2010) 19
  investment returns 188
  and male circumcision 62
  modes of transmission 66–7
  program enablers 194–5
UNAIDS Global Plan 90
UNAIDS Investment Framework analysis 90
UNAIDS MOT (Modes of Transmission) model 81
UNAIDS Strategy (2011–2015) 14–15, 20
UNAIDS (United Nations Joint Programme on HIV/AIDS)
    108–9

UNDP (Joint United Nations Programme on HIV/AIDS)
      346
unexamined metaphors 281–6
UNGASS 189
unintended pregnancies 197
unit costs per country 272–3
United Nations
   General Assembly Political Declaration on HIV/AIDS
      xix, 74
   Security Council Resolution on HIV/AIDS xix
United Nations High-Level Meeting on AIDS, Thematic
      Panel Discussion 214
United Nations Non-Communicable Disease Summit
      (2011) 61
United States, HIV prevalence 153
universal HIV testing 183, 191–2, 206
   adults 193
universal precautions intervention 186

vaccine research and development 7, 299–312, 321–7
   accomplishments to date 300–1
   annual investment in 303–5, 321
   anti-retroviral therapy 330
   benefit-cost analysis 304–9
      of accelerating 309–12
      continued investment 308–9
   benefit-cost ratios 330
   demand creation costs 323
   development history 302–4
   funding sources 300
   infections averted benefits 308
   investment priorities 328–9
   new technologies 328–9
      investments 334
   Nobel Laureate Economist Expert Panel findings on
      337–9
   operational protocols 302
   and productivity levels 311
   prospects 302–4
   R&D 300–4
   research agenda 301–2
   research developments source 313
   secondary infection prevention 311
   and social value 330
   spending 300
varying average costs 294–5
Vassall, Anna 6
VCT (voluntary counseling and testing) see HTC
Vesicular Stomatitis Virus 313
viral load
   and HIV risk 126, 151
   monitoring 179
Voices of the Poor project 196
VSL (Value of Statistical Life) approach 170–1

Watts, Charlotte 6
Whiteside, Alan 4

WHO (World Health Organization)
   on alcohol taxation 243
   Options 5, 162–3
   program 162
women living with HIV, unintended pregnancies 197
World Bank
   decline in benefit-cost analysis 190
   health funding evaluation 233, 235–6
   results-based funding (RBF) programs 202–3
   structural adjustment lending 231–3
   Voices of the Poor 196
   World Development Report 1993, Investing in Health
      203
WTP (willingness to pay) 170–1

ZAC (Zanzibar AIDS Commission) 283
Zambia
   Abuja target 202
   alcohol tax 262–3
   development indicators 227
   health priority survey 230–1
   health worker shortage 196
   HIV epidemic scale 65–6
   HIV incidence/prevalence 12, 13, 34, 66–7, 196
   key indicators 115–16
   life expectancy with/without AIDS 162
   life insurance incentivization 296–7
   male circumcision 23–5
   OIs (opportunistic infections) 76–7, 78
   problems faced by government (Afrobarometer)
      232
   sexually transmitted HIV 11
   unmet need for family planning 165
   Voices of the Poor project 196
Zaric, G. S. 295
ZDV (Zidovudine) program 89, 162–3, 175
zero uptake
   and benefit-cost ratios 151
   counterfactual 135, 136
   simulation results 139
Zimbabwe
   alcohol tax 262–3
   development indicators 227
   health priority survey 230–1
   HIV epidemic scale 65–6
   HIV incidence/prevalence 12, 13, 19, 301, 324
   HIV/AIDS stigma 248–9
   key indicators 115–16
   life expectancy with/without AIDS 162
   male circumcision 23–5
   maternal/infant life expectancy 111
   problems faced by government (Afrobarometer)
      232
   unmet need for family planning 165
   voluntary HIV testing and counseling uptake at
      community level 248
Zuma, Jacob 195